Patents eBook Series

"Topics in Anti-Cancer Research"

Volume 2

Editors

Atta-ur Rahman, FRS
Kings College
University of Cambridge
Cambridge
UK

&

Khurshid Zaman
Bentham Science Publishers
USA

Bentham Science Publishers
Executive Suite Y - 2
PO Box 7917, Saif Zone
Sharjah, U.A.E.
subscriptions@benthamscience.org

Bentham Science Publishers
P.O. Box 446
Oak Park, IL 60301-0446
USA
subscriptions@benthamscience.org

Bentham Science Publishers
P.O. Box 294
1400 AG Bussum
THE NETHERLANDS
subscriptions@benthamscience.org

CONTENTS

FOREWORD

This is the second volume of our Patent eBook Series entitled "Topics in Anti-Cancer Research". The eBook includes updated chapters on important topics of cancer published in the Recent Patents on Anti-Cancer Drug Discovery.

The volume covers scientific and patented novel chemotherapeutic agents and drugs for metastatic castration-resistant prostate cancer and Ras/ Raf /MEK/ERK pathway, P1K, AKT and mTORC1/2 inhibitors, ATPase inhibitors for cancer therapy, and sphingomyelin biosynthesis which regulates cancer cell death and growth.

Tanaka *et al.*, present the latest literature research and strategies on therapeutic agents and patented compounds and improvement of survival for metastatic castration - resistant prostate cancer (CRPC). The role of novel patented compounds *e.g.* N-cadherin, AR splicing variants, PCGEM-1, ELR-CXC chemokine antagonist, dual inhibitor of MET and VEGF as an alternative options for prostate cancer has been discussed in Chapter 1.

Chapter 2 by Ségui *et al.*, focuses on the regulation of cancer cell death, sensitivity and growth by sphingomyelin biosynthesis through a series of metabolic pathways and sphingolipid signaling. Hematological malignancies are also discussed in this chapter

Chapter 3 provides a complete overview of novel patented compounds and patent applications inhibiting the activities of B-Raf/Ras/ERK and MEK signaling pathways. Wong *et al.* present the results of current clinical trials of these inhibitors.

Tabernero *et al.*, in Chapter 4 review new emerging preclinical researches, clinical trials for targeting of P13K, AKT, dual P13K and mTOR inhibitors for treating different types of cancers.

Approaches for studying main stages of cell cycle via biochemical regulatory processes and energy metabolism in cancer cells are presented by Rumjanek *et al.*, in Chapter 5. These pathways are inhibited by synthetic and natural compounds and the involvement of cyclin dependent kinases and phosphatases, oncogenes, mitochondria and histone deacetylases is also discussed.

Hernández *et al.*, in Chapter 6 have given an overview of the origin, structure, function and mechanism of action of patented V-ATPase inhibitors by intraorganellar acidification of membranes for the treatment of cancer.

Chapter 7 describes the use of monoclonal antibodies (MoAbs) used in cancer therapy. Napolioni *et al.* discuss the mechanisms, genetic profiles and interaction of the Fc gamma receptors (FcγRs) with immunotherapeutic drugs.

Sharma *et al.*, present the key role of molecular vascular endothelial growth factor (VEGF) in the treatment of metastatic renal cell carcinoma (RCC) with reference to patents for anti-VEGF drugs for RCC and molecular pathways involved in the development of angiogenesis drugs for renal cancer in Chapter 8.

In the next chapter, Boel De Paepe covers different approaches on tumor neovascularization as a target for cancer therapy. Novel anti-angiogenic agents are also discussed along with relevant biological pathways of neo angiogenesis and its inhibition by natural metabolites, pharmaceutical compounds, and combination therapy.

Cerqueira *et al.* in Chapter 11 review the papers and patents on RNA inhibition, ribonucleotidase reductase inhibitors structure, action mechanism and biochemistry. Rribonucleotidase reductase is clinically used for the control of different specific types of cancers.

Karpel-Massler *et al.* focus on relevant patents for enhancing the anti-cancer activity of erlotinib by combining HER/EGFR- targeted TK inhibitors for the cure of malignant glioblastoma in Chapter 12.

Imran *et al.* present the role of nanodrugs in cancer chemotherapy. Nanodrugs act specifically on cancer cells. Nanodrugs diversity and mechanism, future perspectives, and conventional chemotherapeutic drugs are discussed in Chapter 13.

Chapter 14 by Hsieh *et al.* describe the present status including the literature and patents on nano-sized camptothecin and its analogs for cancer chemotherapy.

In the subsequent chapter, Soria *et al.* discuss the patents on recent developments of redox - chemoprevention by dietary onconutrition and the role and assessment of anticancer functional biomarkers and biomolecules.

Topics in Anti-Cancer Research, is an essential e-book series for oncologists, pharmaceutical scientists, clinicians, scientists, R& D experts and researchers in other cancer related disciplines.

It is hoped that the second volume will be of immense interest to a large number of medicinal chemists, pharmacologists, researchers, clinicians, scientists, R& D experts and medical doctors seeking new targets for the prevention of cancer and new developments for cancer chemotherapy.

The editors wish to express their sincere gratitude to Mr. Mahmood Alam, Ms. Raheela Anjum, Ms. Iffat Shaheen and Mrs. Rafia Rehan, the reviewers, the authors, friends and all colleagues for their assistance in the finalization of eBook.

Atta-ur-Rahman, FRS
Kings College,
University of Cambridge,
Cambridge,
UK

&

Khurshid Zaman
Bentham Science Publishers,
USA

List of Contributors

Ali, Imran	Department of Chemistry, Jamia Millia Islamia (Central University), New Delhi-110025, India
Cerqueira, Nuno M.F.S.A.	REQUIMTE / Faculdade de Ciências do Porto, Rua Campo Alegre, 687, 4169-007 Porto, Portugal
De Paepe, Boel	Ghent University Hospital, Neurology and Pathology, UZ 1K12A, De Pintelaan 185, 9000 Ghent, Belgium
Dhanabal, Mohanraj	EMD Serono Research Institute Inc., 45A Middlesex Turnpike, Billerica, MA 01821, USA
Hernández, Agustín	Instituto de Bioquímica Vegetal y Fotosíntesis, CSIC-Universidad de Sevilla, Avda. Américo Vespucio 49, 41092 Seville, Spain
Hsieh, Ming-Fa	Department of Biomedical Engineering, Chung Yuan Christian University, 200, Chung Pei Rd., Chung Li, Taiwan 32023, R.O.C.
Karpel-Massler, Georg	Department of Neurosurgery, University of Ulm School of Medicine, Albert-Einstein-Allee 23, D-89081 Ulm, Germany
Napolioni, Valerio	School of Biosciences and Biotechnologies, University of Camerino, Via Gentile III da Varano, 62032 Camerino, Italy
Rumjanek, Franklin D.	Instituto de Bioquímica Médica CCS-Universidade Federal do Rio de Janeiro, Ilha do Fundão, Rio de Janeiro, CEP 21941-590, Brazil
Ségui, Bruno	INSERM UMR1037-Cancer Research Center of Toulouse, BP84225, 31432 Toulouse Cedex 4, France

Sharma, Shree G. Department of Pathology, University of Arkansas for Medical Sciences, Little Rock, Arkansas, USA

Soria, Elio A. Instituto de Biología Celular, Enrique Barros S/N, Ciudad Universitaria, Córdoba 5014, Córdoba, Argentina

Tabernero, Josep Medical Oncology Service, Vall d'Hebron University Hospital and Vall d'Hebron Institute of Oncology, Universitat Autonoma de Barcelona, Barcelona, Spain

Tanaka, Tomoaki Department of Urology, Osaka City University Graduate School of Medicine, Osaka, Japan

Wong, Kwong-Kwok Department of Gynecologic Oncology and Reproductive Medicine, The University of Texas M.D. Anderson Cancer Center, 1515 Holcombe Blvd., Houston, TX 77030, USA

INTRODUCTION

This is the second volume of the Patent eBook Series titled **Topics in Anti-Cancer Research**. The eBook includes updated chapters on topics relevant to contemporary cancer research published in the journal, Recent Patents on Anti-Cancer Drug Discovery.

This volume covers scientific and patented novel chemotherapeutic agents and drugs for metastatic castration-resistant prostate cancer and Ras/ Raf /MEK/ERK pathway, P1K, AKT and mTORC1/2 inhibitors, ATPase inhibitors for cancer therapy, and sphingomyelin biosynthesis which regulates cancer cell death and growth.

Other chapters also explain research on biochemical regulation i.e. cell cycle and energy metabolism, the role of genetic variations of FcγRs gamma receptors in monoclonal antibody based anti-cancer therapy and effectiveness of antiangiogenic therapy, endogenous angiogenesis inhibitors and anti-angiogenic drugs for the treatment of renal cell carcinoma, prevention of cancer by ribonucleotide reductase, anticancer activity of Erlotinib in glioblastoma and the mechanisms of action of nanodrugs and nano-sized camptothecin drugs in cancer chemotherapy. The volume also covers recent studies in the field of onconutrition. The broad range of topics covered in this second volume will be of immense interest to clinicians, scientists and R&D experts seeking new targets for the prevention of cancer, novel oncogenic biomarkers, and methods for cancer therapy.

Topics in Anti-Cancer Research, Vol. 2, 2013, 3-34

CHAPTER 1

Emerging Research and Therapeutic Strategies for Castration-Resistant Prostate Cancer

Tomoaki Tanaka* **and Tatsuya Nakatani**

Department of Urology, Osaka City University Graduate School of Medicine, Osaka, Japan

Abstract: Docetaxel has until recently been the only agent with a small survival benefit for metastatic castration-resistant prostate cancer (CRPC). To improve the clinical outcome in CRPC, numerous classes of drugs targeting specific pathways involved in hormone action, bone metabolism, angiogenesis, apoptosis and immune response have recently been investigated for efficacies either as single agents or in combination with docetaxel. Of note, some novel agents or vaccines including cabazitaxel, sipuleucel-T and abiraterone have received US governmental approval to treat patients with CRPC on the evidence of significant improvement of overall survival in CRPC. From the viewpoint of the complex mechanisms implicated in prostate cancer progression, effective therapeutic strategies should be developed by multifaceted approaches, such as the composition of novel agents targeting key molecules, cytotoxic chemotherapy, and immunotherapy. Recently patented molecules (e.g., *N*-cadherin, AR splicing variants, PCGEM-1, ELR-CXC chemokine antagonist, dual inhibitor of MET and VEGF) have strong potential as therapeutic options for CRPC. Here, we review the newest evidence of novel agents and patented compounds and methods for the purpose of future use in CRPC.

Keywords: AR splicing variant, angiogenesis, apoptosis, Bag1-L, cabazitaxel, Castration-resistant prostate cancer, caveolin, chroman-derived compounds, CTL-associated antigen-4, docetaxel, dual inhibitor of MET and VEGF, ELR-CXC chemokine antagonist, hyaluronic acid, microenvironment, *N*-cadherin, novel therapy, patent, PCGEM-1, radium-223-chrolide, target molecule.

INTRODUCTION

Prostate cancer is the second most common cause of cancer-associated death in men in European countries and the United States. In 2009, approximately 25% of the estimated 766,130 men, diagnosed with new cancer, had prostate cancer [1]. Until recently, the incidence of prostate cancer in Asian countries has also

***Address correspondence Tomoaki Tanaka:** Department of Urology, Osaka City University Graduate School of Medicine, 1-4-3, Asahimachi, Abeno-ku, Osaka 545-0051, Japan; Tel: +81 6 6645 3857; Fax: +81 6-6647 4426; E-mail: tomoaki826@msic.med.osaka-cu.ac.jp

Atta-ur Rahman and Khurshid Zaman (Eds)

remarkedly increased. For patients diagnosed with local-stage disease, treatment with surgery or radiation can be curative. However, the majority of cases with locally advanced or metastatic prostate cancer commonly has acquired transient cancer control with androgen ablation therapy and finally developed disease progression regardless of castrate level of serum androgen. This state is characterized as hormone-refractory prostate cancer (HRPC) or currently as castration-resistant prostate cancer (CRPC). No effective therapy based on evidence of prolonged overall survival had been reported until 2004, when two randomized Phase III trials, SWOG 9916 (docetaxel + estramustine) [2] and TAX 327 (docetaxel + prednisone) [3], demonstrated that docetaxel combined with either estramustine or prednisone was able to significantly lengthen the survival period in CRPC compared with mitoxantrone plus prednisone (17.5 vs. 15.6 months in SWOG 9916, and 18.9 vs. 16.5 months in TAX 327). Novel alternatives for treatment of CRPC, with the potential to exceed the clinical benefit of docetaxel, are currently being developed. This review article is initially focused on the highly promising agents that target specific pathways involved in hormonal action, angiogenesis, cell signaling, apoptosis, molecular chaperone, and immune modulation. Several drugs among them are undergoing Phase III trials or have already received US governmental approval. Moreover, we discuss the future strategy for CRPC, including recent patents.

1. ANTIANDROGEN AGENTS

A large number of previous reports demonstrate that prostate cancer, developing under the condition of castration treatment, is continuously dependent on androgen receptor (AR)-mediated signaling via either substitutions in AR such as gene mutation and amplification or enhanced AR transcriptional activity through co-activators and other signal cascades. Although the castration serum level of testosterone is maintained, a minor part of androgens is produced in both the adrenal glands and tumor cells [4]. This is able to accelerate AR transcriptional activity sufficiently in prostate cancer cells. From the view points of these phenomena, novel hormonal therapies have recently been introduced in CRPC [5].

1.1. MDV3100

MDV3100 is a forceful AR antagonist that blocks androgens from binding to the AR, and prevents nuclear translocation of AR, its binding to DNA and co-activator recruitment. As compared with bicalutamide, it has higher affinity for AR, and effectively induces tumor cell apoptosis [6]. In a Phase I/II trial published in 2010 [7], 140 CRPC patients, treated with or without chemotherapy, were administered MDV3100 orally at diverse doses ranging from 30 to 600mg per day in cohorts with dose escalation. After 12 weeks of treatment, the rate of prostate-specific antigen (PSA) response in excess of 50% was significantly higher in patients without chemotherapy than in those with (57%; 37/65 vs. 36%; 27/75). Moreover, the rate of PSA decline (>50% decrease from baseline) was also significantly lower in patients with previous ketoconazole treatment compared to those without (37%; 23/63 vs. 71%; 55/77). The proportion of stable disease was 49% (29/59) in soft tissue masses and 56% (61/109) in bone metastatic lesions. The maximum tolerated dose for sustained treatment was 240 mg. The most common adverse event of grade 3 or 4 was general fatigue (11%; 16/140), which appeared in a dose-dependent manner and was reversed after dose reduction. On the basis of the results shown in this Phase I/II study, a Phase III randomized trial (AFFIRM) is ongoing to examine MDV3100 at 160 mg per day vs. placebo in CRPC patients who have received previous docetaxel administration, with a primary endpoint of overall survival (OS) [8]. The results of a planned interim analysis for AFFIRM showed that MDV3100 achieved 4.8-months longer median OS compared with that in the placebo group (18.4 vs. 13.6 months). Consequently, the Independent Data Monitoring Committee (IDMC) recommended early termination of the AFFIR trial. Furthermore, a current clinical trial (PREVAIL) has been started to determine the benefit of MDV3100 vs. placebo as assessed by the primary endpoints of OS and progression-free survival (PFS) in CRPC patients who have failed androgen ablation therapy but not yet received chemotherapy [9].

1.2. Abiraterone (Johnson & Johnson; Zytiga®)

Ketoconazole, a nonselective inhibitor of CYP 17, has previously shown antitumor effects as secondary hormonal treatment in CRPC patients although severe adverse events appeared [10]. However, it was indicated that insufficient inhibition of production of adrenal androgens was associated with progression of disease in this study. Abiraterone (CB7589) is an oral, selective, irreversible inhibitor of cytochrome P450 (CYP) 17A1 that specifically inhibits both 17α-hydroxylase and C17, 20-lyase enzyme activity. Abiraterone acetate (CB7630) is the prodrug, which is rapidly converted to active metabolite *in vivo*, and is commonly used in clinical settings. Administration of abiraterone acetate has been demonstrated to rapidly reduce the serum testosterone level to an undetectable level (less than 1ng/dL), and was reported to cause a significant the PSA decline, disease repression and amelioration of symptoms in a Phase I trial [11] and a Phase I/II trial [12] enrolling chemotherapy-naïve CRPC patients. The main toxicity of abiraterone acetate administration is hypertension, hypokalemia and lower-limb edema, which are attributable to an excess of mineralcorticoids caused by an increased level of adrenocorticotrophic hormone (ACTH). These adverse events showed no dose-limiting effect, and were reversed by administration of an antialdosterone agent. Furthermore, preliminary analysis of a Phase I/II study demonstrated that the addition of dexamethasone to abiraterone acetate at disease progression reversed resistance to abiraterone in 33% of patients regardless of prior dexamethasone exposure, and the pretreatment serum levels of sexual hormones derived from the adrenal gland, such as androstenedione, dehydroepiandrosterone (DHEA), DHEA sulfate (DHEA-S) and estradiol, were predictive markers of PSA response [12]. Additionally, administration of both abiraterone acetate (1,000mg daily) and prednisone (5mg twice daily) was also effective in docetaxel-pretreated patients who were ketoconazole-naive. From these viewpoints of clinical data, two randomized Phase III studies using abiraterone acetate and prednisone have completed accrual and are ongoing in docetaxel-pretreated CRPC patients [13] and chemotherapy-naive CRPC patients [14]. Recently, administration of abiraterone exhibited a survival benefit in a placebo-controlled Phase III trial in docetaxel-refractory CRPC patients (14.8 months- [abiraterone plus prednisone] vs. 10.9 months- [placebo plus prednisone]) in interim analysis [15]. Based on these data, this agent was approved by the U.S. Food and Drug Administration (FDA) in April 2011.

1.3. TAK-700 (Orteronel)

TAK-700 (also called Orteronel) is an oral, selective, non-steroidal inhibitor of the C17, 20-lyase enzyme, which plays a key role in the production of steroid hormones excreted from both the testis and adrenal gland [16]. In a Phase I/II study that enrolled 26 patients with metastatic CRPC, administration of TAK-700 at ≥ 300mg twice- daily resulted in a PSA decrease with undetectable levels of both DHEA-S and testosterone in all patients [17]. The most common adverse events were fatigue (65%), nausea (42%), constipation (38%), anorexia (35%), and headache (35%). Two large randomized trials composed of placebo plus prednisolone (5mg twice daily) or TAK-700 (400mg twice daily) plus prednisolone (5mg twice daily) are ongoing in chemotherapy-naïve CRPC patients (C21004) [18] and docetaxel-pretreated CRPC patients (C21005) [19] with the primary endpoint of either radiographic PFS and OS or OS, respectively.

1.4. VN/124-1 (TOK-001)

VN/124-1 (now called TOK-001) is a unique 17, 20-lyase inhibitor, which has high structural similarity to abiraterone [20]. In preclinical models of prostate cancer *in vitro* and *in vivo*, this compound has been evaluated as downregulating AR expression as well as competitively blocking androgen binding, in addition to CYP17A1 inhibition. TOK-001 has been shown to have higher affinity for wild-type AR than does bicalutamide in prostate cancer cells [20, 21]. Interestingly, it has been reported that TOK-001 has superior synergistic effects on growth inhibition in combination with everolimus or gefitinib compared with bicalutamide *in vitro* and *in vivo* [22]. TOK-001 is currently being assessed in a Phase I/II open-label trial, namely ARMOR1 (Androgen Receptor Modulation Optimized for Response 1), which Tokai Pharmaceuticals, Inc., initiated in chemotherapy-naïve CRPC patients [23].

2. ENDOTHELIN-RECEPTOR ANTAGONISTS

The endothelin family proteins (endothelin-1, -2, -3), which bind to two types of receptor; endothelin-A (ET_A) and endothelin-B (ET_B), play a crucial role in many biological events, including cell proliferation, angiogenesis, apoptosis and osteogenic bone metastasis. In particular, activation of the ET_A receptor by endothelin-1 (ET-1) is biologically implicated in tumor progression and promotion of osteoblastic activity in bone metastases of prostate cancer [24].

2.1. Atrasentan

Atrasentan is a predominantly ET_A receptor antagonist with low binding-affinity for the ET_B receptor. Thus far, two randomized Phase III studies (atrasentan 10mg daily vs. placebo) have been conducted in 809 patients with metastatic CRPC and 941 patients with non-metastatic CRPC, respectively [25, 26]. However, these two studies showed no significant benefit of atrasentan on time to disease progression

(TTP) and overall survival (OS) despite evidence of effects on PSA and bone alkaline phosphatase (BAP) as surrogate markers of disease burden. Preclinical studies suggest that endothelin-1 reduces docetaxel-induced apoptosis in prostate cancer cells, and inhibition of ET_A activity by atrasentan synergistically enhances tumor regression due to docetaxel administration [27, 28]. On the basis of clinical benefits in a Phase II trial combined with docetaxel (70mg/m^2 every 3 weeks) and atrasentan (10mg daily) [29], this combination regimen is being investigated in an ongoing Phase III trial with the primary end point of OS and PFS in metastatic CRPC patients with addition of either atrasentan or placebo under treatment with docetaxel and prednisone [30].

2.2. Zibotentan (ZD4054)

Zibotentan (ZD4054) is a highly potent, selective ET_A receptor antagonist without inhibitory activity on the ET_B receptor. In a randomized, double-blind, placebo-controlled Phase II trial, a total of 312 bone-metastatic CRPC patients were randomized to once-daily zibotentan 10mg or 15mg or placebo in a 1:1:1 ratio [31]. This study demonstrated no statistically significant difference between zibotentan and placebo on the primary end point of TTP. However, a provisional analysis revealed a promising improvement in OS. Median OS was 17.3, 24.5, and 23.5 months in the placebo, zibotentan 10mg, and zibotentan 15mg treatment group, respectively. This clinical benefit of zibotentan treatment on OS shown in a Phase II study led to three large Phase III trials with approximately 2,500 patients to examine the effects on OS and PFS of once-daily 10 mg zibotentan in CRPC patients with M0 (no evidence of bone metastasis) [32], M1 (bone metastases) [33], and M1c (combination with docetaxel in M1) [34]. Regrettably, the two Phase III studies in CRPC patients with both M1 and M0 have been terminated because of no benefit on OS and PFS in the zibotentan-treated arm (press release on October 2010 and February 2011, respectively) [35].

3. RANK-L INHIBITORS

RANK-L (receptor activator of nuclear factor-κB-ligand) is predominantly synthesized in osteoblasts and activates the downstream pathway via binding to RANK on the cell-surface of osteoclasts. RANKL is also extensively expressed on T lymphocytes and dendritic cells and plays an important role in immune system related to the bone microenvironment [36]. Activation of RANK by RANK-L accelerates cell proliferation and bone resorption of osteoclasts, and ultimately contributes to the appearance of skeletal-related events (SREs) associated with bone metastases. In the microenvironment of bone metastases, RANK-L is highly produced by osteoblasts, which are stimulated by tumor cells, and induces activation of osteoclasts with excessive production of mitogenic factors. Disturbance of this vicious cycle is a potent option for preventing the bone metastasis burden [37]. Bisphosphonates (BPs), which are inhibitors of osteoclast activity and survival, have been shown to be useful compounds to treat prostate cancer bone metastasis and reduce SREs. In a randomized Phase III trial with the third-generation bisphosphonate, zoledronic acid, administration of this agent (4mg every 3 weeks for 24 months) demonstrated a statistically significant decrease in the proportion of patients with SREs and durable pain palliation over 24 months in patients with CRPC and bone metastases [38, 39]. A new agent specific for the RANK/RANK-L pathway has been recently developed.

3.1. Denosumab

Denosumab, a fully human monoclonal antibody directed against RANK-L, inhibits osteoclast-mediated bone resorption via suppression of RANK activation. In a Phase II trial that enrolled patients with bone metastases derived from several types of cancer including prostate cancer, denosumab effectively decreased the elevated levels of urinary N-telopeptide (uNTx) despite previous BPs therapy, and inhibited the incidence of SREs compared with continuous BP treatment [40, 41]. Two large Phase III trials in CRPC patients with or without bone metastases are ongoing to investigate the effects of denosumab on the primary end points of time to first occurrence of either SREs or bone metastasis, and OS, compared with zoledronic acid or placebo, respectively [42, 43]. In the former trial in bone metastatic CRPC patients, interim analysis showed that denosumab significantly delayed the time to first on-study SRE compared with zoledronic acid (median time; 20.7 months for denosumab vs. 17.1 months for zoledronic acid) [44].

4. BONE-SEEKING RADIOPHARMACEUTICALS

Treatment with bone-seeking radiopharmaceuticals selectively carries ionizing radiation to regions of enhanced osteoblastic activity and is capable of aiming at multiple metastases concurrently [45]. The molecular target is hydroxyapatite of metastatic bone sites. β-emitters, derived from the specific radionuclide, have been developed as an effective treatment modality in patients with metastatic bone pain [46]. The radiopharmaceuticals samarium-153-ethylenediaminetetramethylene phosphonic acid (^{153}Sm-EDTMP) and strontium-89-chloride ($^{89}SrCl_2$) are approved worldwide. Phase II clinical studies with ^{89}Sr (Metastron®) have shown effective palliation of pain in most patients (up to 75%) with metastatic prostate cancer [47]. However, a later double-blind randomized Phase III study showed a lower percentage of patients with palliation compared with the Phase II trials [48].

4.1. Alpharadin

Alpharadin (radium-223-chloride) is a promising pharmaceutical containing α-particle emitter. In contrast to β-emitters, α-particle emitters can deliver much more energetic and localized radiation because of relatively heavy charged particles (helium nuclei with two positive charges) [49]. Hence, this particle can produce dense ionizing tracks through target tissues. A large Phase III, randomized, double-blind, placebo-controlled trial (ALSYMPCA) is ongoing with the primary endpoint of OS in CRPC patients with symptomatic bone metastases, administered either Alpharadin plus current standard care or placebo plus current standard care (2:1). Interim analysis of this trial showed that the Alpharadin arm significantly improved OS compared with the placebo arm (14.0 vs. 11.2 months) [50]. The safety and tolerability of Alpharadin were close to those seen in Phase I and II trials. On the basis of the benefit in OS and good tolerability, Alpharadin may be a potent option for the treatment of patients with bone metastatic CRPC.

5. ANGIOGENESIS INHIBITORS

Tumor-associated angiogenesis is essential for the growth of tumors beyond a few millimeters away from the original site. Vascular endothelial growth factor (VEGF), which stimulates the VEGF receptor-2 on the surface of both endothelial cells and tumor cells, is a key molecule in the induction of tumor angiogenesis. The level of VEGF in serum has been found to be higher in patients with CRPC than in patients with localized hormone-sensitive prostate cancer, and to be negatively correlated with outcome [51].

5.1. Bevacizumab

Bevacizumab is a humanized monoclonal antibody that prevents VEGF from binding to its receptor, and has been approved for treatment of metastatic solid tumors, such as colorectal, breast and lung cancer. In a Phase II study that enrolled 20 CRPC patients who had received first-line docetaxel-based chemotherapy, the combination of bevacizumab (10mg/kg) and docetaxel (60mg/m^2) was administered every 3 weeks. Eleven patients (55%) showed a PSA decline greater than 50%, and adverse events were tolerated, with neutropenia (20%) and thrombocytopenia (15%) of grade 3 and 4 [52]. The efficacy of bevacizumab has been investigated in a large randomized Phase III trial (CALGB 90401) of 1050 chemotherapy-naïve metastatic CRPC patients who received either bevacizumab or placebo in addition to docetaxel and prednisone [53]. This study has recently reported that administration of bevacizumab did not affect the primary end point of OS from that of the treatment group with docetaxel and prednisone alone, despite both improvement of PFS and a > 50% PSA decline [54].

5.2. Sunitinib

Sunitinib is a potent inhibitor of several tyrosine kinases, including VEGF-R and platelet-derived growth factor receptor (PDGF-R). In particular, PDGF-R is overexpressed in CRPC with bone metastases, and its inhibition has been shown to reduce tumor growth of prostate cancer in a preclinical model [55]. In a recent Phase II study that enrolled 36 docetaxel-pretreated CRPC patients, administration of sunitinib (50 mg daily for 4 weeks of a 6-week cycle) demonstrated some activity, with extended median PFS (19.4 weeks) and 4 patients (12.1%) showing a ≥ 50% PSA decline despite 52.8% of patients discontinuing treatment because of toxic effects [56]. As a result of these findings, a current Phase III trial in docetaxel-pretreated CRPC patients has employed an altered regimen with sunitinib (continuous daily 37.5mg) with the primary end point of OS [57]. Regrettably, this study has been terminated due to futility on September 2010.

5.3. Aflibercept (ZALTRAP)

Aflibercept (VEGF Trap) is a potent human VEGF-R fusion protein that comprises portions of the extracellular domains of human VEGF-R1 and -R2, fused to the Fc region of human immunoglobulin G_1. In two Phase I studies that enrolled patients with advanced solid tumors excluding prostate cancer, the appropriate administration of aflibercept has proved to be either 4.0mg/kg IV every 2 weeks or 800μg/kg s.c. weekly, based on tolerability and saturation of circulating VEGF [58,

59]. A Phase III trial (VENISE), evaluating the combination of docetaxel and prednisone with or without aflibercept in CRPC, has completed accrual and is currently ongoing [60].

5.4. Tasquinimod (ABR-215050)

Tasquinimod (TASQ) is a quinoline-3-carboxamine derivative which exhibits anti-angiogenic and anti-tumor activities in prostate cancer models *in vitro* and *in vivo* [61, 62]. Although the anti-angiogenic mechanism of action of TASQ remains unclear, it has recently been reported that TASQ induces up-regulation of thrombospondin-1 (TSP1), involving down-regulation of HIF1α and VEGF in a preclinical prostate cancer model [63]. In two Phase I trials in chemotherapy-naïve CRPC patients, the maximum tolerated dose of this compound was determined to be 0.5mg orally once-daily and a dose of 1.0mg was well tolerated under stepwise intra-patient dose escalation [64]. In a randomized, placebo-controlled Phase II trial, a total of 206 metastatic CRPC patients were assigned to receive either oral TASQ once-daily at an initial dose level of 0.25 mg per day escalating to 1.0mg per day over 4 weeks, or placebo, in a 2:1 ratio [65]. This study demonstrated that TASQ significantly improved the disease progression-free rate at 6 months as the primary end point compared with placebo (57% vs. 33%). Common adverse events (> 10%) occurring in patients receiving TASQ included gastrointestinal disorders, fatigue, musculoskeletal pain, and asymptomatic elevation of amylase. CTC grade 3-4 adverse events were reported in 38% of patients on TASQ vs. 10% on placebo. Serious vascular events were more frequent in the TASQ group, including myocardial infarction, heart failure or stroke (3%), and deep vein thrombosis (4%). On the basis of these results, a Phase III trial is ongoing to examine the efficacy in metastatic CRPC patients with mild symptoms as a primary endpoint of PFS [66]. Approximately 1200 eligible patients will be randomized to receive either treatment with TASQ (0.25, 0.5, or 1.0mg per day) or placebo in a 2:1 ratio.

6. SRC INHIBITORS

Src family kinases (SFKs), a major component of non-receptor protein tyrosine kinases, play an essential role in signal transduction associated with diverse cellular functions (e.g., cell proliferation, invasion, migration, differentiation). Activity of SFKs is increased in prostate cancer at various stages, and is also implicated in biological actions of osteoblasts and osteoclasts [67]. Preclinical evidence has revealed that inhibition of SFKs encourages both antitumor effects on prostate cancer and a reduction in bone turnover derived from bone metastases [68, 69].

6.1. Dasatinib

Dasatinib is an oral tyrosine kinase inhibitor with potent activity against various SFKs, BCR-ABL, the PDGF receptor and c-KIT. In a Phase II trial that enrolled 47 chemotherapy-naïve CRPC patients, of whom 41 (87%) had bone metastases, administration of dasatinib (70 or 100mg twice daily) demonstrated a progression-free rate at 12 and 24 weeks of 43% and 19%, respectively [70]. Notably, dasatinib also had inhibitory effects on bone turnover, with a 51% reduction (≥ 40%) in uNTX and 60% decrease in serum BAP. Further analyses revealed that dasatinib administered once daily was better tolerated than a twice daily schedule. An ongoing Phase III randomized trial is evaluating the effects of addition of dasatinib (100mg once daily) to docetaxel and predonisone in chemotherapy-naïve CRPC patients with the primary end point of OS, and secondary end points of reduction in PSA and bone markers [71].

7. CHAPERONE INHIBITORS

Molecular chaperones play a crucial role in preventing cellular proteins from undergoing stress-induced misfolding, aggregation, and denaturation. These actions stabilize the state of cellular functions under diverse environmental stimuli, including treatment with drugs. Chaperone family proteins essentially interfere with multiple pathways involved in tumor progression, invasion and resistance to treatment [72]. Thus, targeting them is a rational strategy in cancer therapy.

7.1. Custirsen (OGX-011)

Secretory clusterin (sCLU) is a cytoprotective chaperone upregulated by a variety of cancer therapies, and confers treatment resistance on tumor cells. In prostate cancer cells, expression of clusterin is increased during the transition from androgen-dependent to CRPC [73]. Custirsen (OGX-011) is an antisense oligonucleotide against sCLU mRNA, which has a long half-life of about 7 days and has been demonstrated to boost antitumor effects of chemotherapy, radiation, and hormone therapy by inhibiting expression of sCLU in preclinical xenograft models [74]. Interestingly, targeted knock-down against sCLU by custirsen has been reported to re-sensitize docetaxel-refractory prostate cancer cells to chemotherapy. In a randomized Phase II trial that enrolled 82 chemotherapy-naïve CRPC patients, the efficacy of custirsen in combination with both docetaxel and prednisone has been evaluated. The arm combined with custirsen had a median OS of 23.8 months compared with 16.9 months in the docetaxel/predonisone alone arm [75]. Two Phase III trials in either chemotherapy-naïve CRPC patients or docetaxel-pretreated CRPC patients with metastases are ongoing to evaluate the efficacy of custirsen in addition to docetaxel and prednisone with the primary end point of OS and rate of durable pain palliation, respectively [76, 77].

8. BCL-2 INHIBITORS

Bcl-2 protein is a key molecule involved in suppression of apoptosis, and plays a crucial role in inhibiting anti-proliferative responses to various treatments [78]. Bcl-2 has been reported to be overexpressed in CRPC and to promote resistance to androgen ablation and chemotherapy [79]. Therefore, strategies targeting Bcl-2 have the potential to promote apoptosis and sensitivity to chemotherapy.

8.1. AT-101

AT-101, a polyphenolic compound derived from the cotton seed plant, inhibits the function of Bcl-2, Bcl-xL, Mcl-1, and Bcl-w, and is a potent activator of proapoptotic factors. In a Phase I/II trial that enrolled chemotherapy-naïve CRPC patients, AT-101 has shown tolerability and efficacy as single-agent therapy [80]. Another Phase I/II trial of AT-101 combined with docetaxel and predonisone in chemotherapy-naïve CRPC patients has recently showed promising responses, such as a 50% PSA decline in 67% of patients and an objective partial response in 42% [81]. Furthermore, a large randomized Phase II trial (n = 220) of docetaxel and prednisone with or without AT-101 has completed accrual [82]. Interestingly, a Phase II trial of AT-101 with androgen deprivation therapy in metatstatic, hormone-sensitive prostate cancer is ongoing on the basis of the rationale that AT-101 interrupts the transition to CRPC through inhibition of the antiapoptotic activity of Bcl-2 family proteins in the preclinical setting [83].

9. CYTOTOXIC AGENTS

Docetaxel has until recently been the main cytotoxic agent that consistently improves survival of CRPC patients to some extent. However, almost half of these patients will be unresponsive to treatment and all will finally develop resistance to chemotherapy. Multiple cellular cascades involving apoptosis, angiogenesis, inflammation, signal transduction, drug efflux pumps and tubulin are involved in the acquirement of resistance to chemotherapy. Particularly, the major signal transducers and transcription activators, STAT1 and STAT3, have been shown to be closely associated with docetaxel-resistance in prostate cancer cells [84, 85]. Furthermore, changes in β-tubulin isotypes, the primary target of taxans, possibly contribute to the resistance to these drugs, based on evidence from pre-clinical models [86, 87].

9.1. Cabazitaxel (XRP6258; Jevtana®)

Cabazitaxel is a novel taxane agent, which has been adopted for clinical use on the basis of low affinity to the ATP-dependent drug efflux pump, P-glycoprotein-1 (P-gp), that is crucial for resistance to docetaxel. In a Phase I trial [88], the maximum tolerated dose of cabazitaxel set as a 1-hour IV 3 weekly dose has been revealed to be 25mg/m^2. In a randomized Phase III trial, 755 CRPC patients with docetaxel- resistance were randomized to receive prednisone 10mg daily with either 3-weekly mitoxantrone 1mg/m^2 or cabazitaxel 25mg/m^2 with the primary end point of OS, and secondary end points of PFS, PSA response, objective response, and pain response [89]. Importantly, the cabazitaxel arm showed significantly improved OS compared with the mitoxantrone arm (median survival; 15.1 vs. 12.7 months, hazard ratio of death, 0.7; 95% CI 0.59, 0.83; $p < 0.0001$). The most common toxicity of cabazitaxel was neutropenia. Grade 3 or higher neutropenia occurred in 82% of cabazitaxel-treated patients, with 8% of patients developing febrile neutropenia. Common nonhematologic toxicity in the cabazitaxel group comprised diarrhea, fatigue, nausea, and asthenia (all grades: 47%, 37%, 34%, and 20%, respectively). In the cabazitaxel group, 7 patients (2%) died of complications associated with neutropenia, while 5 patients (1%) died of cardiac events. Based on this promising evidence, cabazitaxel has emerged as a major second-line chemotherapeutic agent in CRPC.

9.2. Epothilones

Epothilones are macrolide antibiotics that stabilize microtubules, and subsequently induce apoptosis via cell-cycle transition at the G2/M checkpoint. Particularly, these agents are clinically attractive from the standpoint of no linkage to multidrug resistance proteins and β-tubulin mutations that encourage taxane-resistance [90]. Two epothilones, ixabepilone (epothilone B-lactam) [91, 92] and patupilone (epothilone B) [93, 94], have been shown to have significant activity in CRPC patients in some Phase II studies. In chemotherapy-naïve CRPC patients administered ixabepilone (40mg/m^2 every 3 weeks), 72% of PSA responders had a >80% decrease from baseline, and median PFS and survival were 6 months and 18 months, respectively. Predominant toxicity was neutropenia and neuropathy [91]. This marked activity has not been reproduced in another Phase II trial in taxane-resistant CRPC patients [92]. In a recent Phase II trial, patupilone (8 or 10mg/m^2 every 3 weeks) has been evaluated in CRPC patients with progression during 6 months of docetaxel treatment. This study demonstrated a PSA decline greater than 50% in 35 of 78 patients (45%) and pain response in approximately 50% [94]. Interestingly, there was no grade 3 or 4 toxicity of neutropenia or neuropathy. Further investigation of patupilone as second-line chemotherapy will be scheduled in the future.

9.3 Platinum Derivatives

9.3.1. Satraplatin

Satraplatin is an orally active platinum agent that has significant cytotoxic effects on CRPC in preclinical models. In an open label Phase II study with 39 CRPC patients, satraplatin was administered orally at a dose of 120mg/m^2 for 5 days every 4 weeks. This study demonstrated a high proportion of dose delays (77% of courses) and dose reductions (31% of courses) because of myelosuppression. The starting dose of satraplatin in this trial was determined to be too high for prostate cancer patients [95]. In a current, randomized Phase III trial (SPARC) that enrolled 950 chemotherapy-treated CRPC patients, the efficacy of satraplatin (80mg/m^2 for 5 days every 4 weeks) and prednisone was evaluated with the primary end points of OS and PFS compared with placebo and prednisone [96]. Despite a significant delay in disease progression in the satraplatin arm, there was no significant difference in OS between the two treatment arms. Further evaluation of satraplatin in CRPC has been halted.

9.3.2. Picoplatin

Picoplatin is also a potent, third-generation platinum agent that interrupts platinum-resistance and has good tolerability. In a current Phase II trial in 32 chemotherapy-naïve CRPC patients, administration of picoplatin (120mg/m^2 3 weekly) and docetaxel (75mg/m^2 3 weekly) plus prednisone demonstrated a PSA response in 78% of 27 evaluable patients and a median PFS of 32 weeks. The toxicity associated with this regimen was well- tolerated, without $\geq$ grade 2 neuropathy [97]. These results encourage further evaluation of picoplatin in combination with docetaxel for treating CRPC.

10. IMMUNOTHERAPY

Vaccination with prostate-specific antigens, including so-called PSA, prostatic acid phosphatase (PAP), and prostate-specific membrane antigen (PSMA), can promote activity of antigen-specific T cells that have the potential to overcome tumor cells. Immunotherapeutic strategies on the basis of vaccines to increase the proliferation of cytotoxic T lymphocytes against prostate cancer cells have been investigated. T cells can express two types of receptor (CD28 and CTLA-4) on their cell surface, and also bind to the same ligands (CD80 and CD86) that are expressed on antigen-presenting cells. While ligand recruitment of CD28 activates T cells, interfaces between CTLA-4 and these ligands suppress T-cell activation [98]. Blockade of the T-cell inhibitory receptor CTL-associated antigen-4 (CTLA-4) has been shown to increase and prolong T-cell responses, and is a powerful option to obtain anticancer immunity.

10.1. Sipuleucel-T (APC8015; Provenge®)

Sipuleucel-T is a powerful cellular immunotherapy product composed of autologous antigen-presenting cells (APCs), which was shown to encourage immune response against prostate cancer cells as a result of co-culturing with a fusion protein of PAP and granulocyte stimulating factor (GM-CSF) *in vitro*. Sipuleucel-T is produced within 48 hours from APCs isolated from the leukapheresis product, and is administered to patients intravenously every 2 weeks for a total of 3 infusions. In sequential Phase I and Phase II trials in 31 CRPC patients, patients tolerated with the vaccine well, with the most common adverse event of development of fever (14.7%) within 2 hours after infusion [99]. After treatment with sipuleucel-T, 10 (38%) of 26 patients developed a T-cell response to PAP. Three patients had a more than 50% decline in PSA level and another three patients had a 25% to 49% decrease in PSA. The time to disease progression correlated with development of an immune response to PAP and the dose of dendritic cells infused. Two randomized Phase III studies of sipuleucel-T, D9901 [100] and D9902A [101], have been conducted in CRPC patients with progressive disease. The patients were selected based on pretreatment conditions of both positive immunohistochemical staining for PAP in > 25% of tumor cells and > 400 CD4+ T-cells/mm^3. In two trials that recruited 225 men, the group treated with sipuleucel-T showed significantly reduced risk of death compared with the placebo group (hazard ratio, 1.50; 95% CI 1.10, 2.05; $p = 0.01$) despite failure in the primary end point of TTP. This treatment was well- tolerated, with chills, pyrexia, headache, asthenia, dyspnea, vomiting, and tremor of grade 1 or 2. In another Phase III trial (D9902B) with the primary end point of OS, 512 CRPC patients were randomized to either the sipuleucel-T arm or the placebo arm in a 2:1 ratio [102]. This study revealed a relative reduction in the risk of death of 22% (hazard ratio, 0.78; 95% CI, 0.61, 0.98; $P = 0.03$) and a significant improvement in OS as compared with the placebo group (median survival, 25.8 vs. 21.7 months, respectively). On the basis of these results, the use of sipuleucel-T for minimally symptomatic metastatic CRPC was approved by the FDA in USA. However, a recent report has raised severe controversy on scrutiny of the design of the sipuleucel-T trial [103]. Unpublished data from this trial demonstrated worse OS in older (aged > 65 years) vs. younger (aged < 65 years) patients in the placebo group (median survival, 17.3 vs. 28.2 months, respectively). Crucially, two-thirds of the cells harvested from placebo patients were frozen and not reinfused for possible later use. The patients older than 65 years may have been harmed by such cell loss. Furthermore, the older patients gained 5.6-month shorter survival compared with the younger patients in the sipuleucel-T treatment group. The age-dependent impairment of the immune system may have contributed to this deterioration. Thus, the safety and benefits for sipuleucel-T in CRPC patients should be assessed in consideration of all possible interpretations of this trial.

10.2. DCVax-Prostate

DCVax-Prostate is another APC-based vaccine, which is prepared from autologus dendritic cells incubated with a recombinant form of PSMA and GM-CSF. The APCs manufactured in this process are able to be cryopreserved and stored, and are administered by intradermal injection. The results of a Phase I/II trial that enrolled 32 CRPC patients, which were announced by Nothwest Biotherapeutics, indicated a strong T cell response to PSMA in approximately 80% of cases treated with DCVax-Prostate and prolonged TTP [104]. A randomized Phase III trial with 621 CRPC patients without metastasis is ongoing with the primary end point of TTP [104].

10.3. PROSTVAC-VF

PROSTVAC-VF is a vaccine containing two recombinant viral vectors (the vaccinia priming vector and the fowlpox boosting vector) encoding transgenes for PSA and three immune costimulatory molecules, including B7.1 (CD80), ICAM-1 (CD54), and LFA-3 (CD58). Two Phase I studies demonstrated safety of these vectors [105, 106]. In a single-arm Phase II trial, patients with a greater T-cell response to the PSA epitope exhibited a trend toward prolonged OS ($p = 0.055$) [107]. In a Phase II randomized, placebo (empty vector)-controlled trial, a total of 125 chemotherapy-naïve CRPC patients with no narcotic use and a Gleason score of ≤ 7 were randomized to receive either a vaccine or placebo in a 2:1 ratio [108]. Vaccinated patients had a better 3-year OS than controls (30%; 25/82 vs. 17%; 7/40) and a longer median OS (25.1 vs. 16.6 months); estimated hazard ratio 0.56 (95% CI, 0.37 to 0.85; $p = 0.0061$). This vaccine was well tolerated with injection site reactions, including erythema, pain, and swelling. These promising results encourage the development of a larger randomized Phase III study.

10.4. Ipilimumab (Yervoy®)

Ipilimumab (Bristol-Meyers Squibb) is a fully human monoclonal antibody that blocks a negative regulator of T cells, CTL-associated antigen-4 (CTLA-4), resulting in an enhanced anticancer immune response. In early Phase I/II trials evaluating ipilimumab alone [109] and in combination with either GM-CSF [110] or radiotherapy [111], some meaningful immune response activity was observed. Currently, two placebo-controlled Phase III trials to evaluate administration of ipilimumab either following radiotherapy after chemotherapy or in chemotherapy-naïve CRPC patients are ongoing [112, 113].

11. PATENT REVIEW COVERAGE FOR CRPC

Several recent patented strategies target key molecules related to signal transduction, molecular transport, cell adhesion, apoptosis, etc. The methods of knock-down against wild AR or AR splice variants also have an impact on treatment in CRPC. A composition with PCGEM1, prostate-specific non-coding RNA, is a potent candidate to inhibit the progression to CRPC. Recent patented molecules with possible therapeutic application in CRPC are summarized in Table **1**.

Table 1: Recent patented molecules with potent therapeutic application in CRPC.

Target Molecules	**Mechanisms of Action**	**Patent No.**
Hyaluronic acid (HA)	Degradation of HA by hyaluronidase	US0003238
Caveolin	Inhibition of caveolin expression	US7666412
Bag1 peptide	Induction of apoptosis via binding to molecular chaperone	WO2010012452
N-cadherin	Inhibition of *N*-cadherin expression	US0119527
AR splice variants	Regulation of splicing AR genes	US0110926
AR	LNA antagonists against AR sequences	US7737125
PCGEM1	Inhibition of PCGEM1 expression	US7807373
2,2,5,7,8-Pentamethyl-6-chromanol (PMCol)	Anti-inflammatory oxidative stress modulator and androgen antagonist	US7863324
$CXCL8_{(3-72)}$ K11R/G31P (G31P)	ELR-CXC chemokine antagonist	US0070405
Cabozatinib (XL184)	Dual inhibitor of MET and VEGF	WO2012044572

Bag1, Bcl-2 associated athanogene-1; LNA, locked nucleic acid bases; PCGEM1, prostate cancer gene expression marker 1.

US0003238 Frost *et al.* January 7, 2010

The patent is for modified hyaluronidase that degrades hyaluronic acid (HA) [114]. This composition is a potent tool against HA-rich prostate cancer [115].

US7666412 Thompson February 23, 2010

The patent is for treatments with anti-caveolin agents, including vector delivery of antisense caveolin sequences, the use of anti-caveolin antibodies and the use of caveolin-promoters [116]. Caveolin is a major structural component of caveolae, which are specialized plasma membrane invaginations involved in multiple cellular processes such as molecular transport, cell adhesion and signal transduction [117].

WO2010012452 Cato *et al.* February 4, 2010

The patent is for treatment with Bag1 peptide, which inhibits the proliferation of prostate cancer [118]. The nuclear isoform of Bag1 protein, Bag1-L, exhibits pro-apoptotic properties. Bag1-L peptide (68 amino acid sequence), which is correlated with the molecular chaperone GRP75 and GRP78, induces apoptosis in prostate cancer cells [119].

US0119527 Reiter *et al.* May 13, 2010

The patent is for treatment that targets *N*-cadherin in prostate and bladder cancer [120]. The cadherins are a superfamily of calcium-dependent cell adhesion molecules that mediate cell-cell adhesion, cell recognition, and tissue morphology. *N*-cadherin is overexpressed in advanced prostate cancer cells [121].

US0110926 Jun *et al.* May 12, 2011

The patent is for a composition that can be used for the treatment of prostate cancer on the basis of androgen receptor splice variants [122]. These AR variants have been identified to have a role in progression of androgen-independent prostate cancer [123].

US7737125 Worm June 15, 2010

The patent is for a composition comprising oligonucleotide compounds (oligomers) and a method leading to reduced expression of the androgen receptor [124]. Oligonucleotides containing locked nucleic acid bases (LNAs) have increased affinity for complementary DNA sequences (e.g., the promoter sequences of the androgen receptor).

US7807373 Srivastava *et al.* October 5, 2010

This patent is for medical practice such as diagnosis, prevention and treatment, using PCGEM1, a prostate-specific non-coding RNA and regulator of prostate cancer progression [125]. Over expression of PCGEM1 inhibits apoptosis induced by doxorubicin in prostate cancer cells [126]. PCGEM1 expression is upregulated in the progression to CRPC [127].

US7863324 Thompson *et al.* January 4, 2011

This patent is for the treatment of cancer with chroman-derived compounds (2,2,5,7,8-pentamethyl-6-chromanol (PMCol) and 2,2,5,7,8-pentamethylchroman (PMC)) [128]. These compounds basically function as potent anti-inflammatory oxidative stress modulators. PMCol also binds to the AR and acts as a strong androgen antagonist in prostate cancer cells [129].

US0070405 Gordon *et al.* March 22, 2012

This patent is for the use of a modified ELR-CXC chemokine antagonist, $CXCL8_{(3\text{-}72)}$ K11R/G31P (G31P), to treat some cancers including prostate cancer [130]. G31P has been shown to have anti-inflammatory actions that block activation of neutrophils via CXCR1 and CXCR2 [131]. G31P also exhibits suppression of cell proliferation, angiogenesis and migration in prostate cancer cells *in vitro* and in an orthotopic model of prostate cancer [130].

WO2012044572 David *et al.* April 5, 2012

This patent is for the treatment of cancer, particularly castration-resistant prostate cancer and osteoblastic bone metastases, with a dual inhibitor of MET and VEGF [132]. The signaling cascade of the receptor tyrosine kinase MET and its ligand hepatocyte growth factor (HGF) is important for cell growth and motility and is closely linked to the signaling pathway of VEGF, which is a potent factor in angiogenesis and cancer progression [133]. The MET/VEGF axis also plays important roles in osteoblast and osteoclast function [132]. A Phase II study with the current compound, cabozatinib (XL184), in metastatic CRPC patients is ongoing.

CURRENT & FUTURE DEVELOPMENTS

In recent years, treatments with diverse properties with potent antitumor effects on CRPC have been developed (Table **2**). Although docetaxel is a major cytotoxic agent with a survival benefit for CRPC in clinical settings, the further drugs that surpass

Table 2: New target therapies for CRPC in the clinical trials.

Category	Agents	Target Molecules	Mechanisms of Antitumor Effects	Summary of Phase III Trial
Anti-Androgen Agents	MDV3100	Androgen receptor (AR)	AR antagonist	Ongoing (NCT00974311, NCT01212991)
	Abiraterone	17α-Hydroxylase, C17, 20-lyase	CYP 17A1 inhibitor	Docetaxel-pretreated mCRPC Primary end point; OS (median; 14.8 mo Abiraterone vs. 10.9 mo placebo) (HR 0.65; 95% CI: 0.54, 0.77 ; $P < 0.001$)
	TAK-700	C17, 20-lyase	CYP 17A1 inhibitor	Ongoing (C21004, C21005)
	VN/124-1 (TOK-001)	C17, 20-lyase, AR	CYP 17A1 inhibitor, AR antagonist	Ongoing (ARMOR1; Phase I/II trial)
Endothelin Receptor Antagonists	Atrasentan (ABT627)	Endothelin-A (ET_A) receptor	ET_A receptor antagonist	Ongoing (NCT00134056)
	Zibotentan (ZD4054)			Halted (M0; NCT00626548, M1c; NCT00617669)
				Halted (M1; NCT00554229)
RANK-L Inhibitors	Denosumab	RANK-Ligand	Anti-RANK-L MAb	Primary end point; time to first occurrence of either SREs or bone metastasis (median time; 20.7 mo denosumab vs. 17.1 mo zoledronic acid) (HR 0.82; 95% CI: 0.71, 0.95 ; $P = 0.008$)
Bone-Seeking Radiopharmaceuticals	Alpharadin	Hydroxyapatite	α-Particle emitters derived from Radium-223-chrolide	Primary end point; OS (median; 14.0 mo Alpharadin vs. 11.2 mo placebo) (HR 0.695; 95% CI: 0.552, 0.875 ; $P = 0.0018$)
Angiogenesis Inhibitors	Bevacizumab	VEGF	Anti-VEGF Mab	Primary end point; OS (no significant difference between bevacizumab and placebo, in addition to docetaxel and predonisone) (CALGB 90401)
	Sunitinib	VEGF-R, PDGF-R	Tyrosine kinase inhibitor	Halted (NCT00676650)
	Aflibercept	VEGF (decoy)	VEGF trap	Ongoing (NCT00519285)
	Tasquinimod (ABR - 215050)	HIF1α, VEGF	Up-regulation of thrombospondin-1 (TSP1)	A Phase III study is planned

Table 2: contd…

Protein Tyrosine Kinase Inhibitors	Dasatinib	SFKs	Tyrosine kinase inhibitor	Ongoing (NCT00744497)
Molecular Chaperon Inhibitors	Custirsen (OGX-011)	Secretory clusterin (sCLU) mRNA	Antisense oligonucleotides against sSLU	
BCL-2 Inhitibors	AT-101	Bcl-2, Bcl-xL, Mcl-1, Bcl-w	Bcl family proteins inhibitors	Ongoing (NCT00744498; Phase II trial)
Cytotoxic Agents	Cabazitaxel	Microtubules	Stabilization of microtubules without cross-resistance of docetaxel	Primary end point; OS (median; 15.1 mo cabazitaxel vs. 12.7 mo mitoxantrone) (HR 0.7; 95% CI 0.59, 0.83; p < 0.0001)
	Epothilones			A Phase III study will be planned
	(ixabepilone, patupilone)			
	Platinum derivatives	DNA	Inhibition of DNA synthesis to overcome platinum-resistance	No schedule of further study (satraplatin)
	(satraplatin, picoplatin)			A Phase III study with picoplatin and docetavel is planned.
Immunotherapy	Sipuleucel-T	PAP	Induction of cytotoxic T cell acivated by dendric cells	A 33% reduction in the risk of death copmared with placebo (HR 1.50; 95% CI: 1.10, 2.05; p = 0.011) (D9901, D9902A) Primary end point; OS (median; 25.8 mo sipuleucel-T vs. 21.7 mo placebo) (HR 0.751; p = 0.012) (D9902B)
	DCVax-Prostate	PSMA		Ongoing (DCVax-Prostate: Phase III)
	PROSTVAC-VF	PSA		A Phase III study will be planned
	Ipilimumab	CTLA-4	Blockade of a negative T-cell regulator	Ongoing (NCT00861614, NCT01057810)

RANK-L, Receptor activator of nuclear factor-κB-ligand; VEGF, Vascular endothelial growth factor; VEGF-R, VEGF receptor; SFKs, Src family kinases; PAP, protatic acid phosphatase; PSMA, prostate-specific membrane antigen; PSA, prostate-specific antigen; CTLA-4, CTL-associated antigen-4.

the potentials of docetaxel in relation to antitumor activity and tolerability are needed, and to improve the clinical outcome in combination with docetaxel. To date, the cytotoxic cabazitaxel, immunotherapy with sipuleucel-T, and the anti-androgen

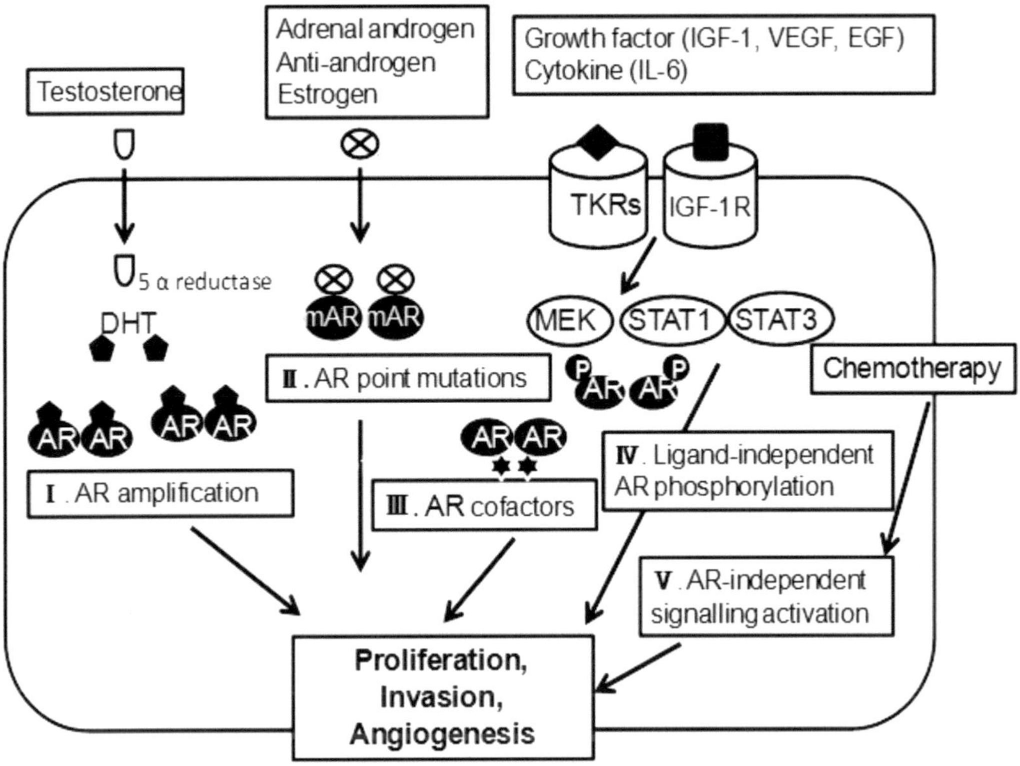

AR, Androgen receptor; DHT, Dihydrotestosterone; IGF-1, Insulin-like growth factor-1; EGF, Epithelial growth factor; TKRs, Tyrosine kinase receptors; IGF-1R, IGF-1 receptor

Figure 1: Schematic multiple cellular pathways related to CRPC.

abiraterone have been evaluated as powerful agents with significant clinical benefits in CRPC, leading to Food and Drug Administration (FDA) approval of these agents. In addition, several attractive endocrine therapies, including MDV3100, TAK700, and TOK-001, have demonstrated extensive efficacy in CRPC patients via strong antagonism of AR or reduction in endocrine production of androgens in the adrenal gland and CRPC cells. On the basis of extensive clinical evidence, a sequential strategy in the first step of CRPC treatment may be applicable to a vaccine-based immune-therapy or novel anti-androgen agents. Next, second-line therapy combined with docetaxel and other agents (e.g., atrasentan, tasquinimod, dasatinib, custirsen) has the potential to enhance the antitumor effects of docetaxel. Moreover, it is also important to focus on interruption of the transition to a CRPC state. Some candidates, such as bcl-2 family proteins, AR splicing variants, and PCGEM1, may be target molecules to prevent androgen-dependent cancer cells from transforming into CRPC. Novel compounds with current patents such as PMCol and G31P are unique with regard to their potential anti-inflammatory and antitumor effects. As for other pharmaceutical mechanisms, both Alpharadin (radium-223-chloride) and cabozatinib (XL184) may be potent agents specific for bone metastases of CRPC. However, multiple cellular pathways implicated in resistance to endocrine therapy or chemotherapy markedly contribute to failure of sequential monotherapy in beating CRPC (Fig. (**1**)). Based on diverse investigations to overcome the development of CRPC (e.g., progression to androgen-independent phase, microenvironment of bone-metastic sites, tumor-surrounding angiogenesis), it is anticipated that novel strategies for the treatment of CRPC will be established in the near future.

ACKNOWLEDGEMENTS

Declared none.

CONFLICT OF INTEREST

The authors confirm that this chapter content has no conflict of interest.

DISCLOSURE

The chapter submitted for Patent eBook Series “Topics in Anti-Cancer Research”, Volume 2 is an update of our article “New Therapeutic Strategies for Castration-Resistant Prostate Cancer”, published in the journal ‘Recent Patents on Anti-Cancer Drug Discovery’, Volume 6, Number 3, September, 2011, Page 373 to 383 with modified title, additional text and references.

REFERENCES

[1] Jemal A, Siegel R, Ward E, Hao Y, Xu J, Thun MJ. Cancer statistics, 2009. CA Cancer J Clin 2009; 59: 225-49.

[2] Petrylak DP, Tangen CM, Hussain MH, Lara PN Jr, Jones JA, Taplin ME, *et al.* Docetaxel and estramustine compared with mitoxantrone and prednisone for advanced refractory prostate cancer. N Engl J Med 2004; 351: 1513-20.

[3] Tannock IF, de Wit R, Berry WR, Horti J, Pluzanska A, Chi KN, *et al.* Docetaxel plus prednisone or mitoxantrone plus prednisone for advanced prostate cancer. N Engl J Med 2004; 351: 1502-12.

[4] Scher HI, Sawyers CL. Biology of progressive, castration-resistant prostate cancer: Directed therapies targeting the androgen-receptor signaling axis. J Clin Oncol 2005; 23: 8253-61.
[5] Attar RM, Takimoto CH, Gottardis MM. Castration-resistant prostate cancer: Locking up the molecular escape routes. Clin Cancer Res 2009; 15: 3251-5.
[6] Tran C, Ouk S, Clegg NJ, Chen Y, Watson PA, Arora V, *et al.* Development of a second-generation antiandrogen for treatment of advanced prostate cancer. Science 2009; 324: 787-90.
[7] Scher HI, Beer TM, Higano CS, Anand A, Taplin ME, Efstathiou E, *et al.* Antitumor activity of MDV3100 in castration-resistant prostate cancer: A Phase 1-2 study. Lancet 2010; 375: 1437-46.
[8] US Institute of Health, Clinical Trials. gov identifier NCT00974311. Available at http://clinicaltrials.gov (Acssesed on: February 6, 2012).
[9] US Institute of Health, Clinical Trials. gov identifier NCT01212991. Available at http://clinicaltrials.gov (Acssesed on: February 6, 2012).
[10] Small EJ, Halabi S, Dawson NA, Stadler WM, Rini BI, Picus J, *et al.* Antiandrogen withdrawal alone or in combination with ketoconazole in androgen-independent prostate cancer patients: A Phase III trial (CALGB 9583). J Clin Oncol 2004; 22: 1025-33.
[11] Ryan CJ, Smith MR, Fong L, Rosenberg JE, Kantoff P, Raynaud F, *et al.* Phase I clinical trial of the CYP17 inhibitor abiraterone acetate demonstrating clinical activity in patients with castration-resistant prostate cancer who received prior ketoconazole therapy. J Clin Oncol 2010; 28: 1481-8.
[12] Attard G, Reid AH, A'Hern R, Parker C, Oommen NB, Folkerd E, *et al.* Selective inhibition of CYP17 with abiraterone acetate is highly active in the treatment of castration-resistant prostate cancer. J Clin Oncol 2009; 27: 3742-8.
[13] US Institute of Health, Clinical Trials. gov identifier NCT00638690. Available at http://clinicaltrials.gov (Acssesed on: February 6, 2012).
[14] US Institute of Health, Clinical Trials. gov identifier NCT00887198. Available at http://clinicaltrials.gov (Acssesed on: February 6, 2012).
[15] de Bono JS, Logothetis CJ, Molina A, Fizazi K, North S, Chu L, *et al.* Abiraterine and increased survival in metastatic prostate cancer. N Engl J Med 2011; 364: 1995-2005.
[16] Yamaoka M, Hara T, Kusaka M. Overcoming persistent dependency on androgen signaling after progression to castration-resistant prostate cancer. Clin Cancer Res 2010; 16: 4319-24.
[17] Dreicer R, Agus DB, MacVicar GR, MacLean D, Zhang T, Stadler WM, *et al.* Safety, pharmacokinetics, and efficacy of TAK-700 in castration-resistant, metastatic prostate cancer: A Phase I/II, open-label study. *American Society of Clinical Oncology Genitourinary Cancers Symposium,* San Francisco, USA (2010).
[18] US Institute of Health, Clinical Trials. gov identifier NCT01193244. Available at http://clinicaltrials.gov (Acssesed on: February 6, 2012).
[19] US Institute of Health, Clinical Trials. gov identifier NCT01193257. Available at http://clinicaltrials.gov (Acssesed on: February 6, 2012).
[20] Vasaitis T, Belosay A, Schayowitz A, Khandelwal A, Chopra P, Gediya LK, *et al.* Androgen receptor inactivation contributes to antitumor efficacy of 17{alpha}-hydroxylase/17,20-lyase inhibitor 3beta-hydroxy-17-(1H-benzimidazole-1-yl) androsta-5,16-diene in prostate cancer. Mol Cancer Ther 2008; 7: 2348-57.

[21] Schayowitz A, Sabnis G, Njar VC, Brodie AM. Synergistic effect of a novel antiandrogen, VN/124-1, and signal transduction inhibitors in prostate cancer progression to hormone independence *in vitro*. Mol Cancer Ther 2008; 7: 121-32.

[22] Schayowitz A, Sabnis G, Goloubeva O, Njar VC, Brodie AM. Prolonging hormone sensitivity in prostate cancer xenografts through dual inhibition of AR and mTOR. Br J Cancer 2010; 103: 1001-7.

[23] US Institute of Health, Clinical Trials. gov identifier NCT00959959. Available at http://clinicaltrials.gov (Acssesed on: February 6, 2012).

[24] Carducci MA, Jimeno A. Targeting bone metastasis in prostate cancer with endothelin receptor antagonists. Clin Cancer Res 2006; 12: 6296s-300s.

[25] Carducci MA, Saad F, Abrahamsson PA, Dearnaley DP, Schulman CC, North SA, *et al.* A Phase 3 randomized controlled trial of the efficacy and safety of atrasentan in men with metastatic hormone-refractory prostate cancer. Cancer 2007; 110: 1959-66.

[26] Nelson JB, Love W, Chin JL, Saad F, Schulman CC, Sleep DJ, *et al.* Phase 3, randomized, controlled trial of atrasentan in patients with nonmetastatic, hormone-refractory prostate cancer. Cancer 2008; 113: 2478-87.

[27] Akhavan A, McHugh KH, Guruli G, Bies RR, Zamboni WC, Strychor SA, *et al.* Endothelin receptor A blockade enhances taxane effects in prostate cancer *in vitro* and *in vivo* molecular evidence for better therapeutic efficacy of ABT-627 and taxotere combination in prostate cancer. Neoplasia 2006; 8: 725-32.

[28] Banerjee S, Hussain M, Wang Z, Saliganan A, Che M, Bonfil D, *et al. In vitro* and *in vivo* molecular evidence for better therapeutic efficacy of ABT-627 and taxotere combination in prostate cancer. Cancer Res 2007; 67: 3818-26.

[29] Armstrong AJ, Creel P, Turnbull J, Moore C, Jaffe TA, Haley S, *et al.* A Phase I-II study of docetaxel and atrasentan in men with castration-resistant metastatic prostate cancer. Clin Cancer Res 2008; 14: 6270-6.

[30] US Institute of Health, Clinical Trials. gov identifier NCT00134056. Available at http://clinicaltrials.gov (Acssesed on: February 7, 2012).

[31] James ND, Caty A, Borre M, Zonnenberg BA, Beuzeboc P, Morris T, *et al.* Safety and efficacy of the specific endothelin-A receptor antagonist ZD4054 in patients with hormone-resistant prostate cancer and bone metastases who were pain free or mildly symptomatic: A double-blind, placebo-controlled, randomised, Phase 2 trial. Eur Urol 2009; 55: 1112-23.

[32] US Institute of Health, Clinical Trials. gov identifier NCT00626548. Available at http://clinicaltrials.gov (Acssesed on: February 7, 2012).

[33] US Institute of Health, Clinical Trials. gov identifier NCT00554229. Available at http://clinicaltrials.gov (Acssesed on: February 7, 2012).

[34] US Institute of Health, Clinical Trials. gov identifier NCT00617669. Available at http://clinicaltrials.gov (Acssesed on: February 7, 2012).

[35] AstraZeneca Press Release. Available at: http://www.astrazeneca.com/ (Accessed on: February 7, 2012).

[36] Narducci P, Bareggi R, Nicolin V. Receptor Activator for Nuclear Factor kappa B Ligand (RANKL) as an osteoimmune key regulator in bone physiology and pathology. Acta Histochem 2009; 17: 17.

[37] Dougall WC, Chaisson M. The RANK/RANKL/OPG triad in cancer-induced bone diseases. Cancer Metastasis Rev 2006; 25: 541-9.

[38] Saad F, Gleason DM, Murray R, Tchekmedyian S, Venner P, Lacombe L, *et al.* A randomized, placebo-controlled trial of zoledronic acid in patients with hormone-refractory metastatic prostate carcinoma. J Natl Cancer Inst 2002; 94:1458-68.

[39] Saad F, Gleason DM, Murray R, Tchekmedyian S, Venner P, Lacombe L, *et al.* Long-term efficacy of zoledronic acid for the prevention of skeletal complications in patients with metastatic hormone-refractory prostate cancer. J Natl Cancer Inst 2004; 96:879-82.

[40] Fizazi K, Bosserman L, Gao G, Skacel T, Markus R, Lipton A, *et al.* Denosumab treatment of prostate cancer with bone metastases and increased urine *N*-telopeptide levels after therapy with intravenous bisphosphonates: Results of a randomized Phase II trial randomized Phase II trial of denosumab in patients with bone metastases from prostate cancer, breast cancer, or other neoplasms after intravenous bisphosphonates. J Urol 2009; 182: 509-15.

[41] Fizazi K, Lipton A, Mariette X, Body JJ, Rahim Y, Gralow JR, *et al.* Randomized Phase II trial of denosumab in patients with bone metastases from prostate cancer, breast cancer, or other neoplasms after intravenous bisphosphonates. J Clin Oncol 2009; 27: 1564-71.

[42] US Institute of Health, Clinical Trials. gov identifier NCT00321620. Available at http://clinicaltrials.gov (Acssesed on: February 7, 2012).

[43] US Institute of Health, Clinical Trials. gov identifier NCT00286091. Available at http://clinicaltrials.gov (Acssesed on: February 7, 2012).

[44] Fizazi K, Carducci MA, Smith MR, Damião R, Brown JE, Karsh L, *et al.* Denosumab versus zoledronic acid for treatment of bone metastases in men with castration-resistant prostate cancer: A randomized, double-blind study. Lancet 2011; 377: 813-22.

[45] Lam MG, de Klerk JM, van Rijk PP, Zonnenberg BA. Bone seeking radiopharmaceuticals for palliation of pain in cancer patients with osseous metastases. Anticancer Agents Med Chem 2007; 7: 381-97.

[46] Tu SM, Lin SH, Podoloff DA, Logothetis CJ. Multimodality therapy: Bone-targeted radioisotope therapy of prostate cancer. Clin Adv Hematol Oncol 2010; 8: 341-51.

[47] Lewington VJ, McEwan AJ, Ackery DM, Bayly RJ, Keeling DH, Macleod PM, *et al.* A prospective, randomised double-blind crossover study to examine the efficacy of strontium-89 in pain palliation in patients with advanced prostate cancer metastatic to bone. J Cancer 1991; 27: 954-8.

[48] Porter AT, McEwan AJ, Powe JE, Reid R, McGowan DG, Lukka H, *et al.* Results of a randomized Phase-III trial to evaluate the efficacy of strontium-89 adjuvant to local field external beam irradiation in the management of endocrine resistant metastatic prostate cancer. Int J Radiat Oncol Biol Phys 1993; 25: 805-13.

[49] Liepe K. Alpharadin, a 223Ra-based alpha-particle-emitting pharmaceutical for the treatment of bone metastases in patients with cancer. Curr Opin Investig Drugs 2009; 10: 1346-58.

[50] Parker C. Overall survival benefit of radium-223 chloride (Alpharadin) in the treatment of patients wirh symptomatic bone metastases in castration-resistant prostate cancer. A Phase III randomized trial (ALSYMPCA). *European Society for Medical Oncology-European Cancer Organization (ESMO-ECCO) Conference,* 2011.

[51] George DJ, Halabi S, Shepard TF, Vogelzang NJ, Hayes DF, Small EJ, *et al.* Prognostic significance of plasma vascular endothelial growth factor levels in patients with hormone-refractory prostate cancer treated on cancer and leukemia Group B 9480. Clin Cancer Res 2001; 7: 1932-6.

[52] Di Lorenzo G, Figg WD, Fossa SD, Mirone V, Autorino R, Longo N, *et al.* Combination of bevacizumab and docetaxel in docetaxel-pretreated hormone-refractory prostate cancer: A Phase 2 study. Eur Urol 2008; 54: 1089-94.
[53] US Institute of Health, Clinical Trials. gov identifier NCT00110214. Available at http://clinicaltrials.gov (Acssesed on: March 16, 2012).
[54] Kelly WK. CALGB90401: Bevacizumab plus docetaxel/predonisone did not increase survival in metastatic CRPC. *American Society of Clinical Oncology Annual Meeting*, Chicago, USA (2010).
[55] Cumashi A, Tinari N, Rossi C, Lattanzio R, Natoli C, Piantelli M, *et al.* Sunitinib malate (SU-11248) alone or in combination with low-dose docetaxel inhibits the growth of DU-145 prostate cancer xenografts. Cancer Lett 2008; 270: 229-33.
[56] Sonpavde G, Periman PO, Bernold D, Weckstein D, Fleming MT, Galsky MD, *et al.* Sunitinib malate for metastatic castration-resistant prostate cancer following docetaxel-based chemotherapy. Ann Oncol 2010; 21: 319-24.
[57] US Institute of Health, Clinical Trials. gov identifier NCT00676650. Available at http://clinicaltrials.gov (Acssesed on: February 7, 2012).
[58] Lockhart AC, Rothenberg ML, Dupont J, Cooper W, Chevalier P, Sternas L, *et al.* Phase I study of intravenous vascular endothelial growth factor trap, aflibercept, in patients with advanced solid tumors. J Clin Oncol 2010; 28: 207-14.
[59] Tew WP, Gordon M, Murren J, Dupont J, Pezzulli S, Aghajanian C, *et al.* Phase 1 study of aflibercept administered subcutaneously to patients with advanced solid tumors. Clin Cancer Res 2010; 16: 358-66.
[60] US Institute of Health, Clinical Trials. gov identifier NCT00519285. Available at http://clinicaltrials.gov (Acssesed on: February 7, 2012).
[61] Isaacs JT, Pili R, Qian DZ, Dalrymple SL, Garrison JB, Kyprianou N, *et al.* Identification of ABR-215050 as lead second generation quinoline-3-carboxamide anti-angiogenic agent for the treatment of prostate cancer. Prostate 2006; 66: 1768-78.
[62] Dalrymple SL, Becker RE, Isaacs JT. The quinoline-3-carboxamide anti-angiogenic agent, tasquinimod, enhances the anti-prostate cancer efficacy of androgen ablation and taxotere without effecting serum PSA directly in human xenografts. Prostate 2007; 67: 790-7.
[63] Olsson A, Bjork A, Vallon-Christersson J, Isaacs JT, Leanderson T. Tasquinimod (ABR-215050), a quinoline-3-carboxamide anti-angiogenic agent, modulates the expression of thrombospondin-1 in human prostate tumors. Mol Cancer 2010; 9: 107.
[64] Bratt O, Haggman M, Ahlgren G, Nordle O, Bjork A, Damber JE. Open-label, clinical Phase I studies of tasquinimod in patients with castration-resistant prostate cancer. Br J Cancer 2009; 101: 1233-40.
[65] Pili R, Haggman M, Stadler WM, Gingrich JR, Assikis VJ, Björk A, *et al.* Phase II randomized, double-blind, placebo-controlled study of tasquinimod in men with minimally symptomatic metastatic castrate-resistant prostate cancer. J Clin Oncol 2011; 29: 4022-8.
[66] US Institute of Health, Clinical Trials. gov identifier NCT01234311. Available at http://clinicaltrials.gov (Acssesed on: February 7, 2012).
[67] Tatarov O, Mitchell TJ, Seywright M, Leung HY, Brunton VG, Edwards J. SRC family kinase activity is up-regulated in hormone-refractory prostate cancer. Clin Cancer Res 2009; 15: 3540-9.
[68] Nam S, Kim D, Cheng JQ, Zhang S, Lee JH, Buettner R, *et al.* Action of the Src family kinase inhibitor, dasatinib (BMS-354825), on human prostate cancer cells. Cancer Res 2005; 65: 9185-9.

[69] Koreckij T, Nguyen H, Brown LG, Yu EY, Vessella RL, Corey E. Dasatinib inhibits the growth of prostate cancer in bone and provides additional protection from osteolysis. Br J Cancer 2009; 101: 263-8.
[70] Yu EY, Wilding G, Posadas E, Gross M, Culine S, Massard C, *et al.* Phase II study of dasatinib in patients with metastatic castration-resistant prostate cancer. Clin Cancer Res 2009; 15: 7421-8.
[71] US Institute of Health, Clinical Trials. gov identifier NCT00744497. Available at http://clinicaltrials.gov (Acssesed on: March 16, 2012).
[72] So A, Hadaschik B, Sowery R, Gleave M. The role of stress proteins in prostate cancer. Curr Genomics 2007; 8: 252-61.
[73] Rizzi F, Bettuzzi S. Clusterin (CLU) and prostate cancer. Adv Cancer Res 2009; 105: 1-19.
[74] Zoubeidi A, Chi K, Gleave M. Targeting the cytoprotective chaperone, clusterin, for treatment of advanced cancer. Clin Cancer Res 2010; 16: 1088-93.
[75] Chi KN, Hotte SJ, Yu EY, Tu D, Eigl BJ, Tannock I, *et al.* Randomized Phase II study of docetaxel and prednisone with or without OGX-011 in patients with metastatic castration-resistant prostate cancer. J Clin Oncol 2010; 28: 4247-54.
[76] US Institute of Health, Clinical Trials. gov identifier NCT01188187. Available at http://clinicaltrials.gov (Acssesed on: March 19, 2012).
[77] US Institute of Health, Clinical Trials. gov identifier NCT01083615. Available at http://clinicaltrials.gov (Acssesed on: March 19, 2012).
[78] Tudor G, Aguilera A, Halverson DO, Laing ND, Sausville EA. Susceptibility to drug-induced apoptosis correlates with differential modulation of Bad, Bcl-2 and Bcl-xL protein levels. Cell Death Differ 2000; 7: 574-86.
[79] McDonnell TJ, Troncoso P, Brisbay SM, Logothetis C, Chung LW, Hsieh JT, *et al.* Expression of the protooncogene bcl-2 in the prostate and its association with emergence of androgen-independent prostate cancer. Cancer Res 1992; 52: 6940-4.
[80] Liu G, Kelly WK, Wilding G, Leopold L, Brill K, Somer B. An open-label, multicenter, Phase I/II study of single-agent AT-101 in men with castrate-resistant prostate cancer. Clin Cancer Res 2009; 15: 3172-6.
[81] MacVicar GR, Greco A, Reeves J, Maleski J, Holmlund J, Leopold L. An open-label, multicenter, Phase I/II study of AT-101 in combination with docetaxel (D) and predonisone (P) in men with castrate-resistant prostate cancer (CRPC). *American Society of Clinical Oncology Annual Meeting*, Orlando, USA (2009).
[82] US Institute of Health, Clinical Trials. gov identifier NCT00571675. Available at http://clinicaltrials.gov (Acssesed on: March 19, 2012).
[83] US Institute of Health, Clinical Trials. gov identifier NCT00666666. Available at http://clinicaltrials.gov (Acssesed on: March 19, 2012).
[84] Patterson SG, Wei S, Chen X, Sallman DA, Gilvary DL, Zhong B, *et al.* Novel role of Stat1 in the development of docetaxel resistance in prostate tumor cells. Oncogene 2006; 25: 6113-22.
[85] Zemskova M, Sahakian E, Bashkirova S, Lilly M. The PIM1 kinase is a critical component of a survival pathway activated by docetaxel and promotes survival of docetaxel-treated prostate cancer cells. J Biol Chem 2008; 283: 20635-44.
[86] Ranganathan S, Benetatos CA, Colarusso PJ, Dexter DW, Hudes GR. Altered beta-tubulin isotype expression in paclitaxel-resistant human prostate carcinoma cells. Br J Cancer 1998; 77: 562-6.

[87] Kamath K, Wilson L, Cabral F, Jordan MA. BetaIII-tubulin induces paclitaxel resistance in association with reduced effects on microtubule dynamic instability. J Biol Chem 2005; 280: 12902-7.
[88] Mita AC, Denis LJ, Rowinsky EK, Debono JS, Goetz AD, Ochoa L, *et al.* Phase I and pharmacokinetic study of XRP6258 (RPR 116258A), a novel taxane, administered as a 1-hour infusion every 3 weeks in patients with advanced solid tumors. Clin Cancer Res 2009; 15: 723-30.
[89] de Bono JS, Oudard S, Ozguroglu M, Hansen S, Machiels JP, Kocak I, *et al.* Prednisone plus cabazitaxel or mitoxantrone for metastatic castration-resistant prostate cancer progressing after docetaxel treatment: a randomised open-label trial. Lancet 2010; 376: 1147-54.
[90] Lee JJ, Kelly WK. Epothilones: Tubulin polymerization as a novel target for prostate cancer therapy. Nat Clin Pract Oncol 2009; 6: 85-92.
[91] Hussain M, Tangen CM, Lara PN, Jr., Vaishampayan UN, Petrylak DP, Colevas AD, *et al.* Ixabepilone (epothilone B analogue BMS-247550) is active in chemotherapy-naive patients with hormone-refractory prostate cancer: A Southwest Oncology Group trial S0111. J Clin Oncol 2005; 23: 8724-9.
[92] Rosenberg JE, Weinberg VK, Kelly WK, Michaelson D, Hussain MH, Wilding G, *et al.* Activity of second-line chemotherapy in docetaxel-refractory hormone-refractory prostate cancer patients: Randomized Phase 2 study of ixabepilone or mitoxantrone and prednisone. Cancer 2007; 110: 556-63.
[93] Hussain A, DiPaola RS, Baron AD, Higano CS, Tchekmedyian NS, Johri AR. Phase II trial of weekly patupilone in patients with castration-resistant prostate cancer. Ann Oncol 2009; 20: 492-7.
[94] Beardsley EK, Saad F, Eigl B, Venner P, Hotte S, Winquist E, *et al.* A Phase II study of patupilone in patients (pts) with metastatic castration-resistant prostate cancer (CRPC) who have progressed after docetaxel. *American Society of Clinical Oncology Annual Meeting*, Orlando, USA (2009).
[95] Latif T, Wood L, Connell C, Smith DC, Vaughn D, Lebwohl D, *et al.* Phase II study of oral bis (aceto) ammine dichloro (cyclohexamine) platinum (IV) (JM-216, BMS-182751) given daily x 5 in hormone refractory prostate cancer (HRPC). Invest New Drugs 2005; 23: 79-84.
[96] Sternberg CN, Petrylak DP, Sartor O, Witjes JA, Demkow T, Ferrero JM, *et al.* Multinational, double-blind, Phase III study of prednisone and either satraplatin or placebo in patients with castrate-refractory prostate cancer progressing after prior chemotherapy: The SPARC trial. J Clin Oncol 2009; 27: 5431-8.
[97] De Jager RL, Roman LD, Lopatkin NA, Karlov PA, Breitz HB, Earhart RH, *et al.* Phase II study of picoplatin with docetaxel and predonisone in first-line treatment of castration-resistant prostate cancer (CRPC). *American Society of Clinical Oncology Genitourinary Cancers Symposium*, San Francisco, USA (2010).
[98] Chambers CA, Krummel MF, Boitel B, Hurwitz A, Sullivan TJ, Fournier S, *et al.* The role of CTLA-4 in the regulation and initiation of T-cell responses. Immunol Rev 1996; 153: 27-46.
[99] Small EJ, Fratesi P, Reese DM, Strang G, Laus R, Peshwa MV, *et al.* Immunotherapy of hormone-refractory prostate cancer with antigen-loaded dendritic cells. J Clin Oncol 2000; 18: 3894-903.

[100] Small EJ, Schellhammer PF, Higano CS, Redfern CH, Nemunaitis JJ, Valone FH, *et al.* Placebo-controlled Phase III trial of immunologic therapy with sipuleucel-T (APC8015) in patients with metastatic, asymptomatic hormone refractory prostate cancer. J Clin Oncol 2006; 24: 3089-94.

[101] Higano CS, Schellhammer PF, Small EJ, Burch PA, Nemunaitis J, Yuh L, *et al.* Integrated data from 2 randomized, double-blind, placebo-controlled, Phase 3 trials of active cellular immunotherapy with sipuleucel-T in advanced prostate cancer. Cancer 2009; 115: 3670-9.

[102] Kantoff PW, Higano CS, Shore ND, Berger ER, Small EJ, Penson DF, *et al.* Sipuleucel-T immunotherapy for castration-resistant prostate cancer. N Engl J Med 2010; 363: 411-22.

[103] Huber ML, Haynes L, Parker C, Iversen P. Interdisciplinary critique of sipuleucel-T as immunotherapy in castration-resistant prostate cancer. J Natl Cancer Inst 2012; 104: 273-9.

[104] Northwest Biotherapeutics. Available at: http://www. nwbio.com/clinical_dcvax_prostate.php. (Accessed on: March 30, 2012).

[105] DiPaola RS, Plante M, Kaufman H, Petrylak DP, Israeli R, Lattime E, *et al.* A Phase I trial of pox PSA vaccines (PROSTVAC-VF) with B7-1, ICAM-1, and LFA-3 co-stimulatory molecules (TRICOM) in patients with prostate cancer. J Transl Med 2006; 4: 1-5.

[106] Arlen PM, Skarupa L, Pazdur M, Seetharam M, Tsang KY, Grosenbach DW, *et al.* Clinical safety of a viral vector based prostate cancer vaccine strategy. J Urol 2007; 178: 1515-20.

[107] Gulley JL, Arlen PM, Madan RA, Tsang KY, Pazdur MP, Skarupa L, *et al.* Immunologic and prognostic factors associated with overall survival employing a poxviral-based PSA vaccine in metastatic castrate-resistant prostate cancer. Cancer Immunol Immunother 2010; 59: 663-74.

[108] Kantoff PW, Schuetz TJ, Blumenstein BA, Glode LM, Bilhartz DL, Wyand M, *et al.* Overall survival analysis of a Phase II randomized controlled trial of a Poxviral-based PSA-targeted immunotherapy in metastatic castration-resistant prostate cancer. J Clin Oncol 2010; 28: 1099-105.

[109] Small EJ, Tchekmedyian NS, Rini BI, Fong L, Lowy I, Allison JP. A pilot trial of CTLA-4 blockade with human anti-CTLA-4 in patients with hormone-refractory prostate cancer. Clin Cancer Res 2007; 13: 1810-5.

[110] Fong L, Kwek SS, O'Brien S, Kavanagh B, McNeel DG, Weinberg V, *et al.* Potentiating endogenous antitumor immunity to prostate cancer through combination immunotherapy with CTLA4 blockade and GM-CSF. Cancer Res 2009; 69: 609-15.

[111] Slovin SF, Beer TM, Higano CS, Tejwani S, Hamid O, Picus J, *et al.* Initial Phase II experience of ipilimumab (IPI) alone and in combination with radiotherapy (XRT) in patients with metastatic castration-resistant prostate cancer (mCRPC). *American Society of Clinical Oncology Annual Meeting*, Orlando, USA (2009).

[112] US Institute of Health, Clinical Trials. gov identifier NCT00861614. Available at http://clinicaltrials.gov (Acssesed on: July 17, 2012).

[113] US Institute of Health, Clinical Trials. gov identifier NCT01057810. Available at http://clinicaltrials.gov (Acssesed on: July 17, 2012).

[114] Frost, G.I., Jiang, P., Thompson, C.B. Modified hyaluronidases and uses in treating hyaluronan-associated diseases and conditions. US0003238 (**2010**) & US20120171153 (**2012**).

[115] Bharadwaj AG, Kovar JL, Loughman E, Elowsky C, Oakley GG, Simpson MA. Spontaneous metastasis of prostate cancer is promoted by excess hyaluronan synthesis and processing. Am J Pathol 2009; 174: 1027-36.

[116] Thompson, T.C. Methods for the treatment of neoplastic disorders with anti-caveolin agents. US7666412 (**2010**).

[117] Thompson TC, Tahir SA, Li L, Watanabe M, Naruishi K, Yang G, *et al.* The role of caveolin-1 in prostate cancer: Clinical implications. Prostate Cancer Prostatic Dis 2010; 13: 6-11.

[118] Cato, A.B.C., Shatkina, L., Jehle, K., Maddalo, D. Bag-1 peptide that inhibits prostate cancer. WO2010012452 (**2010**).

[119] Maddalo D, Neeb A, Jehle K, Shatkina L, Cato A. Heat shock proteins: Distinct peptides derived from the cochaperone Bag-1L inhibit prostate cancer cell growth. *AACR-NCI-EORTC International Conference: Molecular Targets and Cancer Therapeutics*, Boston, USA (2009).

[120] Reiter, R.E. *N*-cadoherin: Target for cancer diagnosis and therapy. US0119527 (**2010**).

[121] Jennbacken K, Tesan T, Wang W, Gustavsson H, Damber JE, Welen K. *N*-cadherin increases after androgen deprivation and is associated with metastasis in prostate cancer. Endocr Relat Cancer 2010; 17: 469-79.

[122] Jun, L., George, S. B., William, I., Thomas, D., Rong, H. Compositions and methods for treating or preventing prostate cancer and for detecting androgen receptor variants. US0110926 (**2011**).

[123] Hu R, Dunn TA, Wei S, Isharwal S, Veltri RW, Humphreys E, *et al.* Ligand-independent androgen receptor variants derived from splicing of cryptic exons signify hormone-refractory prostate cancer. Cnacer Res 2009; 69: 16-22.

[124] Worm, J. LNA antagonists targeting the androgen receptor. US7737125 (**2010**).

[125] Srivastava, S., Moul, J.W., Srikantan, V., Zou, Z. Prostate-specific gene, PCGEM1, and the methods of using PCGEM1 to detect, treat, and prevent prostate cancer. US7807373 (**2010**).

[126] Fu X, Ravindranath L, Tran N, Petrovics G, Srivastava S. Regulation of apoptosis by a prostate-specific and prostate cancer-associated noncoding gene, PCGEM1. DNA Cell Biol 2006; 25: 135-41.

[127] Romanuik TL, Wang G, Morozova O, Delaney A, Marra MA, Sadar MD. LNCaP Atlas: Gene expression associated with *in vivo* progression to castration-recurrent prostate cancer. BMC Med Genomics 2010; 3: 43.

[128] Thompson, T.A. Chroman-derived compounds for the treatment of cancer. US7863324 (**2011**).

[129] Thompson TA, Wilding G. Androgen antagonist activity by the antioxidant moiety of vitamin E, 2,2,5,7,8-pentamethyl-6-chromanol in human prostate carcinoma cells. Mol Cancer Ther 2003; 2: 797-803.

[130] Gordon, J.R., Li, F. Uses of modified ELR-CXC chemokine G31P to treat cancer. US2012070405 (**2012**).

[131] Zhao X, Town JR, Li F, Zhang X, Cockcroft DW, Gordon JR. ELR-CXC chemokine receptor antagonism targets inflammatory responses at multiple levels. J Immunol 2009; 182: 3213-22.

[132] David, S., Maha, H. Dual inhibitors of MET and VEGF for the treatment of castration-resistant prostate cancer and osteoblastic bone metastases. WO2012044572 (**2012**).

[133] Yakes FM, Chen J, Tan J, Yamaguchi K, Shi Y, Yu P, *et al.* Cabozantinib (XL184), a novel MET and VEGFR2 inhibitor, simultaneously suppresses metastasis, angiogenesis, and tumor growth. Mol Cancer Ther 2011; 10: 2298-308.

Send Orders of Reprints at reprints@benthamscience.net
Topics in Anti-Cancer Research, Vol. 2, **2013, 35-62**

CHAPTER 2

Sphingomyelin Biosynthesis Modulates Cancer Cell Death and Growth

Elodie Lafont[1,2], Kazuyuki Kitatani[3], Toshiro Okazaki[4] and Bruno Ségui[1,2]

[1]INSERM UMR1037-Cancer Research Center of Toulouse, BP84225, 31432 Toulouse Cedex 4, France; [2]Department of Cell Biology, Hematology and Immunology, Faculty of Pharmaceutical Sciences, Paul Sabatier University (Toulouse III), 35 Chemin des Maraîchers, 31062, Toulouse, France; [3]Department of Clinical Laboratory, Medicine/Hematology, Faculty of Medicine, Tottori University, Yonago, Tottori 683-8504, Japan; [4]Department of Medicine, Kanazawa Medical University, Uchinada, Ishikawa 920-0293, Japan

Abstract: Resistance to death receptor ligands (such as FasL and TRAIL) and anticancer treatments is a hallmark of cancer cells. Alteration of sphingolipid (SL) metabolism is frequently observed in cancer cells and may contribute to resistance to stress-induced apoptosis. Ceramide, a biologically active sphingolipid, antagonizes cell growth and promotes apoptosis and non-apoptotic forms of cell death. The intracellular levels of ceramide are highly regulated via complex metabolic pathways. Sphingomyelin synthases (SMS) 1 and 2 convert ceramide to sphingomyelin (SM), a ubiquitous phospholipid in mammals. A growing body of evidence in the literature indicates that SMSs likely modulate cell growth and sensitivity to stress-induced apoptosis. On one hand, complete and sustained inhibition of SMS activity likely alters membrane composition and properties through membrane SM depletion, perturbing intracellular signaling pathways and cancer cell growth and conferring partial resistance to death receptor ligands. On the other hand, different patents & reports point to anti-apoptotic functions for SMSs. In patients with chemoresistant leukemia, a decreased intracellular ceramide level was associated with a higher SMS activity. Thus, SMSs and cofactors may constitute original pharmacological targets to treat malignant diseases. This chapter gives an overview on how SM biosynthesis putatively modulates cancer cell death and growth.

Keywords: Anticancer immune response, anticancer treatments, apoptosis, caspases, cell proliferation, cell death, ceramide, ceramidase, CERT, chemoresistance, death receptors, glucosylceramide synthase,

***Adddress correspondence to Bruno Ségui:** INSERM UMR1037-Cancer Research Center of Toulouse, BP84225, 31432 Toulouse Cedex 4, France; Tel: (33)561323531; Fax (33)561322084; E-mail: bruno.segui@inserm.fr and **Toshiro Okazaki:** Department of Medicine, Kanazawa Medical University, Uchinada, Ishikawa 920-0293, Japan; Tel: +81-76-218-8337; Fax: +81-76-286-9290; E-mail: toshiroo@kanazawa-med.ac.jp

Atta-ur Rahman and Khurshid Zaman (Eds)

hematological malignancies, microdomains, plasma membrane, sphingolipids, sphingolipid metabolism, sphingolipid signaling, sphingomyelinase, sphingomyelin synthase.

1. INTRODUCTION

Sphingolipids (SLs) are present in all human cells, in which they play a dual role: i) as modulators of membrane function, and ii) as intracellular signal transducers or extracellular messengers. SLs regulate key events, such as cell growth/survival or cell death [1, 2]. Through modifications in the fine membrane structure, cell-cell or cell-matrix interactions, and/or modulation of intracellular signaling pathways, SLs can affect the tumorigenic potential of numerous cell types. Ceramide and its metabolites can modulate the ability of malignant cells to grow and resist anticancer treatments and immune response. Death receptor (DR) ligands (i.e., CD95L, TRAIL and TNF) play a crucial role in anticancer immune surveillance owing to their ability to induce apoptosis in cancer cells. Anticancer treatments and DR-triggered apoptosis are accompanied by alterations of SL metabolism, leading to increased ceramide levels in sensitive but not resistant cancer cells. Restoring ceramide accumulation through modulation of SL metabolism is a promising therapeutical strategy to overcome cancer resistance to anticancer regimens and immune system [3].

1.1. Sphingolipid Metabolism and Diseases

Most SLs are intracellular and represent key membrane constituents. SL synthesis starts in the endoplasmic reticulum (ER) by several reactions leading to ceramide generation. In the ER, ceramide can be galactosylated by galactosylceramide synthase. However, ceramide is mostly transported to the Golgi apparatus to be metabolized in sphingomyelin (SM), the major sphingophospholipid, and/or glycosphingolipids. Ceramide is transported from the ER via CERT (a ceramide transporter protein) to be converted into SM within the lumen of the Golgi by SM synthases (SMS) [3, 4]. Alternatively, ceramide is transported through vesicular trafficking from the ER to the Golgi to be either converted to SM or glucosylceramide (GlcCer) by SMS and GlcCer synthase (GCS), respectively [5]. Two different mammalian genes encoding SMS have been cloned so far [6, 7] (see paragraph 2.2 for further details). The corresponding proteins, SMS1 and

SMS2, are both localized at the Golgi, SMS2 being also localized at the plasma membrane [6]. In agreement with Ullman and Radin's early observation in mouse liver [8], both SMS1 and 2 transfer the phosphocholine moiety from phosphatidylcholine to ceramide to generate SM and diacylglycerol (DAG) Fig. (**1**). SM as well as GlcCer (or its glycosylated derivatives) are in turn transported by vesicular trafficking to the plasma membrane where they concentrate into microdomains, mostly in the outer leaflet. SL catabolism occurs mainly in the lysosomes. For instance, acidic sphingomyelinase (SMase) and acidic β-glucosylceramidase (GlcCerase) hydrolyse lysosomal SM and GlcCer, respectively. SM breakdown also takes place at the plasma membrane by (neutral or acidic) SMases. In addition, GlcCer may be degraded by a non-lysosomal β-glucosidase [3, 4].

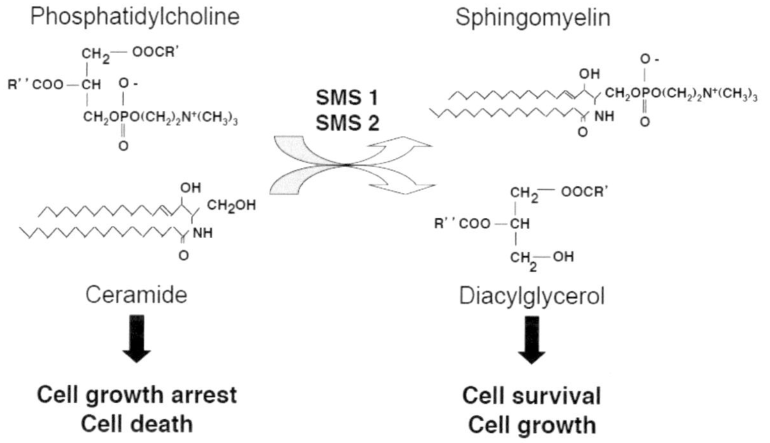

Figure 1: Enzymatic reaction catalyzed by sphingomyelin synthases: SMS1 and 2 can both transfer the phosphocholine moiety from phosphatidylcholine to ceramide, which is a growth inhibitory and pro-apoptotic sphingolipid. Depending on cell type and/or ceramide concentration, ceramide can, on the contrary, trigger cell growth. They concomitantly generate sphingomyelin and the pro-survival and cell growth-promoting diacylglycerol (DAG).

The importance of SLs in health and disease is illustrated by the dramatic consequences of inherited disruption of their normal metabolism (For an exhaustive review on SL metabolism disorders, see [9]). For instance, acid SMase deficiency is responsible for lysosomal SM storage leading to Niemann-Pick disease (type A and B). Acid ceramidase deficiency leads to lysosomal ceramide accumulation in cells derived from Farber disease patients. The most frequent SL metabolism disorder is Gaucher disease, which is characterized by GlcCer accumulation within the lysosomal compartment as a consequence of GlcCerase deficiency [9]. Noteworthy, patients affected with Gaucher disease are predisposed to develop cancers, such as multiple myeloma and hepatocellular carcinoma, with 51.1 and 141.3 relative risks, respectively [10].

1.2. Sphingolipids as Modulators of Cancer Cell Death and Progression

Accumulating evidence indicates that some SLs can facilitate cancer development, for instance by inhibiting cancer cell death or, conversely, by enhancing tumorigenesis, tumor neo-angiogenesis and metastatic potential, or by participating in cancer cell escape from the immune system and chemoresistance [11]. Among those SLs, S1P and gangliosides (i.e., sialic acid-bearing glycosphingolipids) are presently considered to play a major role in tumor biology. For instance, malignant cells display aberrant expression of gangliosides. GD3 expression is increased in melanoma cells as compared to melanocytes and highly metastatic melanoma cells expressed more GD3 than poorly metastatic cells [12]. Targeting glucosylceramide synthase by antisense or pharmacological approaches triggers ganglioside depletion and reduces melanoma progression in mouse [13, 14]. Gangliosides are expressed in the outer leaflet of the plasma membrane and are shed in the tumor microenvironment and circulation. Suppression of gangliosides reduces tumor angiogenesis [15]. Moreover, gangliosides can be considered as tumor weapons against immune cells, inhibiting anti-cancer immune response and promoting cancer progression [16]. S1P negatively modulates cell death and/or promotes cell proliferation and tumor angiogenesis. Also, S1P (and sphingosine kinase over-expression) appears to mediate chemo or radioresistance of solid tumor and leukemia cells [17]. A very recent patent provides siRNAs, which target mRNA encoding sphingosine kinase 1 and potentiate the effect of radiation in the treatment of various cancers [18]. Inventors describe the expression of sphingosine kinase 1 by immunohistochemistry in head and neck squamous cell carcinoma tissue, while the normal tissue does not express this enzyme. Western blotting analysis indicates sphingosine kinase 1 overexpression in primary tumor and lymph node metastases derived from patients affected with head and neck squamous cell carcinoma as compared to normal tissue. Transfection of siRNA targeting sphingosine kinase 1 in various cancer cell types (i.e., head and neck squamous cell carcinoma cell lines SCC-71 and SCC-15, breast cancer cell line MCF-7, prostate cancer cell line PC-3 and colon cancer cell line HT29) reduced cell viability by 20 to 50% 48 hours post-transfection and inhibited SCC-15 tumor growth in athymic mice. Moreover, siRNA transfected cells were highly sensitized to radiation as compared to control cells both *in vitro* and *in vivo* [18]. Thus, targeting sphingosine kinase 1 is a promising strategy to limit cancer progression and sensitize cancer cells to radiotherapy. However, since S1P is also involved in cell growth and survival of normal (not only tumor) cells and plays a critical function in lymphocyte trafficking, targeting S1P-metabolizing enzymes may be toxic for normal cells and impair the establishment of anticancer immune response.

In sharp contrast, ceramide is considered as an anti-proliferative pro-apoptotic SL metabolite for diverse cancer cells derived from solid and hematological malignancies, most likely through its capacity to activate the mitochondrial apoptotic pathway [2, 3, 19]. We have recently provided evidence that exogenously supplied ceramide triggers the increase of mitochondrial membrane permeability, cytochrome c release to the cytosol and caspase-9-dependent apoptosis in Jurkat leukemia T cells [20]. As a matter of fact, whereas wild-type Jurkat cells undergo apoptosis upon treatment with C2-ceramide (from 2.5 to 10μM), caspase-9-deficient Jurkat cells strongly resist. However, at higher concentration (20μM), exogenous ceramide elicits necrosis rather than apoptosis both in wild-type and caspase-9-deficient Jurkat cells [20]. Some exogenous ceramide analogs, which have been covered by patent [21], induce apoptotic and non-apoptotic leukemia cell death that can be inhibited by over-expression of the mitochondrial anti-apoptotic protein Bcl-xL [22]. Moreover, three recent patents provide a method, which associates conventional chemotherapy (i.e., cis-platinum, paclitaxel or gemcitabine) and C6-ceramide for increasing apoptosis in various solid and hematological cancer cells and decreasing tumor progression in mice [23-25]. One should note, however, that ceramide effects on cell fate may depend on cell type and/or ceramide concentration. For instance, C2- or C6-ceramide at low concentration (up to 2.5μM) can promote survival of neural cells, whereas higher concentrations (>10μM) induce cell death [26]. In addition, exogenous ceramide (2.5-5μM C2-ceramide) can trigger cell proliferation of smooth muscle cells, which efficiently convert ceramide into S1P [27].

Failure to generate ceramide in response to chemotherapeutic agents is also a mechanism of resistance that has been reported in various cancer cells [28, 29]. A decreased intracellular ceramide level in chemoresistant leukemia cells has been associated with an altered SL metabolism involving both higher SMS and GCS activities [30]. In addition, the epithelial-mesenchymal transition (EMT), a key process in cancer progression and metastasis [31], has been recently reported to be triggered by pharmacological inhibition of GCS and glycosphingolipid depletion in epithelial cells, including the MCF7 breast carcinoma cell line [32].

Acid ceramidase, which triggers the hydrolysis of ceramide into sphingosine and fatty acid within the lysosomal compartment, is up-regulated in malignant cells, including prostate cancer cells [33]. Enforced expression of acid ceramidase confers resistance to chemotherapy in prostate cancer [34] and melanoma cells [35], whereas acid ceramidase knock-down sensitizes hepatoma cells to chemotherapy [36]. Inhibition of acid ceramidase activity or acid ceramidase knock-down sensitized chronic myelogeneous leukemia (CML) cells to FasL-induced apoptosis. Conversely, overexpression of acid ceramidase decreased CML cells sensitivity to FasL [37]. Pharmacological inhibition of acid ceramidase or acid ceramidase knockdown inhibits tumor growth and metastasis in mouse models [36, 38, 39]. Thus, acid ceramidase, most likely through its ability to catabolize the anti-oncometabolite ceramide, appears to play a critical role in cancer progression and chemoresistance.

DR ligands such as FasL, TNF, and TRAIL all trigger ceramide generation through different mechanisms, including (i) SM breakdown (either by neutral or acid SMase), (ii) increased *de novo* synthesis, or (iii) inhibition of the SMS-mediated conversion of ceramide to SM [3]. Ceramide and/or its metabolites such as ganglioside GD3 or sphingosine are produced in DR signaling and have been suggested to act as second messengers in cell death induction. They indeed may enhance mitochondrial events such as cytochrome c and AIF release from the mitochondria to the cytosol [3, 40]. An attractive hypothesis is to consider that ceramide production regulates the biochemical and biophysical properties of the plasma membrane, enhancing early DR signaling events such as DR translocation to lipid rafts, DR oligomerization and DISC (Death-Inducing Signaling Complex) formation [41]. According to this concept, ceramide would favor early events in DR signaling at the plasma membrane level rather than acting as an intracellular lipid second messenger *per se* [3, 41, 42].

2. A SMS FAMILY

The activity of SM synthesis was reported to be present in mammals [8, 43]. The intracellular SM level is controlled by both its synthetic and catabolic pathways, and its synthesis is catalyzed only by the action of SMS. In 2004, Okazaki and Holthuis' groups discovered the genes encoding mouse and human SMS Table **1** [6, 7], allowing a better understanding of the physiological functions and regulation of SM synthesis in mammalian cells.

Table 1: A family of sphingomyelin synthases.

	Gene Symbol	AA	Cellular Localization	Enzymatic Products	mRNA Abundance
Human SMS1	*SGMS1*	413	GA	SM	Ubiquitous
SMS2	*SGMS2*	365	PM, GA	SM and CPE	Ubiquitous
SMSr	*SAMD8*	414	ER	CPE	
Mouse SMS1	*Sgms1*	419		SM	
SMS2	*Sgms2*	365		SM	
SMSr	*Samd8*	432			

SMS, sphingomyelin synthase; SMSr, sphingomyelin synthase related; AA, the number of amino acids; PM, plasma membrane; GA, Golgi apparatus; ER, endoplasmic reticulum; SM, sphingomyelin; CPE, ceramide phosphoethanolamine

2.1. SM Synthesis

SLs are chemically characterized by the presence of sphingoid bases, and ceramide is a central molecule in SL metabolism. Ceramide serves as a substrate for SMS, which implies that the formation of SM is controlled by the supply of ceramide. There are three major pathways for ceramide formation [19, 44] Fig. (**2**): i) the *de novo* pathway, ii) the "SM-ceramide" pathway, and iii) the salvage pathway. Those pathways are all connected to SM metabolism.

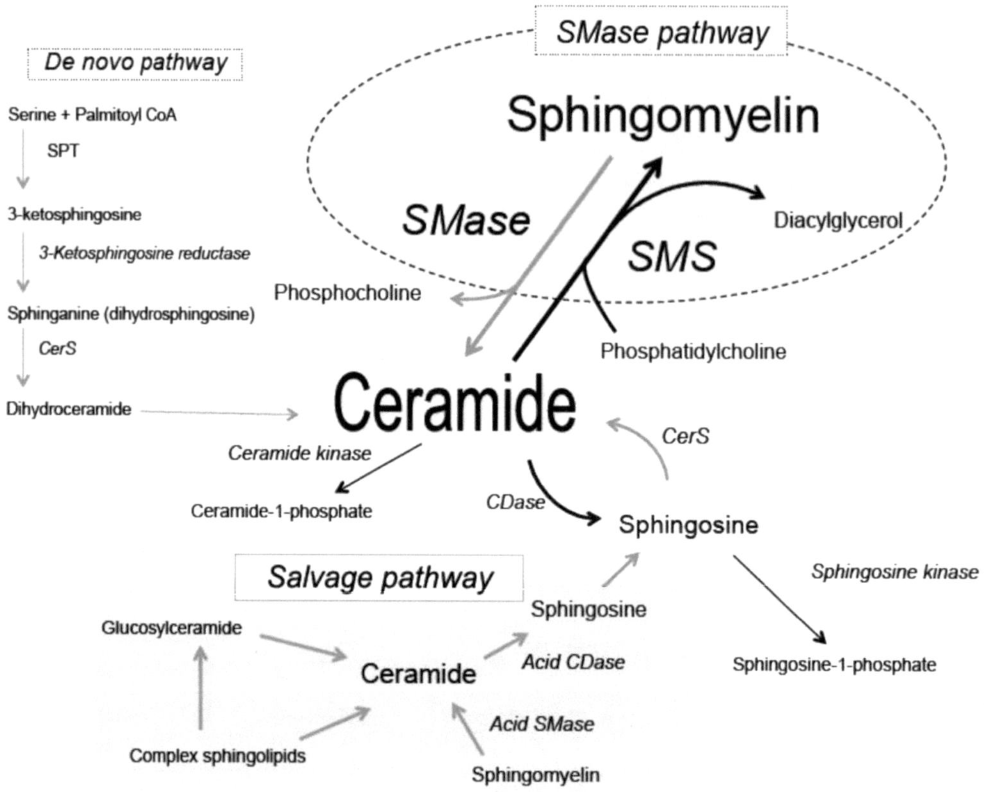

Figure 2: Ceramide synthesis: The scheme shows metabolic pathways for ceramide synthesis composed of the sphingomyelinase pathway, the *de novo* pathway, and the salvage pathway. Gray-colored lines indicate the pathway of ceramide synthesis. CDase, ceramidase; CerS, ceramide synthase; SMase, sphingomyelinase; SMS, sphingomyelin synthase; SPT, serine palmitoyltransferase.

De novo ceramide synthesis begins with the condensation of L-serine and palmitoyl-CoA, yielding 3-keto-dihydrosphingosine. The latter is reduced to dihydrosphingosine that undergoes *N*-acylation followed by desaturation to eventually generate ceramide. Those reactions occur at the cytosolic leaflet of the ER membrane, and CERT subsequently transfers ceramide to the Golgi apparatus to generate *de novo* SM [45].

Two types of SMase enzymes (acid and neutral SMase) are responsible for the "SM-ceramide" pathway, degrading SM to ceramide that modulates cellular signaling [19]. Conversely, SMS can convert back ceramide generated by SMase activation to SM [46]. The successive SM breakdown to ceramide, as a consequence of SMase activation, and SM (re)synthesis from ceramide, as catalyzed by SMS, has been termed the "SM cycle" [47].

The salvage pathway operates first in the acidic compartments by degrading complex sphingolipids to release sphingoid bases that are further metabolized in the ER to ceramide [44], and this salvaged ceramide can be converted to SM by the catalytic action of SMS.

2.2. Mammalian SMS Genes

Progress in understanding the biological roles of SM synthesis and its regulation has long been hampered by the fact that no successful purification of the responsible enzyme (i.e., SMS) was achieved. In 2003, Luberto *et al.*, for the first time, identified the Pseudomonas PlcH as a gene encoding a soluble protein with SMS activity [48]. In 2004, mammalian SMS genes encoding membrane-associated SMS enzymes were cloned [6, 7].

Our group has successfully identified human SMS1 [7]. Methodologically, the SMS molecular cloning began with the isolation of SM-deficient mouse lymphoid cells. Those cells are resistant to cell death induced by the SM-directed cytolytic protein lysenin [7]. Since SM levels play an important role in the retention of cholesterol in the plasma membrane [49], SM-deficient cells are highly sensitive to methyl-β-cyclodextrin, which is capable of inducing cell death by extracting cholesterol from the plasma membrane. SMS1 was cloned by screening a human cDNA library in SM-deficient cells as a suppressor of the toxicity triggered by methyl-β-cyclodextrin [7]. SMS1 expression in the SM-deficient cells restored SM synthesis and sensitivity to lysenin [7]. Consistent with the SMS activity study from Radin and Kennedy's groups [8, 43], SMS1 was able to transfer phosphocholine from phosphatidylcholine to ceramide to generate SM and DAG [6, 7]. The role of SMS1 in SM synthesis in hematological malignant cells was further documented in a Jurkat human T leukemia cell line stably expressing a siRNA targeting SMS1. Indeed, SMS1 knockdown triggered a significant reduction of SM synthesis and SM level and conferred resistance to lysenin-induced toxicity [50].

Holthuis and co-workers identified a family of animal SMS (SMS1, SMS2 and SMSr (SMS related)) using a functional cloning strategy in yeast, an organism lacking SMS activity [6, 46]. Both SMS1 and SMS2, but not SMSr, expression resulted in SM synthesis in yeast [6]. Consistent with the reported enzymatic characterization, SMS1 and SMS2 function as bi-directional lipid choline phosphodiesterases capable of converting phosphatidylcholine and ceramide into SM and DAG, and vice versa [6].

Human SMSr possesses homologs in mouse, nematodes and insects like *Drosophila melanogaster*. *Drosophila* does not synthesize SM but produces the SM analog ceramide phosphoethanolamine (CPE) as a major membrane constituent. Recently, Vacaru *et al.* demonstrated that mammalian SMSr catalyzes the synthesis of this sphingophospholipid in the ER lumen [51]. However, one should note that the CPE intracellular level is very low in mammalian cells, as analysed by mass spectrometry [51]. Another recent study demonstrated that SMS2 can synthesize CPE, indicating that SMS2 has a dual enzyme activity [52].

The nuclear fraction isolated from human leukemia cells has been shown to contain SMS activity [53]. SMS activities were also found in rat liver nuclear membrane and chromatin [54]. Whether or not SMS1 and/or SMS2 are responsible for nuclear SM synthesis remains currently unknown. Because SMS1 is Golgi-localized and SMS2 is mainly located at the plasma membrane [6], it is tempting to speculate that unidentified gene(s) may encode a SMS that specifically synthesizes SM in the nucleus.

2.3. Structure of Animal SMSs

SMS family members were predicted to have distinct domains such as a *N*-terminal sterile α motif (SAM) domain and multiple transmembrane (TM) domains Fig. (**3**) [6].

Both SMS1 and SMSr, but not SMS2, possess a SAM domain at the *N*-terminus part Fig. (**3**). SAM domains are known to be involved in diverse protein-protein interactions [55]. However, no SMS-interacting proteins have been identified so far. Deletion of the SAM domain in SMSr triggered its redistribution from the ER to the Golgi without affecting its enzymatic activity [51]. Neither truncation of

SMS1 SAM domain nor addition of the SAM domain to the *N*-terminus of SMS2 had any effect on their localization and catalytic activities [56]. Thus, the function of SMS SAM domain remains unclear.

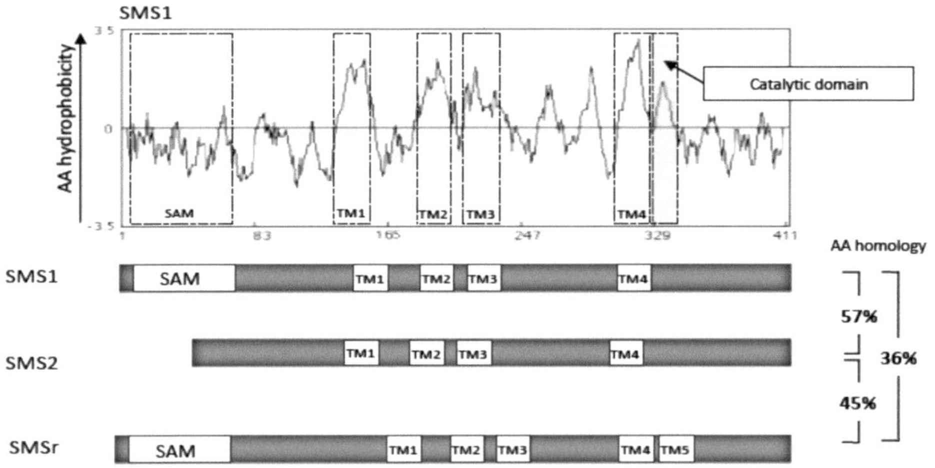

Figure 3: Structure and hydropathy plot of amino acid sequence in human SMS family: AA, amino acids; SAM, sterile alpha motif (SAM) domain; TM, candidate for transmembrane domain; SMS, sphingomyelin synthase; SMSr, sphingomyelin synthase related enzyme.

Both SMS1 and SMS2 contain two histidine and one aspartic acid residues, which are evolutionally conserved within the lipid phosphatase superfamily [6] and account for SMS activity [56]. SMS1 and 2 catalytic domains are located in the lumen of the Golgi [6], where most of SM synthesis takes place. Palmitoylation at the COOH-terminal tail of SMS2 accounts for its localization at the plasma membrane [57], where SMS2 catalytic domain is exposed at the cell surface, possibly allowing SM synthesis in the outer leaflet of the plasma membrane [6].

3. SMS IN CELL GROWTH/SURVIVAL

Several lines of evidence indicate that SMS activity behaves as a critical factor for cell growth and survival.

3.1. Role for SMSs in Cell Proliferation

Up-regulation of SMS activity has been reported to be associated with enhanced proliferation induced by hepatic regeneration [58], SV40-transformation [59] and basic Fibroblast Growth Factor (bFGF) [60]. So far, the mechanisms that promote SMS-dependent cell growth remain poorly understood. By limiting ceramide accumulation and increasing DAG levels, SMS activity likely enhances cell proliferation [61]. Using a fluorescently labelled conventional C1 domain (from protein kinase C (PKC)) for probing cellular DAG *in vivo*, Villani *et al.* demonstrated that SMS1 and SMS2 could substantially modulate subcellular pools of DAG [62]. Tafesse *et al.* have shown that both SMS1 and SMS2 positively modulate human HeLa carcinoma cell growth [61]. As a matter of fact, SMS1 or 2 knockdown in HeLa cells was accompanied by a decreased SM and an increased ceramide intracellular levels and by subsequent cell growth inhibition [61]. Moreover, SM-deficient WR19L mouse lymphoid leukemia did not grow in serum-free medium, which does not contain exogenous SM [7]. Expression of SMS1 not only restored SM synthesis but also cell growth under serum starvation conditions. Of a particular interest was the finding that addition of exogenous SM also restored SM-deficient WR19L cell growth, indicating that SM is an important constituent of cell membranes for optimal cell proliferation [7]. We have also documented the role of SMS1 in clathrin-dependent endocytosis of transferrin and transferrin receptor complexes and subsequent WR19L cell proliferation [63]. Jin *et al.* have recently reported that SMS1 knockdown in Jurkat cells severely impaired T-cell receptor (TCR) signaling, reducing LAT (Linker for activation of T cells)-dependent signaling complex formation in plasma membrane microdomains [50]. Similar findings have been documented in CD4+ T cells derived from SMS1 knockout mice [64]. Moreover, SMS1 knockout mice were more resistant to concanavalin A-induced hepatitis than their wild-type littermates most likely as a consequence of reduced CD4+ T cell proliferation and cytokine (IL-2 and IFNγ) production [64]. Thus, membrane SM appears to be critical for TCR signaling, leading to T cell proliferation and activation.

The increase in SMS activity is not always associated with an augmented cell proliferation rate. First, SMS activity and SM contents seem to be reduced in some cancer cells [65]. Second, the antitumor compound 2-hydroxyoleic acid (2OHOA) triggers SMS activity increase and growth arrest in human U118 glioma cells. Since pharmacological inhibition of SMS (by D609) attenuates the effect of 2OHOA on cell growth and SM synthesis, the authors concluded that the increased SMS activity was the cause of the observed anti-proliferative effect [65]. However, D609 can trigger anti-proliferative and/or cytotoxic effects in different cell types [66, 67], including in leukemia cells [68]. In addition, in a model of transient middle cerebral artery occlusion in rat, D609 reduced cerebral infarction [69]. This was associated with ceramide increase and up-regulation of Cdk inhibitor p21 and down-regulation of phospho-retinoblastoma (pRb) expression [69]. Thus, the D609 effects may depend on the cell type and/or pathophysiological context as well as D609 concentration. Moreover, one should note that D609 is unlikely a specific SMS inhibitor (see chapter 4.2) [66]. Thus, the sole use of this pharmacological inhibitor should not be considered as a sufficient experimental proof to implicate SMS in a given phenomenon.

SMS enzymes likely contribute to the modulation of phosphatidylcholine, ceramide, SM and DAG intracellular levels. Depending on the cell type and/or experimental conditions, SMS enzymes may differently modulate the balance between those lipids, which are also regulated by other lipid-metabolizing enzymes, the activity of which likely differs according to cell type and/or experimental conditions. The equilibrium between phospholipids (i.e., SM, phosphatidylcholine) and lipid bioactive molecules (i.e., DAG and ceramide), which are regulated by SMS, may govern the ability of SMS to favor or inhibit cell growth.

3.2. SMS Activity in the Survival of Normal and Cancer Cells

Interleukin-2 (IL-2) is a key cytokine for the clonal expansion and functional differentiation in natural killer (NK) cells. Human KHYG-1 NK cells require IL-2 for cell growth and survival. Experimentally, IL-2 deprivation from cell culture medium caused reduction of SMS activity, generation of ceramide and subsequent cell death [70]. Considering the function of ceramide as a pro-apoptotic molecule, inhibition of ceramide conversion to SM by down-regulation of SMS activity may favor ceramide accumulation and ceramide-dependent cell death. Thus, SMS activation in response to IL-2 likely limits ceramide accumulation and participates to the pro-survival effects triggered by IL-2 in NK cells [70].

Ceramide serves as a substrate for SMS and GCS, forming SM and GlcCer, respectively. The latter has been implicated in drug resistance because GCS up-regulation promotes the conversion of ceramide to GlcCer and blocks ceramide accumulation [71]. Drug-resistant HL-60/ADR cells have been established from human leukemic HL-60 cells, and doxorubicin treatment increased the ceramide levels and apoptosis in drug-sensitive HL-60 cells but not drug-resistant HL-60/ADR cells [30]. HL-60/ADR cells displayed an up-regulation of SMS and GCS activities as compared with the parental cells. Consistently, those enzyme activities were also up-regulated and ceramide was decreased in leukemic cells from chemoresistant patients. Those results might imply that the coordination of ceramide consumption by those enzymes is involved in chemoresistance of leukemia.

Recently, Swanton *et al.* identified CERT gene influencing sensitivity of different cancer cell types to chemotherapeutic agents, and showed that CERT expression is increased in drug-resistant cell lines [72]. As CERT delivers ceramide to the sites of SMS activity, CERT up-regulation might increase the availability of ceramide for SM synthesis and eventually suppress ceramide accumulation that leads to cell death. This CERT-SMS cooperation may influence the sensitivity of cancer cells to chemotherapeutic agents. Taken together, inhibiting SM biosynthesis may represent an interesting strategy to sensitize cancer cells to chemotherapy.

4. SM SYNTHESIS IN STRESS-INDUCED APOPTOSIS

SM is the most abundant SL in human cell (plasma) membranes [73, 74]. SM synthesis is known to modulate apoptosis, and may represent a pivotal element in tuning the response of cancer cells to insults such as DR ligands and chemotherapeutics. First, a growing body of evidence indicates that inhibition of SM synthesis may be responsible, at least in part, for stress-induced ceramide increase. Second, as a substrate for SMases, SM constitutes a main source of ceramide production in stress-induced apoptosis. Third, SM is a key microdomain component and may therefore regulate biophysical and biochemical plasma membrane properties, modulating stress-induced proximal apoptotic signaling events [3, 74, 75].

4.1. Inhibition of SM Synthesis in Stress-Induced Apoptosis

Various stress stimuli, including FasL (or agonistic anti-Fas antibody), TNF, staurosporine, UVB and photodynamic therapy, inhibit SM synthesis [53, 75-79].

For instance, CD95/Fas engagement is accompanied by (i) the activation of a neutral SMase activity, (ii) the inhibition of a SMS activity, and (iii) ceramide increase within the nucleus in Jurkat leukemia T cells [53]. All these events occurred in a caspase-dependent manner since they were prevented by the caspase inhibitor DEVD-cmk [53]. Thus, together with SMase activation, the inhibition of SMS activity likely enhances ceramide production in Fas signaling. More recently, we provided evidence that FasL-induced apoptosis is accompanied by caspase-dependent cleavage and inhibition of SMS1, which is the most expressed isoform in Jurkat leukemic cells [75]. Furthermore, we demonstrated that SMS1 is a novel caspase substrate, which was cleaved in a cell free system by various caspases including caspase-2, -7, -8 and -9, but not caspase-3 and -10. FasL-triggered SMS1 cleavage and inhibition were abolished by zVAD-fmk, a broad-spectrum caspase inhibitor [75]. *In vitro*, SMS specific activity, as measured in protein extracts derived from Jurkat cells, was decreased in a time- (as early as 15 min) and caspase-dependent manner in Fas signaling [75], further indicating that SMS1 is directly cleaved and inactivated by caspases Fig. (**4**).

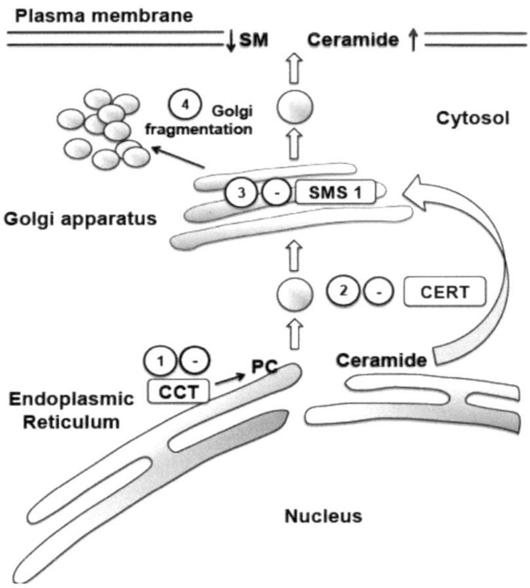

Figure 4: Different ways to inhibit *de novo* SM synthesis: (1) the inhibition of *de novo* PC synthesis, as a consequence of caspase-dependent CTP:phosphocholine cytidylyltransferase (CCT) cleavage and inhibition, (2) the inhibition of vesicular- or CERT-dependent ceramide transfer from the endoplasmic reticulum to the Golgi apparatus, (3) the caspase-dependent SMS1 cleavage and inhibition, (4) the caspase-dependent Golgi apparatus fragmentation.

Caspase-dependent cleavage of SMS1 is unlikely to be the only mechanism that accounts for the inhibition of SM synthesis in Fas signaling. Indeed, Golgi dismantling rapidly occurs after Fas ligation [80]. Golgi fragmentation may be responsible for the alteration of specific catalytic activity of Golgi-located enzymes. Accordingly, we have shown that SMS1, which is Golgi-localized in untreated cells, relocates throughout the cytoplasm upon FasL treatment [75]. Moreover, one can speculate that Golgi alteration and consequently, SMS1 relocation, may decrease SMS substrates (i.e., ceramide and PC) delivery and accessibility and, in turn, could reduce SM synthesis. In addition, stress-induced apoptosis is associated with caspase-dependent cleavage and inhibition of CTP:phosphocholine cytidylyltransferase (CCT), the rate-limiting enzyme of *de novo* PC synthesis [81]. Hence, CCT inhibition results in the decrease of synthesis of PC, a direct substrate of SMS and thus, likely impairs *de novo* SM synthesis [3]. Indeed, we observed that *de novo* PC synthesis was significantly reduced in Fas signaling [75]. The other substrate of SMS is ceramide. Whereas, stress-induced apoptosis triggers *de novo* ceramide synthesis, the transport of ceramide from the ER to the Golgi may be impaired as a consequence of the inhibition of CERT activity [3] and/or vesicular trafficking [5]. Interestingly, inhibition of SM synthesis in response to UVB was associated with the homotrimerization of CERT, indicating that the alteration of CERT-dependent ceramide trafficking may constitute an alternative mechanism for SM synthesis inhibition [79] Fig. (**4**). More recently, CERT has been described as a novel caspase substrate that is cleaved and mislocalized, inhibiting SM synthesis in TNF-induced apoptosis [82].

4.2. Does SMS Inhibition Modulate Apoptotic Signaling?

To evaluate whether SMS inhibition may be a causal event in stress-induced ceramide generation and apoptosis rather than a mere consequence of cell death, SMS activity and expression in malignant cells were inhibited by pharmacological and silencing strategies, respectively.

Jaspine B, a phytosphingosine derived from marine sponge, which displayed toxicity towards various cancer cells [83], has been recently reported to trigger SM synthesis inhibition, ceramide increase and cell death in melanoma cells [84]. In addition, the CERT inhibitor *N*-(3-hydroxy-1-hydroxymethyl-3-phenylprol)alkaneamide 12

(HPA-12), which impairs SM synthesis [85, 86], restored paclitaxel-induced cell death in resistant ovarian cancer cells [72]. Thus, pharmacological inhibition of SM synthesis in cancer cells may trigger apoptosis and/or sensitize cells to chemotherapy, most likely by perturbing the ceramide-SM equilibrium.

D609 is a compound that has been widely used as an inhibitor of phosphatidylcholine-specific phospholipase C (PC-PLC) and, indirectly, acidic SMase. For instance, D609 impairs TNF- and anti-Fas-induced activation of a PC-PLC (the molecular identity of which remains unknown) and acidic SMase [87-90]. In this context, PC-PLC stimulation leads to the rise of DAG, which enhances acidic SMase activity and hence ceramide levels [87, 88]. Although in the literature, D609 was used as acidic SMase inhibitor, it cannot be considered as a specific inhibitor of this enzyme. Indeed, D609 has been shown to inhibit SMS [6, 53, 59]. Noteworthy, D609 and derivatives, which inhibit SMS activity and display cytotoxicity towards cancer cells, including leukemic cells, have been recently patented [91].

D609 has been reported to modulate cell death signaling initiated by death receptors. D609 can prevent TNF-induced cytotoxicity in various cell types both *in vitro* and *in vivo* [90, 92]. However, D609 has been shown to sensitize U937 leukemic cells to TNF and an agonistic anti-Fas antibody [93]. Controversy exists as to the effect of D609 in Fas signaling. D609 inhibits a nuclear SMS activity and enhances Fas cross-linking-induced ceramide production and cell death in Jurkat cells [53]. More recently, it has been published that D609 impaired HeLa cell death in response to an agonistic anti-Fas antibody whereas it had no effect in SKW6.4 cells [94]. Thus, one can speculate that the ability of D609 to modulate death receptor-induced cell death is cell type-dependent. However, it should be noted that opposite findings were reported using the same cell type, i.e., Jurkat cells, in response to Fas engagement [53, 94]. In our hands, D609 triggers ceramide increase as well as caspase-dependent and caspase-independent cell death in Jurkat and PHA-activated T cells [68]. Moreover, sub-toxic D609 concentrations significantly enhance FasL-induced cell death and overcome, to some extent, the resistance to FasL conferred by caspase-8 or RIP deficiency [68].

The conflicting findings observed using D609 might be related to the lack of specificity of this inhibitor [66]. As a matter of fact, we have recently shown that not only SMS activity but also, albeit to a lesser extent, GCS activity is decreased in Jurkat and PHA-activated T cells incubated in the presence of D609 [68]. Thus, D609 cannot be considered as a specific inhibitor of PC-PLC and SMS and is likely able to inhibit other lipid-metabolizing enzymes such as GCS or phospholipases including PC-PLD and PE-PLC [95]. Hence, D609 probably acts on multiple metabolic and signaling pathways, and the molecular mechanisms involved are not fully established. Further studies are needed to elucidate the mode of action of this compound.

Based on an epigenetic strategy, we have recently reported that, in Jurkat cells, the inhibition of SMS1 expression by RNA interference triggered 40% SMS activity reduction and significantly enhanced FasL-triggered ceramide generation, caspase cascade activation and apoptosis [75]. Conversely, FasL neither increased ceramide levels nor efficiently induced cell death in SMS1-overexpressing HeLa cells, exhibiting 150% SMS activity increase. Finally, SMS1 knockdown not only sensitized HeLa cells to FasL but also overcame the resistance conferred by SMS1 overexpression. Moreover, SMS2, which is expressed in HeLa cells, may also negatively regulate FasL-induced apoptosis, albeit to a lesser extent as compared to SMS1 [75]. Thus, our findings argue for an anti-apoptotic function of SMS enzymes in Fas signaling, SMS1 displaying the highest anti-apoptotic activity. Because SMS1 is Golgi-located whereas SMS2 is mostly localized at the plasma membrane, it is tempting to speculate that the conversion of ceramide to SM in the Golgi apparatus, rather than at the plasma membrane, is critical for apoptosis inhibition. This notion is supported by different reports, indicating the compartimentalization of ceramide metabolism likely contributes to the ceramide function in cell signaling pathways [96].

The anti-apoptotic function of SMS is unlikely restricted to Fas signaling. Indeed, different studies indicate that SMS inhibits apoptosis under various stress conditions. In *Saccharomyces cerevisiae*, which do not express endogenous SMS, expression of mouse SMS1 suppressed the growth-inhibitory effect of Bax and other cytotoxic stimuli including hydrogen peroxide, heat shock, osmotic stress and exogenous ceramide [97]. In Jurkat cells, whereas SMS1 or SMS2 knockdown sensitized cells to phototherapy-induced cell death, SMS1 over-expression was protective [77, 78]. Finally, SMS1 overexpression inhibits staurosporine-triggered apoptosis in oligodendroglioma cells [98]. Thus, under various stress conditions, SMSs behave as anti-apoptotic enzymes, likely through their ability to metabolize the pro-apoptotic ceramide into non-apoptotic (inert) SM. Alternatively, SMS activity may increase the Golgi level of DAG [62], thereby inhibiting stress-induced apoptosis via recruitment and activation of DAG-binding protein, such as PKC.

Other reports, however, may indicate a pro-apoptotic function of SMS. A S49 mouse lymphoma cell line, which was completely deficient for SMS1 expression and SMS activity, resisted alkyl-lysoPC (edelfosine)-induced cell death [99]. SMS1-knockdown in parental S49 cells triggered SM deficiency and conferred resistance to edelfosine. In this study, it was concluded that SMS1 downregulation impairs lipid raft composition, and, in turn, inhibits edelfosine uptake [99]. Of note, different patents covered the use of various exogenous SLs, including SM analogs, for increasing chemotherapeutic drug delivery and/or cytotoxicity effect in cancer cells [21, 100, 101]. Moreover, it has been reported that edelfosine-resistant S49 cells display decreased Fas expression and resist FasL-induced apoptosis [102]. Interestingly, addition of exogenous short-chain SM partially restored Fas expression into microdomains and FasL sensitivity. Thus, SM, which is enriched in plasma membrane microdomains, likely stabilizes Fas expression at the cell surface, facilitating FasL-induced cell death [102]. In another SM-deficient murine leukemia cell line (WR19L), CD95 relocation into microdomains, DISC formation and apoptosis were significantly impaired upon treatment with an agonistic anti-CD95 antibody [103]. Overexpression of SMS1 restored DISC formation, full caspase activation and cell death in SM-deficient WR19L cells upon CD95 engagement [103]. In addition, SMS1 expression in SM-deficient WR19L cells significantly enhanced DISC formation and cell death in response to cisplatin combined to anti-Fas antibody [104]. These results seem at odds with our recent observations in HeLa and Jurkat cells, in which SMS1 knockdown enhanced FasL-induced apoptosis [75]. However, one should note that, under our experimental conditions, SM level was minimally affected by SMS1 knockdown. Thus, partial SMS1 inhibition does not drastically impair SM content and significantly enhanced FasL-induced cell death most likely by limiting ceramide conversion to SM. In sharp contrast, membrane SM depletion, as a consequence of complete and sustained inhibition of SMS activity, may alter microdomain composition and properties and impair proximal events in CD95 signaling such as DISC formation, thereby conferring partial resistance to CD95 agonists [3].

In addition, TNF-triggered pro-apoptotic and pro-inflammatory cell signaling is likely modulated by SM synthesis. Whereas overexpression of SMS1 or 2 in Chinese hamster ovarian cells enhanced apoptosis in response to TNF [105], SMS2 knockdown in HEK293 cells decreased by 50% *de novo* SM synthesis and impaired TNF-triggered recruitment of TNF-R1 to lipid rafts, TNF-R1 internalization and NF-κB activation [106]. The same group reported that SMS1 or 2 knockdown in THP1-derived macrophages reduced intracellular SM level by 20% and sensitivity to lipopolysaccharide (LPS)-mediated apoptosis [105]. Finally, LPS-triggered NF-κB activation was altered in macrophages derived from SMS2-knockout mice, which displayed reduced *de novo* SM synthesis [106]. SMS silencing or deficiency resulted in the impairment of membrane recruitment of TLR4 signaling complexes, altering LPS signaling in macrophages [105, 106]. Thus, the two latter studies further support the notion that plasma membrane SM is important to modulate proximal events in cell signaling, enabling formation of macromolecular signaling complexes upstream of cascade pathway activation.

5. CURRENT & FUTURE DEVELOPMENTS

Different studies demonstrate that SM synthesis is important for cell growth. First, cell growth is significantly reduced in SM-deficient cells, including in leukemia cells [7]. Second, SMS1 or SMS2 knockdown slows down cell growth in HeLa cells [61]. Third, two different reports indicate that SM synthesis is likely increased in chemoresistant cancer cells. SMS activity, along with GCS activity, was higher in chemoresistant leukemia cells as compared to chemosensitive cells. Accordingly, ceramide levels were lower in chemoresistant cells, indicating that ceramide is metabolized into complex sphingolipids (i.e., SM and glycosphingolipids) [30]. In addition, the expression of CERT, which is required for efficient SM synthesis, was increased in paclitaxel-resistant cell lines and ovarian tumors [72]. Interestingly, CERT knockdown significantly sensitized cancer cells to multiple anticancer drugs [72]. Thus, inhibiting SM synthesis through blockade of CERT-dependent ceramide trafficking or SMS activity, may constitute an interesting strategy to increase intracellular levels of ceramide and sensitize cancer cells to chemotherapy. One should note however that SM depletion as a consequence of SMS1 or SMS2 gene knockout enhanced SV40-transformed mouse embryonic fibroblast migration in response to CXCL12 [107], a chemokine being chemoattractant towards different leukocytes, including lymphocytes, and involved in tumor angiogenesis and metastasis [108]. Two recent patents indicate that SMS1 expression is downregulated during cancer progression [109, 110]. The expression of SMS1 is decreased in metastatic melanoma relative to non-metastatic melanoma samples [109]. Moreover, the deletion of chromosome 10 region 51.9 - 54.2, containing the *SGMS1* gene, is associated with a poor disease outcome in non-small cell lung cancer [110]. Thus, more studies are needed to clarify the role of SMS in cancer progression and to evaluate the putative therapeutic benefit of modulating SMS expression and/or activity to fight cancer.

ACKNOWLEDGEMENTS

We are grateful to Drs. T. Levade and H. Benoist for critical reading of the chapter. This study has been funded by Paul Sabatier University, INSERM (to EL and BS) and was supported in part by the Sapporo Biocluster "Bio-S", the Knowledge Cluster Initiative of the Ministry of Education, Sports, Science and Technology (Japan), and the Japan Society for the Promotion of Science (Grant-in-Aid for Young Scientists Start-up 21890144 to K.K.).

CONFLICT OF INTEREST

Authors declare no conflict of interest.

DISCLOSURE

The chapter submitted for Patent eBook Series "Topics in Anti-Cancer Research", Volume 2 is an update of our article "Regulation of Death and Growth Signals at the Plasma Membrane by Sphingomyelin Synthesis: Implications for Hematological Malignancies", published in the journal 'Recent Patents on Anti-Cancer Drug Discovery', Volume 6, Number 3, September 2011, Page 324 to 333 with modified title, additional text and references.

REFERENCES

1] Hannun YA, Obeid LM. The ceramide-centric universe of lipid-mediated cell regulation: Stress encounters of the lipid kind. J Biol Chem 2002; 277(29): 25847-50.

[2] Hannun YA. Functions of ceramide in coordinating cellular responses to stress. Science 1996; 274(5294):1855-9.

[3] Segui B, Andrieu-Abadie N, Jaffrezou JP, Benoist H, Levade T. Sphingolipids as modulators of cancer cell death: Potential therapeutic targets. Biochim Biophys Acta 2006; 1758(12): 2104-20.

[4] Futerman AH, Hannun YA. The complex life of simple sphingolipids. EMBO Rep 2004; 5(8): 777-82.

[5] Giussani P, Colleoni T, Brioschi L, Bassi R, Hanada K, Tettamanti G, *et al.* Ceramide traffic in C6 glioma cells: Evidence for CERT-dependent and independent transport from ER to the Golgi apparatus. Biochim Biophys Acta 2008; 1781(1-2): 40-51.

[6] Huitema K, van den Dikkenberg J, Brouwers JF, Holthuis JC. Identification of a family of animal sphingomyelin synthases. Embo J 2004; 23(1): 33-44.

[7] Yamaoka S, Miyaji M, Kitano T, Umehara H, Okazaki T. Expression cloning of a human cDNA restoring sphingomyelin synthesis and cell growth in sphingomyelin synthase-defective lymphoid cells. J Biol Chem 2004; 279(18): 18688-93.

[8] Ullman MD, Radin NS. The enzymatic formation of sphingomyelin from ceramide and lecithin in mouse liver. J Biol Chem 1974; 249(5): 1506-12.

[9] Sabourdy F, Kedjouar B, Sorli SC, Colie S, Milhas D, Salma Y, *et al.* Functions of sphingolipid metabolism in mammals-lessons from genetic defects. Biochim Biophys Acta 2008; 1781(4): 145-83.

[10] de Fost M, Vom Dahl S, Weverling GJ, Brill N, Brett S, Haussinger D, *et al.* Increased incidence of cancer in adult Gaucher disease in Western Europe. Blood Cells Mol Dis 2006; 36(1): 53-8.

[11] Ogretmen B, Hannun YA. Biologically active sphingolipids in cancer pathogenesis and treatment. Nat Rev Cancer 2004; 4(8): 604-16.

[12] Birkle S, Zeng G, Gao L, Yu RK, Aubry J. Role of tumor-associated gangliosides in cancer progression. Biochimie 2003; 85(3-4): 455-63.

[13] Deng W, Li R, Guerrera M, Liu Y, Ladisch S. Transfection of glucosylceramide synthase antisense inhibits mouse melanoma formation. Glycobiology 2002; 12(3): 145-52.

[14] Guerrera M, Ladisch S. *N*-Butyldeoxynojirimycin inhibits murine melanoma cell ganglioside metabolism and delays tumor onset. Cancer Lett 2003; 201(1): 31-40.

[15] Zeng G, Gao L, Birkle S, Yu RK. Suppression of ganglioside GD3 expression in a rat F-11 tumor cell line reduces tumor growth, angiogenesis, and vascular endothelial growth factor production. Cancer Res 2000; 60(23): 6670-6.

[16] Potapenko M, Shurin GV, de Leon J. Gangliosides as immunomodulators. Adv Exp Med Biol 2007; 601: 195-203.

[17] Pyne NJ, Pyne S. Sphingosine 1-phosphate and cancer. Nat Rev Cancer 2010; 10(7): 489-503.

[18] Sinha, U.K., Masood, R. Compositions and methods of sphingosine kinase inhibitors in radiation therapy of various cancers. US20100331393 (**2010**) & US20120259150 (**2012**).

[19] Hannun YA, Obeid LM. Principles of bioactive lipid signaling: Lessons from sphingolipids. Nat Rev Mol Cell Biol 2008; 9(2): 139-50.

[20] Lafont E, Dupont R, Andrieu-Abadie N, Okazaki T, Schulze-Osthoff K, Levade T, *et al.* Ordering of ceramide formation and caspase-9 activation in CD95L-induced Jurkat leukemia T cell apoptosis. Biochim Biophys Acta 2012; 1821(4): 684-93.

[21] Dagan, A., Gatt, S. Sphingolipids. US6756504 (**2004**).

[22] Granot T, Milhas D, Carpentier S, Dagan A, Segui B, Gatt S, *et al.* Caspase-dependent and -independent cell death of Jurkat human leukemia cells induced by novel synthetic ceramide analogs. Leukemia 2006; 20(3): 392-9.

[23] Wanebo, H.J., Mehta, S. Combinations of ceramide and chemotherapeutic agents for inducing tumor cell death. US7015251 (**2006**).

[24] Wanebo, H.J. Combination of ceramide and gemcitabine for inducing cell death and uses thereof in treating cancer. US20090246271 (**2009**).

[25] Wanebo, H.J., Mehta, S. Combinations of ceramide and chemotherapeutic agents for inducing cell death and uses thereof in treating cancer. US7820718 (**2010**).

[26] Luberto C, Kraveka JM, Hannun YA. Ceramide regulation of apoptosis versus differentiation: A walk on a fine line. Lessons from neurobiology. Neurochem Res 2002; 27(7-8): 609-17.

[27] Auge N, Nikolova-Karakashian M, Carpentier S, Parthasarathy S, Negre-Salvayre A, Salvayre R, *et al.* Role of sphingosine 1-phosphate in the mitogenesis induced by oxidized low density lipoprotein in smooth muscle cells via activation of sphingomyelinase, ceramidase, and sphingosine kinase. J Biol Chem 1999; 274(31): 21533-8.

[28] Kolesnick R. The therapeutic potential of modulating the ceramide/sphingomyelin pathway. J Clin Invest 2002; 110(1): 3-8.

[29] Saddoughi SA, Song P, Ogretmen B. Roles of bioactive sphingolipids in cancer biology and therapeutics. Subcell Biochem 2008; 49: 413-40.

[30] Itoh M, Kitano T, Watanabe M, Kondo T, Yabu T, Taguchi Y, *et al.* Possible role of ceramide as an indicator of chemoresistance: Decrease of the ceramide content via activation of glucosylceramide synthase and sphingomyelin synthase in chemoresistant leukemia. Clin Cancer Res 2003; 9(1): 415-23.

[31] Hugo H, Ackland ML, Blick T, Lawrence MG, Clements JA, Williams ED, *et al.* Epithelial-mesenchymal and mesenchymal-epithelial transitions in carcinoma progression. J Cell Physiol 2007; 213(2): 374-83.

[32] Guan F, Handa K, Hakomori SI. Specific glycosphingolipids mediate epithelial-to-mesenchymal transition of human and mouse epithelial cell lines. Proc Natl Acad Sci USA 2009; 106(18): 7461-6.

[33] Seelan RS, Qian C, Yokomizo A, Bostwick DG, Smith DI, Liu W. Human acid ceramidase is overexpressed but not mutated in prostate cancer. Genes Chromosomes Cancer 2000; 29(2): 137-46.

[34] Saad AF, Meacham WD, Bai A, Anelli V, Elojeimy S, Mahdy AE, *et al.* The functional effects of acid ceramidase overexpression in prostate cancer progression and resistance to chemotherapy. Cancer Biol Ther 2007; 6(9): 1455-60.

[35] Bedia C, Casas J, Andrieu-Abadie N, Fabrias G, Levade T. Acid ceramidase expression modulates the sensitivity of A375 melanoma cells to dacarbazine. J Biol Chem 2011; 286(32): 28200-9.

[36] Morales A, Paris R, Villanueva A, Llacuna L, Garcia-Ruiz C, Fernandez-Checa JC. Pharmacological inhibition or small interfering RNA targeting acid ceramidase sensitizes hepatoma cells to chemotherapy and reduces tumor growth *in vivo*. Oncogene 2007; 26(6): 905-16.

[37] Hu X, Yang D, Zimmerman M, Liu F, Yang J, Kannan S, *et al.* IRF8 regulates acid ceramidase expression to mediate apoptosis and suppresses myelogeneous leukemia. Cancer Res 2011; 71(8): 2882-91.
[38] Selzner M, Bielawska A, Morse MA, Rudiger HA, Sindram D, Hannun YA, *et al.* Induction of apoptotic cell death and prevention of tumor growth by ceramide analogues in metastatic human colon cancer. Cancer Res 2001; 61(3): 1233-40.
[39] Samsel L, Zaidel G, Drumgoole HM, Jelovac D, Drachenberg C, Rhee JG, *et al.* The ceramide analog, B13, induces apoptosis in prostate cancer cell lines and inhibits tumor growth in prostate cancer xenografts. Prostate 2004; 58(4): 382-93.
[40] Siskind LJ. Mitochondrial ceramide and the induction of apoptosis. J Bioenerg Biomembr 2005; 37(3): 143-53.
[41] van Blitterswijk WJ, van der Luit AH, Veldman RJ, Verheij M, Borst J. Ceramide: Second messenger or modulator of membrane structure and dynamics? Biochem J 2003; 369(Pt 2): 199-211.
[42] Segui B, Legembre P. Redistribution of CD95 into the lipid rafts to treat cancer cells? Recent Pat Anticancer Drug Discov 2010; 5(1): 22-8.
[43] Voelker DR, Kennedy EP. Cellular and enzymic synthesis of sphingomyelin. Biochemistry 1982; 21(11): 2753-9.
[44] Kitatani K, Idkowiak-Baldys J, Hannun YA. The sphingolipid salvage pathway in ceramide metabolism and signaling. Cell Signal 2008; 20(6): 1010-8.
[45] Hanada K, Kumagai K, Yasuda S, Miura Y, Kawano M, Fukasawa M, *et al.* Molecular machinery for non-vesicular trafficking of ceramide. Nature 2003; 426(6968): 803-9.
[46] Tafesse FG, Ternes P, Holthuis JC. The multigenic sphingomyelin synthase family. J Biol Chem 2006; 281(40): 29421-5.
[47] Hannun YA. The sphingomyelin cycle and the second messenger function of ceramide. J Biol Chem 1994; 269(5): 3125-8.
[48] Luberto C, Stonehouse MJ, Collins EA, Marchesini N, El-Bawab S, Vasil AI, *et al.* Purification, characterization, and identification of a sphingomyelin synthase from *Pseudomonas aeruginosa*. PlcH is a multifunctional enzyme. J Biol Chem 2003; 278(35): 32733-43.
[49] Fukasawa M, Nishijima M, Itabe H, Takano T, Hanada K. Reduction of sphingomyelin level without accumulation of ceramide in Chinese hamster ovary cells affects detergent-resistant membrane domains and enhances cellular cholesterol efflux to methyl-beta - cyclodextrin. J Biol Chem 2000; 275(44): 34028-34.
[50] Jin ZX, Huang CR, Dong L, Goda S, Kawanami T, Sawaki T, *et al.* Impaired TCR signaling through dysfunction of lipid rafts in sphingomyelin synthase 1 (SMS1)-knockdown T cells. Int Immunol 2008; 20(11): 1427-37.
[51] Vacaru AM, Tafesse FG, Ternes P, Kondylis V, Hermansson M, Brouwers JF, *et al.* Sphingomyelin synthase-related protein SMSr controls ceramide homeostasis in the ER. J Cell Biol 2009; 185(6): 1013-27.
[52] Ternes P, Brouwers JF, van den Dikkenberg J, Holthuis JC. Sphingomyelin synthase SMS2 displays dual activity as ceramide phosphoethanolamine synthase. J Lipid Res 2009; 50(11): 2270-7.
[53] Watanabe M, Kitano T, Kondo T, Yabu T, Taguchi Y, Tashima M, *et al.* Increase of nuclear ceramide through caspase-3-dependent regulation of the "sphingomyelin cycle" in Fas-induced apoptosis. Cancer Res 2004; 64(3): 1000-7.
[54] Albi E, Magni MV. Sphingomyelin synthase in rat liver nuclear membrane and chromatin. FEBS Lett 1999; 460(2): 369-72.

[55] Kim CA, Bowie JU. SAM domains: Uniform structure, diversity of function. Trends Biochem Sci 2003; 28(12): 625-8.

[56] Yeang C, Varshney S, Wang R, Zhang Y, Ye D, Jiang XC. The domain responsible for sphingomyelin synthase (SMS) activity. Biochim Biophys Acta 2008; 1781(10): 610-7.

[57] Tani M, Kuge O. Sphingomyelin synthase 2 is palmitoylated at the COOH-terminal tail, which is involved in its localization in plasma membranes. Biochem Biophys Res Commun 2009; 381(3): 328-32.

[58] Miro-Obradors MJ, Osada J, Aylagas H, Sanchez-Vegazo I, Palacios-Alaiz E. Microsomal sphingomyelin accumulation in thioacetamide-injured regenerating rat liver: Involvement of sphingomyelin synthase activity. Carcinogenesis 1993; 14(5): 941-6.

[59] Luberto C, Hannun YA. Sphingomyelin synthase, a potential regulator of intracellular levels of ceramide and diacylglycerol during SV40 transformation. Does sphingomyelin synthase account for the putative phosphatidylcholine-specific phospholipase C? J Biol Chem 1998; 273(23): 14550-9.

[60] Riboni L, Viani P, Bassi R, Giussani P, Tettamanti G. Basic fibroblast growth factor-induced proliferation of primary astrocytes: Evidence for the involvement of sphingomyelin biosynthesis. J Biol Chem 2001; 276(16): 12797-804.

[61] Tafesse FG, Huitema K, Hermansson M, van der Poel S, van den Dikkenberg J, Uphoff A, *et al.* Both sphingomyelin synthases SMS1 and SMS2 are required for sphingomyelin homeostasis and growth in human HeLa cells. J Biol Chem 2007; 282(24): 17537-47.

[62] Villani M, Subathra M, Im YB, Choi Y, Signorelli P, Del Poeta M, *et al.* Sphingomyelin synthases regulate production of diacylglycerol at the Golgi. Biochem J 2008; 414(1): 31-41.

[63] Shakor AB, Taniguchi M, Kitatani K, Hashimoto M, Asano S, Hayashi A, *et al.* Sphingomyelin synthase 1-generated sphingomyelin plays an important role in transferrin trafficking and cell proliferation. J Biol Chem 2011; 286(41): 36053-62.

[64] Dong L, Watanabe K, Itoh M, Huan CR, Tong XP, Nakamura T, *et al.* CD4+ T-cell dysfunctions through the impaired lipid rafts ameliorate concanavalin A-induced hepatitis in sphingomyelin synthase 1-knockout mice. Int Immunol 2012; 24(5): 327-37.

[65] Barcelo-Coblijn G, Martin ML, de Almeida RF, Noguera-Salva MA, Marcilla-Etxenike A, Guardiola-Serrano F, *et al.* Sphingomyelin and sphingomyelin synthase (SMS) in the malignant transformation of glioma cells and in 2-hydroxyoleic acid therapy. Proc Natl Acad Sci USA 2011; 108(49): 19569-74.

[66] Adibhatla RM, Hatcher JF, Gusain A. Tricyclodecan-9-yl-xanthogenate (D609) mechanism of actions: A mini-review of literature. Neurochem Res 2012; 37(4): 671-9.

[67] Gusain A, Hatcher JF, Adibhatla RM, Wesley UV, Dempsey RJ. Anti-proliferative effects of tricyclodecan-9-yl-xanthogenate (D609) involve ceramide and cell cycle inhibition. Mol Neurobiol 2012; 45(3): 455-64.

[68] Milhas D, Andrieu-Abadie N, Levade T, Benoist H, Ségui B. The tricyclodecan-9-yl-xanthogenate D609 triggers ceramide increase and enhances FasL-induced caspase-dependent and -independent cell death in T lymphocytes. Int J Mol Sci 2012; 13(7): 8834-52.

[69] Adibhatla RM, Hatcher JF. Protection by D609 through cell-cycle regulation after stroke. Mol Neurobiol 2010; 41(2-3): 206-17.

[70] Taguchi Y, Kondo T, Watanabe M, Miyaji M, Umehara H, Kozutsumi Y, *et al.* Interleukin-2-induced survival of natural killer (NK) cells involving phosphatidylinositol-3 kinase-

dependent reduction of ceramide through acid sphingomyelinase, sphingomyelin synthase, and glucosylceramide synthase. Blood 2004; 104(10): 3285-93.

[71] Gouaze-Andersson V, Cabot MC. Glycosphingolipids and drug resistance. Biochim Biophys Acta 2006; 1758(12): 2096-103.

[72] Swanton C, Marani M, Pardo O, Warne PH, Kelly G, Sahai E, *et al.* Regulators of mitotic arrest and ceramide metabolism are determinants of sensitivity to paclitaxel and other chemotherapeutic drugs. Cancer Cell 2007; 11(6): 498-512.

[73] Merrill AH, Jr., Jones DD. An update of the enzymology and regulation of sphingomyelin metabolism. Biochim Biophys Acta 1990; 1044(1): 1-12.

[74] Milhas D, Clarke CJ, Hannun YA. Sphingomyelin metabolism at the plasma membrane: Implications for bioactive sphingolipids. FEBS Lett 2009; 584(9): 1887-94.

[75] Lafont E, Milhas D, Carpentier S, Garcia V, Jin ZX, Umehara H, *et al.* Caspase-mediated inhibition of sphingomyelin synthesis is involved in FasL-triggered cell death. Cell Death Differ 2010; 17(4): 642-54.

[76] Bourteele S, Hausser A, Doppler H, Horn-Muller J, Ropke C, Schwarzmann G, *et al.* Tumor necrosis factor induces ceramide oscillations and negatively controls sphingolipid synthases by caspases in apoptotic Kym-1 cells. J Biol Chem 1998; 273(47): 31245-51.

[77] Separovic D, Hanada K, Maitah MY, Nagy B, Hang I, Tainsky MA, *et al.* Sphingomyelin synthase 1 suppresses ceramide production and apoptosis post-photodamage. Biochem Biophys Res Commun 2007; 358(1): 196-202.

[78] Separovic D, Semaan L, Tarca AL, Awad Maitah MY, Hanada K, Bielawski J, *et al.* Suppression of sphingomyelin synthase 1 by small interference RNA is associated with enhanced ceramide production and apoptosis after photodamage. Exp Cell Res 2008; 314(8): 1860-8.

[79] Charruyer A, Bell SM, Kawano M, Douangpanya S, Yen TY, Macher BA, *et al.* Decreased ceramide transport protein (CERT) function alters sphingomyelin production following UVB irradiation. J Biol Chem 2008; 283(24): 16682-92.

[80] Ouasti S, Matarrese P, Paddon R, Khosravi-Far R, Sorice M, Tinari A, *et al.* Death receptor ligation triggers membrane scrambling between Golgi and mitochondria. Cell Death Differ 2007; 14(3): 453-61.

[81] Lagace TA, Miller JR, Ridgway ND. Caspase processing and nuclear export of CTP: Phosphocholine cytidylyltransferase alpha during farnesol-induced apoptosis. Mol Cell Biol 2002; 22(13): 4851-62.

[82] Chandran S, Machamer CE. Inactivation of ceramide transfer protein during pro-apoptotic stress by Golgi disassembly and caspase cleavage. Biochem J 2012; 442(2): 391-401.

[83] Higa, T., Tanaka, J., Garcia-Gravalos, D. Oxy- and amino-substituted tetrahydrofuryl derivatives with antitumor activity. US6864283 (**2005**).

[84] Salma Y, Lafont E, Therville N, Carpentier S, Bonnafe MJ, Levade T, *et al.* The natural marine anhydrophytosphingosine, Jaspine B, induces apoptosis in melanoma cells by interfering with ceramide metabolism. Biochem Pharmacol 2009; 78(5): 477-85.

[85] Kobayashi, S., Hanada, K. Sphingolipid synthesis inhibitor. US6888015 (**2005**).

[86] Hanada, K., Nishijima, M., Kumagai, K. Drug promoting ceramide transport, base sequence for producing the drug, method of measuring activity of promoting ceramide release and method of measuring activity of promoting intermembrane ceramide transfer. US20080085859 (**2008**).

[87] Schutze S, Potthoff K, Machleidt T, Berkovic D, Wiegmann K, Kronke M. TNF activates NF-kappa B by phosphatidylcholine-specific phospholipase C-induced "acidic" sphingomyelin breakdown. Cell 1992; 71(5): 765-76.

[88] Wiegmann K, Schutze S, Machleidt T, Witte D, Kronke M. Functional dichotomy of neutral and acidic sphingomyelinases in tumor necrosis factor signaling. Cell 1994; 78(6): 1005-15.

[89] Cifone MG, Roncaioli P, De Maria R, Camarda G, Santoni A, Ruberti G, *et al.* Multiple pathways originate at the Fas/APO-1 (CD95) receptor: Sequential involvement of phosphatidylcholine-specific phospholipase C and acidic sphingomyelinase in the propagation of the apoptotic signal. Embo J 1995; 14(23): 5859-68.

[90] Machleidt T, Kramer B, Adam D, Neumann B, Schutze S, Wiegmann K, *et al.* Function of the p55 tumor necrosis factor receptor "death domain" mediated by phosphatidylcholine-specific phospholipase C. J Exp Med 1996; 184(2): 725-33.

[91] Meier, G.P., Bai, A., Zhou, D. Site and rate selective prodrug formulations of D609 with antioxidant and anticancer activity. US20070244076 (**2007**).

[92] Thon L, Mohlig H, Mathieu S, Lange A, Bulanova E, Winoto-Morbach S, *et al.* Ceramide mediates caspase-independent programmed cell death. FASEB J 2005; 19(14): 1945-56.

[93] Porn-Ares MI, Chow SC, Slotte JP, Orrenius S. Induction of apoptosis and potentiation of TNF- and Fas-mediated apoptosis in U937 cells by the xanthogenate compound D609. Exp Cell Res 1997; 235(1): 48-54.

[94] Zhang L, Shimizu S, Tsujimoto Y. Two distinct Fas-activated signaling pathways revealed by an antitumor drug D609. Oncogene 2005; 24(18): 2954-62.

[95] Kiss Z, Tomono M. Compound D609 inhibits phorbol ester-stimulated phospholipase D activity and phospholipase C-mediated phosphatidylethanolamine hydrolysis. Biochim Biophys Acta 1995; 1259(1): 105-8.

[96] Hannun YA, Obeid LM. Many ceramides. J Biol Chem 2011; 286(32): 27855-62.

[97] Yang Z, Khoury C, Jean-Baptiste G, Greenwood MT. Identification of mouse sphingomyelin synthase 1 as a suppressor of Bax-mediated cell death in yeast. FEMS Yeast Res 2006; 6(5): 751-62.

[98] Kilkus JP, Goswami R, Dawson SA, Testai FD, Berdyshev EV, Han X, *et al.* Differential regulation of sphingomyelin synthesis and catabolism in oligodendrocytes and neurons. J Neurochem 2008; 106(4): 1745-57.

[99] Van der Luit AH, Budde M, Zerp S, Caan W, Klarenbeek JB, Verheij M, *et al.* Resistance to alkyl-lysophospholipid-induced apoptosis due to downregulated sphingomyelin synthase 1 expression with consequent sphingomyelin- and cholesterol-deficiency in lipid rafts. Biochem J 2007; 401(2): 541-9.

[100] Veldman, R.J., Van Blitterswijk, W.J., Verheij, M., Koning, G.A. Pharmaceutical formulations employing short-chain sphingolipids and their use. WO046637 (**2005**).

[101] Modrak, D. Sphingomyelin enhancement of tumor therapy. US6541462 (**2003**).

[102] van Blitterswijk WJ, Klarenbeek JB, van der Luit AH, Alderliesten MC, van Lummel M, Verheij M. Fas/CD95 down-regulation in lymphoma cells through acquired alkyllysophospholipid resistance: Partial role of associated sphingomyelin deficiency. Biochem J 2010; 425(1): 225-34.

[103] Miyaji M, Jin ZX, Yamaoka S, Amakawa R, Fukuhara S, Sato SB, *et al.* Role of membrane sphingomyelin and ceramide in platform formation for Fas-mediated apoptosis. J Exp Med 2005; 202(2): 249-59.

[104] Huang CR, Jin ZX, Dong L, Tong XP, Yue S, Kawanami T, *et al.* Cisplatin augments FAS-mediated apoptosis through lipid rafts. Anticancer Res 2010; 30(6): 2065-72.

[105] Ding T, Li Z, Hailemariam T, Mukherjee S, Maxfield FR, Wu MP, *et al.* SMS overexpression and knockdown: Impact on cellular sphingomyelin and diacylglycerol metabolism, and cell apoptosis. J Lipid Res 2008; 49(2): 376-85.

[106] Hailemariam TK, Huan C, Liu J, Li Z, Roman C, Kalbfeisch M, *et al.* Sphingomyelin synthase 2 deficiency attenuates NFkappaB activation. Arterioscler Thromb Vasc Biol 2008; 28(8): 1519-26.

[107] Asano S, Kitatani K, Taniguchi M, Hashimoto M, Zama K, Mitsutake S, *et al.* Regulation of cell migration by sphingomyelin synthases: Sphingomyelin in lipid rafts decreases responsiveness to signaling by the CXCL12/CXCR4 pathway. Mol Cell Biol 2012; 32(16): 3242-52.

[108] Domanska UM, Kruizinga RC, Nagengast WB, Timmer-Bosscha H, Huls G, de Vries EG, *et al.* A review on CXCR4/CXCL12 axis in oncology: No place to hide. Eur J Cancer 2012; 49(1): 219-30.

[109] Riker, A., Enkemann, S. Melanoma gene signature. US20080113360 (**2008**).

[110] Semizarov, D., Lu, X., Zhang, K., Lesniewski, R., Coon, J. Diagnostic methods for determining prognosis of non-small cell lung cancer. US20110105341 (**2011**) & EP2494360 (**2012**).

Send Orders of Reprints at reprints@benthamscience.net
Topics in Anti-Cancer Research, Vol. 2, 2013, 63-94

CHAPTER 3

The Therapeutic Promise of Anti-Cancer Drugs Against the Ras/Raf/MEK/ERK Pathway

Erin K. Crane and Kwong-Kwok Wong*

Department of Gynecologic Oncology and Reproductive Medicine, The University of Texas M.D. Anderson Cancer Center, Houston, Texas, USA

Abstract: The Ras/Raf/MEK/ERK mitogen-activated protein kinase (MAPK) pathway mediates cellular responses to different growth signals and is frequently deregulated in cancer. There are three Raf kinases-A-Raf, B-Raf, and C-Raf; however, only B-Raf is frequently mutated in various cancers. The most common B-Raf mutation involves a substitution of a glutamic acid residue to a valine moiety at codon 600. Subsequently, the MAPK pathway is constitutively activated, even in the absence of any growth signals. Although early attempts to target Ras have not yielded any viable drug candidates, many novel compounds inhibiting the activities of B-Raf and MEK have been developed and investigated in clinical trials in recent years and have shown promising result. The first MEK inhibitor (CI-1040) lacked efficacy in clinical trials, but its low toxicity encouraged the search for novel compounds-now there are over a hundred open clinical trials employing various B-Raf and MEK inhibitors. Several of these trials are now in Phase III. In this chapter, we will discuss new patents and patent applications related to inhibitors of the Ras/Raf/MEK/ERK pathway and some recent clinical trial results.

Keywords: ARQ736, AS703026, B-Raf inhibitors, dabrafenib, ERK, GDC-0879, heterocyclic compounds, imidazole derivatives, MEK inhibitors, MEK162, RAF265, refametinib, regorafenib, RO4987655, selumetinib, sorafenib, TAK-733, trametinib, vemurafenib, XL281.

INTRODUCTION

The Ras/Raf/MEK/ERK signaling pathway regulates the expression of a large number of proteins involved in the control of cell proliferation, differentiation, and apoptosis. In response to the binding of growth factors, cytokines, and hormones to cell surface receptors [1, 2], the level of Ras-guanosine triphosphate

***Address correspondence to Kwong-Kwok Wong:** Department of Gynecologic Oncology and Reproductive Medicine, The University of Texas M.D. Anderson Cancer Center, 1515 Holcombe Blvd., Houston, TX 77030, USA; Tel: 713-792-0229; Fax: 713-745-5099; E-mail: kkwong@mdanderson.org

Atta-ur Rahman and Khurshid Zaman (Eds)

(GTP) increases in cells, which in turn promotes kinase activation. The GTP-bound forms of Ras directly bind and thus recruit cytosolic dimers of the Raf kinases to the plasma membrane. Once localized at the membrane, Raf is activated through phosphorylation by other kinases or by autophosphorylation [3]. Activated and membrane-associated Raf assembles a mitogen-activated protein kinase (MAPK) signaling complex that consists of two kinase classes: extracellular signal-regulated kinase (ERK) and MAPK/ERK (MEK) [4]. The MAPK cascade initiates with the phosphorylation and activation of MEK by Raf and, subsequently, the phosphorylation and activation of ERK by MEK. Activated ERK dissociates from the Ras/Raf/MEK/ERK complex and phosphorylates a number of cytoskeletal proteins, kinases, and transcription factors, such as nuclear factor NF-κB [5], AP-1, ETS-1, c-Jun, and c-Myc [2, 6, 7]. The functional consequences of substrate-level phosphorylation by ERK include changes in cellular motility and gene expression changes that promote proliferation, differentiation, cellular survival, immortalization, and angiogenesis [7, 8].

Aberrant activation of the Ras/Raf/MEK/ERK pathway is common and is observed in one third of all cancers [9]. Thus, therapeutic targeting of individual components of the Ras/Raf/MEK/ERK pathway has attracted much attention in the development of anti-cancer drugs. In addition, inhibitors targeting "active" protein kinases have demonstrated potential utility in anti-cancer drug activity, as is the case with B-Raf mutations. These mutations are especially prevalent in melanomas, thyroid cancers, and colorectal carcinomas, and are the focus of many clinical trials evaluating B-Raf inhibitors. Several drugs targeting B-Raf mutation or the Ras/Raf/MEK/ERK pathway are either in development or are currently in clinical trial and have shown promising results. The purpose of this chapter is to provide an update on the drugs currently in development that target the Ras/Raf/MEK/ERK pathway.

B-RAF ACTIVATING MUTATION

B-Raf is a serine/threonine kinase and a primary target of oncogenic Ras [10]. The identification of *B-Raf* gene mutations in various human cancers has stimulated numerous studies [11]. More than 80% of *B-Raf* mutations are single amino acid substitutions of glutamic acid for valine at codon 600 (previously thought to be at 599) within the kinase domain. *B-Raf* mutations have been identified in a wide variety of human cancers, such as melanomas, ovarian borderline tumors, sporadic colorectal carcinomas, and thyroid carcinomas Table **1** [11-15]. The data were extracted from "The Catalogue of Somatic Mutations in Cancer" (COSMIC) database [16]. The B-Raf mutated protein, referred as B-Raf^{V600E}, has increased kinase activity compared to wild-type B-Raf [11]. B-Raf^{V600E} activates the downstream MEK/ERK signaling pathway independently of Ras-GTP and its expression is required to maintain the proliferative and oncogenic characteristics of B-Raf^{V600E}-expressing human tumor cell lines [14-16]. Recent evidence suggests that mutant B-Raf also causes chromosome instability via phosphorylation of Mps1; up-regulates GLUT-1 which enhances glucose metabolism in tumor cells; and causes DNA strand breakage and damage [17, 18]. Mutated B-Raf^{V600E} is also no longer repressed by SPRY2-an inhibitor of MAPK signaling in epithelial and fibroblast cell lines [19] which only binds to wild-type B-Raf to initiate the inhibition of MEK/ERK signaling, but will not bind to B-Raf^{V600E} [20]. Thus, specifically targeting the mutated B-Raf^{V600E} protein without inhibiting the wild-type B-Raf is one of the goals of anti-cancer drug development to improve anti-tumor cell activities while minimizing toxicity.

Table 1: Frequency of mutated B-Raf genes in various tumor locations.

Primary Tumor Location	**Total Number of Samples**	**Number of Mutated Samples (%)**
Skin	10885	4550 (42%)
Thyroid	22408	8547 (38%)
Large Intestine	46321	5596 (12%)
Eye	526	2865 (12%)
Ovary	2022	236 (12%)
Small Intestine	137	10 (7%)
Biliary Tract	490	29 (6%)
Hematopoietic and Lymphoid Tissue	1645	107 (7%)
Prostate	1188	42 (4%)
Central Nervous System	1572	70 (4%)
Endometrium	848	30 (4%)
Soft Tissue	1191	30 (3%)
Breast	603	14 (2%)

Table 1: contd...

Lung	6261	135 (2%)
Upper Aerodigestive Tract	769	12 (2%)
Pancreas	563	10 (2%)
Oesophagus	203	3 (1%)
Cervix	451	5 (1%)
Liver	175	2 (1%)
Stomach	1128	11 (1%)

DRUGS TARGETING THE RAS/RAF/MEK/ERK PATHWAY CURRENTLY IN CLINICAL TRIAL

Several anti-cancer drugs targeting Raf or downstream MEK have been developed and are in various Phases of clinical trials (Table **2**), including PLX4032 Fig. (**1A**) (also known as Vemurafenib, RG7204, R7204 & RO5185426, specifically targets B-Raf^{V600E}), RAF265 Fig. (**1B**) (targets both Raf and vascular endothelial growth factor receptor [VEGFR]-2, sorafenib tosylate Fig. (**1C**) (targets multiple kinases), regorafenib (targets multiple kinases), XL281 (targets Raf kinases, structure not disclosed), and AZD6244 (Selumetinib) Fig. (**1D**) (specifically targets MEK).

Table 2: Clinical trials of B-Raf and downstream MEK inhibitors.

NCT ID	Trial Name	Tumor Type	Drug Name (Target)	Trial Phase
Examples of Phase II Clinical Trials with Raf Inhibitors				
NCT01400451	Ph I/II Ipilimumab vemurafenib combo	Metastatic Melanoma	PLX4032 and Iplimumab (CTLA-4)	Phase I/II
NCT01512251	BKM120 combined with vemurafenib (PLX4032) in B-RafV600E/K mutant advanced melanoma	Metastatic Melanoma	PLX4032 and BKM120 (PI3K)	Phase I/II
NCT01286753	A study of RO5185426 (vemurafenib) in patients with metastatic or unresectable papillary thyroid cancer positive for the B-Raf V600 mutation	Papillary Thyroid Cancer	PLX4032	Phase II
NCT01378975	A study of vemurafenib in metastatic melanoma patients with brain metastases	Metastatic Melanoma	PLX4032	Phase II

Table 2: contd…

NCT01474551	Vemurafenib (R05185426) in poor performance status patients with unresectable locally advanced or metastatic melanoma harboring a V600EB-Raf mutation	Metastatic Melanoma	PLX4032	Phase II
NCT01495988	Trial of vemurafenib with or without bevacizumab in patients with stage IV B-RafV600 mutant melanoma	Metastatic Melanoma	PLX4032 with or without bevacizumab (VEGF)	Phase II
NCT01524978	A study of vemurafenib in patients with B-Raf V600 mutation-positive cancers	Solid tumors and multiple myeloma, except melanoma and papillary thyroid cancer	PLX4032	Phase II
NCT01352273	MEK162 and RAF265 in adult patients with advanced solid tumors harboring RAS or B-RafV600E mutations	Solid Tumors	RAF265 and MEK 162 (MEK1/2)	Phase I/II
NCT01336634	A Phase II study of the selective B-Raf kinase inhibitor GSK2118436 in subjects with advanced non-small cell lung cancer and B-Raf mutations	Non-Small Cell Lung Cancer	SB-590885	Phase II
Examples of Phase II Clinical Trials with MEK Inhibitors				
NCT01029418	AZD6244 and sorafenib in advanced hepatocellular carcinoma	Hepatocellular carcinoma	AZD6244 and Sorafenib (multiple kinase)	Phase I/II
NCT01242605	ABC-04 a study of cisplatin, gemcitabine and selumetinib in patients with advanced biliary tract cancer	Biliary tract cancer	AZD6244 and Cisplatin/Gemcitabine	Phase I/II
NCT01143402	Phase II randomized study of temozolomide *vs.* MEK inhibitor AZD6244 (selumetinib) in patients with metastatic uveal melanoma	Uveal melanoma	AZD6244 vs. Temozolomide	Phase II
NCT01160718	Fulvestrant with or without AZD6244 in treating patients with advanced breast cancer that progressed after aromatase inhibitor therapy	Breast cancer	AZD6244 with or without fulvestrant	Randomized Phase II
NCT01206140	Study of MEK inhibitor AZD6244 with *vs.* without temsirolimus in patients with metastatic, recurrent, or locally advanced unresectable soft tissue sarcomas	Sarcomas	AZD6244 and/or temsirolimus (mTOR)	Phase II

Table 2: contd…

NCT01222689	Phase II study of MEK inhibitor AZD6244 and erlotinib hydrochloride for second-line treatment in patients with locally advanced or metastatic pancreatic adenocarcinoma	Pancreatic cancer	AZD6244 and erlotinib (EGFR)	Phase II
NCT01239290	Phase II randomized study of selumetinib and erlotinib hydrochloride in patients with K-RAS wild type or mutant K-RAS advanced non-small cell lung cancer	Non-small cell lung cancer	AZD6244 and erlotinib (EGFR)	Randomized Phase II
NCT01256359	Docetaxel with or without AZD6244 in melanoma	Melanoma	AZD6244 with or without docetaxel	Phase II
NCT01306045	Molecular profiling and targeted therapy for advanced non-small cell lung cancer, small cell lung cancer, and thymic malignancies	Lung and thymic cancer	AZD6244, erlotinib (EGFR), MK-2206 (Akt), lapatinib (ERBB2), or sunitinib (multiple kinase), based on molecular profiling of tumor	Phase II
NCT01333475	MK-2206 and AZD6244 in Patients with advanced colorectal carcinoma	Colorectal carcinoma	AZD6244 and MK-2206 (Akt)	Phase II
NCT01519427	Phase II randomized study of selumetinib with vs. without akt inhibitor MK2206 in patients with B-Raf V600E mutant stage III or IV melanoma who failed prior therapy with vemurafenib or dabrafenib	Melanoma	AZD6244 and/or MK2206 (Akt)	Randomized Phase II
NCT00551070	AZD6244 in treating woman with recurrent low-grade ovarian cancer	Ovarian cancer	AZD6244	Phase II
NCT01553851	GSK1120212 in surgically resectable oral cavity squamous cell cancer	Oral squamous cell carcinoma	GSK1120212	Phase II
NCT01362296	An open-label study of GSK1120212 compared with docetaxel in stage IV KRAS-mutant non-small cell lung cancer	Non-small cell lung cancer	GSK1120212 vs. docetaxel	Phase II

Table 2: contd…

NCT00920140	Open-label study to evaluate the safety, PK, and PD of MEK inhibitor GSK1120212 in subjects with relapsed or refractory leukemia's	Leukemia	GSK1120212	Phase II
NCT01251640	Combination with gemcitabine in advanced pancreatic cancer	Pancreatic cancer	BAY86-9766	Phase I/II
NCT01016483	Trial of gemcitabine with or without MSC1936369B in pancreatic cancer	Pancreatic cancer	AS703026 and/or gemcitabine	Phase I/II
NCT00957580	Trial of mitogen-activated protein/extracellular signal-regulated kinase kinase (MEK) inhibitor	Advanced hematologic malignancies	AS703026	Phase I/II
NCT01266967	A study of GSK2118436 in B-Raf mutant metastatic melanoma to the brain (Break MB)	Metastatic melanoma to the brain	SB-590885	Phase II
Examples of Phase III Clinical Trials with Sorafenib or Regorafenib				
NCT00111007	A treatment combination for patients with unresectable stage III or stage IV melanoma	Melanoma	Sorafenib tosylate with paclitaxel/carboplatin vs. paclitaxel/carboplatin	Phase III
NCT00492258	Phase III randomized study of sorafenib tosylate in patients with resected primary renal cell carcinoma at high- or intermediate-risk of relapse	Renal cell carcinoma	Sorafenib tosylate	Phase III
NCT00541021	Phase III randomized study of gemcitabine hydrochloride and sorafenib tosylate in patients with locally advanced or metastatic adenocarcinoma of the pancreas	Pancreatic cancer	Sorafenib tosylate and gemcitabine	Phase III
NCT01015833	Phase III randomized study of sorafenib tosylate with vs. without doxorubicin hydrochloride in patients with locally advanced or metastatic hepatocellular carcinoma	Hepatocellular carcinoma	Sorafenib tosylate and/or doxorubicin	Phase III
NCT01223027	Study of dovitinib vs. sorafenib in patients with metastatic renal cell carcinoma	Renal cell carcinoma	Sorafenib tosylate vs. dovitinib (VEGFR and FGFR)	Phase III
NCT01234337	Phase III trial comparing capecitabine in combination with sorafenib or placebo in the treatment of locally advanced or metastatic HER2-negative breast cancer	Metastatic breast cancer	Sorafenib tosylate and/or capecitabine	Phase III

Table 2: contd…

NCT01189903	Clinical evaluation - A Phase IIA proof of concept study of regorafenib (Bayer 73-4506) in biopsy-amenable asian colorectal cancer patients	Colorectal cancer	Regorafenib	Phase II/III
NCT01298570	Regorafenib+FOLFIRI vs. placebo+FOLFIRI as 2nd line Tx in K-RAS/B-Raf mutant metastatic colorectal cancer	Colorectal cancer	FOLFIRI (Leucovorin, 5-fluorouracil, irinotecan, and cetuximab) with or without regorafenib	Phase II

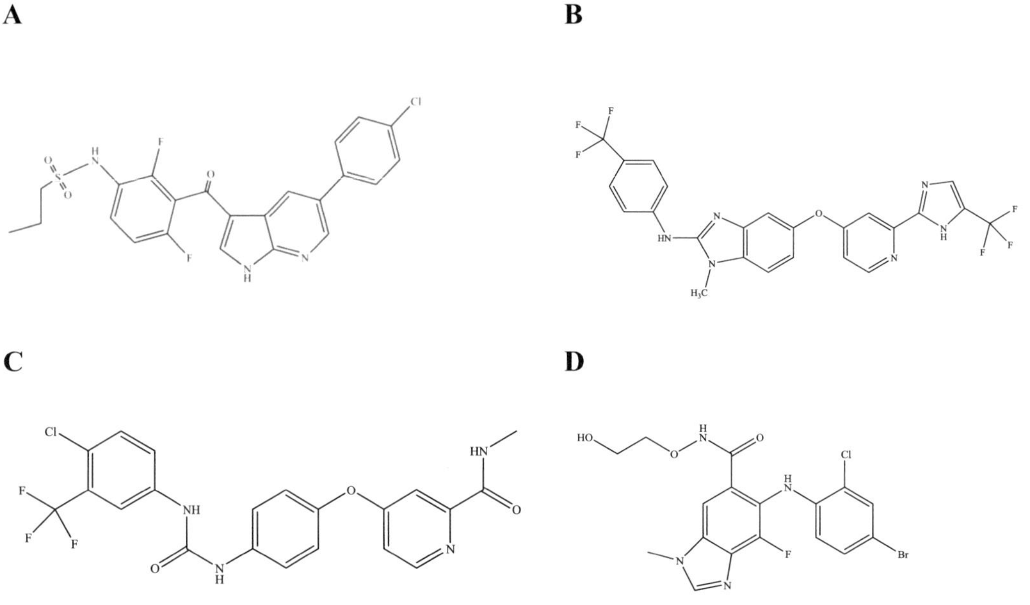

Figure 1: Chemical structures of (A) PLX4032, (B) RAF265, (C) Sorafenib, and (D) AZD6244.

PLX4032 (Vemurafenib, Plexxikon, Inc., Berkeley, CA) is a highly selective inhibitor of B-Raf kinase activity with an IC_{50} of 44nM against mutant B-Raf^{V600E}. The IC_{50} of PLX4032 is the lowest among a panel of 65 non-Raf kinases tested [21]. This small molecule was identified from Plexxikon's proprietary Scaffold-based Drug Discovery platform [22]. Most of the other kinases tested have a more than 100-fold higher IC_{50}, except Brk (also known as PTK6), which has an IC_{50} of 240nmol/L. PLX4032 specifically targets B-Raf^{V600E}; however, inhibition of tumor cell proliferation and MEK phosphorylation was only observed in colorectal tumor cell lines harboring B-Raf^{V600E} but not wild-type B-Raf [23]. Clinically, this compound has had profound effects on melanoma patients who previously had a very grim prognosis. Several Phase I-III clinical trials have evaluated the efficacy of vemurafenib, especially in the setting of melanoma. In one hundred and thirty two patients with previously treated B-Raf^{V600E}-mutant metastatic melanoma enrolled in a multicenter Phase II trial of vemurafenib, overall response rate was 53% with a median duration of response of 6.7 months and median overall survival of 15.9 months [24]. A randomized Phase III trial also showed improved overall and progression-free survival in melanoma as a first-line agent when compared to dacarbazine in 675 patients with metastatic melanoma [25]. At 6 months, 84% of the vemurafenib group was still alive, compared to 64% of the dacarbazine group. This data led to FDA approval of vemurafenib for use in B-Raf^{V600E}-positive melanoma in 2011. While highly efficacious in melanoma, unfortunately, the same activity has not been observed in colorectal carcinoma. In a Phase I study of 21 patients with B-Raf^{V600E}-positive metastatic colorectal carcinoma, there was only one partial response and 4 minor responses [26]. Toxicity of vemurafenib is generally mild: The most common adverse events in the clinical trials were rash, nausea, diarrhea, arthralgia, photosensitivity, fatigue, and alopecia. However, paradoxical activation of the Ras pathway leads to formation of keratoacanthomas and squamous cell carcinomas in these patients-a significant side effect which requires routine screening [27].

RAF265 (CHIR-265; Novartis Pharmaceuticals, Basel, Switzerland), an orally bioavailable small molecule, is a potent inhibitor of Raf with a highly selective profile and is a derivative of benzazoles (Chiron, a subsidiary of Novartis) [28]. RAF265 binds and inhibits Raf kinases, which results in apoptosis and reduction in tumor proliferation. In addition, RAF265 inhibits VEGFR-2, thereby disrupting tumor angiogenesis [29]. A preclinical study found that RAF265 inhibits all three isoforms of Raf, as well as B-Raf^{V600E}, with high potency. RAF265's antitumor activity has also been seen in preclinical xenograft models [30]. In a Phase I first-in-human trial of RAF265 in 76 patients with advanced melanoma, overall response rate was 16% for patients with B-Raf mutations and 13% for wild-type/unknown mutations [31]. A major side effect was dose-limiting hematologic toxicity. Phase II trials are currently ongoing.

Sorafenib (BAY43-9006; Bayer Schering Pharma, Pittsburgh, PA) is a bi-aryl urea which was initially identified as an adenosine triphosphate competitive inhibitor of the C-Raf kinase (from now on referred to as the Raf1 kinase). *In vitro* biochemical assays confirmed that sorafenib is a potent *in vitro* inhibitor of the Raf1 kinase (IC_{50} = 6nM) [32]. Sorafenib has also been shown to inhibit Raf1 and, thus, tumor cell proliferation and tumor growth in several human tumor xenograft models [33]. Subsequently, sorafenib was shown to have multikinase inhibition activities, which is likely responsible for sorafenib's clinical efficacy [32]. Sorafenib targets two kinase classes known to be involved in both tumor proliferation and angiogenesis [34]. These include the enzyme Raf kinase, a critical component of the Ras/Raf/MEK/ERK signaling pathway; and the VEGFR-2/platelet-derived growth factor receptor (PDGFR)-beta signaling cascade, thereby blocking tumor growth and angiogenesis. It also inhibits c-Kit and fibroblast growth factor receptor 1 (FGFR1) [35]. Sorafenib has been evaluated as a single-therapy agent and in combination with various chemotherapy drugs in a number of clinical trials [36-38]. In a study that compared sorafenib with placebo, treatment with sorafenib prolonged progression-free survival in patients with advanced clear-cell renal cell carcinoma for whom previous therapy had failed. Subsequently, sorafenib was approved by the U.S. Food and Drug Administration for the treatment of advanced renal cell carcinoma and advanced hepatocellular carcinoma and has since performed well in Phase III trials [39]. Over 200 clinical trials are currently ongoing, and a few studies are investigating the correlation between clinical response and B-Raf mutation status. Interestingly, the most clinically beneficial function of sorafenib arises from its anti-angiogenicity; the Raf inhibition seems less potent, as evidenced by Phase II and III trials in melanoma patients, where sorafenib had limited efficacy even when response was analyzed according to B-Raf mutation status [37, 40].

Regorafenib (BAY73-4506; Bayer Schering Pharma, Pittsburgh, PA) is a more potent derivative of sorafenib formed by adding a fluorine atom to the phenyl group. Similar to sorafenib, it inhibits multiple kinases, including VEGFR 1-3,

TIE2, PDGFR, FGFR1, cKIT, RET, and B-Raf, with an IC_{50} ranging from 4 to 311nM [41]. In xenograft models, it inhibited tumor growth in glioblastoma, breast, renal cell, and colorectal carcinomas [41]. A recent Phase I trial demonstrated acceptable activity and toxicity in 53 patients with solid tumors, three of 47 patients achieved a response and the most common side effects were dermatologic manifestations, hypertension, and diarrhea [42]. In Phase II trials, regorafenib has performed well: In pretreated gastrointestinal stromal tumors (GIST), 19 of 22 patients were without progression after 4 cycles [43]. In a Phase III trial in patients with metastatic colorectal cancer, a statistically significant benefit in progression-free survival (PFS) and overall survival (OS) was observed in the regorafenib group vs. supportive care, such that the control group was allowed crossover into regorafenib treatment [44]. Phase II and III trials are ongoing.

XL281 (Exelixis, San Francisco, CA) is an orally active small molecule with potential antineoplastic activity that specifically inhibits Raf kinases, including Raf1, B-Raf, and activated B-Raf^{V600E} [45]. XL281 has shown activity in tumor xenograft models [46]. A Phase I clinical trial concluded that XL281 had acceptable activity and toxicity in adult patients with solid tumors [47]; however, there are currently no open clinical trials evaluating this compound.

AZD6244 (ARRY-142886, Selumetinib; AstraZeneca, London, England) is an oral, highly selective allosteric inhibitor of MEK [48]. AZD6244 was the second MEK inhibitor to enter clinical trials after the first MEK inhibitor, CI-1040, demonstrated poor clinical efficacy. However, the encouraging safety profile of CI-1040 provided the momentum to search for more potent analogues [49]. AZD6244 is a benzimidazole derivative with reported nanomolar activity against the purified MEK1 enzyme [50]. Through a series of studies using preclinical cell cultures and animal models, it was shown that AZD6244 suppresses the growth of melanoma cells through the induction of cytostasis, but AZD6244 has a limited ability to induce apoptosis or block angiogenesis [51]. In a Phase I study in patients with advanced cancer, AZD6244 was well tolerated with demonstrable clinical activity [35], with rash being the most common dose-limiting toxicity. This prompted several Phase II studies which have now evaluated AZD6244. Overall, AZD6244 has displayed modest antineoplastic activity in iodinerefractory papillary thyroid cancer [52] and metastatic biliary cancer [53], while results in hepatocellular cancer patients were less robust [54]. In the papillary thyroid patient population, patients with B-Raf^{V600E} mutations had longer median PFS [52]. Phase II studies have also compared single-agent AZD6244 to other antineoplastics, and have found that AZD6244 is effective but not superior to standard chemotherapeutics. Compared to temozolomide in 200 advanced-stage melanoma patients [55], AZD2644 was active, but there was no difference in progression free survival between the two drugs. However, 5 of 6 partial responders to AZD6244 had B-Raf mutations. Compared to permextred in 84 heavily-pretreated patients with advanced non-small cell lung cancer, AZD6244 was again active, but there was no difference in disease progression between both groups [56]. Finally, in patients with advanced pancreatic cancer who had progressed through treatment with gemcitabine, there was no difference in overall survival in patients treated with AZD6244 compared to capecitabine [57]. Common side effects of AZD6244 in the above clinical trials included nausea, rash, peripheral edema, and diarrhea.

DERIVATIVES OF INITIAL LEAD COMPOUNDS IMPROVE SPECIFICITY AND POTENCY

Patents issued and patent applications published in recent years have identified numerous lead compounds that target Raf, MEK, or multiple tyrosine kinases [58-66]. Many of these compounds are derived from aromatic heterocyclic compounds, such as imidazole, quinazoline, phenethylamide, malonamide, and benzazoles Tables **3-4**. Using these compounds as the initial scaffolds for modifications, more potent inhibitors have been identified. For example, to improve the bioavailability and potency of CI-1040 [67], a derivative, PD0325901, was developed [68]. PD0325901 was derived by replacing the cyclopropylmethoxy group with a (*R*)-2,3-dihydroxypropoxy group and replacing the 2-chloro substituent with a 2-fluoro group on the second aromatic ring of CI-1040 Fig. (**2A**). Such small structural changes resulted in a more than 100-fold target potency as reflected by PD0325901's ability to inhibit both purified MEK, as well as cellular activation of MAPK, at concentrations in the nanomolar range. Moreover, the activity of PD0325901 has also been observed against a panel of B-Raf^{V600E} xenografts [69]. A Phase I trial investigated PD0325901 in 13 patients with metastatic melanoma, colorectal, or breast cancer at doses of 20 mg and 15 mg orally twice daily [70]. Although one patient had a complete response and 5 had stable disease, the study was terminated early due to an unexpected high incidence of musculoskeletal and neurological toxicity. However, another Phase I trial (NCT01347866) is examining a PI3K/mTOR inhibitor in combination with PD0325901 or irinotecan. Given its untoward neurologic side effects, modifications of PD0325901 have led to the development of two new more specific, stable compounds: RO4987655 (CH4987655; Hoffman-La Roche, Basel, Switzerland) and TAK-733 (Takeda Pharmaceutical, Osaka, Japan), both of which are less susceptible to hydrolyzation than PD0325901. TAK-733 is a novel 5-phenylamino-8-methylpyrido[2,3-*d*]pyrimidine-4,7(3*H*,8*H*)-dione with a bicyclic pyridopyrimidinione core and a dihydroxypropane side chain. It is highly selective, performing in the nanomolar range with an IC_{50} of 3.2nM against MEK1/2, and antitumor activity in xenograft models of melanoma, non-small cell lung, breast, pancreatic, and colorectal carcinoma [71]. A Phase I study is underway evaluating TAK-733 in advanced nonhematologic malignancies (NCT00948467). RO4987655 was developed with a unique 3-oxo-[1,2]oxazinan-2-ylmethyl group at the 5-position, and inhibits MEK at an IC_{50} of 5nM. In xenograft models with colorectal, non-small cell lung, and pancreatic carcinomas, RO4987655 potently inhibited MEK activity [72].

Table 3: Recently issued patents.

Patent Number	Title	Assignee
US7737152	6-Carboaryl-oxy-pyrazin-2-yl-carboaryl-amines and compositions comprising said compounds	The Wellcome Trust, Ltd.
US7772246	Pyrazole compounds as RAF inhibitors	Pfizer, Inc.
7795249	Certain pyrazoline derivatives with kinase inhibitory activity	Millenium Pharmaceuticals, Inc.
US7799827	Macrocyclic compounds useful as pharmaceuticals	Eisai Co., Ltd.
US7807672	Compounds that are ERK inhibitors	Schering Corporation
US7951819	Imidazo[4, 5-B]pyridin-2-one and oxazolo[4, 5-B] pyridin-2-one compounds and analogs thereof as cancer therapeutic compounds	Astex Therapeutics, Ltd.
US7968536	Heterocyclic compounds useful as RAF kinase inhibitors	Millenium Pharmaceuticals, Inc.
US7968554	Pyrazolo[3,4-d]pyrimidine derivatives	Hoffman La Roche, Inc.
US7994321	Substituted thieno[3,2-C]pyridine-7-carboxylic acid derivatives	Hoffman La Roche, Inc.

Table 3: contd...

US8044049	Fused heterocyclic derivative and use thereof	Takeda Pharmaceutical Co., Ltd.
US8063066	MAPK/ERK kinase inhibitors	Takeda Pharmaceutical Co., Ltd.
US8076486	Heteroaryl-substituted arylaminopyridine derivatives as MEK inhibitors	Merck Sorono S.A.
US8110687	Bicyclic compounds with kinase inhibitory activity	Millenium Pharmaceuticals, Inc.
US8119637	Substituted pyrrolo[2,3-b]pyrazines and methods for kinase modulation, and indications therefor	Plexxikon, Inc.
US8129394	Heteroaryl-substituted imidazole compounds and uses thereof	Novartis AG
US8129404	Compounds and uses thereof	Plexxikon, Inc.
US8143258	Benzothiazole compounds useful for Raf inhibition	Takeda Pharmaceutical Co., Ltd.
US8143271	Compounds and methods for kinase modulation, and indications therefor	Plexxikon, Inc.

Table 4: Recent patent applications.

Patent Application Number	Title	Target	Applicants	Reference
US20110306625	Compounds and compositions as protein kinase inhibitors	B-Raf	Novartis, Inc.	Huang *et al.* 2011 [122]
US20120053177	Compounds and methods for kinase modulation, and indications therefor	B-Raf	Plexxikon, Inc.	Ibrahim *et al.* 2012 [58]
US20110003859	*N*- (6-Aminopyridin-3-yl) -3- (sulfonamido) benzamide derivatives as B-Raf inhibitors for the treatment of cancer	B-Raf	Array Bio Pharma, Inc.	2011 [61]
US2011051297	Substituted azaindoles	B-Raf	Concert Pharmaceuticals, Inc.	2011 [65]
US20110166191	3-(2-Amino-ethyl)-5-(3-cyclohexyl-propylidene)-thiazolidine-2,4-dione and its derivatives as multiple signaling pathway inhibitors and for the treatment of cancer	Dual Raf/PI3K	N/A	2011 [123]

Table 4: contd…

WO2012036997	Fused pyrazole derivatives as novel ERK inhibitors	ERK	Schering Corporation	2011 [62]
WO2012030685	Indazole derivatives useful as ERK inhibitors	ERK	Schering Corporation	2011 [66]
US20100240613	Pyrimidine compound and medical use thereof	MEK	Japan Tobacco, Inc.	Kawasaki *et al.* 2010 [63]
US20110158971	Compositions comprising N3 alkylated benzimidazole derivatives as MEK inhibitors and methods of use thereof	MEK	Array Bio Pharma, Inc.	2011 [92]
US20100234435	Cycloalkylamino acid derivatives	Multiple kinases	Pfizer, Inc.	Bhattacharya *et al.* 2010 [121]
US20110294806	Azaindole derivatives as kinase inhibitors	Multiple kinases	ARIAD Pharmaceuticals, Inc.	Qi *et al.* 2011 [64]
US20110257165	Bicyclic pyrazoles as protein kinase inhibitors	Multiple kinases	Nerviano Medical Sciences S.R.I.	2011 [60]
US20100330069	Heterocyclic compounds and methods of use	Raf	TargeGen, Inc.	Wrasidlo *et al.* 2010 [59]
US20100234394	Substituted benzimidazoles and methods of their use	Raf	Novartis, Inc.	Aikawa *et al.* 2010 [90]
US20110118245	Raf kinase modulator compounds and methods of use thereof	Raf	Plexxikon, Inc.	2011 [119]
US20110257207	Raf inhibitors	Raf	Agennix USA, Inc.	2011 [120]
US20110110889	Raf inhibitor compounds and methods of use thereof	Raf	Array Bio Pharma, Inc.	2011 [124]

In continuing to improve specificity and circumvent undesirable neurologic side effects, BAY86-9766 (RDEA119, refametinib; Bayer Schering Pharma, Pittsburgh, PA) was developed. It binds noncompetitively to MEK1/2 adjacent to the Mg-ATP binding region and inhibits MEK1/2 activity at an IC_{50} of 19 and 47nM, respectively [73]. It inhibits colorectal carcinoma and melanoma tumor xenografts without neurologic penetration [73], and Phase I trials have confirmed safety. A Phase II trial evaluating refametinib in combination with gemcitabine in pancreatic cancer patients is ongoing (NCT01251640).

A

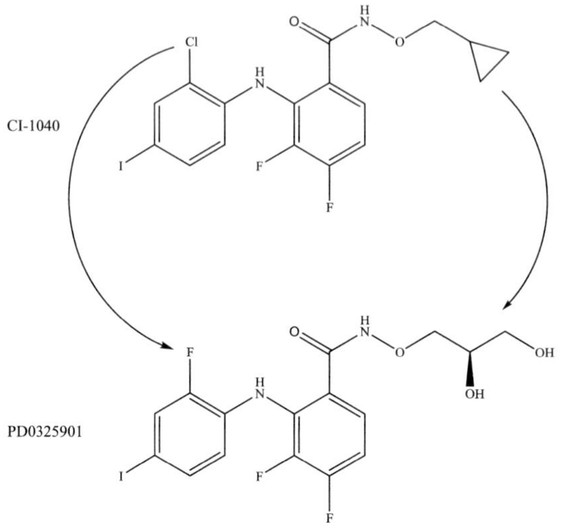

B

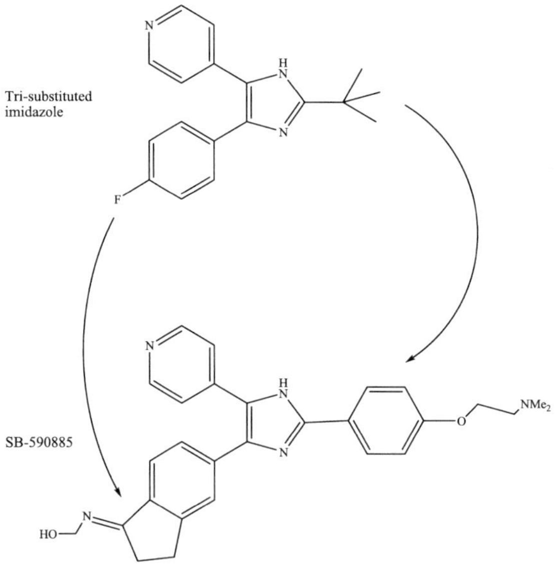

Figure 2: Derivatives of lead compounds with enhanced target potency. (A) PD0325901 is derived by replacing the cyclopropylmethoxy group with a (*R*)-2,3-dihydroxypropoxy group and replacing the 2-chloro substituent with a 2-fluoro group on the second aromatic ring of CI-1040. (B) SB-590885 is a triarylimidazole derivative with a 2,3-dihydro-1H-inden-1-one oxime substituent from a derivative of imidazole.

A derivative of imidazole was identified from the SmithKline Beecham compound bank as a submicromolar inhibitor of B-Raf [74, 75]. Structural modification of imidazole resulted in the formation of GSK2118436 (SB-590885, dabrafenib; SmithKline Beecham, Middlesex, England), which is a triarylimidazole derivative with a 2,3-dihydro-1*H*-inden-1-one oxime substituent Fig. (**2B**). Is a potent and extremely selective inhibitor of the B-Raf kinase in the nanomolar range [76]. Unlike the multikinase inhibitor BAY43-9006, dabrafenib seems to target cells that express oncogenic B-Raf [77]. A Phase I trial displayed encouraging results in melanoma patients, with 24 of 32 patients with a partial response and 2 patients exhibiting a complete response. Median progression-free survival was over 7 months [78]. Perhaps most excitingly, preliminary results from a Phase II clinical trial (NCT01266967) in metastatic melanoma with brain involvement revealed a 90% response rate. Clinical trials are now examining this compound in the setting of lung and thyroid cancer, and B-Raf mutant-positive tumors.

Further modification of GSK2118436 has also resulted in the identification of a series of furan-based derivatives with enhanced central nervous system penetration and B-Raf inhibitory activity [79, 80]. Such B-Raf inhibitors may be of value in the treatment of specific types of pediatric gliomas (*e.g.*, low-grade astrocytomas), as MAPK pathway activation was discovered in low-grade astrocytomas as a result of *B-Raf* gene duplication [81]. GSK1120212 (Trametinib) was created with a pyrido-pyrimidin core and an N-phenylacetamide substituent. It inhibits MEK1/2 enzymatic activity at an IC_{50} of 10nM, with a particularly long circulating half-life and p-ERK suppression for over 24 hours. It also displayed potent activity in melanoma and colorectal cancer xenograft models [82], which has led to several Phase I trials confirming its safety and efficacy. The first Phase I trial investigated trametinib in 84 patients, and in 20 evaluable melanoma patients of known B-Raf status there were 5 partial responses, three of whom have stayed $\geq$ 30 weeks on study [83]. There are now several Phase II studies.

AS703026 (Merck KGaA, Darmstadt, Germany) is yet another imidazole derivative, with an *N*-substitution and the chemical formula (*N*-[(2*S*)-2,3-dihydroxypropyl]-3-[(2-fluoro-4-iodophenyl)amino] isonicotinamide hydrochloride).

Preclinical testing yielded effective and specific MEK1/2 inhibition in multiple myeloma and colorectal tumors [84, 85], which prompted several clinical trials. A Phase I trial in advanced solid tumors with AS703026 resulted in two confirmed partial responses prior to reaching the maximum tolerated dose [86]. Common side effects were asthenia, diarrhea, skin reactions, nausea, and vomiting. There are currently 6 Phase I or combination Phase I/II trials open evaluating the compound as a single agent or in combination with other antitumor drugs.

By using a structure-guided discovery approach [22], a small-molecule 7-azaindole was found to bind the ATP-binding site of kinases with weak affinity. Subsequently, a group of mono- and disubstituted 7-azaindoles with increased affinity was synthesized. Screening of these compounds revealed a set of compounds containing a difluoro-phenylsulfonamide substructural motif that demonstrated excellent potency for oncogenic B-Raf. Co-crystallization of these compounds with engineered forms of B-Raf^{V600E} and wild-type B-Raf provided co-crystal structures for subsequent optimization chemistry, which led to the discovery of propane-1-sulfonic acid [3-(5-chloro-1*H*-pyrrolo[2,3-*b*]pyridine-3-carbonyl)-2,4-difluoro-phenyl]-amide (PLX4720). PLX4720 inhibits B-Raf^{V600E} kinase activity *in vitro*, with an IC_{50} of 13 nM, which is 10-fold lower than the concentration needed to inhibit wild-type B-Raf. Furthermore, in B-Raf^{V600E}-dependent tumor xenograft models, oral PLX4720 significantly reduced tumor growth and even caused tumor regression, without evidence of toxicity [87]. PLX4032 is a structurally distinct analog of PLX4720. PLX3603, another derivative of PLX4032, is under evaluation in a Phase I clinical trial.

MEK162 (ARRY162, Novartis Pharmaceuticals, Basel, Switzerland) is another new oral MEK inhibitor, initially developed for rheumatoid arthritis, which functions through noncompetitive allosteric inhibition against MEK1/2 (IC_{50} 12nM) and ERK (IC_{50} 11nM), as well as IL-1, TNF, and IL-6, with activity against pancreatic, colorectal, and non-small cell lung carcinoma, as well as fibrosarcoma [88]. Phase I studies have been completed with tolerable efficacy and toxicity, and several Phase I/II studies are examining its efficacy in combination with other targeted agents (AMG479, an IGF-1R inhibitor, NCT01562899; RAF265, NCT01352273; BEZ235, a PIK/mTOR inhibitor,

NCT01337765). Another Phase II trial is investigating MEK162 as a single agent in melanoma (NCT01320085).

ARQ 736 (ArQule, Woburn, Massachusetts) is an allosteric inhibitor which specifically targets B-Raf^{V600E} kinase and functions at nanomolar concentrations. It is under investigation in humans in NCT01225536, a Phase I dose escalation study with ARQ 736, in patients with advanced solid tumors harboring B-Raf and/or NRAS mutations.

Other recently-developed inhibitors currently in Phase I trials include GDC-0879 (B-Raf inhibitor; Genentech, San Francisco, CA), GDC-0623 (MEK1/2 inhibitor; Genentech, San Francisco), AZD8330 (MEK1/2 inhibitor; AstraZeneca, London, England), RO5126766 (dual Raf and MEK1/2 inhibitor; Hoffman La Roche, Basel, Switzerland), RO5212054 (B-Raf inhibitor, Hoffman La Roche, Basel, Switzerland), RO5068760 (MEK inhibitor, Hoffman La Roche, Basel, Switzerland), and PD318088 (MEK inhibitor, Pfizer, New York, New York).

CURRENT & FUTURE DEVELOPMENTS

Targeting the Ras/Raf/MEK/ERK cascade has provided novel opportunities for the development of new anti-cancer drugs that are less toxic than conventional chemotherapeutic drugs. Several promising compounds have been developed to inhibit the activities of B-Raf, MEK, or multiple kinases Fig. (**3**). Continued efforts aimed at structural optimization of the chemical scaffolds of compounds such as imidazole and quinazoline have resulted in more potent inhibitors in nanomolar or even subnanomolar ranges [89-92]. Multikinase inhibitors or B-Raf-specific inhibitors can have been developed from similar chemical scaffolds. For example, derivatives of quinazoline may have multiple tyrosine kinase [93] or B-Raf-specific [94] inhibition activities. (E)-α-benzylsulfonyl chalcone derivatives have also been identified as B-Raf inhibitors [95].

While MEK inhibitors harbor anticancer activity, they have generally not outperformed standard chemotherapy in Phase II and III trials. However, more specific compounds which preferentially target B-Raf mutations, such as SB-590885 and PLX4032, have had a profound effect on melanoma patients, extending lifespan in B-Raf^{V600E}-positive patients by an average of seven months [24]. Targeting specific oncogenic mutated kinases will theoretically allow specific inhibition or elimination of tumor cells, depending on the mutated kinases, without introducing too much toxicity in the subjects, since the normal physiological function of wild-type kinases provides an essential role in normal regulation of cell growth.

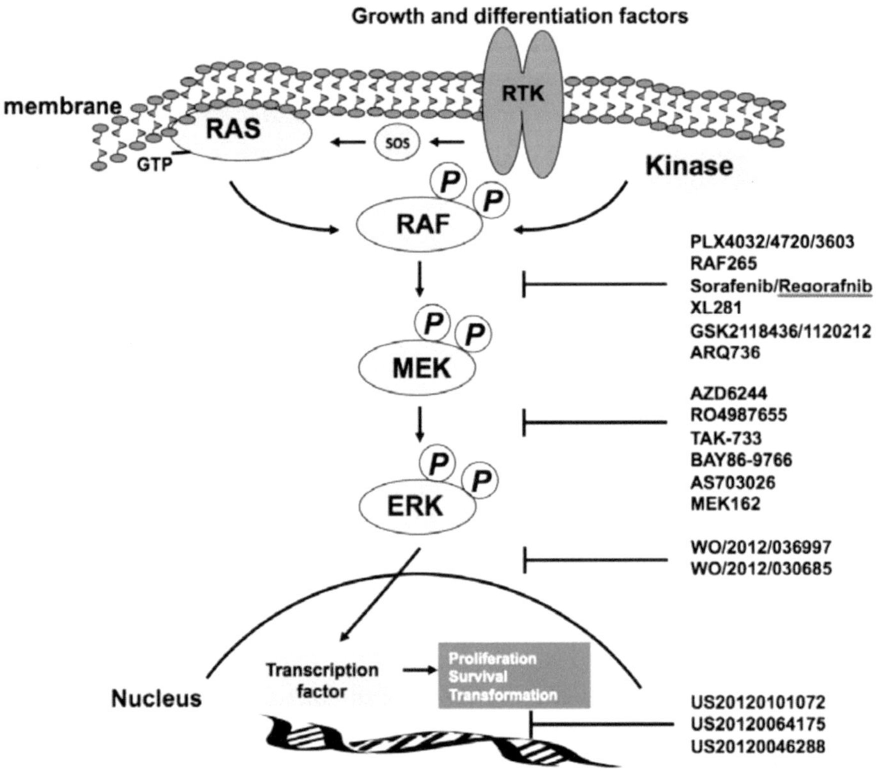

Figure 3: Intracellular signaling pathways that mediate ERK activation and are targeted by anti-cancer drugs currently in development.

However, the clinical success of sorafenib and other multikinase inhibitors has provoked a debate regarding the pros and cons of highly specific *vs.* broadly specific kinase inhibitors [96]. Indeed, drug resistance to B-Raf inhibitors has emerged, stemming from both intrinsic and extrinsic pathways. Resistance has been associated with increased Akt signaling in the presence of PTEN loss [97], as well as increased insulin-like growth factor-1 (IGF-1) signaling [98]. On the other hand, resistant mechanism to MEK inhibitors involves the amplification or up-regulation of B-Raf or KRAS has also been found [99]. Logically, attention has turned towards co-targeting multiple pathways in an effort to improve efficacy. *In vitro,* increased Akt signaling and B-Raf inhibitor resistance were attenuated with the combination of a PI3K and B-Raf inhibitor [97]. Similarly, in the case of colorectal carcinoma, where B-Raf^{V600E} inhibition was less effective than in melanoma, Prahallad and colleagues [100] discovered that dual inhibition with PLX4032 and an EGFR inhibitor (cetuximab, gefitinib, or erlotinib), overcame B-Raf-mediated resistance in colorectal carcinoma cell lines. Co-targeting MEK, the IGF-1 receptor, and PI3K in combination with B-Raf inhibition has also overcome resistance preclinically [101]. Indeed, several patents combining MEK and B-Raf inhibition with other agents have recently emerged [102-105], as have clinical trials. Preliminary results from a Phase I/II trial combining the MEK 1/2 inhibitor GSK1120212 with the B-Raf inhibitor GSK2118436 in patients with stage IV previously-untreated melanoma revealed an objective response rate of 77%, and a decrease in the incidence of keratoacanthomas [106].

Multikinase inhibitors such as sorafenib and regorafenib are therefore attractive owing to their multitarget activity. Fortuitously, sorafenib was found to have activity against multiple protein kinases, yet the original goal in developing sorafenib was to identify a Raf inhibitor. It remains uncertain whether Raf inhibition alone provides adequate clinical efficacy. Therefore, future clinical trials of more specific and potent Raf kinase inhibitors are warranted. The clinical success of highly selective protein kinase inhibitors, in particular monoclonal antibody-based drugs (e.g., trastuzumab and bevacizumab) [107, 108], demonstrates that there is clinical value for both highly selective and multiple-target inhibitors.

Along the same lines, additional interest has developed in heat shock protein 90 (Hsp90) inhibitors in targeting B-Raf and attenuating resistance. Hsp90 is a "chaperone" molecule for proteins such as HER2, EGFR, mutant ER, HIF1α, Raf-1, AKT and mutant p53, the inhibition of which blocks several signaling pathways [109]. It also specifically binds mutant but not wild-type B-Raf, and early evidence suggests that Hsp90 inhibitors may overcome drug resistance

[110]. While a clinical trial with the Hsp90 inhibitor 17-allylamino-17-demethoxygeldanamycin (17-AAG) in melanoma patients yielded no objective clinical responses [111], novel non-benzoquinone small molecule Hsp90 inhibitors may prove more effective with their improved solubility and specificity [110]. Accordingly, several patents exploiting Hsp90 inhibition have surfaced in the past two years [112-114].

Patient selection also plays an important role in targeted therapeutics; patients with a B-Raf^{V600E} mutation are more likely to derive clinical benefit than those with wild-type B-Raf, therefore mutation analysis is an important component of screening prior to clinical trial entry. Additional new patents are aimed at determining which patients will respond to therapy [115, 116].

Important advances have been achieved in expanding our knowledge of how to make highly potent and selective MAPK pathway inhibitors. More drugs are currently in the pipeline, such as GDC-0879, GDC-0623, AZD8330, RO5126766, RO5212054, RO5068760, and PD318088. These drugs all promise increased potency and specificity, with less toxicity. The clinical oncology field will be anxious to evaluate these and other B-Raf and MEK inhibitors, and other MAPK inhibitors, including those targeting ERK, which were reported in recent patent applications [66, 117-124]. Although there is still a paucity of published data, the novel ERK inhibitors AEZS-131 (Æterna Zentaris, Frankfurt, Germany) and SCH772984 (Bayer Schering Pharma, Pittsburgh, PA) are currently in preclinical evaluation. Determining which cancer patients will receive the most benefit and with what regimens or combinations of inhibitors targeting multiple pathways to overcome drug resistance will be a challenge as we move forward to more individualized cancer therapies.

ACKNOWLEDGEMENTS

Author Erin R. King is supported by the National Cancer Institute-Department of Health and Human Services-National Institutes of Health Training of Academic Oncologists Grant (T32 CA101642). This research is also supported in part by the Sara Brown Musselman Fund for Serous Ovarian Cancer Research and the National Institutes of Health, The University of Texas MD Anderson Cancer

Center Specialized Program of Research Excellence in Ovarian Cancer (P50 CA08369).

CONFLICT OF INTEREST

The authors confirm that this chapter content has no conflict of interest.

DISCLOSURE

The chapter submitted for Patent eBook Series "Topics in Anti-Cancer Research", Volume 2 is an update of our article "Recent Developments in Anti-Cancer Agents Targeting the Ras/Raf/MEK/ERK Pathway", published in the journal 'Recent Patents on Anti-Cancer Drug Discovery', Volume 4, Number 1, January 2009, Page 28 to 35 with additional text and references.

ABBREVIATIONS

AP-1	=	Activator protein 1 (JUN)
c-Myc	=	Cellular myelocytomastosis oncogene
COSMIC	=	Catalogue of somatic mutations in cancer
b.i.d.	=	"Bis in die" which Latin means twice a day
ERK	=	Extracellular signal-regulated kinase
ETS-1	=	Erythroblastosis virus E26 oncogene homolog 1
GTP	=	Guanosine-5′-triphosphate
IC_{50}	=	Inhibition concentration which is required for 50% inhibition *in vitro*
MAPK	=	Mitogen-activated protein kinase
MEK	=	MAPK/ERK kinase 1

NF-κB = Nuclear factor-kappaB

nM = Nanomolar

PDGFR = Platelet-derivated growth factor receptor

Raf1 = Murine leukemia viral oncogene homolog 1

B-Raf = V-Raf murine sarcoma viral oncogene homolog B1

KRAS = V-Ki-ras2 Kirsten rat sarcoma viral oncogene homolog

SPRY2 = Sprouty homolog 2

VEGFR-2 = Vascular endothelial growth factor receptor-2

REFERENCES

[1] Peyssonnaux C, Eychene A. The Raf/MEK/ERK pathway: New concepts of activation. Biol Cell 2001; 93: 53-62.

[2] Matallanas D, Birtwistle M, Romano D, Zebisch A, Rauch J, von Kriegsheim A, *et al.* Raf family kinases: Old dogs have learned new tricks. Genes Cancer 2011; 2: 232-60.

[3] Rushworth LK, Hindley AD, O'Neill E, Kolch W. Regulation and role of Raf-1/B-Raf heterodimerization. Mol Cell Biol 2006; 26: 2262-72.

[4] Ahearn IM, Haigis K, Bar-Sagi D, Philips MR. Regulating the regulator: Post-translational modification of RAS. Nat Rev Mol Cell Biol 2011; 13: 39-51.

[5] Palona I, Namba H, Mitsutake N, Starenki D, Podtcheko A, Sedliarou I, *et al.* BRAFV600E promotes invasiveness of thyroid cancer cells through nuclear factor kappaB activation. Endocrinology 2006; 147: 5699-707.

[6] Pratilas CA, Solit DB. Targeting the mitogen-activated protein kinase pathway: Physiological feedback and drug response. Clin Cancer Res 2010; 16: 3329-34.

[7] Wortzel I, Seger R. The ERK cascade: Distinct functions within various subcellular organelles. Genes Cancer 2011; 2: 195-209.

[8] Gough NR. Focus issue: Recruiting players for a game of ERK. Sci Signal 2011; 4: eg9.

[9] Santarpia L, Lippman SM, El-Naggar AK. Targeting the MAPK-RAS-RAF signaling pathway in cancer therapy. Expert Opin Ther Targets 2012; 16: 103-19.

[10] Marais R, Light Y, Paterson HF, Mason CS, Marshall CJ. Differential regulation of Raf-1, A-Raf, and B-Raf by oncogenic Ras and tyrosine kinases. J Biol Chem 1997; 272: 4378-83.

[11] Davies H, Bignell GR, Cox C, Stephens P, Edkins S, Clegg S, *et al.* Mutations of the BRAF gene in human cancer. Nature 2002; 417: 949-54.

[12] Cohen Y, Xing M, Mambo E, Guo Z, Wu G, Trink B, *et al.* BRAF mutation in papillary thyroid carcinoma. J Natl Cancer Inst 2003; 95: 625-7.

[13] Kimura ET, Nikiforova MN, Zhu Z, Knauf JA, Nikiforov YE, Fagin JA. High prevalence of BRAF mutations in thyroid cancer: Genetic evidence for constitutive activation of the RET/PTC-RAS-BRAF signaling pathway in papillary thyroid carcinoma. Cancer Res 2003; 63: 1454-7.

[14] Singer G, Oldt R, 3rd, Cohen Y, Wang BG, Sidransky D, Kurman RJ, *et al.* Mutations in BRAF and KRAS characterize the development of low-grade ovarian serous carcinoma. J Natl Cancer Inst 2003; 95: 484-6.

[15] Wong KK, Gershenson D. The continuum of serous tumors of low malignant potential and low-grade serous carcinomas of the ovary. Dis Markers 2007; 23: 377-87.

[16] Forbes SA, Bhamra G, Bamford S, Dawson E, Kok C, Clements J, *et al.* The catalogue of somatic mutations in cancer (COSMIC). Curr Protoc Hum Genet 2008; Chapter 10: Unit 10 1.

[17] Liu J, Cheng X, Zhang Y, Li S, Cui H, Zhang L, *et al.* Phosphorylation of MPS1 by BRAF(V600E) prevents MPS1 degradation and contributes to chromosome instability in melanoma. Oncogene 2013; 32(6): 713-23.

[18] Sheu JJ, Guan B, Tsai FJ, Hsiao EY, Chen CM, Seruca R, *et al.* Mutant BRAF induces DNA strand breaks, activates DNA damage response pathway, and up-regulates glucose transporter-1 in nontransformed epithelial cells. Am J Pathol 2012; 180: 1179-88.

[19] Gross I, Bassit B, Benezra M, Licht JD. Mammalian sprouty proteins inhibit cell growth and differentiation by preventing ras activation. J Biol Chem 2001; 276: 46460-8.

[20] Tsavachidou D, Coleman ML, Athanasiadis G, Li S, Licht JD, Olson MF, *et al.* SPRY2 is an inhibitor of the Ras/extracellular signal-regulated kinase pathway in melanocytes and melanoma cells with wild-type BRAF but not with the V599E mutant. Cancer Res 2004; 64: 5556-9.

[21] Sala E, Mologni L, Truffa S, Gaetano C, Bollag GE, Gambacorti-Passerini C. BRAF silencing by short hairpin RNA or chemical blockade by PLX4032 leads to different responses in melanoma and thyroid carcinoma cells. Mol Cancer Res 2008; 6: 751-9.

[22] Artis, D.R., Bremer, R.E., Gillette, S.J., Hurt, C.R., Ibrahim, P.L., Zuckerman, R.L. Molecular scaffolds for kinase ligand development. US20050164300 (**2005**).

[23] Su F, Yang H, Higgins B, Chen J, Kolinsky K, Packman K, *et al.* PLX4032, a selective B-Raf V600E inhibitor, has potent anti-tumor activity in B-Raf V600E-bearing colorectal xenografts and shows additive effect with other chemoagents. *19th EORTC-NCI-AACR Symposium on Molecular Targets and Cancer Therapeutics*. California, USA (2007).

[24] Sosman JA, Kim KB, Schuchter L, Gonzalez R, Pavlick AC, Weber JS, *et al.* Survival in BRAF V600-mutant advanced melanoma treated with vemurafenib. N Engl J Med 2012; 366: 707-14.

[25] Chapman PB, Hauschild A, Robert C, Haanen JB, Ascierto P, Larkin J, *et al.* Improved survival with vemurafenib in melanoma with BRAF V600E mutation. N Engl J Med 2011; 364: 2507-16.

[26] Kopetz S, Desai J, Chan E, Hecht JR, O'Dwyer PJ, Lee RJ, *et al.* PLX4032 in metastatic colorectal cancer patients with mutant BRAF tumors. 2010 ASCO Annual Meeting. Chicago, USA (2010).

[27] Su F, Viros A, Milagre C, Trunzer K, Bollag G, Spleiss O, *et al.* RAS mutations in cutaneous squamous-cell carcinomas in patients treated with BRAF inhibitors. N Engl J Med 2012; 366: 207-15.

[28] Amiri, P., Fantl, W., Hansen, T., Levine, H.B., McBride, C., Poon, D.J., Ramurthy, S., Renhowe, P.A., Shafer, C.M., Subramanian, S., Sung, L. Substituted benz-azoles and methods of their use as inhibitors of Raf kinase. US7728010 (**2010**).

[29] Amiri P, Aikawa ME, Dove J, Stuart DD, Poon D, Pick T, *et al.* CHIR-265 is a potent selective inhibitor of c-Raf/B-Raf/mutB-Raf that effectively inhibits proliferation and survival of cancer cell lines with Ras/Raf pathway mutations. 97th AACR Annual Meeting. Washington DC, USA (2006).

[30] Venetsanakos E, Stuart D, Tan N, Ye H, Salangsang F, Aardalen K, *et al.* CHIR-265, a novel inhibitor that targets B-Raf and VEGFR, shows efficacy in a broad range of preclinical models. 97th AACR Annual Meeting. Washington DC, USA (2006).

[31] Sharfman WH, Hodi FS, Lawrence DP, Flaherty KT, Amaravadi RK, Kim KB, *et al.* Results from the first-in-human (FIH) Phase I study of the oral RAF inhibitor RAF265 administered daily to patients with advanced cutaneous melanoma. 2011 ASCO Annual Meeting. Chicago, USA (2011).

[32] Wilhelm S, Carter C, Lynch M, Lowinger T, Dumas J, Smith RA, *et al.* Discovery and development of sorafenib: A multikinase inhibitor for treating cancer. Nat Rev Drug Discov 2006; 5: 835-44.

[33] Kim S, Yazici YD, Calzada G, Wang ZY, Younes MN, Jasser SA, *et al.* Sorafenib inhibits the angiogenesis and growth of orthotopic anaplastic thyroid carcinoma xenografts in nude mice. Mol Cancer Ther 2007; 6: 1785-92.

[34] Adnane L, Trail PA, Taylor I, Wilhelm SM. Sorafenib (BAY 43-9006, Nexavar), a dual-action inhibitor that targets RAF/MEK/ERK pathway in tumor cells and tyrosine kinases VEGFR/PDGFR in tumor vasculature. Methods Enzymol 2006; 407: 597-612.

[35] Wilhelm SM, Carter C, Tang L, Wilkie D, McNabola A, Rong H, *et al.* BAY 43-9006 exhibits broad spectrum oral antitumor activity and targets the RAF/MEK/ERK pathway and receptor tyrosine kinases involved in tumor progression and angiogenesis. Cancer Res 2004; 64: 7099-109.

[36] Egberts F, Kahler KC, Livingstone E, Hauschild A. Metastatic melanoma: Scientific rationale for sorafenib treatment and clinical results. Onkologie 2008; 31: 398-403.

[37] Eisen T, Ahmad T, Flaherty KT, Gore M, Kaye S, Marais R, *et al.* Sorafenib in advanced melanoma: A Phase II randomised discontinuation trial analysis. Br J Cancer 2006; 95: 581-6.

[38] Gupta-Abramson V, Troxel AB, Nellore A, Puttaswamy K, Redlinger M, Ransone K, *et al.* Phase II trial of sorafenib in advanced thyroid cancer. J Clin Oncol 2008; 26: 4714-9.

[39] Escudier B, Eisen T, Stadler WM, Szczylik C, Oudard S, Siebels M, *et al.* Sorafenib in advanced clear-cell renal-cell carcinoma. N Engl J Med 2007; 356: 125-34.

[40] Hauschild A, Agarwala SS, Trefzer U, Hogg D, Robert C, Hersey P, *et al.* Results of a Phase III, randomized, placebo-controlled study of sorafenib in combination with carboplatin and paclitaxel as second-line treatment in patients with unresectable stage III or stage IV melanoma. J Clin Oncol 2009; 27: 2823-30.

[41] Wilhelm SM, Dumas J, Adnane L, Lynch M, Carter CA, Schutz G, *et al.* Regorafenib (BAY 73-4506): A new oral multikinase inhibitor of angiogenic, stromal and oncogenic receptor tyrosine kinases with potent preclinical antitumor activity. Int J Cancer 2011; 129: 245-55.

[42] Mross K, Frost A, Steinbild S, Hedbom S, Buchert M, Fasol U, *et al.* A Phase I dose-escalation study of regorafenib (BAY 73-4506), an inhibitor of oncogenic, angiogenic and

stromal kinases, in patients with advanced solid tumors. Clin Cancer Res 2012; 18(9): 2658-67.

[43] George S, von Mehren M, Heinrich MC, Wang Q, Corless CQ, Butrynski JE, *et al.* A multicenter Phase II study of regorafenib in patients (pts) with advanced gastrointestinal stromal tumor (GIST), after therapy with imatinib (IM) and sunitinib (SU). 2011 ASCO Annual Meeting. Chicago, USA (2011).

[44] Grothey A, Sobrero AF, Siena S, Falcone A, Ychou M, Lenz HJ, *et al.* Results of a Phase III randomized, double-blind, placebo-controlled, multicenter trial (CORRECT) of regorafenib plus best supportive care (BSC) *vs.* placebo plus BSC in patients (pts) with metastatic colorectal cancer (mCRC) who have progressed after standard therapies. 2012 Gastrointestinal Cancers Symposium. San Francisco, USA (2012).

[45] Anand, N.K., Blazey, C.M., Bowles, O.J., Bussenius, J., Costanzo, S., Curtis, J.K., Dubenko, L., Kennedy, A.R., Defina, S.C., Kim, A.I., Manalo, J.-C.L., Peto, C.J., Rice, K.D., Tsang, T.H., Joshi, A.A. Raf modulators and methods of use. US20080009488 (**2008**).

[46] Malek S. Selective Inhibition of RAF results in downregulation of the RAS/RAF/MEK/ERK pathway and inhibition of tumor growth *in vivo*. 18th EORTC-NCI-AACR Symposium on Molecular Targets and Cancer Therapeutics. Prague, Czech Republic (2006).

[47] Schwartz GK, Robertson S, Shen A, Wang E, Pace L, Dials H, *et al.* A Phase I study of XL281, a selective oral RAF kinase inhibitor, in patients (Pts) with advanced solid tumors. 2009 ASCO Annual Meeting. Chicago, USA (2009).

[48] Wallace, E.M., Lyssikatos, J.P., Marlow, A.L., Hurley, T.B., Koch, K. N3 alkylated benzimidazole derivatives as MEK inhibitors. US20070299063 (**2007**) & SI2130537 (**2013**).

[49] Allen LF, Sebolt-Leopold J, Meyer MB. CI-1040 (PD184352), a targeted signal transduction inhibitor of MEK (MAPKK). Semin Oncol 2003; 30: 105-16.

[50] Davies BR, Logie A, McKay JS, Martin P, Steele S, Jenkins R, *et al.* AZD6244 (ARRY-142886), a potent inhibitor of mitogen-activated protein kinase/extracellular signal-regulated kinase kinase 1/2 kinases: Mechanism of action *in vivo*, pharmacokinetic/pharmacodynamic relationship, and potential for combination in preclinical models. Mol Cancer Ther 2007; 6: 2209-19.

[51] Haass NK, Sproesser K, Nguyen TK, Contractor R, Medina CA, Nathanson KL, *et al.* The mitogen-activated protein/extracellular signal-regulated kinase kinase inhibitor AZD6244 (ARRY-142886) induces growth arrest in melanoma cells and tumor regression when combined with docetaxel. Clin Cancer Res 2008; 14: 230-9.

[52] Hayes DN, Lucas AS, Tanvetyanon T, Krzyzanowska MK, Chung CH, Murphy BA, *et al.* Phase II efficacy and pharmacogenomic study of selumetinib (AZD6244; ARRY-142886) in iodine-131 refractory papillary thyroid carcinoma with or without follicular elements. Clin Cancer Res 2012; 18: 2056-65.

[53] Bekaii-Saab T, Phelps MA, Li X, Saji M, Goff L, Kauh JS, *et al.* Multi-institutional Phase II study of selumetinib in patients with metastatic biliary cancers. J Clin Oncol 2011; 29: 2357-63.

[54] O'Neil BH, Goff LW, Kauh JS, Strosberg JR, Bekaii-Saab TS, Lee RM, *et al.* Phase II study of the mitogen-activated protein kinase 1/2 inhibitor selumetinib in patients with advanced hepatocellular carcinoma. J Clin Oncol 2011; 29: 2350-6.

[55] Kirkwood JM, Bastholt L, Robert C, Sosman J, Larkin J, Hersey P, *et al.* Phase II, open-label, randomized trial of the MEK1/2 inhibitor selumetinib as monotherapy vs. temozolomide in patients with advanced melanoma. Clin Cancer Res 2012; 18: 555-67.

[56] Tzekova V, Cebotaru C, Ciuleanu TE, Damjanov D, Ganchev H, Kanarev HV, *et al.* Efficacy and safety of AZD6244 (ARRY-142886) as second/third-line treatment of patients (pts) with advanced non-small cell lung cancer (NSCLC). 2008 ASCO Annual Meeting. Chicago, USA (2008).

[57] Bodoky G, Timcheva C, Spigel DR, La Stella PJ, Ciuleanu TE, Pover G, *et al.* A Phase II open-label randomized study to assess the efficacy and safety of selumetinib (AZD6244 [ARRY-142886]) vs. capecitabine in patients with advanced or metastatic pancreatic cancer who have failed first-line gemcitabine therapy. Invest New Drugs 2012; 30(3): 1216-23.

[58] Ibrahim, P.N., Artis, D.R., Bremer, R., Zhang, C., Zhang, J., Zhu, Y.-L., Tsai, J., Hirth, K.-P., Bollag, G., Cho, H. Compounds and methods for kinase modulation, and indications therefor. US8143271 (**2012**).

[59] Wrasidlo, W., Dneprovskaia, E. Heterocyclic compounds and methods of use. US8084618 (**2011**).

[60] Pulici, M., Marchionni, C., Piutti, C., Gasparri, F. Bicyclic pyrazoles as protein kinase inhibitors US20110257165 (**2011**).

[61] Ahrendt, K. *N*- (6-Aminopyridin-3-YL) -3- (sulfonamido) benzamide derivatives as B-Raf inhibitors for the treatment of cancer. US20110003859 (**2011**).

[62] Shipps, G., Deng, Y., Cooper, A.B., Sun, B., Wang, J., Zhu, L. Fused pyrazole derivatives as novel ERK inhibitors. WO2012036997 (**2012**).

[63] Kawasaki, H., Abe, H., Hayakawa, K., Iida, T., Kikuchi, S., Yamaguchi. T., Nanayama, T., Kurachi, H., Tamaru, M., Hori, Y., Takahashi, M., Yoshida, T., Sakai, T. Pyrimidine compound and medical use thereof. US20100240613 (**2010**).

[64] Qi, J., Wang, Y., Li, F., Shakespeare, W.C., Kohlmann, A., Dalgarno, D.C., Zhu, X. Azaindole derivatives as kinase inhibitors. US20110294806 (**2011**).

[65] Tung R. Substituted azaindoles. US2011051297 (**2011**).

[66] Deng Y, Shipps G, Lo SM, Zhu L, Cooper AB, Muppala K. Indazole derivatives useful as ERK inhibitors. WO2012030685 (**2011**).

[67] Rinehart J, Adjei AA, Lorusso PM, Waterhouse D, Hecht JR, Natale RB, *et al.* Multicenter Phase II study of the oral MEK inhibitor, CI-1040, in patients with advanced non-small-cell lung, breast, colon, and pancreatic cancer. J Clin Oncol 2004; 22: 4456-62.

[68] Thompson N, Lyons J. Recent progress in targeting the Raf/MEK/ERK pathway with inhibitors in cancer drug discovery. Curr Opin Pharmacol 2005; 5: 350-6.

[69] Solit DB, Garraway LA, Pratilas CA, Sawai A, Getz G, Basso A, *et al.* BRAF mutation predicts sensitivity to MEK inhibition. Nature 2006; 439: 358-62.

[70] Boasberg PD, Redfern CH, Daniels GA, Bodkin D, Garrett CR, Ricart AD. Pilot study of PD-0325901 in previously treated patients with advanced melanoma, breast cancer, and colon cancer. Cancer Chemother Pharmacol 2011; 68: 547-52.

[71] Dong Q, Dougan DR, Gong X, Halkowycz P, Jin B, Kanouni T, *et al.* Discovery of TAK-733, a potent and selective MEK allosteric site inhibitor for the treatment of cancer. Bioorg Med Chem Lett 2011; 21: 1315-9.

[72] Isshiki Y, Kohchi Y, Iikura H, Matsubara Y, Asoh K, Murata T, *et al.* Design and synthesis of novel allosteric MEK inhibitor CH4987655 as an orally available anticancer agent. Bioorg Med Chem Lett 2011; 21: 1795-801.

[73] Iverson C, Larson G, Lai C, Yeh LT, Dadson C, Weingarten P, *et al.* RDEA119/BAY 869766: A potent, selective, allosteric inhibitor of MEK1/2 for the treatment of cancer. Cancer Res 2009; 69: 6839-47.

[74] Dean, D.K., Takle, A.K., Wilson, D.M. Imidazole derivatives as Raf kinase inhibitors. US7199137 (**2007**).

[75] Steadman, J.G., Takle, A.K. Imidazole derivatives as Raf kinase inhibitors. US7235658 (**2007**).

[76] Takle AK, Brown MJ, Davies S, Dean DK, Francis G, Gaiba A, *et al.* The identification of potent and selective imidazole-based inhibitors of B-Raf kinase. Bioorg Med Chem Lett 2006; 16: 378-81.

[77] King AJ, Patrick DR, Batorsky RS, Ho ML, Do HT, Zhang SY, *et al.* Demonstration of a genetic therapeutic index for tumors expressing oncogenic BRAF by the kinase inhibitor SB-590885. Cancer Res 2006; 66: 11100-5.

[78] Flaherty KT, Puzanov I, Kim KB, Ribas A, McArthur GA, Sosman JA, *et al.* Inhibition of mutated, activated BRAF in metastatic melanoma. N Engl J Med 2010; 363: 809-19.

[79] Takle AK, Bamford MJ, Davies S, Davis RP, Dean DK, Gaiba A, *et al.* The identification of potent, selective and CNS penetrant furan-based inhibitors of B-Raf kinase. Bioorg Med Chem Lett 2008; 18: 4373-76.

[80] Dean, D.K., Takle, A.K., Wilson, D.M. Pyridine substituted furan derivatives as Raf kinase inhibitors. US7375105 (**2008**).

[81] Pfister S, Janzarik WG, Remke M, Ernst A, Werft W, Becker N, *et al.* BRAF gene duplication constitutes a mechanism of MAPK pathway activation in low-grade astrocytomas. J Clin Invest 2008; 118: 1739-49.

[82] Gilmartin AG, Bleam MR, Groy A, Moss KG, Minthorn EA, Kulkarni SG, *et al.* GSK1120212 (JTP-74057) is an inhibitor of MEK activity and activation with favorable pharmacokinetic properties for sustained *in vivo* pathway inhibition. Clin Cancer Res 2011; 17: 989-1000.

[83] Infante JR, Fecher JA, Nallapareddy S, Gordon MS, Flaherty KT, Cox DS, *et al.* Safety and efficacy results from the first-in-human study of the oral MEK 1/2 inhibitor GSK1120212. 2010 ASCO Annual Meeting. Chicago, USA (2010).

[84] Kim K, Kong SY, Fulciniti M, Li X, Song W, Nahar S, *et al.* Blockade of the MEK/ERK signalling cascade by AS703026, a novel selective MEK1/2 inhibitor, induces pleiotropic anti-myeloma activity *in vitro* and *in vivo*. Br J Haematol 2010; 149: 537-49.

[85] Yoon J, Koo KH, Choi KY. MEK1/2 inhibitors AS703026 and AZD6244 may be potential therapies for KRAS mutated colorectal cancer that is resistant to EGFR monoclonal antibody therapy. Cancer Res 2011; 71: 445-53.

[86] Delord J, Houede N, Awada A, Taamma A, Faivre SJ, Besse-Hammer T, *et al.* First-in-human Phase I safety, pharmacokinetic (PK), and pharmacodynamic (PD) analysis of the oral MEK-inhibitor AS703026 (two regimens [R]) in patients (pts) with advanced solid tumors. 2010 ASCO Annual Meeting. Chicago, USA (2010).

[87] Tsai J, Lee JT, Wang W, Zhang J, Cho H, Mamo S, *et al.* Discovery of a selective inhibitor of oncogenic B-Raf kinase with potent antimelanoma activity. Proc Natl Acad Sci USA 2008; 105: 3041-6.

[88] Winski S, Anderson D, Bouhana K, Rhodes S, Impastato R, Roessner R, *et al.* MEK162 (ARRY-162), a Novel MEK 1/2 Inhibitor, Inhibits Tumor Growth Regardless of KRas/Raf Pathway Mutations 2010 EORTC-NCI-AACR Annual Meeting. Brussels, Belgium (2010).

[89] James J, Ruggeri B, Armstrong RC, Rowbottom MW, Jones-Bolin S, Gunawardane RN, *et al.* CEP-32496: A novel orally active BRAFV600E inhibitor with selective cellular and *in vivo* antitumor activity. Mol Cancer Ther 2012; 11: 930-41.

[90] Aikawa, M.E., Amiri, P., Dove, J.H., Levine, B.H., McBride, C., Pick, T.E., Poon, D.J., Ramurthy, S., Renhowe, P.A., Shafer, C., Stuart, D., Subramanian, S. Substituted benzimidazoles and methods of their use. US20100234394 (**2010**).

[91] Rowbottom MW, Faraoni R, Chao Q, Campbell BT, Lai AG, Setti E, *et al.* Identification of 1-(3-(6,7-dimethoxyquinazolin-4-yloxy)phenyl)-3-(5-(1,1,1-trifluoro-2-methylpropa n-2-yl)isoxazol-3-yl)urea hydrochloride (CEP-32496), a highly potent and orally efficacious inhibitor of V-RAF murine sarcoma viral oncogene homologue B1 (BRAF) V600E. J Med Chem 2012; 55: 1082-105.

[92] Wallace, E.M., Lyssikatos, J.P., Marlow, A.L., Hurley, T.B. Compositions comprising N3 alkylated benzimidazole derivatives as MEK inhibitors and methods of use thereof. US20110158971 (**2011**).

[93] Cockerill, G.S., Lackey, K.E. Anilinoquinazolines as protein tyrosine kinase inhibitors. US7189734 (**2007**).

[94] Aquila, B., Lyne, P., Pontz, T. Quinazolinone derivatives having b-raf inhibitory activity. WO2007113558 (**2007**).

[95] Li QS, Li CY, Lu X, Zhang H, Zhu HL. Design, synthesis and biological evaluation of novel (E)-alpha-benzylsulfonyl chalcone derivatives as potential BRAF inhibitors. Eur J Med Chem 2012; 50: 288-95.

[96] Sebolt-Leopold JS, English JM. Mechanisms of drug inhibition of signalling molecules. Nature 2006; 441: 457-62.

[97] Paraiso KH, Xiang Y, Rebecca VW, Abel EV, Chen YA, Munko AC, *et al.* PTEN loss confers BRAF inhibitor resistance to melanoma cells through the suppression of BIM expression. Cancer Res 2011; 71: 2750-60.

[98] Gopal YN, Deng W, Woodman SE, Komurov K, Ram P, Smith PD, *et al.* Basal and treatment-induced activation of AKT mediates resistance to cell death by AZD6244 (ARRY-142886) in Braf-mutant human cutaneous melanoma cells. Cancer Res 2010; 70: 8736-47.

[99] Little AS, Balmanno K, Sale MJ, Newman S, Dry JR, Hampson M, *et al.* Amplification of the driving oncogene, KRAS or BRAF, underpins acquired resistance to MEK1/2 inhibitors in colorectal cancer cells. Sci Signal 2011; 4: ra17.

[100] Prahallad A, Sun C, Huang S, Di Nicolantonio F, Salazar R, Zecchin D, *et al.* Unresponsiveness of colon cancer to BRAF(V600E) inhibition through feedback activation of EGFR. Nature 2012; 483: 100-3.

[101] Villanueva J, Vultur A, Lee JT, Somasundaram R, Fukunaga-Kalabis M, Cipolla AK, *et al.* Acquired resistance to BRAF inhibitors mediated by a RAF kinase switch in melanoma can be overcome by cotargeting MEK and IGF-1R/PI3K. Cancer Cell 2010; 18: 683-95.

[102] Jure-Kinkel, M., Wiggington, J.M., Gupta, A.K. Combinations of anti-CTLA4 antibody with BRAF inhibitors for the synergistic treatment of proliferative diseases. WO2012027536 (**2012**).

[103] Coopersmith, R., Lehrer, R. Method to treat melanoma in BRAF inhibitor-resistant subjects. US20120053185 (**2012**).

[104] Lane, H. Pharmaceutical combinations comprising a MTOR inhibitor and a RAF kinase inhibitor. US20110301184 (**2011**).

[105] Wang, Y., Pachter, J.A., Bishop, W.R. Anti-IGFR1 antibody therapeutic combinations. US8017735 (**2011**).

[106] Infante JR, Falchook GS, Lawrence DA, Weber JS, Kefford RF, Bendell JC, *et al.* Phase I/II study of the oral MEK1/2 inhibitor GSK1120212 dosed in combination with the oral BRAF inhibitor GSK2118436. 2011 ASCO Annual Meeting. Chicago, USA (2011).

[107] Schilling G, Bruweleit M, Harbeck N, Thomssen C, Becker K, Hoffmann R, *et al.* Phase II trial of vinorelbine and trastuzumab in patients with HER2-positive metastatic breast cancer. A prospective, open label, non-controlled, multicenter Phase II trial (to investigate efficacy and safety of this combination chemotherapy). Invest New Drugs 2008; 27: 166-72.

[108] Caprioni F, Fornarini G. Bevacizumab in the treatment of metastatic colorectal cancer. Future Oncol 2007; 3: 141-8.

[109] Porter JR, Fritz CC, Depew KM. Discovery and development of Hsp90 inhibitors: A promising pathway for cancer therapy. Curr Opin Chem Biol 2010; 14: 412-20.

[110] Paraiso KH, Haarberg HE, Wood E, Rebecca VW, Chen YA, Xiang Y, *et al.* The HSP90 inhibitor XL888 overcomes BRAF inhibitor resistance mediated through diverse mechanisms. Clin Cancer Res 2012; 18(9): 2502-14.

[111] Solit DB, Osman I, Polsky D, Panageas KS, Daud A, Goydos JS, *et al.* Phase II trial of 17-allylamino-17-demethoxygeldanamycin in patients with metastatic melanoma. Clin Cancer Res 2008; 14: 8302-7.

[112] Burlison, J.A., Zhang, S., Ying, W., Chimmanamada, D.U., Song, M., Chae, J., Schweizer, S.M. Triazole compounds that modulate Hsp90 activity. US20120101072 (**2012**).

[113] Vukovic, V., Teofilovici, F. HSP90 inhibitors for treating non-small cell lung cancer in wild-type EGFR and/or KRAS patients. WO2012037072 (**2012**).

[114] Burlison, J.A., Chimmanamada, D.U., Ying, W., Zhang, S., James, D. Hydrazonamide compounds that modulate Hsp90 activity. US20120046288 (**2012**).

[115] Borthakur, G., Kadia, T.M. Biomarkers useful to predict MEK inhibitor drug efficacy. WO2012048106 (**2012**).

[116] Clark, D. P., Schayowitz, A., Cabradilla, C.D. Compositions and methods for prediction of drug sensitivity, resistance, and disease progression. US20120094853 (**2012**).

[117] Deng, Y., Shipps, Jr. G.W., Cooper, A., Nan, Y., Wang, T., Siddiqui, M.A., Zhu, H., Sun, R., Kelly, J.M., Doll, R., Desai, J., Wang, J.J.-S., Dong, Y., Madison, V., Xiao, L., Hruza, A., Shih, N.-Y. Novel compounds that are ERK inhibitors. US20070232610 (**2007**).

[118] Cooper, A.B., Nan, Y., Deng, Y., Shipps, Jr. G.W., Shih, N.-Y., Zhu, H.Y., Kelly, J.M., Gudipati, S., Doll, R.J., Patel, M.F., Desai, J.A., Wang, J.J.-S., Paliwal, S., Tsui, H.-C., Bga, S.B., Alhassan, A.-B., Gao, X., Zhu, L., Yao, X. Novel compounds that are ERK inhibitors. US20110189192 (**2011**).

[119] Abraham, S., Bhagwat, S.S., Campbell, B.T., Chao, Q., Faraoni, R., Holladay, M.W., Lai, A.G., Rowbottom, M.W., Setti, E., Sprankle, K.G. Raf kinase modulator compounds and methods of use thereof. US20110118245 (**2011**).

[120] Backes, A., Vogt, J., Amon, P., Ivanov, I., Hannus, S., Borgmann, M., Hansen, K., Casaubon, R., Smith, C., Murthi, K., Kluge, A., Schoop, A., Neumann, L., Eickhoff, J. Raf inhibitors. US20110257207 (**2011**).

[121] Bhattacharya, S.K., Brown, M.F., Dorff, P.H., LaGreca, S.D., Mickelson, J.W., Cornicelli, J.A., Brown, D.L., Rex, J., Walker, J.K., Huff, R., Strohbach, J.W., Maguire, R.J. Cycloalkylamino acid derivatives. US20100234435 (**2010**).

[122] Huang, S., Jin, X., Liu, Z., Poon, D., Tellew, J., Wan, Y., Wang, X., Xie, Y. Compounds and compositions as protein kinase inhibitors. US20110306625 (**2011**).

[123] Zhang, S., Guo, T. 3-(2-Amino-ethyl)-5-(3-cyclohexyl-propylidene)-thiazolidine-2,4-dione and its derivatives as multiple signaling pathway inhibitors and for the treatment of cancer. US20110166191 (**2011**).

[124] Ahrendt, K.A., Buckmelter, A.J., Grina, J., Hansen, J.D., Laird, E.R., Moreno, D., Newhouse, B., Ren, L., Wenglowsky, S.M., Feng, B., Gunzner, J., Malesky, K., Mathieu, S., Rudolph, J., Wen, Z., Young, W.B. Raf inhibitor compounds and methods of use thereof. US20110110889 (**2011**).

Send Orders of Reprints at reprints@benthamscience.net
Topics in Anti-Cancer Research, Vol. 2, 2013, 95-196

CHAPTER 4

Recent Developments in Anticancer Agents Targeting PI3K, AKT and mTORC1/2

Irene Brana[1], Sara De Dosso[2], Rodrigo Dienstmann[3], Jordi Rodon[3], Josep Tabernero[3] and Ben Markman[4]

[1]Drug Development Program.Princess Margaret Cancer Center, UHN-Division of Medical Oncology & Hematology, Post-Graduate Medical Education, University of Toronto; [2]Clinical Research Unit, Oncology Institute of Southern Switzerland, Bellinzona, Switzerland; [3]Medical Oncology Service, Vall d'Hebron University Hospital and Vall d'Hebron Institute of Oncology, Universitat Autonoma de Barcelona, Barcelona, Spain; [4]Centre for Cancer Research, Monash Institute of Medical Research, Monash University, Victoria, Australia

Abstract: Inappropriate phosphoinositide 3-kinase (PI3K) signaling is one of the most frequent occurrences in human cancer and is critical for tumor progression. Various genetic mutations and amplifications have been described affecting key components of this pathway, with implications for tumorigenesis and also for resistance to targeted agents. Emerging preclinical research has significantly advanced our understanding of the PI3K pathway and its complex downstream signaling, interactions and crosstalk. This knowledge, combined with the limited clinical antitumor activity of mTOR complex 1 inhibitors, has led to the development of rationally designed drugs targeting key elements of this pathway, such as pure PI3K inhibitors (both pan-PI3K and isoform-specific), dual PI3K/ mTOR inhibitors, AKT inhibitors, and mTOR complexes 1 and 2 catalytic site inhibitors. This chapter will focus primarily on an analysis of newly developed inhibitors of this pathway that have entered clinical trials, and recently registered patents in this field.

Keywords: AKT inhibitors, antineoplastic-agent, biological marker, clinical trial, drug combination, drug design, drug mechanism, gene mutation, human, mammalian target of rapamycin, mammalian target of rapamycin inhibitors, molecularly targeted therapy, neoplasm, patents, phosphoinositide 3-kinase, phosphoinositide 3-kinase inhibitors, pre-clinical experiment, pre- hyperglycemia, proto-oncogene proteins c-AKT, rash.

***Address correspondence to Josep Tabernero:** Medical Oncology Service, Vall d'Hebron University Hospital and Vall d'Hebron Institute of Oncology , P. Vall d'Hebron 119-129, 08035 Barcelona Spain; Tel: +34 93 274 6077; Fax: +34 93 274 6059; E-mail: jtabernero@vhebron.net

Atta-ur Rahman and Khurshid Zaman (Eds)

INTRODUCTION

1. PI3K/ AKT/ mTOR pathway

The phosphoinositide 3-kinases (PI3K) are a family of lipid kinases whose primary biochemical function is to phosphorylate the 3-hydroxyl group of phosphoinositides. Phosphorylation results in activation of second messengers, the most important being the serine-threonine kinase AKT, with consequent signal transduction and stimulation of various physiological cellular metabolic and survival functions. PI3Ks are grouped into three classes (I-III) with varying structure and substrate preference [1].

Class I PI3Ks regulate glucose homeostasis, metabolism, growth, proliferation, motility and cell survival. Class IA PI3K molecules, most commonly implicated in human cancer, are heterodimers comprising a regulatory subunit (p85) and a catalytic subunit (p110). Three mammalian genes, *PIK3R1*, *PIK3R2*, and *PIK3R3*, encode p85alpha, p85beta, and p55gamma regulatory subunits, respectively. The catalytic isoforms, p110alpha, p110beta, and p110delta, are the products of three genes, *PIK3CA*, *PIK3CB*, and *PIK3CD*. Mutations in *PIK3CA* and *PIK3R1* promote activation of the PI3K pathway and are commonly observed in cancer. There are three isoforms in class IA PI3K, namely PI3Kalpha, PI3Kbeta, and PI3Kdelta, with the respective p110 catalytic subunit bound to the p85 regulatory subunit. Conversely, class IB molecules (PI3Kgamma) form a heterodimer between p110gamma, a catalytic subunit similar to class IA p110, with a distinct regulatory subunit, p101 or p84. The ubiquitously expressed PI3Kalpha and PI3Kbeta influence cellular proliferation and insulin signaling, whereas PI3Kgamma and PI3Kdelta are mostly involved in immune function and inflammation, being primarily expressed in leukocytes. As other tissues also express PI3Kgamma and delta, they could play a role in solid tumors [1, 2].

Class II PI3Ks comprise three monomeric catalytic isoforms (C2alpha, C2beta and C2gamma) without regulatory proteins. They phosphorylate phosphatidylinositol (PI) and phosphatidylinositol 3-monophosphate (PIP) and are involved in the regulation of membrane trafficking, receptor internalization, smooth muscle cell contraction and apoptosis. Class II PI3K is usually located in intracellular membranes and, to a lesser extent, in the cytosol. Several factors induce PI3K class II relocalization and activation: tyrosine kinase receptors (RTK) ligands, G protein-coupled receptor (GPCR) ligands, and membrane-bound GTPases, such as TC10. These factors do not interact directly with PI3K Class II; the activation of PI3K Class II requires membrane-associated adaptor proteins, such as GRB2, or other structural proteins, such as clathrin, acting as intermediaries [3]. Class III PI3K is composed of a regulatory subunit (p150) and a catalytic subunit (Vps34) that phosphorylates PI to phosphatidylinositol 3-phosphate and has been implicated in endocytosis, vesicular trafficking, regulation of autophagy and phagocytosis [4]. In mammals, Vps34 interacts with several protein complexes, such as the suppressor protein Beclin 1, the ultraviolet radiation resistance-associated gene protein (UVRAG), or the Bax-interacting factor 1 (BIF1). The interaction of Vps34 with these protein complexes regulates its function [3]. The roles of class II and III PI3Ks in cancer need to be established with development of specific inhibitors, using genetic and pharmacological tools.

Activation of the class IA PI3K is initiated when a growth factor or ligand binds to its cognate receptor tyrosine kinase (RTK), as shown in Fig. (**1**). These receptors include members of the human epidermal growth factor receptor (HER) family, platelet-derived growth factor receptor and the insulin and insulin-like growth factor 1 (IGF1) receptors [5]. Subsequent RTK dimerization and autophosphorylation enable the PI3K heterodimer to interact with its intracellular portion via p85. This is particularly the case for HER3, which has multiple docking sites for p85, as opposed to HER2, which is unable to directly bind PI3K, thus stressing the importance of HER2-HER3 heterodimer formation for transmission of tumorigenic signals via PI3K [6]. The binding of growth factors to RTK relieves the intermolecular inhibition of the p110 catalytic subunit by p85 and localizes PI3K to the plasma membrane. PI3K phosphorylates phosphatidylinositol 4,5-bisphosphate (PIP2) on the 3′OH position to produce phosphatidylinositol 3,4,5-trisphosphate (PIP3) [1]. Additionally, GPCR and RAS can activate class I PI3K. The GPCRs interact directly with the p110beta and p110gamma subunits. In addition, all the class I catalytic subunits can interact with RAS, as they have a RAS biding domain; however, while RAS has been associated with p110alpha, 110delta and p110gamma activation, the role of RAS on the p110beta isoform activation remains controversial [3].

For further propagation of intracellular signaling, PIP3 directly binds pleckstrin homology (PH) domains of various signaling proteins. PIP3 brings two PH domain-containing serine/ threonine kinases, phosphoinositide-dependent kinase 1 (PDK1) and AKT (also known as protein kinase B, PKB), into close proximity. To date, three members of the AKT family, AKT1, AKT2, and AKT3, have been identified, referred to as PKBalpha, PKBbeta, and PKBgamma, respectively. They are the products of three distinct genes (human homologue of the viral oncogene v-AKT) but are closely related as they exhibit greater than 80% homology at the amino acid level within the catalytic kinase domain [7]. PDK1 exerts its growth-promoting effects by phosphorylating and activating downstream protein kinases, including isoforms of AKT at threonine-308 [8-10]. Phospho-AKT^{T308} is able to activate some of its substrates [11, 12]; however, a second phosphorylation event at serine-473 in the helical domain of AKT by the mTOR-rictor complex (mTORC2) is necessary for full AKT activation [10, 13]. In mammalian cells, mTORC2 controls the actin cytoskeleton [14]. Fully activated AKT then translocates to the cytosol or to the nucleus to phosphorylate its downstream substrates involved in cell cycle progression, survival, apoptosis and translation, as shown in Fig. (**1**) [15].

The PI3K/ AKT pathway promotes cell growth and survival through several mechanisms. PI3K signaling studies have mainly focused on AKT and its downstream targets. AKT activation is usually concomitant with PI3K activation but this is not always the case. In addition, recent data indicate the potential for differential signaling outputs downstream of specific PI3K isoforms, in parallel with a possibly more universal AKT activation [3]. AKT influences cellular proliferation by inactivating CDK (cyclin dependent kinase) cell cycle inhibitors, such as p27 and p21; this inactivation could be accomplished through direct phosphorylation of p27 [16, 17] and p21[18] or indirectly through the inhibitory effect of AKT on FOXO (forkhead box O, a subfamily of the forkhead transcription factor family). FOXO is retained in the cytosol and is not able to trigger the transcription of pro-apoptotic genes (Fas ligand, Bim and BAD) [19]. In addition, AKT phosphorylates BAD and releases it from the complex with Bcl-2 or Bcl-X_L, enabling the anti-apoptotic function [20]. Phosphorylation of MDM2 by AKT antagonizes p53-mediated apoptosis [21]. In addition, through activation of IKK (inhibitor of kappaB kinase) and further phosphorylation of IkappaB-alpha (inhibitor of kappaB alpha), AKT impedes negative regulation of the transcription factor NF-kappaB (nuclear factor kappaB), allowing it to translocate to the nucleus and stimulate transcription of pro-survival genes [22]. Furthermore, AKT promotes cell cycle progression by inhibiting glycogen synthesis kinase 3 (GSK3), leading to stabilization of cyclin D1 and c-Myc [23]. Finally, AKT controls cell growth by phosphorylation of the downstream serine/threonine mTOR-raptor complex (mTORC1). AKT can phosphorylate and activate mTORC1 either directly at threonine-2446 and serine-2448 residues, or indirectly by phosphorylation and inactivation of TSC2 (tuberous sclerosis complex 2, also called tuberin), which normally inhibits mTOR through the guanosine triphosphate (GTP)-binding protein Rheb (Ras homolog enriched in brain) [24, 25]. Subsequently, mTORC1 phosphorylates the ribosomal protein S6 kinases (S6K1 and S6K2) and the eukaryotic initiation factor 4E (eIF4E)-binding protein 1 (4E-BP1), components involved in ribosomal biogenesis and messenger RNA translation, determinants of growth and cell size [26, 27]. Phosphorylation of 4E-BPs and S6Ks is reduced by overexpression of a component of mTORC1 termed PRAS40 (Proline Rich AKT Substrate 40kDa) [28]. PRAS40 binds to raptor via a TOR signaling motif (commonly found in other mTORC1 targets) and functions as a downstream target of mTORC1 that inhibits its signaling by competing with 4E-BPs and S6Ks for binding and phosphorylation [29]. In addition, hypoxia-inducible factor 1alpha (HIF-1alpha) is upregulated downstream of mTORC1, and then promotes angiogenesis by enhancing transcription of vascular endothelial growth factor (VEGF) [30].

PI3K signaling has a central role in mediating the effects of insulin on cellular metabolism that is conserved throughout eukaryotic evolution [4]. Noninsulin-dependent diabetes mellitus, marked by insulin insensitivity, is associated with diminished PI3K response to insulin signaling [31]. While both PI3Kalpha and PI3Kbeta appear to play specific roles in insulin signaling, studies suggest that PI3Kalpha predominantly mediates glucose homeostasis [32-34]. PI3Kbeta inactivation has only a mild effect on insulin action, which fits with the observation that this isoform, despite high homology with PI3Kalpha, is not primarily activated by tyrosine kinase receptors, but rather via GPCRs [3].

Inhibition of p110alpha, but not p110beta or p110delta, has been shown to inhibit insulin-stimulated glucose uptake in adipocytes and to block insulin-mediated glucose regulation in mice [33].

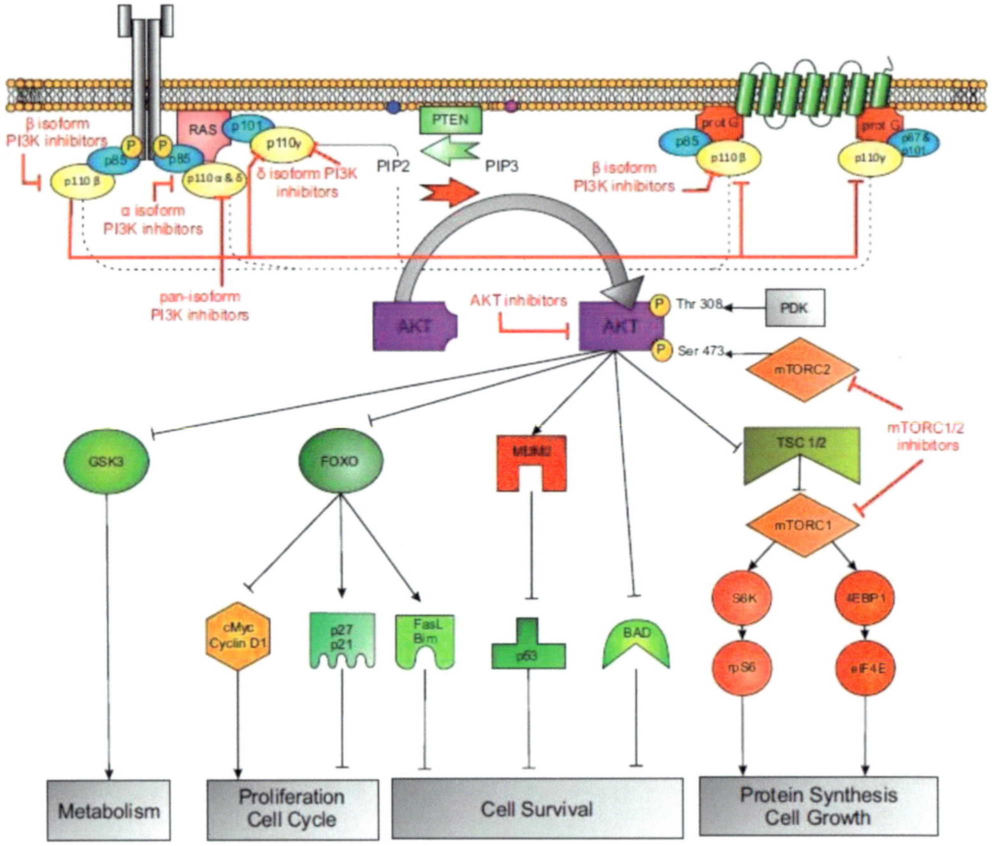

Figure 1: PI3K/ AKT/ mTOR pathway and recently developed inhibitors.

1.1. Downregulation of the PI3K/ AKT/ mTOR pathway

The most important mechanism for downregulating pathway activity occurs through Phosphatase and TENsin homolog deleted on chromosome ten (PTEN). *PTEN* was originally identified as a tumor suppressor gene and mapped to chromosome 10q23. It is a dual-specificity phosphatase that dephosphorylates both protein and lipid substrates. PTEN dephosphorylates cytoplasmic PIP3, forming the inactive PIP2 [35]. Thus, PTEN antagonizes PI3K function and negatively regulates AKT activities [36]. PTEN also acts in the nucleus in a phosphatase-independent manner to further impact cell cycle activity, apoptosis and chromosomal integrity [37]. Germline and somatic deregulations of this critical protein both occur, the latter frequently seen in human cancer.

Additionally, another control mechanism exists in the PI3K pathway. S6K, one of the key effectors of mTORC1, can exert feedback that downregulates IRS1 (insulin receptor substrate 1), the adapter molecule linking the IGF1 receptor and PI3K. This effect appears to be direct and impedes the ability of IRS1 to associate with the insulin receptor, resulting in reduced input into the PI3K pathway in the presence of ongoing stimulation of insulin/IGF1R [38].

The mTOR binding protein DEPTOR, a product of the *DEPDC6* gene, has been identified as another mTORC1 regulator [35]. DEPTOR normally functions to inhibit the mTORC1 and mTORC2 pathways and its depletion results in increased *in vitro* kinase activity towards S6K1 and 4E-BP1. When highly overexpressed, DEPTOR inhibited mTORC1, and, unexpectedly, this led to the activation of the PI3K/mTORC2/AKT pathway in a subset of multiple myeloma cell lines. Overexpression of DEPTOR caused an increase in the phosphorylation of AKT at serine-473 and at threonine-308, the PDK1-catalyzed site that serves as a read-out of PI3K activity [39].

In addition to the complexity of the PI3K pathway, extensive crosstalk exists with other cellular signaling networks. Activation of the tumor suppressor p53 causes both increased PTEN and decreased p110 expression. Further, p53 degradation is reduced indirectly by PTEN via its antagonism of PI3K [40, 41]. Finally, activated GTP-bound RAS proteins are capable of activating the PI3K pathway by binding directly to p110 [42]. Downstream of RAS, in the mitogen-activated protein kinase (MAPK) pathway, extracellular signal-regulated kinase (ERK) has been shown to negatively regulate TSC2 [43]. To corroborate the crosstalk between these two important cascades, MAPK pathway activation has been identified as a consequence of mTORC1 inhibition [44].

1.2. PI3K Pathway Signaling and Cancer

With the exception of the p53 tumor suppressor pathway, the PI3K pathway is the most highly mutated in human cancer. Deregulation of this cascade can be due to a host of genetic aberrations, resulting in either decreased expression of PTEN, amplification or mutation of *PIK3CA*, amplification or mutation of *AKT* and other less frequent events. Not only is pathway activation prevalent in myriad human cancers but its status also has prognostic and predictive relevance.

1.2.1. Germline Mutations and Clinical Syndromes

Genetic mutations and aberrations affecting various components of the PI3K pathway have been described. The consequences of each alteration depend on a host of factors such as which pathway element is affected and whether other tumor genes or proteins are concomitantly deregulated. The most common genetic alteration of the PI3K signaling pathway found in human cancer is inactivation of the *PTEN* tumor suppressor gene. A group of overlapping clinical syndromes, with hamartoma formation being the common clinical feature, is described in association with germline mutations affecting the *PTEN* gene locus - Cowden syndrome (80%), Lhermitte-Duclos disease, Bannayan-Riley- Ruvalcaba syndrome (60%), Proteus syndrome (20%) and Proteus-like syndrome (50%). In addition to hamartomas in the skin, breast, thyroid and intestine, the autosomal dominant Cowden syndrome is associated with a predisposition to cancer, especially breast (30% - 50%), thyroid (10%) and endometrial cancers [45]. Other tumor suppressor genes exert inhibitory effects on PI3K signaling, in particular restricting mTOR activity, by acting through the TSC complex. Germline mutations, with consequent loss of function of *LKB1* and *TSC1/2* tumor suppressor genes, give rise to Peutz-Jeghers syndrome and tuberous sclerosis, respectively. In neurofibromatosis, mutations in the *NF1* tumor suppressor gene lead to increased RAS cascade signaling action and activity of its downstream effectors, such as the PI3K pathway. These entities are characterized by hamartomas and increased risk of certain malignancies, such as neuroendocrine tumors. Together with Cowden syndrome, they result in chronic activation of mTOR signaling. However, the potential for developing overt malignancy is considerable in Cowden syndrome, but rare in the other conditions, reflecting constitutively active AKT in Cowden syndrome but attenuated AKT activity due to of feedback inhibition in the other syndromes [46].

1.2.2. PI3K

PIK3CA, encoding p110alpha, is commonly mutated or amplified in several human cancers. Mutations occur with highest frequency in breast, colon, endometrial and hepatocellular cancers and in glioblastomas, while amplifications are most often encountered in cervical, lung, gastric, ovarian and head and neck cancers [4, 47-60]. Approximately 80% of the mutations have been localized to three "hot spots", resulting in single amino acid substitutions: E545K and E542K in the helical domain and H1047R in the catalytic domain [47, 54]. They increase enzymatic function, enhance downstream signaling elements including AKT and promote oncogenic transformation *in vitro* and *in vivo* with high efficiency in the absence of growth factors and, therefore, seem to obviate the usual obligate interactions with tyrosine phosphorylated RTKs and/or adapters [61]. Exon 9 encodes the helical domain of p110alpha, and mutations in this domain de-repress an inhibitory interaction between the *N*-terminal SH2 (Src Homology 2) domain of p85 and the p110alpha catalytic subunit. Exon 20 encodes the catalytic domain of p110alpha, and mutations in this domain may constitutively activate its enzymatic activity and affect specificity or affinity of p110alpha toward its substrates [5, 61-63]. In addition to these activating mutations, amplification of *PIK3CA* is observed frequently in ovarian cancer and other tumors, but how amplification affects PI3K activation is less clear [64].

Mutations in the p85alpha regulatory subunit *PIK3R1* are observed in a variety of human cancers, including glioblastomas, ovarian cancers, and colorectal cancers [65, 66]. Mutations in *PIK3R1* generally produce either truncations or in-frame deletions that often localize to the inter-SH2 domain of p85alpha. Structural analyses suggest that the inter-SH2 domain of p85 interacts with the C2 domain of p110 [61]. Thus, it seems likely that these p85aplha mutations also activate PI3K signaling by relieving the inhibitory effect of p85 on p110 [67].

While activating mutations in *PIK3CA* are frequently identified in human cancers, no oncogenic mutations have been verified in p110beta, p110delta, or the class IB catalytic isoform p110gamma. However, increased p110beta and p110delta have been identified in some colon, endometrial and bladder cancers, as well as in glioblastomas [68-71]. Amplification/ overexpression of *PIK3CB* is capable of acting as an oncogene in model systems [72]. In addition, p110delta appears to provide the critical PI3K activity in acute myelogenous leukemia, while p110gamma is upregulated by the *BCR-ABL* oncogene in chronic myelogenous leukemia [73, 74]. On the other hand, PI3K-independent activation of downstream effectors of the mTORC1 pathway has been observed in some hematologic malignancies. A recent study identified the Pim-2 serine/threonine kinase as mainly responsible for 4E-BP1 phosphorylation and subsequent protein translation control in acute myeloid leukemia [75].

1.2.3. AKT

Mutations in *AKT* family genes encoding for *AKT1*, *AKT2*, and *AKT3* have also been identified in human cancers. A missense mutation at E17K of *AKT1* with transforming potential has recently been identified in a small proportion of breast, colorectal, ovarian and endometrial cancers [76-78]. This amino acid change alters AKT1 lipid binding, leading to constitutive membrane localization in the absence of PIP3. However, although phosphorylation on serine-473 was constitutive in this mutant, threonine-308 phosphorylation was still responsive to PI3K activation [77]. Thus, it is unclear if PI3K inhibitors will effectively decrease AKT signaling in cancers with these mutations. Despite the confirmed oncogenic function of the *AKT1* E17K, the rare incidences of the mutation suggest that it may not play a crucial role in the development of the most common types of human cancers. Additionally, mutations affecting the kinase domain of AKT2 have been found in colorectal, gastric and lung carcinomas [79, 80]. The E17K mutation has also been identified in *AKT3* in some melanomas [81]. Amplification of AKT is seen most often in head and neck, gastric, pancreatic and ovarian cancers [4, 52, 82-84].

Recently, a MAGI3-AKT3 rearrangement has been described predominantly in triple negative breast cancers. The fusion protein that results from this rearrangement has AKT constitutively activated, inducing phosphorylation of their downstream targets. The activity of this fusion protein can be blocked by specific AKT inhibitors [57].

1.2.4. mTOR

Recently, mTOR activating mutations were identified in the human cancer genome database. Two different point mutations, S2215Y (colon adenocarcinoma) and R2505P (renal cell carcinoma), conferred constitutive activation of mTOR signaling even under nutrient starvation conditions [85]. Their frequency in human cancer appears low.

1.2.5. PTEN

Homozygous and hemizygous deletions, as well as epigenetic silencing of *PTEN*, are also observed in human cancers [86, 87]. Loss of heterozygosity (LOH) 10q occurs when the remaining copy of *PTEN* is haploinsufficient and thus unable to prevent the malignant phenotype. LOH rates are highest in glioblastoma, endometrial, gastric, prostate and breast cancers and melanoma, whereas a PTEN mutation is most prevalent in endometrial cancers (especially the endometroid subtype in 80% to 90%) and glioblastomas [88-98]. LOH occurs with greater frequency than mutation alone due the presence of alternate mechanisms such as homozygous deletion and epigenetic silencing via promoter hypermethylation. Because there are both genetic and epigenetic causes for *PTEN* loss, accurate assessment of a cancer's PTEN status remains challenging and may ultimately require reliable measurements of protein expression.

Functional PTEN loss appears to be important in cancer progression [99]. PTEN mutation is associated with earlier stage and a more favorable survival in endometrial cancer [97]. In prostate cancer, loss of PTEN expression is correlated with high Gleason grade and advanced stage [100, 101]. In gliomas, PTEN mutation is more frequent in primary high-grade than in low-grade gliomas and is associated with reduced survival [102, 103]. Alteration in PTEN expression is associated with an increased Breslow thickness and ulceration in melanomas [104, 105]. In breast cancer, loss of PTEN expression is associated with lymph node metastasis, loss of estrogen receptor expression and poor outcome [106]. Interestingly, largely mutually exclusive mutations of PTEN and RAS family members are described in tumor types including endometrial cancer and glioblastoma [107, 108]. A similar relationship between PI3K and RAS pathway mutations and between PTEN and TP53 mutations has been noted in breast cancers [109, 110]. These findings indicate that mutation of either *RAS* or *TP53* may often provide a sufficient impetus for tumorigenesis so as to remove any selective pressure for additional PTEN mutations to occur. On the other hand, some studies indicate that functional PTEN loss and PIK3CA mutations can coexist in breast, endometrial and colon cancers [111].

Recent data also suggest a prominent role for PI3Kbeta in PTEN-deficient tumors. In preclinical studies with PTEN-deficient prostate and colorectal cancer cell lines, down-regulation of p110beta, but not p110alpha, resulted in PI3K pathway inactivation and subsequent inhibition of growth in both cell-based and *in vivo* settings [32, 112]. However, in cells with mutations in both *PTEN* and *PIK3CA*, downregulation of p110alpha activity, but not p110beta activity, results in PI3K pathway inactivation and cell growth inhibition [112, 113]. As stated by Jia *et al.*, it is perhaps best to consider PTEN as the brake that modulates PI3K signaling. In a given tumor driven by PTEN loss, the most relevant question in determining p110 isoform dependence is which receptors are providing the input signals that are amplified by the loss of PTEN. If these signals arise from GPCRs, p110beta will be the major isoform carrying the load. Conversely, if stronger signals come from coexisting mutant RTKs, RAS or p110alpha, which potentiate total PI3K activity caused by PTEN loss, the isoform dependency may be switched to p110alpha [114].

2. RATIONALE FOR TARGETING THE PI3K PATHWAY IN CANCER THERAPEUTICS

Preclinical studies have shown that PI3K pathway inhibitors may have significant single-agent activity in cancers with *PIK3CA* mutations and PTEN deficiency [115-126]. In mismatch repair-deficient colorectal cell lines, activity of PI3K pathway inhibitors has also been preferential [127]. In HER2-overexpressing breast cancer, trastuzumab requires intact PTEN for its therapeutic response and PTEN loss predicts trastuzumab resistance [128]. The HER2-amplified breast cancer cell lines with *PIK3CA* mutations are also resistant to trastuzumab, and this can be reversed with treatment with PI3K inhibitors [129, 130]. Similarly, PTEN loss, or activating mutations in *PIK3CA,* confers resistance to lapatinib, which can be overcome by treatment with a PI3K inhibitor [131]. In colorectal cancer, *PIK3CA* mutation and PTEN loss renders cells resistant to the anti-EGFR monoclonal antibody cetuximab [132]. In these scenarios, inhibition of PI3K may provide one alternate avenue for treatment in cases of trastuzumab, lapatinib or cetuximab resistance due to abnormal PTEN/ PI3K status. Additionally, constitutively active AKT contributes to tumor cell survival and therapeutic resistance to a range of cytotoxic agents and radiation in lung cancer and glioblastoma, to carboplatin and paclitaxel in ovarian cancer and to doxorubicin, tamoxifen and trastuzumab in breast cancer. In each case, the use of PI3K inhibitors increases the apoptotic effects of these therapies when used in combination, thus laying the foundation for possible future treatment strategies [133-142].

Most models of cancers that are sensitive to single-agent PI3K pathway inhibitors have demonstrated tumor stasis rather than frank regressions *in vivo* [117, 118, 143]. Consequently, it may be necessary to combine PI3K pathway inhibitors with other agents to induce dramatic responses. Furthermore, there may be cancers that show no response to single-agent PI3K pathway inhibitors that will respond to PI3K pathway inhibitors combined with other therapies. Data suggest that cancers with *KRAS* mutations may be resistant to PI3K pathway inhibitors [115, 116]. Consequently, it seems likely that the presence of *KRAS* mutations will limit the efficacy of single-agent PI3K pathway inhibitors in cancers harboring both *KRAS* and *PIK3CA* mutations, such as colon cancers. However, combined PI3K and MAPK pathway inhibition by treatment with a PI3K/mTOR inhibitor and a MEK inhibitor led to marked tumor regression in a *KRAS* lung cancer model [116]. As indicated by Courtney *et al.* PI3K pathway inhibitors may be effective agents for treating cancers that acquire resistance to RTK inhibitors [144]. Cancers that are sensitive to receptor tyrosine kinase inhibitors (TKIs) have PI3K pathway signaling under the exclusive control of that RTK [128]. When a TKI works, it leads to downregulation of PI3K activity. When cancers that were initially sensitive to TKIs (i.e., oncogeneaddicted to an RTK) subsequently develop resistance, they invariably find a way to maintain PI3K signaling in the presence of the TKI [145]. These cancers may therefore be susceptible to adding a PI3K pathway inhibitor to the TKI to re-induce remission.

Similarly, tumors addicted to certain PI3K isoforms and, therefore, potentially susceptible to PI3K isoform-specific inhibitors, could develop resistance through a PI3K-dependent or independent mechanism. More specifically, Met overexpression leads to tumor survival dependent on PI3K pathway reactivation, and represents an example of a PI3K-dependent mechanism of resistance, whereas Myc induction, contributing to oncogene independence, is an example of PI3K-independent resistance.

2.1. Biomarker Development

Biomarkers (BMs) are measurable characteristics of physiological or pathological states. Thus, BMs aim to serve varied functions during drug development, including provision of proof-of principle, refinement of patient selection, assessment of responders versus non-responders early in treatment and facilitation of optimal biological dose determination [146]. To date, BMs reflecting PI3K and mTOR pathway activity or inhibition have been investigated in preclinical and clinical settings. Although, they do not yet have a definitive role in the clinic, emerging data are showing promise in this field. In a recent study, authors generated phosphospecific antibodies against drug-regulated phosphorylation sites that could be suitable as BM tools for PI3K pathway inhibitors. In a PTEN-deficient prostate tumor model and triple-negative breast tumor tissues, an antibody against phospho-PRAS40 (threonine-246) showed positive correlation with PI3K pathway activation and predicted AKT inhibitor sensitivity. In contrast to phosphorylation of AKT (threonine-308), the phospho-PRAS40 (threonine-246) epitope was highly stable in tissue samples and thus ideal for immunohistochemistry [147]. Additionally, in a Phase I study of the mTOR inhibitor everolimus, a strong correlation was noted between the degree of mTOR inhibition in skin and tumor (through evaluation of phospho-S6 and phospho-eIF-4G levels), indicating that skin might serve as a valuable surrogate tissue reflecting pathway modulation [148]. Further, modulation of PI3K pathway elements has also been shown in hair follicles [149, 150]. Sampling convenience and the high basal pathway activity in this tissue make it a good candidate for continued development.

The assessment of *PIK3CA* mutation and PTEN loss as BMs of response to PI3K pathway inhibitors requires availability of tumor tissue. However, measuring free nucleic acids in plasma may detect mutations (such as *PIK3CA*) in circulating tumor DNA. It is highly tumor specific and has the potential to be used to monitor tumor burden with the advantage of compartment accessibility [151].

Finally, positron emission tomography (PET) is being employed as a potential pharmacodynamic BM and also as a potential BM of response when using PI3K inhibitors. As these drugs may affect the glucose metabolism, 18 fluorodeoxyglucose (FDG)-PET may be useful as a pharmacodynamic marker of pathway inhibition. Plasma glucose, fructosamine, C-peptide and insulin levels are also being evaluated as BMs. Preliminary results of the first-in-human studies with PI3K inhibitors show minimal changes in glucose levels but a trend to increased insulin levels in an exposure-dependent manner [152]. Use of these strategies continues to evolve and effectively incorporating BM studies into clinical trials of new PI3K-pathway inhibitors is a challenge for investigators.

2.2. Studies with mTORC1 Inhibitors

The mTOR pathway is a validated target for cancer therapeutics. mTORC1 is a master regulator of cell mass and metabolism, which is in part regulated by growth factor signaling through the PI3K-AKT axis. In this context, mTORC1 blockade with rapamycin derivatives is also expected to lead to significant antineoplasic effects in tumor cells in which the PI3K pathway is constitutively active. As single agents, temsirolumis and everolimus have provided significant clinical benefit in treating patients with advanced renal cell carcinoma [153, 154]. In pancreatic neuroendocrine tumors, everolimus has shown a promising progression-free survival benefit in a recently reported placebo-controlled trial [152]. As single agents the activity of mTOR inhibitors in breast cancer has been modest [155]; however, the combination of everolimus and exemestane has produced a relevant improvement in disease-free survival. This result has led to the approval of everolimus in this setting [156]. In the subset of patients with HER2 positive refractory disease, promising activity was observed with the combination of everolimus and trastuzumab [157, 158].

Everolimus also showed encouraging single-agent clinical efficacy in pretreated patients with recurrent endometrial cancer [159]. In this study, loss of PTEN expression was predictive of clinical benefit. Molecular mechanisms responsible for differences in sensitivity to mTOR inhibition have not been clearly elucidated. As previously discussed, evidence exists showing that mTORC1 inhibition can lead to pathway reactivation through abrogation of the negative feedback loop that is normally initiated by the direct mTORC1 substrate S6K on IRS proteins [44]. In addition, everolimus can cause ERK pathway reactivation in a PI3K-dependent manner [44]. Moreover, rapamycin derivatives cannot inhibit mTORC2, which is one of the two AKT upstream kinases [160]. Altogether, these data suggest that pathway activation and reactivation could be avoided by PI3K, AKT or concomitant PI3K and mTOR catalytic inhibition (that would target both mTORC1 and mTORC2).

3. PI3K PATHWAY INHIBITORS

The first generation of PI3K inhibitors includes the viridin soil bacteria product Wortmannin, isolated from Penicillium wortmanni in 1957, and LY294002, a synthetic compound derived from quercetin [161]. These compounds have been used widely as pharmaceutical tools to provide evidence for the involvement of the PI3K pathway in various biological systems. Both of these inhibitors are characterized by the ability to target the ATP (adenosine triphosphate)-binding site of PI3K, albeit with differing mechanisms, and to achieve significant growth inhibition across a broad spectrum of cancer cell lines when administered as single agents, especially under the circumstances of excess PI3K activity [139]. However, neither Wortmannin nor LY294002 have progressed to clinical trials. Wortmannin shows poor stability and targets many other PI3K-related molecules and thus showed considerably toxicity in animal models at low doses. LY294002 has superior stability, but is poorly soluble and shares the same undesirable characteristic of poor selectivity [162, 163]. Regardless, invaluable knowledge of the PI3K/AKT pathway has been gained through their use, adding momentum to the pursuit of more specific and tolerable agents.

Significant investment in rational drug development has been underway in recent times due to an enormous potential therapeutic benefit from targeting the PI3K pathway. Consequent to the extensive and intensive efforts of the pharmaceutical industry and scientific community alike, several novel compounds have been developed with the intention of improving pharmacokinetic profiles, achieving superior target specificity and thus minimizing toxicity [164]. The three-dimensional structure of p110alpha in association with its regulatory subunit p85alpha has been solved, and co-crystals of PI3K in complex with inhibitors from distinct chemical scaffolds have been obtained [33, 165]. These data, together with the original co-crystal structures obtained with PI3Kgamma, have been crucial for identifying key interactions needed to improve specificity and potency against the different class I PI3Ks, and fuelled the use of structure-based drug-design approaches to identify new molecular entities [166-169]. In addition, the establishment of robust biochemical and cellular assays has been critical to determine the activity and selectivity profile of PI3K inhibitors [170].

The PI3K inhibitors can be divided into pan-PI3K inhibitors that target all class IA PI3Ks or isoform-specific inhibitors. As the catalytic domains of the p110 subunits and mTOR are structurally similar, dual inhibitors of both PI3K and mTOR are also emerging. The varying target specificities of these agents promote diverse safety and efficacy profiles. A number of potential therapeutic agents targeting the PI3K signaling pathway have been generated. Here, we review four different classes: dual PI3K-mTOR inhibitors, pan-PI3K and isoform-specific PI3K inhibitors (that do not inhibit mTOR), AKT inhibitors, and mTOR catalytic site inhibitors. Table **1** summarizes PI3K pathway inhibitors in clinical trials [150, 171-278].

3.1. PI3K-mTOR Inhibitors in Clinical Development

SF1126 (Semafore Pharmaceuticals) is a small-molecule prodrug, a conjugate of LY294002 linked to an integrin-binding component designed to enhance delivery to the tumor and its associated vasculature, where cleavage leads to release of the active drug. Compared with the parent drug LY294002, SF1126 has better pharmacokinetic properties and higher distribution in tumor tissues, indicating a more favorable *in vivo* antitumor efficacy [279]. SF1126 is a pan-class IA PI3K-mTOR inhibitor with anti-angiogenic activity, partly attributed to targeting of integrins and reduction of HIF-1alpha [279]. It is administered intravenously, unlike most other PI3K inhibitors currently in clinical use. In a Phase I study, mTORC1 inhibition in several neoplasms was demonstrated by decreased S6 phosphorylation [172]. In particular, in a solid tumor cohort of the Phase I clinical trial, no responses were observed; however, 19 of 33 evaluated patients (57%) had stable disease [173]. Among them, a patient with GIST and one with renal cell carcinoma achieved a prolonged stabilization of 48 and 84 weeks, respectively. An expansion cohort in B-cell malignancies was utilized based on the encouraging preclinical activity previously observed in chronic lymphocytic leukemia (CLL), mantle cell lymphoma or diffuse large B-cell lymphoma (DLBCL) [280]. Data from 5 patients with hematological malignancies (4 CLL and 1 DLBCL), were reported: 1 CLL patient achieved a partial response, while the other 2 obtained some benefit in terms of decreased white cell counts or improved symptoms. In addition, the DLBCL patient had a reduction of more than 40% of the lymph nodes.

Table 1: PI3K, AKT and mTORC1/2 inhibitors in clinical trials.

Target	Agent	Phase	Study Population	Monotherapy/ Combination	Clinical Trial	Results Presented (Reference)
PI3K/mTOR	SF1126 (Semafore Pharmaceuticals)	I	Advanced solid tumors	Monotherapy	NCT00907205	[173]
	BEZ235 (Novartis)	I	Advanced solid tumors	Monotherapy	NCT00620594	[174-176]
		I	Advanced breast cancer HER2 +	Combination with trastuzumab		[177]
		I	Advanced solid tumors	Monotherapy (twice daily)	NCT01343498	[178]
		I/II	Renal cell carcinoma	Monotherapy	NCT01453595	-
		0	Breast cancer	Monotherapy	NCT01513356 *	-
		I	Advanced solid tumors	Combination with paclitaxel +/- trastuzumab	NCT01285466 *	-
		I	Metastatic breast cancer	Combination with capecitatine	NCT01300962 *	-
		I	Hormone receptor-positive metastatic breast cancer	Combination with letrozole	NCT01248494 *	-
		I	Advanced solid tumors	Combination with MEK162 (preselected by mutation)	NCT01337765	-
		Ib/II	HER2-positive breast cancer (after trastuzumab failure)	Randomized; BEZ235 + trastuzumab *vs* lapatinib-capecitabine	NCT01471847	-
		I	Advanced solid tumors	Combination with everolimus	NCT01482156	[179]
		I	Metastatic prostate cancer	Combination with abiraterone	NCT01634061 *	-
	BGT226 (Novartis)	I	Advanced solid tumors	Monotherapy	NCT00600275	[180]
	SAR245409 (Sanofi-Aventis) Previously known as XL765 (Exelixis)	I	Advanced solid tumors and lymphomas	Monotherapy	NCT00485719	
		I	Advanced solid tumors and non-small cell lung cancer	Combination with erlotinib	NCT00777699	[185, 186]
		I	High-grade gliomas	Combination with temozolomide	NCT00704080	[187, 188]
		I/II	Metastatic breast cancer	Combination with letrozole	NCT01082068►	[189]

Table 1: contd….

		I	Glioblastoma multiforme (candidates for surgical resection)	Monotherapy	NCT01240460▶	-
		I	Advanced solid tumors	Combination with MSC1936369B (MEK inhibitor)	NCT01390818	-
		II	Certain lymphoma or leukemia	Monotherapy	NCT01403636	-
		I	Indolent Lymphoma Mantle cell lymphoma Chronic lymphocytic leukemia	Combination with bendamustine and/or rituximab	NCT01410513	-
		I	Advanced solid tumors	Continuation trial	NCT01587040	-
		I	Advanced solid tumor or Lymphoma	Single agent Tablet formulation	NCT01596270	-
	GDC-0980 (Genentech/ Piramed Pharma)	I	Advanced solid tumors and Non-Hodgkin lymphomas	Monotherapy once daily	NCT00854152	[190-192]
				Monotherapy once weekly	NCT00854126	[192-196]
		I	Locally recurrent or metastatic breast cancer	Combination paclitaxel +/- bevacizumab	NCT01254526	-
		I	Healthy volunteer	Food and drug-drug interaction (rabeprazole)	NCT01287091	-
		I	Advanced solid tumors	Combination with carboplatin and paclitaxel +/- bevacizumab	NCT01301716	-
		I	Advanced solid tumors	Combination mFOLFOX6 and bevacizumab Combination with XELOX and bevacizumab	NCT01332604	-
		II	Recurrent or persistent endometrial carcinoma	Monotherapy	NCT01455493	-
		I	Healthy volunteer	Drug-Drug interaction study (ketokonazole)	NCT01473316	-
		II	Castration resistant prostate cancer	Randomized: GDC-0068-abiraterone GDC-0980-abiraterone abiraterone	NCT01485861■	[197]

Table 1: contd…

		II	Metastatic breast cancer	Combination with fulvestrant	NCT01437566╧	-
		I	Healthy volunteer (postmenopausal female)	[14C]-GDC-0980	NCT01487239	-
	PF-04691502 (Pfizer)	I	Advanced solid tumors	Monotherapy	NCT00927823	[198, 199]
		I	Advanced solid tumors	Combination with PD-0325901 (MEK inhibitor) Combination with irinotecan	NCT01347866●	-
		Ib	Advanced breast cancer	Combination with letrozole	NCT01430585	-
			Early breast cancer	Randomized letrozole PF-04691502		[200]
		II		PF-04691502+letrozole	NCT01430585	
		II	Endometrial neoplasms	Monotherapy. Randomized PF-04691502 PF-05212384	NCT01420081●	-
	PF-05212384 [previously known as PKI-587] (Pfizer)	I	Advanced solid tumors	Monotherapy	NCT00940498	[201, 202]
		I	Advanced solid tumors	Combination with PD-0325901 (MEK inhibitor) Combination with irinotecan	NCT01347866●	-
		II	Endometrial neoplasms	Monotherapy. Randomized PF-04691502 PF-05212384	NCT01420081●	-
	GSK2126458 (GlaxoSmithKline)	I	Advanced solid tumors	Monotherapy	NCT00972686	[204]
		I	Advanced solid tumors	Combination with GSK1120212 (MEK inhibitor)	NCT01248858	[205]
pan-PI3K	BKM120 (Novartis)	I	Advanced solid tumors	Monotherapy	NCT01068483	[206-210]
		I	Breast cancer HER2 +	Combination with trastuzumab	NCT01132664	[211]

Table 1: contd…

		I	Advanced solid tumors (Japanese population)	Monotherapy	NCT01283503	-
		I	Leukemia	Monotherapy	NCT01396499	-
		I	Advanced solid tumors (Chinesse population)	Monotherapy	NCT01626209	-
		I	Selected advanced solid tumors	Combination with GSK1120212 (MEK inhibitor)	NCT01155453	[212]
		I	Hormone receptor-positive metastatic breast cancer	Combination with letrozole	NCT01248494 *	[213]
		I	Metastatic renal cell carcinoma	Combination with bevacizumab	NCT01283048	-
		I	Refractory solid tumors Glioblastoma	Combination wit bevacizumab	NCT01349660	-
		I	Advanced solid tumors	Combination with paclitaxel +/- trastuzumab	NCT01285466 *	-
		I	Metastatic breast cancer	Combination with capecitatine	NCT01300962 *	-
		I	Advanced solid tumors	Combination with carboplatin-paclitaxel	NCT01297452	-
		I	Advanced colorectal cancer	Combination with irinotecan	NCT01304602	-
		I	Estrogen receptor-positive stage IV breast cancer (postmenopausal)	Combination with fulvestrant	NCT01339442	[214]
		I	Selected advanced solid tumors	Combination with MEK162	NCT01363232	-
		0	Breast cancer	Monotherapy	NCT01513356 *	-
		II	Advanced endometrial cancer	Monotherapy	NCT01289041	-
		I	GIST (third line)	Combination with imatinib	NCT01468688	-
		I	Advanced solid malignancies	Combination with everolimus	NCT01470209	-
		I	Newly diagnosed glioblastoma	Combination with temozolamide	NCT01473901	-
		I	NSCLC previously sensitive to erlotinib	Combination with erlotinib	NCT01487265	-
		I	Advanced solid tumors	Combination with docetaxel	NCT01540253	-

Table 1: contd…

		I	Metastatic NSCLC Enrichment: PI3K pathway alteration or EGFR overexpression	Combination with gefinitinb	NCT01570296	-
		I	Metastatic colorectal cancer KRAS wt	Combination with mFOLFOX6	NCT01571024	-
		I	Advanced solid tumors	Combination with LDE225	NCT01576666	-
		I	Metastatic prostate cancer	Combination with abiraterone	NCT01634061 *	-
		I	Breast cancer or High-grade serous ovarian cancer	Combination with olaparib	NCT01623349	-
		I/II	Metastatic melanoma	Combination with vemurafenib	NCT01512251	[215]
		I/II	HER2 positive, PI3K activated, trastuzumab resistant advanced breast cancer	Combination with lapatinib	NCT01589861	-
		I/II	Metastatic or advanced RAS wild-type colorectal cancer	Combination with panitumumab	NCT01591421	-
		II	Recurrent glioblastoma	Monotherapy	NCT01339052	-
		II	Metastatic castration resistant prostate cancer	Monotherapy	NCT01385293	-
		II	Initial or recurrent endometrial cancer	Monotherapy	NCT01397877	-
		II	Cancers with PIK3CA mutations	Monotherapy	NCT01501604	-
		II	Advanced head and neck carcinoma	Monotherapy	NCT01527877	-
		II	Advanced endometrial cancer	Monotherapy	NCT01550380	-
		II	Metastatic transitional cell carcinoma of the urothelium	Monotherapy	NCT01551030	-
		II	Metastatic or locally advanced cervical cancer	Monotherapy	NCT01613677	-
		II	Metastatic squamous cell carcinoma of the lung	Monotherapy *vs.* docetaxel	NCT01297491	-
		II	Metastatic adenocarcinoma of the lung	Monotherapy *vs.* docetaxel *vs.* pemetrexed		-
		II	Locally advanced or metastatic HER2 negative breast cancer (with and without PIK3CA mutation)	Randomized: Paclitaxel + BKM120 Paclitaxel + placebo	NCT01572727	-
		III	HER2 negative breast cancer refractory to aromatase inhibitor (postmenopausal)	Randomized: Fulvestrant-BKM120 Fulvestrant-placebo	NCT01610284	-

Table 1: contd...

		III	HER2 negative breast cancer refractory to aromatase inhibitor Who has progressed to a mTOR inhibitor	Randomized: Fulvestrant-BKM120 Fulvestrant-placebo	NCT01633060	-
	SAR245408 (Sanofi-Aventis) Previously known as XL147 (Exelixis)	I	Advanced solid tumors and lymphomas	Monotherapy	NCT00486135	[216, 217]
		I	Advanced solid tumors	Combination with Erlotinib	NCT00692640	[218, 219]
		I	Advanced solid tumors	Combination with Paclitaxel and Carboplatin	NCT00756847	[220]
		I	Advanced solid tumors	Combination with XL647 (EGFR, HER2, VEGFR and EphB4 inhibitor)	NCT00704392	-
		I	Glioblastoma (candidates for surgical resection)	Monotherapy	NCT01240460▶	-
		I	Advanced solid tumors	Combination with MSC1936369B (MEK inhibitor)	NCT01357330	-
		I/II	Advanced breast cancer HER2 +	Combination with trastuzumab or paclitaxel + trastuzumab	NCT01042925	[221]
		I/II	Advanced breast cancer HR +	Combination with letrozole	NCT01082068	[189]
		II	Advanced endometrial cancer	Monotherapy	NCT01013324	-
	PX-866 (Oncothyreon Inc.)	I	Advanced solid tumors	Monotherapy	NCT00726583	[222-225]
		I	Healthy volunteers	Monotherapy (different formulations)	NCT01408316	-
		I/II	NSCLC SCCHN	Randomized: Docetaxel Docetaxel+PX-866	NCT01204099	[226, 227]
		I/II	Metastatic colorectal cancer SCCHN	Randomized: Cetuximab Cetuximab +PX866	NCT01252628	[323]
		I/II	Advanced melanoma	Combination with vemurafenib	NCT01616199	-

Table 1: contd…

		II	Glioblastoma	Monotherapy	NCT01259869	[228]
		II	Recurrent or metastatic prostate cancer	Monotherapy	NCT01331083	-
	GDC-0941 (Genentech/ Piramed Pharma)	I	Advanced solid tumors	Monotherapy	NCT00876109	[229, 230]
		I	Advanced solid tumors and non-Hodgkin lymphomas	Monotherapy	NCT00876122	[231-233]
		I	Advanced solid tumors and Non-small cell lung cancer	Combination with e	NCT00975182	-
		I	Non-small cell lung cancer	Combination with paclitaxel and carboplatin with or without bevacizumab	NCT00974584	[234]
				Combination with cisplatin, pemetrexed and bevacizumab	NCT00974584	-
		II	Non-small cell lung cancer	Combination with paclitaxel and carboplatin with or without bevacizumab	NCT01493843	-
		I	Advanced breast cancer HER2 +	Combination with trastuzumab-MCC-DM1	NCT00928330	[235]
		I	Advanced breast cancer	Combination with paclitaxel and bevacizumab	NCT00960960	[236]
		I	Advanced solid tumors	Combination with GDC-0973 (MEK inhibitor)	NCT00996892	[237-239]
		II	Metastatic breast cancer	Combination with fulvestrant	NCT01437566	-
		I	Healthy volunteers	Food effect and proton pump inhibitor	NCT00999128	-
		I	Healthy volunteers	Drug-drug interaction (ketoconazole)	NCT01240226	-
		I	Healthy volunteers	Monotherapy Metabolism study	NCT01474668	-
	GSK1059615 (GlaxoSmithKline)	I	Advanced solid tumors and lymphomas	Monotherapy	NCT00695448	[240]
	BAY 80-9646 (Bayer)	I	Advanced solid tumors	Monotherapy	NCT00962611	[241, 242]
		I	Advanced solid tumors (Japanesse population)	Monotherapy	NCT01404390	-

Table 1: contd…

		I/II	Advanced solid tumors	Combination gemcitabine with or without cisplatin	NCT01460537	-
		I	Advanced solid tumors	Combination with paclitaxel	NCT01411410	-
		I	Advanced solid tumors	Combination with BAY86-9766 (MEK inhibitor)	NCT01392521	-
	CH5132799 (Chugai Pharmaceutical)	I	Advanced solid tumors	Monotherapy	NCT01222546	[243]
	ZSTK474 (Zenyaku Kogyo)	I	Advanced solid tumors	Monotherapy	NCT01280487	-
PI3K alpha	BYL719 (Novartis)	I	Advanced solid tumors PIK3CA gene altered	Monotherapy	NCT01219699	[244]
		I	Advanced solid tumors	Monotherapy	NCT01387321	-
		I	Advanced gastric cancer	Combination with AUY922 (HSP90 inhibitor)	NCT01613950	-
		I/II	Recurrent or metastatic Head and Neck Squamous Cell Carcinoma	Combination with cetuximab	NCT01602315	-
		II	Advanced solid tumors	Combination with MEK162 (MEK inhibitor)	NCT01449058	-
	INK-1117 (Intellikine)	I	Advanced solid tumors	Monotherapy	NCT01449370	
	GDC-0032 (Genentech)	I	Advanced solid tumors	Monotherapy	NCT01296555	-
PI3K beta	GSK2636771 (Glaxo-Smith-Kline)	I	Advanced solid tumors with PTEN deficiency	Monotherapy	NCT01458067	-
	SAR260301 (Sanofi-Aventis)	I	Advanced solid tumors		pending	-

Table 1: contd…

PI3K delta	GS-1101 (Gilead) Previously known as CAL-101 (Calistoga Pharmaceuticals)	I	Hematologic malignancies	Monotherapy	NCT00710528	[245-248]
		I	Indolent B-cell Non-Hodgkin Lymphoma or Chronic Lymphocytic Leukemia	Several combinations: Rituximab Bendamustine and rituximab Bendamustine Ofatumumab Fludarabine Bortezomib Chlorambucil Rituximab-Chlorambucil	NCT01088048	[249-252]
		I	Recurrent follicular non-Hodgkin lymphoma	Combination with lenalidomide and rituximab	NCT01644799	-
		I/II	Previously treated Low-grade lymphoma	Monotherapy	NCT01306643	-
		II	Indolent B-Cell non-Hodgkin lymphoma	Monotherapy	NCT01282424	-
		II	Relapsed or refractory Hodgkin Lymphoma	Monotherapy	NCT01393106	-
		II	Untreated CLL or small lymphocytic leukemia	Combination with rituximab	NCT01203930	-
		III	Previously treated CLL	Randomized; Rituximab + placebo Rituximab+GS-1101	NCT01539512	-
		III	Previously treated CLL	Randomized: bendamustine-Rituximab +placebo bendamustine-Rituximab + GS-1101	NCT01569295	-
	AMG 319 (Amgen)	I	Relapsed or refractory lymphoid malignancies	Monotherapy	NCT01300026	-
AKT	MK-2206 (Merck)	I	Advanced solid tumors	Monotherapy	NCT00670488	[253-257]
		I	Advanced solid tumors	Combination with erlotinib or paclitaxel + carboplatin or docetaxel	NCT00848718	[260]

Table 1: contd…

		I	Advanced breast cancer HER2 +	Combination with rtastuzumab and lapatinib	NCT00963547	[261]
		I	Advanced solid tumors	Combination with AZD6244 (MEK inhibitor)	NCT01021748	[262, 263]
		I	Advanced solid tumors	Monotherapy (weekly administration) Japanese population	NCT01071018	-
		I	NSCLC	Combination with gefinitinb	NCT01147211	-
		I	Pediatric recurrent solid tumors or leukemia	Monotherapy	NCT01231919	-
		I	HER2 overexpressing malignancies	Combination with paclitaxel and trastuzumab	NCT01235897	-
		I	Hormone receptor-positive breast cancer	Combination with exemestane with or without goserelin	NCT01240928	-
		I	Solid tumors	Combination of: MK-2206-Dalotuzumab MK-0752-Dalotuzumab MK-8669-Dalotuzumab	NCT01243762	[264]
		I	Advanced or metastatic breast cancer	Combination with lapatinib	NCT01245205	-
		I	Advanced solid tumors and breast cancer	Combination with paclitaxel	NCT01263145	-
		I	Metastatic breast cancer	Combination with lapatinib	NCT01281163	-
		I	Advanced solid tumors	Combinations: Ridaforolimus-MK-2206 Ridaforolimus-MK-0752	NCT01295632	-
		I	Metastatic breast cancer (postmenopausal)	Combination with anastrozole, letrozole, exemestane or fulvestrant	NCT01344031	-
		I	Advanced solid tumors Prostate cancer Renal cell carcinoma	Combination with hydroxychloroquine	NCT01480154	-
		I/II	CLL and SLL	Combination with bendamustine and rituximab	NCT01369849	-

Table 1: contd…

		II	I-SPY TRIAL: neoadjuvant, adaptative breast cancer	Evaluation of different targeted agents as neoadjuvant treatment: Neratinib ABT-888 AMG 386 Ganitumab + metfomin MK-2206+/- trastuzumab	NCT01042379	-
		II	Neuroendocrine tumors	Monotherapy	NCT01169649	-
		II	KRAS wild type, *PIK3CA*-mutant colorectal cancer	Monotherapy	NCT01186705	-
		II	Refractory kidney cancer	Randomized: everolimus *vs.* MK-2206	NCT01239342	-
		II	Hepatocellular carcinoma	Monotherapy	NCT01239355	-
		II	Hormone receptor-positive Breast Cancer	Combination with exemestane with or without goserelin	NCT01240941	-
		II	BATTLE-2: NSCLC	Randomized : erlotinib erlotinib + MK-2206 AZD-6244 + MK-2206 sorafenib	NCT01248247	-
		II	Recurrent glioma	Monotherapy	NCT01249105	-
		II	Previously treated prostate cancer	Randomized: bicalutamide bicalutamide + MK-2206	NCT01251861	-
		II	Refractory acute myeloid leukemia	Monotherapy	NCT01253447	-
		II	Relapsed lymphoma	Monotherapy	NCT01258998	-
		II	Advanced gastric or gastroesophageal junction cancer	Monotherapy	NCT01260701	-
		II	Advanced breast cancer harboring PIK3CA mutation and/or PTEN loss	Monotherapy	NCT01277757	-
		II	Recurrent platinum resistant ovarian, fallopian tube or peritoneal cancer	Monotherapy	NCT01283035	-

Table 1: contd…

		II	NSCLC previously responder to erlotinib	Combination with erlotinib	NCT01294306	-
		II	NSCLC, SCLC and thymic malignancies	Assigned to several treatment groups based on molecular profile: AZD6244 MK-2206 Lapatinib Erlotinib Sunitinib	NCT01306045	-
		II	Advanced endometrial cancer	Monotherapy	NCT01307631	-
		II	Advanced endometrial cancer	Monotherapy (stratified by PIK3CA mutation)	NCT01312753	-
		II	Pharmacodynamic study operable breast cancer	Monotherapy	NCT01319539	[265]
		II	Colorectal carcinoma	Combination with AZD6244	NCT01333475	[266]
		II	Recurrent or metastatic head and neck cancer	Monotherapy	NCT01349933	-
		II	Recurrent nasopharyngeal carcinoma	Monotherapy	NCT01370070	-
		II	Unresectable Advanced refractory biliary cancer	Monotherapy	NCT01425879	-
		II	Relapsed or refractory diffuse B Cell lymphoma	Monotherapy	NCT01466868	-
		II	Relapsed or refractory diffuse B Cell lymphoma	Monotherapy	NCT01481129	-
		II	Relapsed BRAF mutant advanced melanoma	Combination with AZD6244	NCT01510444	-
		II	Advanced melanoma after failure to vemurafeninb or dabrafenib	Randomized: AZD6244 AZD6244 +MK-2206	NCT01519427	-
		II	Progressive, recurrent or metastatic adenoid cyst carcinoma	Monotherapy	NCT01604772	-
	GSK690693 (GlaxoSmithKline)	I	Advanced solid tumors and lymphomas	Monotherapy	NCT00493818	-
	GSK2141795 (GlaxoSmithKline)	I	Advanced solid tumors and lymphomas	Monotherapy	NCT00920257	[267]
		I	Ovarian cancer	Monotherapy (pharmacodynamic)	NCT01266954	[268]

Table 1: contd…

		I	Advanced solid tumors Pancreatic cancer, endometrial cancer or colorectal cancer	Combination with GSK1120212 (MEK inhibitor)	NCT01138085	[269]
	GSK2110183 (Octagon Research Solutions)	I	Hematologic malignancies	Monotherapy	NCT00881946	-
		I	Multiple myeloma	Combination with bortezomib and dexamethasone	NCT01428492	-
		I	Multiple myeloma and solid tumors	Combination with GSK1120212 (MEK inhibitor)	NCT01476137	-
		II	Langerhans cell hstiocytosis	Monotherapy	NCT01395004	-
		II	Multiple myeloma	Monotherapy	NCT01445587	-
		II	Several tumor types	Continuation trial	NCT01531894	-
		II	Refractory CLL	Combination with ofatumumab	NCT01532700	-
	GDC-0068 (Genentech)	I	Advanced solid tumors	Monotherapy	NCT01090960	[270]
		I	Advanced solid tumors	Combination with docetaxel or FOLFOX	NCT01362374	[271]
		I	Advanced solid tumors	Combination with GDC-0973 (MEK inhibitor)	NCT01562275	-
		II	Castration resistant prostate cancer	Randomized: GDC-0068-abiraterone GDC-0980-abiraterone Abiraterone	NCT01485861	[197]
	LY2780301 (Eli Lilly and Company)	I	Advanced solid tumors	Monotherapy	NCT01115751	[272]

Table 1: contd…

mTORC1/2	MLN0128 (Millenium) Previously INK128 (Intellikine)	I	Advanced solid tumors	Monotherapy	NCT01058707	[273, 274]
		I	Multiple myeloma or Waldenstrom Macroglobulinemia	Monotherapy	NCT01118689	-
		I	Advanced solid tumors	Combination with paclitaxel with or without trastuzumab	NCT01351350	-
	AZD8055 (AstraZeneca)	I	Advanced solid tumors	Monotherapy	NCT00731263	[275, 383]
		I	Advanced solid tumors (Japanese population)	Monotherapy	NCT00973076	-
		I	Hepatocellular carcinoma	Monotherapy	NCT00973076	-
		I	Glioma	Monotherapy	NCT01316809	-
	OSI-027 (OSI Pharmaceuticals)		Advanced solid tumors	Monotherapy	NCT00698243	[276]
	AZD2014	I	Advanced solid tumors	Monotherapy	NCT01026402	[277]
		I	Metastatic breast cancer	Combination with fulvestrant	NCT01597388	-
	CC-223	I	Advanced solid tumors, lymphoma or multiple myeloma	Monotherapy	NCT01177397	[278]
		I	Metastatic NSCLC	Combination with erlotinib or azacitidine	NCT01545947	-

HER2: human epidermal growth factor receptor 2, HR: hormone receptor

BEZ235 (Novartis) is an imidazoquinoline derivative, optimized for PI3K inhibition [281], whose function also blocks VEGF-induced angiogenesis and tumor vascular permeability, suggesting anti-angiogenic activity secondary to inhibition of the PI3K pathway [282].

In preclinical models, BEZ235 was critical to understand the role of the PI3K pathway in several tumor types [283]. BEZ235 showed antitumor activity in a variety of cell lines and mouse models including breast [284-286], prostate [287], ovarian [288-290], endometrial [291, 292], gastric [293], colon [293], pancreatic [294], renal [295] or non-small cell lung cancer [296, 297], as well as lymphoma [298, 299], leukemia [300-304] or plasmocytoma [305]. The presence of *PIK3CA* mutations has been described as one of the most relevant predictors of response in different tumor types [283, 286, 293]. Another molecular factor associated with sensitivity to BEZ235 has been *HER2* amplification [286, 306], Actually, activation of the PI3K pathway has been described as a major resistance factor to anti-HER2 therapy [129, 131, 307, 308] the resistance to anti-hormonal therapy and anti-HER2 targeted therapy. This result supports the assessment of BEZ235 in patients with p110alpha mutations, who are often resistant to trastuzumab. In addition, BEZ235 was further demonstrated to induce apoptosis in estrogen-deprived estrogen receptor-positive breast cancer cells harboring either *PIK3CA* mutations or *PIK3CB* amplification [309].

Preliminary data from several Phase I clinical trials investigating BEZ235 as a single agent or in combination have already been presented. A Phase I trial with BEZ235 orally administered is still accruing patients with promising results. Early data from 51 patients showed 2 partial responses (1 Cowden syndrome patient and 1 breast cancer patient), 16 minor responses and 14 cases of disease stabilization [174]· Adverse events observed were: nausea, vomiting, diarrhea, fatigue/asthenia, anemia, and anorexia, usually mild to moderate. Based on the bioavailability issues of the initial formulation, a special drug delivery system of BEZ235 was evaluated, achieving a more predictable pharmacokinetic profile. Stable disease was observed in 6 of 15 evaluable patients treated with this formulation [176], and the drug is currently being evaluated in subsequent clinical trials. Moreover, schedule for drug delivery is also an important factor and, so far, a twice a day program is being investigated. Recent data report similar pharmacokinetic and toxicity profiles in the once a day administration schedule. Overall, among the 15 patients enrolled so far, only 1 patient with endometrial carcinoma had prolonged disease stabilization and stayed in the trial after more than 34 weeks of treatment. The expansion cohort evaluating 400mg twice a day is still ongoing [178].

Recently, *Krop et al.* recently reported results from the Phase I/IB trial of BEZ235 in combination with trastuzumab demonstrating that the combination of BEZ235 and trastuzumab was feasible and had a toxicity profile similar to that expected based on the single-agent profiles. Among the 27 patients enrolled so far, 2 patients achieved a partial response and 4 had prolonged stable disease for more than 6 months (1 of them for more than 2 years), while 7 were still receiving treatment. The dose expansion arm of the trial evaluating the estimated maximum tolerated dose (MTD) of 600mg daily is still ongoing [177].

In addition, the results from the first cohort of patients enrolled in a clinical trial evaluating the combination of BEZ235 and everolimus has been presented, although the dose escalation Phase was still ongoing. Once the MTD is achieved, this combination will be also considered in hepatocellular carcinoma, neuroendocrine tumors and glioblastoma multiforme [179].

BEZ235 is currently being investigated as a single agent in renal cell carcinoma (NCT01453595) and in a preoperative pharmacodynamic study in early breast cancer (NCT01513356). Several combinations, including capecitabine (NCT01300962), letrozole (NCT01248494) and trastuzumab with or without paclitaxel (NCT01285466, NCT01471847), are being evaluated in patients with metastatic breast cancer. Other combinations under evaluation include the Phase I clinical trial investigating BEZ235 in combination with the MEK inhibitor MEK162 (NCT01337765) in solid tumors and a Phase I evaluating BEZ235 in combination with abiraterone in patients with metastatic prostate cancer (MCT01634061).

BGT226 is the second PI3K-mTOR inhibitor from Novartis to have entered clinical trials. Preclinically, BGT226 has shown activity in myeloma [310], leukemia [301, 311], head and neck [312], breast [313] and pancreatic cancer cell lines [314, 315]. In the clinical setting, 57 patients were enrolled in the Phase I clinical trial, with no partial responses, but with 9 patients achieving prolonged disease stabilization longer than 16 weeks. The most common side effects were diarrhea, nausea, vomiting, decreased appetite and fatigue. Pharmacokinetic analysis revealed a significant variability and the achieved plasma levels were lower than expected based on the preclinical data. There was no consistent reduction in pS6 and pAKT in paired tumor samples [180], and no further development of this drug is described.

SAR245409 (Sanofi-Aventis), previously known as XL765 is a potent, specific, ATP competitive and reversible dual inhibitor of class I PI3K isoforms and of mTOR. Tumor stabilization or shrinkage has been observed with XL765 in a variety of mouse xenograft models of human cancer, including breast, ovary, lung, prostate and brain cancers [316]. In solid tumors, the Phase I trial with oral administration of this agent reported as the most common related adverse events: nausea and vomiting, diarrhea, anorexia, elevated liver enzymes and skin disorders. Meanwhile, no significant changes in serum glucose were noted. Robust pharmacodynamic modulation of PI3K signaling was evident in tumors and surrogate tissues. Even if there were no radiological responses among the patients with solid tumors, disease stabilization longer than 14 weeks was observed in 12 of the 83 patients enrolled (14%), 4 of them for more than 6 months (1 renal cell carcinoma, 1 sarcoma, 1 mesothelioma and 1 appendiceal adenocarcinoma). Interestingly, an additional patient with estrogen receptor positive breast cancer harboring an *AKT* and a *PIK3CA* mutation, not evaluable by RECIST criteria, experienced clinical improvement of skin metastasis [184].

In the expansion cohort in patients with lymphoma, 3 out of 13 patients achieved a partial response [183].

A combination of SAR245409 and erlotinib in patients with lung cancer refractory to anti-EGFR therapy was investigated and reported several patients with prolonged disease stabilization, 3 of them in patients who had previously progressed on erlotinib. [186]. Moreover, in a clinical trial combining SAR245409 and temozolomide in glioblastoma patients having completed chemoradiation treatment, the MTD was not already reached. Of note, a patient with a *PTEN* mutation, EGFR amplification and MGMT methylation continued treatment after 62 weeks [219].

At the 2011 San Antonio Breast Cancer Symposium, Baselga *et al.* presented data from 17 patients enrolled in the Phase I portion of the Phase I/II trial testing SAR245408 or the combination of SAR245409 with letrozole. The MTD for both arms was already established and the only dose-limiting toxicity observed was grade 3 rash in the SAR245409 arm. No antitumor activity data were presented at that time [189]. The Phase II part of the study is ongoing. Phase I/II trials of SAR245409 in glioblastoma are currently being evaluated as a single agent (NCT01240460) in lymphoma and leukemia (NCT01403636) or in combination with bendamustine with or without rituximab (NCT01410513), and in patients with advanced solid tumors in combination with the MEK inhibitor MSC1936369B (NCT01390818).

GDC-0980 (Genentech/ Piramed Pharma) is a potent, highly selective, oral, dual inhibitor of class I PI3K and mTOR kinase, which demonstrates broad preclinical activity in breast, ovarian, lung, and prostate cancer models [317].

Two distinct drug schedules were evaluated in two different Phase I clinical trials: once daily and once weekly. Wagner *et al.* presented the data from the Phase I clinical trial of the daily administration of GDC-0980; 58 patients were enrolled in the clinical trial at the time of the analysis. An overall adequate inhibition of pAKT in platelet-rich plasma was achieved. The most frequent side effects were fatigue, gastrointestinal symptoms and hyperglycemia. In addition, 3 patients experienced reversible pneumonitis and 1 patient experienced a grade 5 colitis. As far as antitumor activity, 1 patient with adrenal carcinoma achieved a partial response and continued on trial after a year of treatment. Moreover, a relevant activity on mesothelioma was observed and, in particular, 3 patients experienced more than 20% tumor shrinkage. Additionally, although it did not fulfill partial response criteria, 1 of those patients, diagnosed with a peritoneal mesothelioma, remained on treatment more than a year. Interestingly, another 4 patients with renal cell carcinoma, mesothelioma and sarcoma, had a prolonged stabilization that lasted more than six months [195].

GDC-0980 is being studied as a single agent in endometrial cancer (NCT01455493). Several combinations are currently being evaluated in Phase I clinical trials; in solid tumors, some combinations used include FOLFOX-bevacizumab (NCT01332604), paclitaxel and carboplatin with or without bevacizumab (NCT01301716), while in metastatic breast cancer combinations of fulvestrant or paclitaxel with or without bevacizumab (NCT01254526) are administered. An additional trial combining GDC-0980 or the AKT inhibitor GDC-0068 with abiraterone in patients with prostate cancer is also under evaluation (NCT01485861).

PF-04691502 (Pfizer) is a potent oral dual pan-isoform PI3K and mTOR inhibitor. It has shown preclinical activity in breast, glioblastoma and ovarian cancer cell lines with *PIK3CA* mutations or PTEN deletion [318].

In the preliminary analysis of the single-agent Phase I clinical trial, 33 patients were enrolled so far. The main side effects observed were: fatigue, gastrointestinal discomfort, rash and hyperglycemia. No partial responses were observed, but 5 patients (15%) experienced stable disease lasting greater than 16 weeks. Their primary diagnoses were ovarian cancer, HER2- positive breast cancer, melanoma, non-small cell lung cancer and colorectal cancer. The MTD was defined and the expansion cohort was ongoing at the time of the presentation [199].

Currently, PF-04691502 and its intravenous counterpart PF-05212384 are being tested as single agents in endometrial carcinoma (NCT01420081). They are also being evaluated in combination with irinotecan or a MEK inhibitor (PD-0325901) in advanced solid tumors (NCT01347866). A randomized, neoadjuvant clinical trial in postmenopausal patients with hormone-receptor positive breast cancer investigating letrozole with or without PF-04691502 is ongoing (NCT01430585).

PF-05212384 (Pfizer), previously known as PKI-587, is an intravenous pan isoform PI3K and mTOR inhibitor. Preclinically, it has shown activity in cell lines with an active PI3K pathway, including glioma, breast, colon, prostate, pancreas, renal and non-small cell lung cancer [319].

The preliminary analysis of the Phase I clinical trial included 53 patients in the dose escalation Phase, with reported side effects such as mucositis, nausea, anorexia, rash and fatigue. Two patients, 1 with ovarian cancer and 1 with an EGFR-mutated non-small cell lung cancer (NSCLC), achieved a partial response. The compound is also being tested in the previously described trials for patients with endometrial cancer (NCT01420081) and in combination with irinotecan or PD-0325901 in solid tumors (NCT01347866).

GSK2126458 (GlaxoSmithKline) is a dual pan-isoform PI3K and mTOR inhibitor, with preclinical activity previously described in breast cancer cell lines. In the Phase I clinical trial, including the dose escalation and the dose expansion Phase, 129 patients were enrolled. The most common side effects were fatigue, gastrointestinal symptoms and hyperglycemia. In the expansion cohort, 2 out of 25 patients with renal cell carcinoma and 2 out of 20 patients with *PIK3CA* mutated urothelial carcinoma, achieved a partial response [204]. Moreover, an ongoing trial is combining GSK2126458 with the MEK inhibitor (GSK1120212) in patients with solid tumors. In the first interim report, 34 patients had been enrolled. The most common adverse events were rash, diarrhea and nausea/vomiting. No partial response was observed, but 2 patients, one with renal cell carcinoma and other with a colorectal cancer, remained on stable disease for more than 6 months [205].

3.2. Pan-PI3K Inhibitors in Clinical Development

BKM120 (Novartis) is a potent and highly specific oral pan-class I PI3K inhibitor. In the single-agent Phase I clinical trial, only one patient, with a triple negative breast cancer, out of 31 evaluable, achieved a partial response. Overall, data showed that 16 patients had stable disease for more than 6 weeks. In the expansion cohort, 2 of the 31 patients demonstrated a partial response: one with hormone receptor-positive breast cancer and a *PIK3CA* mutation and the other with *PIK3CA* mutant and null *PTEN* salivary gland cancer. Eighteen patients had stable disease for more than 16 weeks. Dose-limiting toxicities included hyperglycemia, diarrhea and upper abdominal pain, skin rash and mood alteration.

There is an ongoing Phase I/II trial utilizing the combination of BKM120 and trastuzumab in HER2-positive metastatic breast cancer. The preliminary analysis of the first 17 patients showed a tolerable toxicity profile and encouraging antitumor activity. Two partial responses were observed. The Phase II part of this study is still in progress [211]. Results for the combination of BKM120 and letrozole in hormone receptor positive breast cancer were recently presented; among 20 patients enrolled in the continuous schedule of BKM120, one patient, not previously exposed to hormone therapy, achieved a complete response, while another one had a partial response and 4 patients had prolonged stable disease (more than 6 months). In the intermittent schedule, no patient reached a partial response, but 9 of the 31 enrolled patients had a prolonged stabilization of their disease [320].

Recently, results of the escalation portion of the Phase I clinical trial studying the combination of BKM120 and the MEK inhibitor GSK1120212 in 66 enrolled patients were also presented. The main side effects reported were skin and gastrointestinal toxicities, creatine kinase elevation, hyperglycemia, stomatitis, and elevated liver enzymes. More specifically, skin toxicity, including acneiform or maculopapular rash and dry skin, occurred in 88% of the enrolled patients, however, it was grade 3 or 4 in only in 20% of the patients. The pattern of toxicity was similar at the MTD dose: 94% patients had skin toxicity of any kind and 25% had grade 3 or 4 toxicity. Three patients, all with *KRAS* mutated ovarian cancer, achieved a partial response. Although not qualified as a partial response, tumor shrinkage was observed in *BRAF* and *NRAS* mutated melanomas; however, no significant activity was observed in colorectal cancer [212]. This drug combination is currently being evaluated in the expansion cohort in *RAS* or *BRAF* mutated pancreatic, ovarian and non-small cell cancer.

Currently, several Phase II clinical trials are ongoing, evaluating the activity of BKM120 in several solid tumors, such as NSCLC, glioblastoma, and endometrial cancer among others. Several Phase I clinical trials are evaluating the combination of BKM120 with the standard chemotherapeutic or targeted agents utilized in specific solid tumors, such as breast, prostate, colon or NSCLC. In conclusion, there are two randomized controlled Phase III clinical trials evaluating the activity of the combination of fulvestrant and BKM120, which are still ongoing (Table **1**).

SAR245408 (Sanofi-Aventis), previously known as XL147, is another oral pan-PI3K inhibitor. Tumor stabilization or shrinkage was observed with SAR245408 in a variety of mouse xenograft models of human cancer, including breast, lung and prostate. Further, enhanced antitumor effects have been demonstrated when XL147 was combined with cytotoxic chemotherapy (paclitaxel or carboplatin) or with rapamycin.

Data from the Phase I trial revealed prolonged disease stabilization in 9 out of 68 patients (13%) with advanced solid tumors, while a partial response was observed in a lung cancer patient [216]. The most common drug-related toxicity was skin rash, whereas plasma glucose levels were minimally affected by the treatment. Specifically, SAR245408 reduces PI3K pathway signaling and phosphorylation of MEK and ERK in tumor tissues exhibiting diverse molecular alterations, resulting in an associated reduction in Ki67 and an increase in apoptosis. Recently, safety data from the expansion cohort in patients with lymphoma demonstrated that SAR245408 has adequate tolerability in this particular patient subpopulation [217]. However, activity of SAR245408 in this cohort has not been presented yet.

Several Phase I clinical trials are evaluating combinatorial treatment with SAR245408 (Table **1**). In the specific study utilizing the combination of SAR245408 and erlotinib, at the time of the interim analysis 28 patients were enrolled: 1 of those patients achieved a partial response and 8 remained on stable disease for more than 16 weeks [218].

Another trial, combining SAR245408 and carboplatin and paclitaxel, reported one patient with Merkel cell carcinoma with a complete response, and four patients achieved a partial response (2 head and neck cancers, 1 cervical cancer, and 1 esophageal) [220]. The combination study of SAR245408 or SAR245409 with letrozole has been previously described [189].

Currently, in glioblastomas, in addition to the single agent, other combinations with targeted agents (XL647 and MSC19363698) are under investigation (Table **1**).

PX-866 (Oncothyreon Inc.), a semi-synthetic agent with a mechanism similar to Wortmannin, is another class IA and B PI3K inhibitor. PX-866 showed higher stability and reduced liver toxicity than Wortmannin [321]. Recently published *in* *vivo* studies demonstrate that *PIK3CA*-mutant or PTEN-null xenografts were sensitive to treatment with PX-866. However, mutant oncogenic RAS was reported as a dominant predictor of resistance to this agent [321, 322].

Results of a Phase I trial with oral administration of PX-866 showed disease stabilization in various patients with heavily pretreated solid tumors. The most common adverse events included nausea, vomiting, diarrhea and liver enzyme elevations, and no relevant changes were identified in blood glucose or insulin levels [225].

On the other hand, results of the Phase I trial with a combination of PX-866 and docetaxel were presented. Two patients (one with ovarian cancer and another with NSCLC), out of a total of 32 evaluable patients, achieved a partial response. A trend was noted in a longer median time in studies of patients with *PIK3CA* mutated tumors [227].

Results from the Phase I portion of the Phase I clinical trial evaluating PX-866 and cetuximab were presented this year. The most common adverse events (AEs) included were diarrhea, hypomagnesaemia, nausea, vomiting, dehydration, fatigue, and rash. Four of the 8 evaluable patients achieved a partial response, one of them had previously received cetuximab treatment [323].

PX-866 is being evaluated as single agent in glioblastoma in a two-stage Phase II. By the time of the presentation, 18 patients were enrolled. The most common side effects listed were diarrhea and fatigue. There was an unconfirmed partial response and several patients with stable disease. Based on this anticancer activity, the second stage of the trial started and enrollment has just begun.

Lastly, PX-866 is also being evaluated in prostate cancer as a single agent (NCT01616199) and in combination with vemurafenib in melanoma (NCT01616199).

GDC-0941 (Genentech/ Piramed Pharma) is a selective and potent inhibitor of class I PI3Ks with weaker activity against mTOR [324]. As an orally administered agent, GDC-0941 exhibited significant *in vivo* antitumor efficacy against human cancer xenografts [325]. Furthermore, a combination of GDC-0941 with docetaxel or gemcitabine enhanced their chemotherapeutic effects without obvious toxicities being observed [326].

Several drug administration schedules were planned in two separate Phase I clinical trials, daily (intermittent or continuously) and twice a day [230, 233]. Preliminary results identified a decrease in pS6 staining of > 50% in paired tumor biopsies in addition to decreases of > 90% in pAKT levels assayed in platelet-rich plasma from patients treated at the higher dose levels [231]. Gastrointestinal side effects, fatigue and rash were common adverse events in both studies; however, the incidence of hyperglycemia was higher in the North American trial [230]. The English study enrolled 42 patients; among them, one patient with melanoma obtained a partial response and remained in the study for 9.5 months. Moreover, a patient with GIST had a prolonged stabilization and a patient with ovarian cancer had a biological response (decreased CA125 by 86%) [233]. In the North American trial, 97 patients were enrolled (61 with a single daily dosage and 36 with twice a day administration). Overall, there were two partial responses, on was in a patient with a *PIK3CA*-mutant endocervical cancer and the other in a patient with a hormone-positive breast cancer. Two patients, ovarian and ampullary carcinoma, remained on the study for over a year. In addition, there were signs of activity, where CA125 decreased in patients with ovarian cancer [230].

Clinical trials are testing several drug combinations, in NSCLC (Phase I: NCT00974584; Phase II: NCT01493843), breast cancer (NCT00928330, NCT00960960 or NCT01437566) or in solid tumors (NCT00996892). Some preliminary results have already been presented.

Moreover, a Phase I clinical trial is evaluating the combination of GDC-0941 and the MEK inhibitor GDC-0973, in patients with solid tumors. In this study a drug dosage was administered continuously for 21 days followed by 28 days without treatment. The preliminary analysis identified 78 patients. The expected toxicity profile was based on the single-agent toxicities, and the most common side effects reported were gastrointestinal symptoms, rash, fatigue, dysgeusia and elevated creatine kinase. Of 46 evaluable patients, only 3 (6%) partial responses were observed, from a BRAF mutated melanoma, BRAF mutated pancreatic cancer and a KRAS mutated endometrioid carcinoma. In addition, five patients (10%) had prolonged stable disease (more than 5 months) [239]

The Phase I trial testing the combination of GDC-0941 with carboplatin and paclitaxel, with or without bevacizumab in NSCLC demonstrated efficacy, and the toxicities were those expected from the toxicity profile of each single agent. By the time of the presentation of the results, 22 patients were enrolled, 17 with non-squamous and 5 with squamous cell carcinoma, resulting in 6 (out of 17) partial responses in the non-squamous group and 1 complete and 2 partial responses (out of 5) in the squamous group [234]. A Phase II clinical trial with this combination is currently enrolling patients.

In breast cancer patients, preliminary data of the combination with T-DM1 and in combination with carboplatin, paclitaxel and bevacizumab have already been presented. More specifically, in the T-DM1 combination study, 13 patients were enrolled so far. Three out of 6 patients at the first dose level experienced a dose-limiting toxicity (thrombocytopenia and fatigue); none presented relevant toxicities at a reduced dose level. Patient recruitment is still active, since signs of activity were observed.

The combination with paclitaxel and bevacizumab was well tolerated. Of the 25 patients enrolled, one had a complete response and 9 achieved a partial response.

GSK1059615 (GlaxoSmithKline), a thiazolidinedione, is another orally dosed pan-isoform PI3K inhibitor that entered Phase I clinical trial evaluation in patients with solid tumors and lymphomas. Unfortunately, the Phase I study was interrupted due to the limited bioavailability of the compound [240].

BAY 80-9646 (Bayer) is a highly selective, reversible, pan-class I inhibitor. In preclinical models BAY 80-9646 induced apoptosis in 60 (out of 140) different cell lines, and preferentially in cell lines with *PIK3CA* mutations [327]. Preclinical activity was also observed *in vivo* [126].

Two preliminary reports of the Phase I clinical trial have been presented so far: the first with 17 patients and a second one with 40 patients [242], which, in the expansion cohort, included 24 patients with solid tumors and 5 patients with non-

Hodgkin lymphoma [241]. The main side effects described were diarrhea, nausea, fatigue, mucositis, hyperglycemia and hypertension. Two partial responses were observed in two patients with breast cancer, both hormone receptor-positive tumors, one HER2-positive and the other HER2-negative. All 5 patients with non-Hodgkin lymphoma achieved a partial response [241].

The compound is currently being tested combined with gemcitabine with or without cisplatin (NCT01460537), with paclitaxel (NCT01411410) and with a MEK inhibitor (NCT01392521). The results are awaited.

CH5132799 (Chugai Pharmaceutical) is a class I, pan isoform PI3K inhibitor. Preclinically, the compound has shown activity in a broad panel of cell lines, especially those harboring *PIK3CA* mutations [120].

At the time of interim analysis, 31 patients had been enrolled, describing the most common adverse events as similar to other compounds of the same class: gastrointestinal symptoms, rash, fatigue, mucositis and liver function test alteration. No partial response was observed by RECIST, but one patient with clear cell ovarian cancer had a 75% decrease in her CA125 level [243].

ZSTK474 (Kenyaku Kogyo) is a pan-isoform PI3K inhibitor that has shown preclinical activity in several cell lines and xenografts [328, 329]. Currently, ZSTK474 is being investigated in a Phase I clinical trial in patients with advanced solid tumors (NCT01280487).

3.3. Isoform-Specific PI3K Inhibitors in Clinical Development

3.3.1. PI3K α-Specific Inhibitors

BYL719 (Novartis) is a 2-Aminothiazole with specific selectivity against the PI3K α-isoform (IC_{50} 4.6nm) and the most common mutant variants (IC_{50}: E545K: 4nM, H1047R 5nM), but it has weak potency against the PI3K β-isoform (IC_{50} 1156nM), delta-isoform (IC_{50} 290nM), gamma (IC_{50}250), Vps34 ($IC_{50} >$ 9100nM) and mTOR ($IC_{50} >$ 9100nM) [330]. Its preclinical activity was evaluated in the Cancer Cell Line Encyclopedia, which includes a large panel of molecularly characterized cell lines. As expected, BYL719 sensitivity was associated with

PIK3CA mutations, but also with *ERBB2* amplification and *PIK3CA* amplification, whereas *PTEN* and *BRAF* mutation were not [124].

The data of the dose escalation Phase of the Phase I clinical trial evaluating BYL719 has been recently presented [244]. For the first time, this clinical trial investigated a PI3K inhibitor in which a molecular prescreening was performed from the dose escalation part of the trial; only patients whose tumors harbored *PIK3CA* mutations could take part in the study. Thirty-five patients had been recruited before the interim analysis. The toxicity profile was similar to those observed with the pan-isoform PI3K inhibitors, and the most frequently observed adverse events were hyperglycemia, nausea, fatigue, rash and gastrointestinal toxicities

Three out of the 35 patients (8%) achieved a partial response; a patient with hormone receptor-positive breast cancer, a patient with cervical cancer and a patient with *KRAS*-mutant colon cancer. Furthermore, in 10 patients (28%) the disease remained stable for more than 4 months. This group included a variety of primary tumors: colon cancer, estrogen receptor-positive breast cancer or head and neck tumors.

The expansion cohort of this clinical trial is still under investigation. In addition, BYL is being evaluated in combination with the MEK inhibitor MEK162 in patients with solid tumors (NCT01449058), cetuximab in patients with head and neck cancers (NCT01602315) and with the HSP90 inhibitor AUY922 in patients with gastric cancer (NCT01613950).

INK1117 (Intellikine) is a potent and selective PI3K α-isoform inhibitor, which shows more than 100-fold selectivity against the α-isoform in comparison to other the other isoforms or mTOR. Preclinically, INK1117 has showed activity in cell lines and xenografts with *PIK3CA* mutations, while PTEN deficiency or *KRAS* mutation was associated with lack of response [123]. INK1117 is currently being investigated in a Phase I clinical trial in patients with advanced solid tumors (NCT01449370).

GDC-0032 (Genentech) is a PI3K α-isoform specific inhibitor which is currently under evaluation in a Phase I clinical trial (NCT01296555).

3.3.2. PI3K β-Specific Inhibitors

GSK2636771(Glaxo-Smith-Kline) is an oral PI3K β-isoform specific inhibitor [331], which is currently being assessed in a Phase I clinical trial in patients with PTEN deficient tumors (NCT01458067) [332].

3.3.3. PI3K δ-Specific Inhibitors

GS-1101 (Gilead), previously known as CAL-101 (Calistoga Pharmaceuticals), is a PI3Kdelta-specific inhibitor. Pharmacological investigations on GS-1101 were originally focused on its effect against inflammation and autoimmune diseases.

In preclinical models, GS-1101 has shown activity against different lymphoid malignancies including acute myeloid leukemia [333, 334], B-cell acute lymphoblastic leukemia [335], chronic lymphocytic leukemia [335, 336], mantle cell lymphoma [337], Hodgkin lymphoma [338], and multiple myeloma [339]. In addition, GS-1101 seems to have a synergic effect with everolimus in mantle cell lymphoma [337] and with bortezomib in multiple myeloma [339]. GS-1101 may potentially have a role reverting, at least partially, the resistance to chemotherapy in chronic lymphocytic leukemia [340, 341].

In the Phase I clinical trial of GS-1101 patients with a variety of relapsed or refractory hematologic malignancies: 54 patients with chronic lymphocytic leukemia [246, 342], 24 patients with indolent lymphoma, 16 patients with mantle cell lymphoma, 9 patients with diffuse B-cell lymphoma [248] and 7 patients with acute myeloid leukemia [343].

In the chronic lymphocytic cohort [246, 342], 80% of the 54 patients had lymphadenopathy shrinkage greater than 50% and the response rate by the 2008 International Workshop on Chronic Lymphocytic Leukemia (IWCLL) response criteria [344] was 26%. In this cohort, the most relevant grade 3 or higher adverse events were pneumonia, neutropenia (in 7% of patients also with febrile neutropenia), thrombocytopenia, anemia, and transaminase elevation [246, 342]. There were no responses among the patients with acute myeloid leukemia [247].

In patients with non-Hodgkin lymphoma, 62% of the patients with indolent non-Hodgkin lymphoma (15 of 24) and 10 of 16 patients with mantle cell lymphoma achieved a partial response. However, there were no responses among the 9 patients with diffuse large B-cell lymphoma. The toxicity profile in this cohort was similar to that seen in chronic lymphocytic lymphoma [248].

Encouraged by the activity observed with the single agent, GS-1101 is being evaluated in a Phase I clinical trial in combination with different anticancer compounds active in hematological malignancies. The data from the combination arms of GS-1101 with rituximab with or without bendamustine [249, 251] and in combination with ofatumumab [252] have been recently reported. A relevant antitumor activity, with an adequate toxicity profile, expected by the single agents' toxicities, was observed.

Currently, the combination arms of this trial with fludarabine, chlorambucil, everolimus and bortezomib arms have not yet been presented (NCT01088048). The combination of GS-1101 with rituximab (NCT01539512) and with rituximab and bendamustine (NCT01569295) in patients with previously treated chronic lymphocytic leukemia are currently being evaluated in two Phase III clinical trials. There are also Phase II clinical trials in indolent non-Hodgkin lymphoma (NCT01282424) and in relapsed Hodgkin lymphoma (NCT01393106), as well as in chronic lymphocytic lymphoma as a first line of treatment (NCT01203930).

AMG-319 (Amgen) is a PI3K δ-specific inhibitor also under development. Preclinically it has shown activity against B-cell malignancies and synergy with vincristine [345, 346]. A Phase I clinical trial with this agent in patients with relapsed or refractory lymphoid malignancies is ongoing (NCT01300026).

3.4. AKT Inhibitors in Clinical Development

AKT inhibitors hold the promise of being broadly effective agents in combination therapy with various standard chemotherapeutics. The study of AKT as a potential therapeutic target for cancer therapy has been hampered by a lack of small molecule kinase inhibitors specific for AKT. Due to the high degree of homology in the ATP binding pocket between AKT, protein kinase A (PKA) and protein kinase C (PKC), many typical PKA and PKC inhibitors have been identified as inhibitors of AKT. Due to high sequence identity, the development of AKT specific and isozyme selective inhibitors was predicted to be difficult. Despite these expectations, novel AKT inhibitors that display an unprecedented level of specificity have been reported. Not only are they specific with respect to other kinases, but some are also isozyme specific, most of them inhibiting AKT1 and AKT2 [347]. Phenotypic analyses of AKT isoform knockout mice documented AKT isoform-specific functions in the regulation of cellular growth and glucose metabolism. Those studies establish that the functions of the different AKT kinases are not completely overlapping and that isoform-specific signaling contributes to the diversity of AKT activities [348]. However, despite these important advances, a thorough understanding of the specific roles of each AKT family member will be essential to elucidate the complexity of AKT regulated cellular processes and how AKT isoform-specific deregulation might contribute to disease states. Isoform-specific AKT inhibitors serve as valuable tools to assess the role of the three isoenzymes in tumor formation and maintenance.

AKT has a number of specific binding pockets that can be targeted with small molecules. The most clearly described pockets are the PIP3 binding pocket on the PH domain, the phosphorylated carboxy terminus binding hydrophobic pocket and the ATP/substrate pocket [347]. Both ATP catalytic site AKT inhibitors and non-catalytic site (allosteric) AKT inhibitors are in active clinical development [349]. There are ongoing efforts to identify other AKT inhibitors with acceptable pharmaceutical properties. Cancers with *AKT1* mutations and *AKT1* and *AKT2* amplifications may be expected to be among the most sensitive to AKT inhibitors. It has been recently shown that *PIK3CA* mutant cancer cell lines exhibit only minimal AKT activation and a diminished reliance on AKT for anchorage-independent growth. Instead, these cells retain robust PDK1 activation and membrane localization and exhibit dependency on the PDK1 substrate SGK3 [350]. Despite these findings, a recent study demonstrated that a non-catalytic site AKT1/AKT2 inhibitor was effective against breast cancer cell lines with *PIK3CA* mutations and *HER2* amplifications [119]. In addition, another study demonstrated that tumors with *PIK3CA* mutations were the most sensitive to an AKT PH domain inhibitor, and *KRAS*-mutant tumors were the least sensitive [351].

Non-specific inhibitors of AKT have previously been evaluated in cancer patients. Those targeting the PH domain of AKT prevent its translocation to the plasma membrane. Preclinical activity was observed in breast, ovarian and prostate cancer models; this activity usually correlated with the degree of AKT activation previous to treatment. Downregulation of the downstream targets of AKT after treatment with perifosine was observed in these preclinical models [352].

Despite preliminary activity being observed in sarcoma in a Phase I clinical trial [353], perifosine has failed to show activity in Phase II clinical trials in this patient population [258]. Perifosine has shown lack of activity in other solid tumors [259, 354-360]. Even in patients with colorectal cancer with encouraging activity in combination with capecitabine as second or third line of treatment [361], perifosine ultimately failed to produce improvement in overall survival and progression-free survival in addition to capecitabine in the randomized controlled Phase III clinical trial [362].

Nevertheless, promising activity has been observed in patients with multiple myeloma and Waldenstrom´s macroglobulinemia with perifosine used as a single agent [363, 364], in combination with bortezomib [365] and more recently in combination with lenalidomide [366]. A randomized, controlled Phase III clinical trial evaluating perifosine, bortezomib, and dexamethasone is currently recruiting patients (NCT01002248).

Triciribine (API-2) is a cell-permeable and reversible tricyclic nucleoside that selectively inhibits the cellular phosphorylation/activation of AKT1/2/3 and exhibits little effect towards cellular signaling pathways mediated by PKC, PKA, SGK, Stat3, p38, ERK1/2, or JNK. Triciribine preferentially induces apoptosis and growth arrest in cancer cells with aberrant AKT activity both *in vitro* and *in vivo* [367]. Phase I trials observed severe hyperglycemia, hypertriglyceridemia, hepatoxicity, mucositis and fatigue as major adverse events [368, 369]. Efficacy in Phase II trials has been limited, compromising further development of this compound [370, 371].

MK-2206 (Merck) is a first-in-class, potent, allosteric non-catalytic site AKT1/2/3 inhibitor with wide preclinical antitumor activity. Results from the Phase I clinical trial evaluating single-agent MK-2206 have been recently published [254]. Thirty-three patients were enrolled in the dose escalation part using an alternate day schedule. The recommended Phase II dose was 60mg on alternate days. Common reversible drug-related toxicities included rash, nausea, mucositis, fatigue and hyperglycemia. Serial tumor biopsies demonstrated pAKT inhibition following MK-2206 in most patients. This correlated with sustained falls in pAKT in platelet-rich plasma and pPRAS40 in hair follicles. Overall, the best response was prolonged stable disease (more than 4 months) in 4 patients. A patient with PTEN-negative pancreatic cancer experienced a tumor shrinkage of 23%. Another two patients with pancreatic cancer achieved tumor shrinkage of 13% and 17%, respectively. A weekly schedule was also evaluated in this Phase I clinical trial. The recommended Phase II dose ranged between 135 and 200mg weekly.

The interim analyses of several Phase I combination trials have been presented so far: the combination with the MEK inhibitor selumetinib (AZD6244) in patients with solid tumors (NCT01021748) or with colorectal cancer (NCT01333475), the combination with trastuzumab and lapatinib in HER2-positive solid tumors (NCT00963547), the combination with carboplatin-paclitaxel, docetaxel or erlotinib in solid tumors (NCT00848718), and a parallel Phase I clinical trial in which one of the evaluated arms was the combination of dalotuzumab and MK-2206 (NCT01243762).

The first interim analysis of the Phase I clinical trial combining MK-2206 with selumetinib was presented, with 42 patients included. The main dose-limiting toxicities observed were rash, diarrhea, stomatitis and ocular toxicities. Two patients (4%) achieved a partial response; a patient with a *KRAS*-mutated serous ovarian carcinoma and a patient with NSCLC, while 4 patients (9%) experienced sustained disease stabilization [263]. In a more recent update, including 51 patients overall, a third partial response was observed in a pancreatic cancer patient. The recommended Phase II dose was established for MK-2206 at 135mg weekly and selumetinib 100mg daily [262].

The combination of MK-2206 and selumetinib is still under investigation in patients with metastatic colorectal cancer in concert with a pharmacodynamic analysis of changes in pERK and pAKT expression. The first 12 patients received a dose of MK-2206 90mg weekly and selumetinib 100mg daily, that was considered the recommended dose at the time of the first preliminary analysis. In these patients downregulation of one of the markers was observed in 4 of 8 evaluable patients, but none had simultaneous downregulation of the two markers. The patients currently enrolled are being evaluated at the updated recommended Phase II dose, but no data are available yet [266].

In the Phase I clinical trial evaluating MK-2206 with carboplatin-paclitaxel, docetaxel or erlotinib, 72 patients have been enrolled so far. The weekly administration had less hematological toxicity and was selected for the recommended Phase II dose. In the erlotinib combination arm the DLTs were mucositis and rash. Globally, the main adverse events were hematological, hyperglycemia and rash. In the carboplatin-paclitaxel arm, 1 complete response was observed along with 3 partial responses. Six patients had prolonged disease stabilization [260].

The Phase I clinical trial combining MK-2206 and lapatinib included 31 patients at the time of the interim analysis. The main toxicities reported were those observed with the single agent administration: fatigue, hyperglycemia, gastrointestinal toxicities and rash. One breast cancer patient achieved a complete response and 2 more patients had a partial response. All 3 of these patients had previously experienced disease progression with trastuzumab. Moreover, several prolonged disease stabilizations were also reported (one in a gastric cancer patient). The addition of lapatinib is speculated to further increase efficacy and is currently being tested [261].

In the Phase I trial evaluating MK-2206 and dalotuzumab, an anti-IGFR-1 monoclonal antibody,18 patients were enrolled in the dose-escalation part. The adverse events were similar to those observed with the single agents: fatigue, rash, gastrointestinal toxicities and hyperglycemia. For the preliminary recommended Phase II dose, both drugs were administered at the single agent recommended Phase II doses [264].

MK-2206 has been also evaluated in pediatric patients. The recommended Phase II dose for the weekly and the every other day schedule have been established.

The most common dose-limiting toxicity was rash. No activity data have yet been provided [372].

MK-2206 is currently being evaluated in multiple tumor types, including hematological malignancies and solid tumors, both as a single agent and in combination. Some of the approaches include the evaluation of MK-2206 as single agent in the neoadjuvant setting in patients with breast cancer (NCT01042379). In the metastatic setting, MK-2206 is being investigated with aromatase inhibitors (NCT01240928, NCT01344031, NCT01240941) and in combination with lapatinib (NCT01245205, NCT01281163) or trastuzumab with paclitaxel (NCT01235897). In patients with lung cancer, MK-2206 is being assessed with gefitinib (NCT01147211) or erlotinib (NCT01248247). The combination with the MEK inhibitor selumetinib is also being evaluated in this setting (NCT01248247). The combination of MK-2206 and selumetinib is also being investigated in patients with colorectal cancer or melanoma. Other currently active clinical trials are summarized in Table **1**.

GSK690693 (GlaxoSmithKline) is an intravenous potent ATP-competitive AKT inhibitor that also inhibited the phosphorylation of the downstream target GSK3 in cells [373]. In the interim analysis of the Phase I trial in 14 patients with solid tumors, the most relevant adverse event was hyperglycemia. The enrollment was still active at the time of the data presentation. The study aimed to evaluate GSK690693 in patients with hematological malignancies was discontinued prior to enrollment.

GSK2141795 (GlaxoSmithKline) is a reversible, selective, ATP-competitive inhibitor of all three AKT isoforms. In the Phase I clinical trial evaluating the single agent, 76 patients had been enrolled: 45 in the dose escalation Phase and 31 in the expansion cohort, which included three cohorts: prostate cancer, endometrial cancer, and tumors of any histology harboring an alteration in the AKT pathway. The main side effects were gastrointestinal toxicities, fatigue, and hyperglycemia. One patient with anal carcinoma achieved a partial response, and sustained disease stabilization was observed in several patients with prostate and endometrial carcinoma.

GSK2141795 has been also evaluated in ovarian cancer, using [17F] FDG PET as a pharmacodynamic marker. At the time of the interim analysis, 12 patients were included. Although, no partial responses according to RECIST criteria were recorded, 2 of 10 patients achieved a response according to CA125 GCIG criteria [374]. One of these patients had a *PIK3CA* mutation. The analysis of potential sensitivity and resistance predictive factors has been recently presented [268].

GSK2110183 (Octagon Research Solutions) is a potent, oral, ATP competitive inhibitor of all AKT isoforms. The preliminary report of the Phase I clinical trials evaluating GSK2110183 in hematological malignancies, summarizes the data of 73 patients enrolled so far. The main side effects were gastrointestinal toxicities and fatigue. The dose-limiting toxicities were liver enzyme elevation and memory loss. The main focus of the expansion cohort was multiple myeloma. Of 32 patients with multiple myeloma treated at the recommended Phase II dose, 3 achieved a partial response and another 3 achieved a minor response [375].

These results have encouraged pursuing the evaluation of GSK2110183 in multiple myeloma as a single agent (Phase II: NCT01445587), in combination with bortezomib and dexamethasone (Phase I: NCT01428492) and in combination with the MEK inhibitor GSK1120212 (NCT01476137). In addition, the combination of GSK2110183 with ofatumumab is under investigation in patients with relapsed or refractory chronic lymphocytic leukemia (NCT01532700).

GDC-0068 (Genentech) is an ATP-competitive inhibitor of AKT. It exerts its activity against the three AKT isoforms, as well as activating AKT mutations such E17K. GDC-0068 inhibited viability of cancer cell lines with a PTEN deficiency, *PIK3CA* mutations or *HER2* amplification [376].

The preliminary data of the single-agent Phase I clinical trial have been presented. Among the 22 patients enrolled, one patient with PTEN null colon cancer had stable disease for more than 8 cycles (32 weeks) The most common adverse events were fatigue, nausea, diarrhea and hyperglycemia [270]. At the time of the data presentation, an intermediate dose of 600mg daily was being evaluated, which finally was considered the MTD [271]. The data of the expansion cohort in patients with PTEN null/PIK3CA mutant breast cancer or prostate cancer have not been reported so far.

Recently, the preliminary data of the Phase I study combining docetaxel or mFOLFOX with GDC-0068 have been presented. The dose escalation part is still ongoing and no dose-limiting toxicity has yet been observed. Two of the 23 patients enrolled achieved a partial response, a cervical cancer and a PTEN-deficient colon cancer patient.

LY2780301 (Eli Lilly and Company) is an oral potent selective AKT and p70S6 kinase. Thirty-two patients were enrolled in a Phase I clinical trial. No serious adverse events were recorded. The most common grade 1 or 2 toxicities were gastrointestinal symptoms and fatigue. The pharmacokinetic profile favored daily dosing. No partial responses were observed, but one patient with mesothelioma, achieved disease stabilization for 8 months.

Preliminary results with an antisense oligonucleotide with a sequence complementary to AKT-1 mRNA, **RX-0201,** have been presented [377]. The drug is administered as a continuous infusion and the dose-limiting toxicity was fatigue. No efficacy data are available.

3.5. mTOR Catalytic Site Inhibitors in Clinical Development

Rapamycin and its analogues partially inhibit mTOR through allosteric binding to mTORC1 but not mTORC2, an emerging player in cancer. The discovery of the direct involvement of mTORC2 in the activation of AKT, combined with the limited clinical antitumor activity of mTORC1-directed agents have led to the development of ATP-competitive catalytic site inhibitors of the mTOR kinase that inhibit the function of both mTORC1 and mTORC2 [173]. Preclinical studies demonstrate stronger inhibition of cancer cell growth. Feldman *et al.* demonstrated that two mTOR kinase domain inhibitors, PP242 and PP30, inhibit both mTORC1 and mTORC2. Unlike acute rapamycin treatment, PP242 administration to mice suppressed AKT activation in tissues. PP242 was also a more effective inhibitor of proliferation than rapamycin [174]. In models of acute leukemia harboring the Philadelphia chromosome translocation, Janes *et al.* compared rapamycin with PP242 and demonstrate that the mTORC1/2 inhibitor, but not rapamycin, caused death of mouse and human leukemia cells [175]. Three additional ATP-competitive mTOR inhibitors, -WAY-600, WYE-687, and WYE-354, have been shown to inhibit proliferation of a variety of cancer cell lines more effectively than rapamycin [176].

Based on these promising preclinical data, several mTORC1/2 inhibitors have been developed in the clinical setting.

MLN0128, previously known as INK128 (Intellikine), is an oral potent inhibitor of mTORC1 and mTORC2 [378]. It has shown preclinical activity in several models as a single agent and also in combination with chemotherapy or other targeted agents [378-382]. In the single agent Phase I trial, two administration schedules were evaluated: once daily continuously and intermittent.

In the intermittent cohort, several dose schedules were assessed: weekly, 3 days a week or 5 days a week. The toxicity profile was similar in the 3 arms, with a slight higher rate of grade 3 events in the 3 days a week schedule. The most common side effects were nausea and vomiting, hyperglycemia, mucositis and fatigue. In terms of activity, only 1 patient (with renal cell carcinoma) out of the 52 enrolled, achieved a partial response, and a NSCLC patient experienced a 25% tumor shrinkage [274].

Twenty-five patients were enrolled in the daily dosing schedule. The most common side effects were hyperglycemia, rash, gastrointestinal symptoms and fatigue. Pharmacodynamic studies showed a dose-dependent inhibition of pS6, p4EBP1 and PRAS40. Twenty-four percent of patients demonstrated stable disease for at least 4 cycles, and 12% remained on study for at least 6 cycles [273].

MNL0128 is currently being evaluated in patients with solid tumors in combination with paclitaxel with or without trastuzumab (NCT01351350).

AZD8055 (Astra Zeneca) is also a dual mTORC1/mTORC2 inhibitor. The data from the Phase I clinical trial included 49 patients enrolled at the time of analysis. Despite having a short half-life of 2.4 hours, AZD8055 induced pharmacodynamic changes in peripheral blood mononuclear cells [275, 383]. The dose-limiting toxicity was transaminase elevation. Other common adverse events were fatigue and gastrointestinal toxicities. No RECIST responses were observed, but 7 patients had stable disease longer than 4 months [275].

OSI-027 (OSI Pharmaceuticals) is entering early clinical trials [276, 384]. So far, preliminary results of the Phase I trial with OSI-027 have been presented [276]. Major toxicities were fatigue and decreased left ventricular ejection fraction. Pharmacodynamic data indicate that substantial decreases in 4E-BP1 phosphorylation were observed in peripheral blood mononuclear cells from 13 of 23 patients following OSI-027 treatment. Disease stabilization was found in patients with various tumor types.

AZD2014 is close analogue of AZD8055 that selectively targets mTORC1 and mTORC2. Its potency *in vitro* is 5-fold lower in comparison to AZD8055, but its pharmacokinetic profile is more favorable. It has shown preclinical activity against several cancer models, including an estrogen receptor-positive breast cancer xenograft [385]. In addition, it has also demonstrated synergy with paclitaxel in ovarian cancer models [386].

The results of a Phase I clinical trial with AZD 2014 have been recently presented; 54 patients were enrolled, 23 in the dose escalation part, 31 in the dose expansion (breast cancer). The most common side effects were fatigue, nausea, mucositis, anorexia and rash. Reduction in pS6 and pAKT was observed in paired biopsies. There was a partial response in a pancreatic cancer patient and two patients remained on treatment for 273 and 365 days, respectively [277].

CC-223 is a potent selective ATP-competitive mTORC1 and mTORC2 inhibitor. The preliminary results of the Phase I clinical trials have been recently presented. The study has an accelerated dose escalation Phase followed by a dose expansion with different cohorts evaluating several selected tumor types: NSCLC, glioblastoma, hepatocellular carcinoma, breast cancer, neuroendocrine tumors, diffuse large B-cell lymphoma and myeloma. By the time of the presentation, 28 patients were enrolled in the dose escalation part. The most common side effects were fatigue, nausea, diarrhea, hyperglycemia and mucositis. One patient (with breast cancer) out of a total of 19 evaluable patients obtained a partial response.

There were 5 patients with prolonged disease stabilization for at least 4 cycles, in breast cancer, salivary, adrenal, pancreatic, and NSCLC cancer [278].

4. RECENTLY ISSUED PATENTS OF PI3K/ AKT/ MTORC1/2 INHIBITORS

As the PI3K/AKT/ mTOR pathway is one of the most intriguing targets for cancer therapeutics, development of inhibitors has become an area of intense interest in both academia and the pharmaceutical industry in recent years. More than two decades have been spent optimizing the chemical structures of these compounds in the quest to find candidates having acceptable pharmacological, pharmacokinetic and selectivity profiles. Driven by efforts in computer-based drug design and synthetic structure-activity relationship studies, dozens of promising PI3K/ AKT/ mTORC1/2 inhibitors have been developed. Their chemical structures and important features are summarized in Table **2** [387-405]. Novel therapeutics targeting different components of this pathway are demonstrating efficacy in an array of human cancer types in preclinical studies, and many of these drugs are being carried forward into clinical trials.

5. CHALLENGES IN THE DEVELOPMENT OF PI3K, AKT AND MTORC1/2 INHIBITORS

As more therapeutic options targeting the PI3K/AKT/mTOR pathway become available, important issues need further evaluation for the development and clinical use of this class of agents in cancer patients. It is still unknown if certain tumors or tumor subtypes would benefit more from upstream inhibition-PI3K inhibition-or downstream inhibition-AKT or mTOR inhibition-in the PI3K-AKT-mTOR pathway. A first step would be to compare the effect of PI3K inhibitors, AKT inhibitors and mTORC1/2 inhibitors in preclinical settings. The use of models most accurately mirroring the molecular complexity of the patients' tumors, such as patient-derived tumor xenografts, is of special interest [406]. The results from these preclinical studies would help optimize the design of clinical trials to compare the anticancer effects and toxicities of the different drug classes. Another unresolved question is whether certain tumors would be more dependent

Table 2: Recently Issued Patents PI3K/ AKT/ mTORC1/2 Inhibitors.

Patent Number	Chemical Structure	Feature	Reference
PI3K Inhibitors			
US20130029984 Intellikine LLC Infinity Pharmaceuticals Inc.	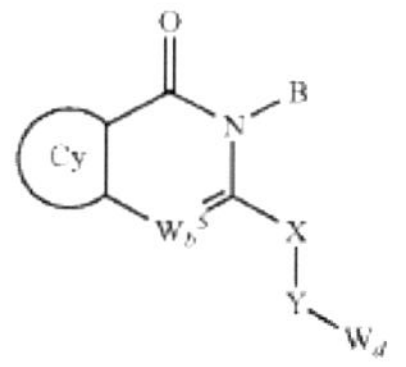	Compounds capable of selectively inhibiting certain isoform(s) of class I PI3K without substantially affecting the activity of the remaining isoforms of the same class. For example, non-limiting examples of inhibitors, capable of selectively inhibiting PI3K-δ and/or PI3Kγ, but without substantially affecting the activity of PI3K-β are disclosed. Such inhibitors can be effective in ameliorating disease conditions associated with PI3K-δ/γ activity	[387]
WO2012151525 Rhizen Pharmaceuticals SA	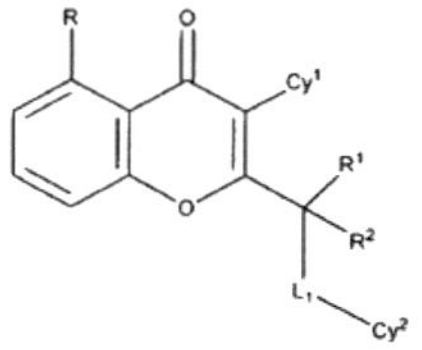	The present invention provides PI3K protein kinase modulators, methods of preparing them, pharmaceutical compositions containing them and methods of treatment, prevention and/or amelioration of kinase mediated diseases or disorders with them	[388]
PI3K-mTOR Inhibitors			
EP2524918 Centro Nacional de Investigaciones Oncologicas (CNIO)	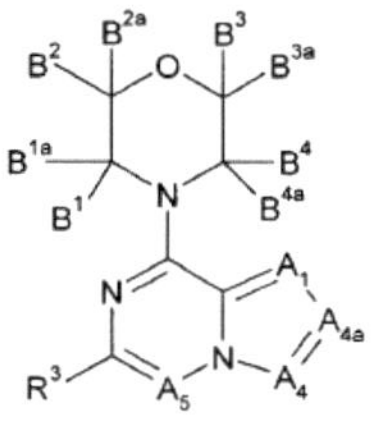	There is provided compounds of the previously described formula, wherein A1, A4, A4a, A5, B1, B1a, B2, B2a, B3, B3a, B4, B4a and R3 have meanings given in the description, and pharmaceutically-acceptable esters, amides, solvates or salts thereof, which compounds are useful in the treatment of diseases in which inhibition of a protein or lipid kinase (*e.g.* a PI3-K and/or mTOR) and, additionally, HDAC, is desired and/or required, and particularly in the treatment of cancer or a proliferative disease	[389]

Table 2: contd….

US20130029967 Centro Nacional de Investigaciones Oncologicas (CNIO)	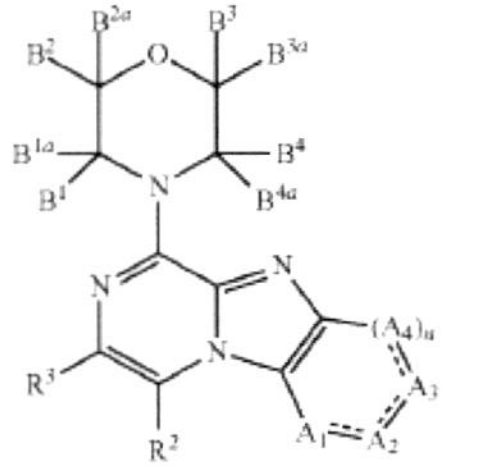	There is provided compounds of the previously described formula, wherein A1, A2, A3, A4, n, the dotted lines, B1, B1a, B2, B2a, B3, B3a, B4, B4a, R2 and R3 have meanings given in the description, and pharmaceutically-acceptable esters, amides, solvates or salts thereof, which compounds are useful in the treatment of diseases in which inhibition of a protein kinase (*e.g.* a PI3-K and/or mTOR) is desired and/or required, and particularly in the treatment of cancer or a proliferative disease	[390]
US8314103 Piramal Enterprises Limited	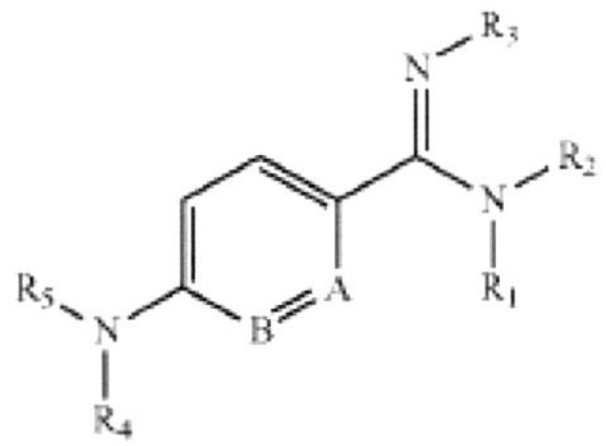	The present invention relates to pyridyl derivatives capable of inhibiting phosphatidylinositol-3-kinase (PI3k), mammalian target of rapamycin (mTOR) and/or hypoxia inducible factor 1α (HIF-1α) mediated signaling. Also disclosed are processes for preparation of the pyridyl derivatives, and their use in the manufacture of pharmaceutical compositions for the treatment of clinical conditions caused by deregulation of signaling pathways selected from one or more of PI3K, mTOR and HIF-1α pathways. The pyridyl derivatives are also useful for the treatment of conditions or disorders mediated by TNF-α	[391]
WO2012154608 Intellikine LLC	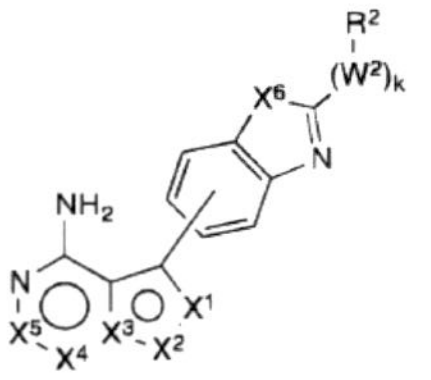	The present invention provides for a compounds and methods for treating a disease condition associated with mTor and PI3-kinases in a subject	[392]

Table 2: contd….

WO2012154610 Intellikine LLC	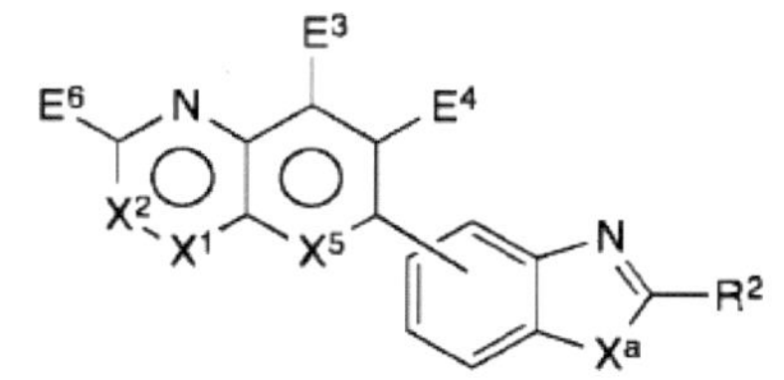 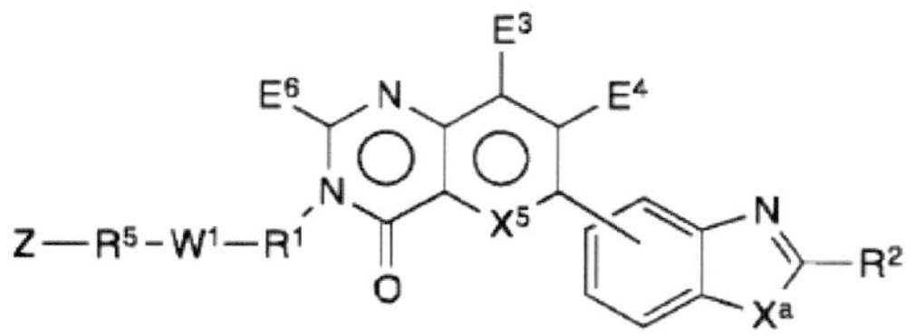	The present invention provides for bicyclic heterocyclic compounds as PI3 kinase inhibitors e.g., PI3 kinase alpha, capable of covalently reacting with the kinase protein through binding to a PI3'kinase cysteine residue leading to the formation of a conjugate product, as well as methods utilizing such PI3 kinase inhibitors for treating a disease condition associated with the PI3-kinase in a subject	[393]
WO2012148540	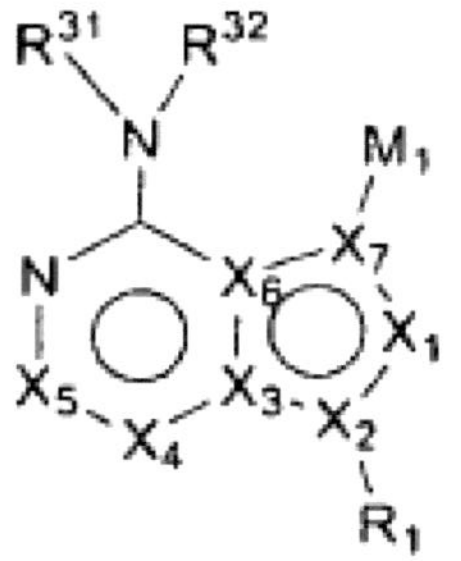	The present invention provides for a method for treating a disease condition associated with PI3 -kinase α and/or mTOR in a subject. In another aspect, the invention provides for a method for treating a disease condition associated with PI3 -kinase α and/or mTOR in a subject. In yet another aspect, a method of inhibiting phosphorylation of both AKT (S473) and AKT (T308) in a cell is set forth	[394]

Table 2: contd….

AKT Inhibitors			
US20120329808 Array Biopharma Inc.	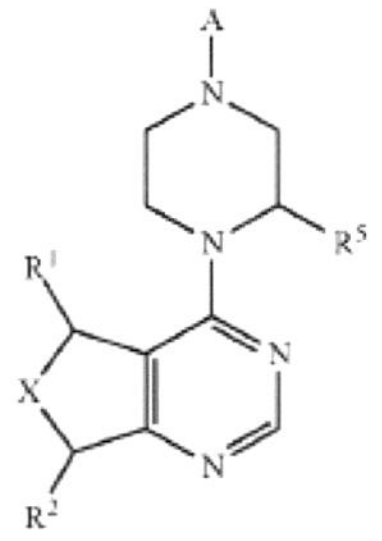 	**Dihydrothienopyrimidines as AKT protein kinase inhibitors** The present invention provides compounds, including resolved enantiomers, diastereomers, solvates and pharmaceutically acceptable salts thereof, comprising the previously described formula	[395]
EP2240455 Array Biopharma, Inc. Genentech, Inc.	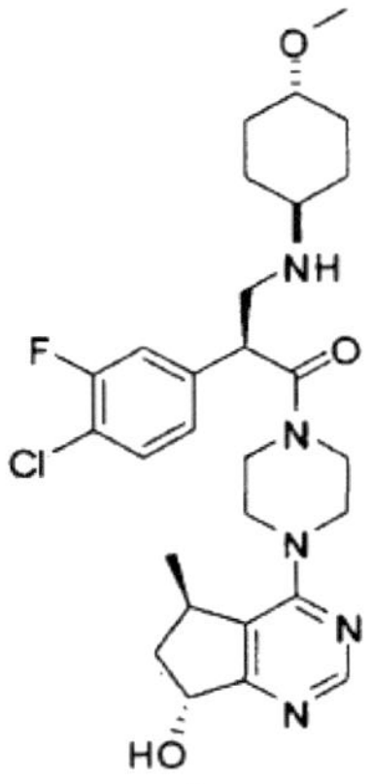 **I**	**Hydroxylated Pyrimidyl Cyclopentane as AKT protein kinase inhibitor** This invention provides a novel compound that inhibits AKT protein kinases. The compound of the present invention has utility as a therapeutic agent for diseases and conditions that can be treated by the inhibition of AKT protein kinases	[396]

Table 2: contd….

US8338434 GlaxoSmithKline LLC	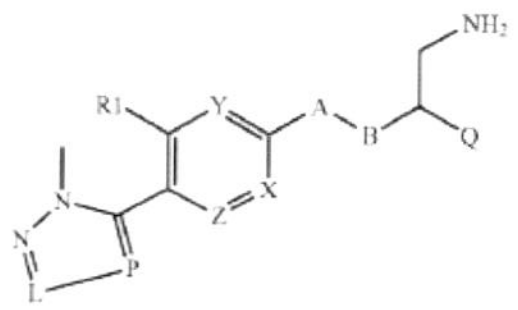	Invented are novel pyrazole compounds, the use of such compounds as inhibitors of protein kinase B activity and in the treatment of cancer and arthritis	[397]
US8329709 Genentech, Inc. Array BioPharma Inc.	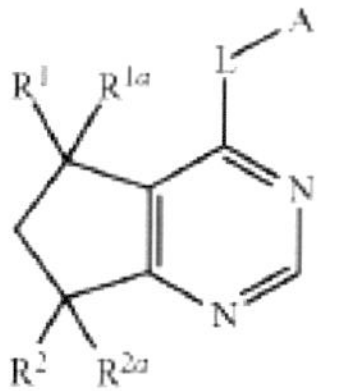	**5H-cyclopenta[D]pyrimidines as AKT protein kinase inhibitors** Compounds derived from previously described formula are useful for inhibiting AKT protein kinases. Methods using compounds of previously described formula and stereoisomers and pharmaceutically acceptable salts thereof, for *in vitro*, *in situ*, and *in vivo* diagnosis, prevention or treatment of such disorders in mammalian cells, or associated pathological conditions are disclosed	[398]
US8329701 Array Biopharma Inc.	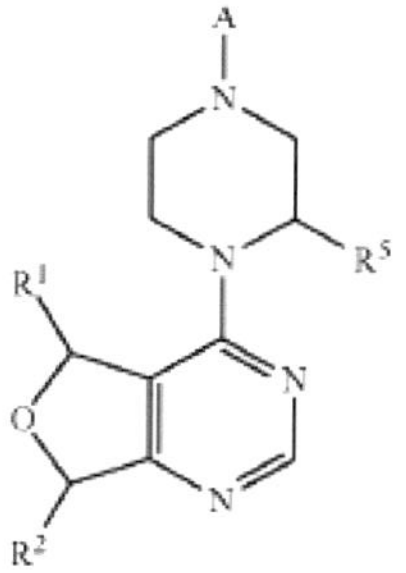	**Dihydrofuro pyrimidines as AKT protein kinase inhibitors** The present invention provides compounds, including resolved enantiomers, diastereomers, solvates and pharmaceutically acceptable salts thereof, comprising thepreviously described formula; also provided are methods of using the compounds of this invention as AKT protein kinase inhibitors and for the treatment of hyperproliferative diseases such as cancer	[399]

Table 2: contd….

US8324221 Array Biopharma Inc.	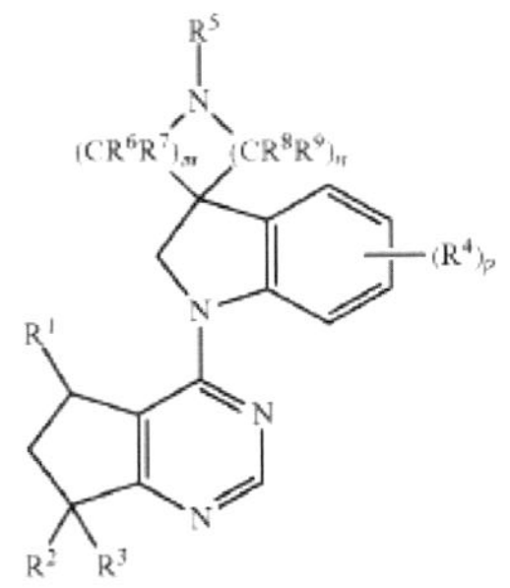	**Pyrimidyl cyclopentanes as AKT protein kinase inhibitors** The present invention provides compounds of previously described formula including tautomers, resolved enantiomers, resolved diastereomers, solvates, metabolites, salts and pharmaceutically acceptable prodrugs thereof. Also provided are methods of using the compounds of this invention as AKT protein kinase inhibitors and for the treatment of AKT-mediated diseases, for example, hyperproliferative diseases such as cancer	[400]
WO2012089633 Sanofi	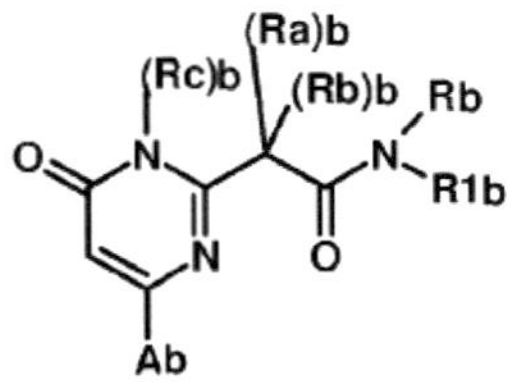	The present invention relates to novel chemical compounds derived from pyrimidines, to the method for preparing same, to the novel intermediates obtained, to the use thereof as drugs, to the pharmaceutical compositions containing same, and to the therapeutic use thereof as AKT inhibitors	[401]
US20120270867 Sanofi	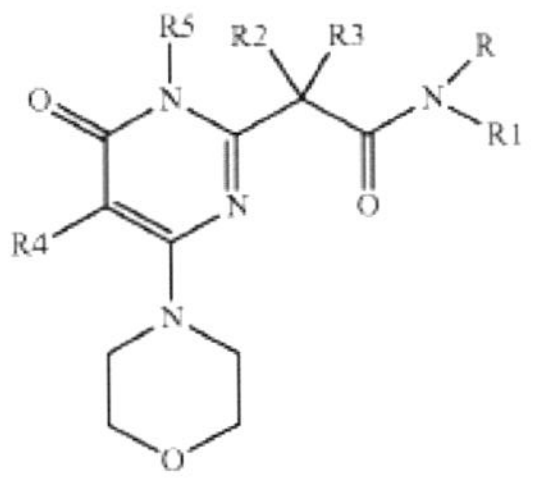	New (6-oxo-1,6-dihydro-pyrimidin-2-yl)-amide derivatives are AKT phosphorylation inhibitors useful for treating e.g. gastric cancers, glioblastoma, thyroid cancers, bladder cancers, breast cancers, melanoma, sarcoma and hamartoma	[402]

Table 2: contd….

WO2012158197 Lyndor Biosciences LLC	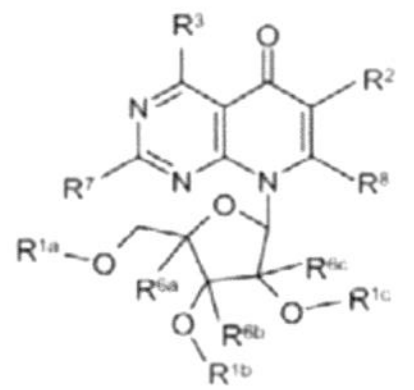	Compounds, and pharmaceutical compositions, and formulations thereof, are disclosed that have formula (I): where R1a, R1b, R1c, R2, R3, R6a, R6b, R6c, R7, and R8 are as defined herein. The compounds, pharmaceutical compositions, and pharmaceutical formulations thereof are useful for the prevention and treatment of a variety of conditions in mammals including humans, including by way of non-limiting example, cancer, and others. The manufacturing and analytical methods for LD- 101 are also disclosed	[403]
mTOR Inhibitors			
US20120289481	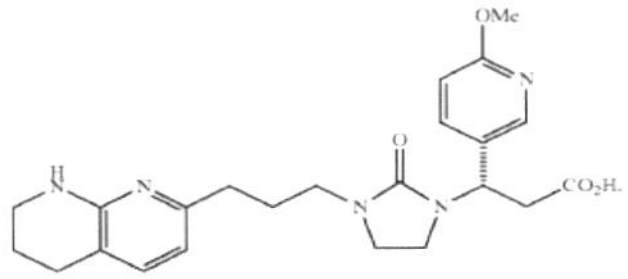	The instant invention provides a method of treating a cancer selected from the group consisting of non-small cell lung cancer and breast cancer with an mTOR inhibitor and an αvβ3 integrin antagonist, wherein the mTOR inhibitor is ridaforolimus, everolimus, temsirolimus or a combination thereof	[404]
P70S6K Inhibitors			
US8343953 Astex Therapeutics Limited The Institute of Cancer Research: Royal Cancer Hospita Cancer Research Technology Limited	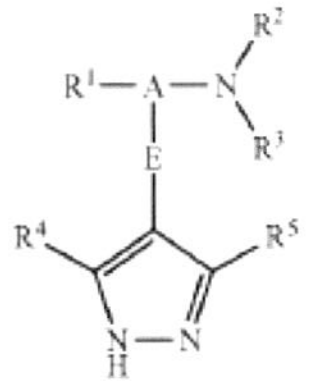	The invention provides compounds of the formula (I) having ROCK kinase and/or protein kinase p70S6K inhibiting activity: wherein A is a saturated hydrocarbon linker group containing from 1 to 7 carbon atoms, the linker group having a maximum chain length of 5 atoms extending between R1 and NR2R3 and a maximum chain length of 4 atoms extending between E and NR2R3, wherein one of the carbon atoms in the linker group may optionally be replaced by an oxygen or nitrogen atom; and wherein the carbon atoms of the linker group A may optionally bear one or more substituents selected from oxo, fluorine and hydroxy, provided that the hydroxy group when present is not located at a carbon atom ± with respect to the NR2R3 group and provided that the oxo group when present is located at a carbon atom ± with respect to the NR2R3 group; E is a monocyclic or bicyclic carbocyclic or heterocyclic group; R1 is an aryl or heteroaryl group; and R2, R3, R4 and R5 are as defined in the claims	[405]

on a single PI3K or AKT isoform or on several ones [407]. This question is relevant to decide whether an isoform-specific or a pan-isoform inhibitor would be preferable [408]. Another key point in the development of drugs targeting the PI3K/AKT/mTOR pathway is designing an appropriate drug combination. The PI3K/AKT/mTOR pathway has a relevant role in the resistance to several targeted agents, such as anti-EGFR[60, 409-411] or anti-HER2[284, 412, 413] therapies. Combining these targeted agents with drugs targeting PI3K/AKT/mTOR is a promising approach. On the other hand, other pathways, such as the MAPK[296] pathway, have shown to participate in the resistance to PI3K/AKT/mTOR inhibitors; thus, combining agents targeting each pathway is another attractive strategy currently being evaluated.

5.1. Isoform Selective Inhibition versus Pan-Isoform Inhibition

Because each PI3K isoform has a discrete function and is correspondingly involved in various diseases, isoform selectivity is likely a key consideration in developing PI3K inhibitors. Discovery of isoform-specific PI3K inhibitors was pursued on the basis of the understanding that a non-selective PI3K inhibitor would lead to deleterious side effects. Most PI3K inhibitors currently under development as antitumor agents are pan-PI3K isoform inhibitors, and clinical data have shown that they are generally well tolerated without major toxicities; however, the minimum target inhibition required in a clinical setting to achieve a response, and whether PI3K isoform-specific inhibitors lead to a more effective target blockade, remains unclear.

PI3Kalpha-specific inhibitors were originally pursued for cancer therapy based on the knowledge that only p110alpha gene mutations and amplification were observed in human cancers. However, accumulating evidence has demonstrated that in addition to PI3Kalpha, the three other known PI3K isoforms are also involved in tumorigenesis. Even in tumors that are initially addicted to a specific PI3K isoform, a PI3K-depedent mechanism of resistance could be subsequently developed; as a result, a pan-PI3K inhibitor, through a complete blockade of the entire pathway, might potentially offer enhanced therapeutic benefit, compared with a PI3Kalpha-specific inhibitor [407]. For that reason, it is still unclear in which cases a PI3K alpha-specific inhibitor would be superior than a pan-isoform

PI3K inhibitor or in which cases a complete inhibition all the isoform with a pan-isoform PI3K inhibitor will be preferred.

As always in the field of drug discovery, the definite answer to this question will have to wait for the results from clinical trials. Drugs targeting particular isoforms could avoid particular side effects. For example, PI3Kalpha/beta inhibitors that do not hit PI3Kgamma and PI3Kdelta would likely spare immune cells. PI3Kdelta-selective inhibitors may be advantageous in some leukemias and lymphomas and avoid possible metabolic effects on PI3Kalpha/beta. Preferential activity on PI3Kalpha may be desirable in cancers with mutant or amplified *PIK3CA*. In addition, activity of selective PI3Kalpha isoform inhibitors has been described in cell lines harboring HER2 amplification [124]. Though a number of recent studies have shown that p110beta plays a key role in transformation driven by loss of PTEN, it is likely that this reliance is dependent on the signaling input and genetic context of the tumor.

Regarding AKT inhibitors, our understanding of AKT biology, mechanisms of inhibition and the design of small molecule AKT inhibitors has grown tremendously. However, key issues regarding AKT specificity and AKT isozyme selectivity remain unanswered. With the recent discovery of allosteric AKT kinase inhibitors, these issues have begun to be addressed. Several series of allosteric and PH domain-dependent inhibitors have demonstrated specificity for AKT versus other kinases. Data obtained from the use of these inhibitors indicate that a candidate slated for development should inhibit both AKT1 and AKT2. It remains to be determined if a compound that only inhibits AKT1 and AKT2 will have an improved therapeutic profile compared to an inhibitor of all three AKT isoenzymes. In addition, AKT inhibitors hold the promise of being broadly effective agents in combination therapy with various standard chemotherapeutic agents.

5.2. Targeted Agent Combinations to Enhance Anticancer Activity

The clinical efficacy of PI3K inhibitors, AKT inhibitors and mTORC1/2 inhibitors as single agents has been limited and, in many cases, short-lived. Combining the PI3K, AKT, or mTORC1/2 inhibitors with agents targeting resistance pathways is an innovative strategy for improving results. Another relevant strategy is combining

PI3K, AKT or mTOR1/2 inhibitors with targeted agents, such as anti-EGFR or anti-HER2 therapies, in which the PI3K/AKT/mTOR pathway has a key role in the development of resistance (Fig. (**2**)).

The role of the PI3K/AKT/mTOR pathway as a mechanism of resistance to anti-EGFR [60, 409-411] and anti-HER2 therapy [284, 412, 413] has been extensively described. Currently several clinical trials are evaluating the combination of anti-EGFR or anti-HER2 therapies in combination with PI3K, AKT or mTOR inhibitors (Table **1**). As expected, the tumor sites in which this strategy is being investigated are those in which the anti-EGFR and anti-HER2 has proved to be beneficial; for example, combinations with erlotinib or gefinitinib in NSCLC, with cetuximab or panitumumab in KRAS wild-type colorectal cancer or head and neck cancers, or trastuzumab or lapatinib in HER2-positive breast cancer. The first results from some of these studies have been already reported, showing some promising preliminary data [177, 185, 186, 211, 218, 219, 260, 261, 323].

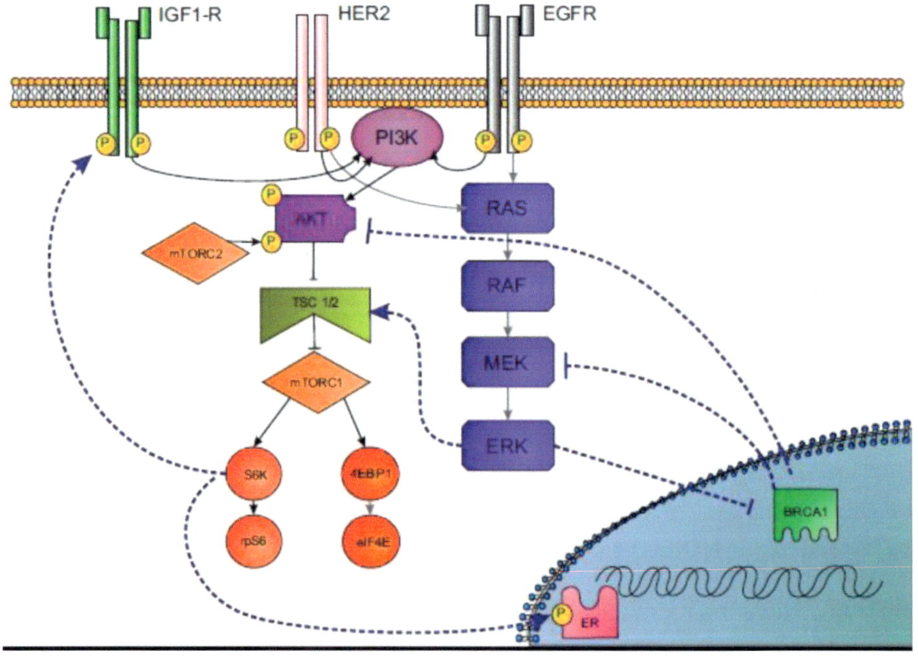

Figure 2: Cross-talk among PI3K and other cellular pathways PI3K is a known mechanism of resistance against anti-EGFR, anti-HER2 or anti-hormonal therapies. Several pathways are involved on resistance to PI3K pathway inhibition including the MAPK pathway and the IGF-1R pathway.

The PI3K/AKT/mTOR pathway plays a relevant role in resistance to hormonal therapy [414, 415]. A recently published study evaluating the combination of the aromatase inhibitor exemestane and the mTORC1 inhibitor everolimus has improved the overall survival of patients with hormone receptor-positive breast cancer [156]. Several clinical trials evaluating the combination of anti-hormonal therapy and PI3K and AKT inhibitors in breast and prostate cancer are ongoing (Table **1**).

The MAPK pathway is the most commonly associated with resistance to PI3K/AKT/mTOR inhibition [296]. Thus, several clinical trials are evaluating the simultaneous inhibition of both pathways. Although most of these clinical trials are still Phase I clinical trials in patients with solid tumors, some of these studies are selecting patients with tumors harboring *KRAS* or *BRAF* mutations. In the Phase I clinical trials that have already reported data, several partial responses have been observed [212, 237, 239, 262, 263], including patients with *BRAF*-mutant melanoma, pancreatic cancer, *KRAS*-mutant NSCLC, *KRAS*-mutant endometrioid adenocarcinoma and *KRAS*-mutant ovarian cancer.

Another described mechanism of resistance to PI3K/AKT/mTOR pathway inhibition is IGF1-R upregulation [160, 416, 417]. The combination of ridaforolimus, a mTORC1 inhibitor, and dalotuzumab, an anti-IGF1-R monoclonal antibody, has shown promising activity in a Phase I clinical trial, especially in patients with hormone-positive breast cancer [418]. Currently, a similar approach is being evaluated in a Phase I clinical trial in which dalotuzumab is combined with the AKT inhibitor MK-2206. An expansion cohort in patients with ovarian cancer is evaluating the activity of this combination in this tumor type [264].

Another potential synergy is the one observed with the simultaneous inhibition of PARP and PI3K inhibition [419, 420]. Currently, the combination of BKM120 and olaparib is under evaluation in patients with breast cancer or high-grade ovarian cancer (Table **1**).

CONCLUSIONS

Early clinical data with PI3K/ AKT/ mTORC1/2 inhibitors show promising activity in unselected patient populations. Many of the current trials with PI3K pathway inhibitors will carry out retrospective analyses of the mutational status of enrolled patients. Many early clinical trials exploring the novel PI3K isoform-specific inhibitors are pre-selecting patients with tumors with the molecular alteration of interest, such as PIK3CA mutation or amplification for PI3K α-isoform inhibitors or PTEN deficiency for PI3K β, for the dose escalation Phase [244]. The preliminary results of the dose escalation Phase of one of these compounds have been already presented, showing a promising response rate that would encourage the use of this approach in further clinical trials [244, 332].

However, it is important to remember that in several patients experiencing a clinical benefit from a PI3K inhibitor, no activating mutations or recognized PI3K pathway alterations were found. Molecular characterization of these tumors becomes instrumental to investigate the underlying reason for their addiction to the PI3K pathway and to identify further patients that can potentially benefit from the treatment with PI3K inhibitors in the future. As technology continues to be developed, such as next-generation sequencing and the use of circulating DNA, and a greater number of genes are routinely assessed in tumor tissue, the picture and potential for efficacious targeted therapy will improve.

The assessment of PI3K pathway activation in cancer specimen remains an important obstacle for BM-based treatment with PI3K pathway inhibitors. In the ideal situation, one test should be able to assay activation of the pathway and should preferably distinguish upstream (RTK activation) from downstream (*PIK3CA* mutation, PTEN loss) activation, which would guide the decision between RTK-targeting agents and downstream inhibitors. Attempts to find an expression signature for PI3K pathway activation thus far have failed and the detection of PTEN loss in cancer tissue remains problematic. Despite some exciting successful examples, meaningful clinical progress for drugs targeting a single kinase or a single molecular pathway has been rare, especially in the cancers responsible for the largest proportion of cancer deaths. Even though some cancers seem to be addicted to signaling in one molecular pathway, inhibition of such a pathway is often not enough for a meaningful clinical response. In addition, molecular pathways may influence the downstream PI3K targets and could affect the sensitivity to inhibition of members of the PI3K pathway. It is currently not known which pathways are primarily responsible for the antiproliferative and apoptotic effects of PI3K pathway inhibition; alterations in these downstream pathways could cause resistance in response to PI3K, AKT or mTOR inhibition.

Experience with modern targeted molecular cancer therapeutics suggests that the presence of multiple genetic abnormalities and the induction of feedback loops and other resistance mechanisms is likely to mean that PI3K pathway inhibitors will need to be given in combination with other agents, such as anti-HER2 agents and MEK inhibitors. Recognizing that these pathways likely operate in complex networks in which the outcomes of pharmacologic modulation may be difficult to predict is of paramount importance. There is also a need for further research to determine whether doses that are biologically active according to BM studies, properly reflect the optimal dose for all patient populations and subgroups. Currently, there are still too many uncertainties in this respect and it seems prudent not to omit establishing the highest achievable dose of each PI3K pathway inhibitor, as this may be useful in the future.

ACKNOWLEDGEMENTS

Irene Brana is supported by a “Spanish Society of Medical Oncology (SEOM) translational grant” and a “Conquer Cancer Foundation of ASCO Young Investigator Award”.

CONFLICT OF INTEREST

No financial interest in any of the companies or patents reviewed in this chapter.

DISCLOSURE

The chapter submitted for Patent Series eBook entitled "Topics in Anti-Cancer Research", Volume 2 is an update of our article "**Recent Developments in Anti-Cancer Agents Targeting PI3K, AKT and mTORC1/2**", published in the journal ‘Recent Patents on Anti-Cancer Drug Discovery’, Volume 6, Number 2, May 2011, Page 210 to 236 with additional text and references.

ABBREVIATIONS

4E-BP1	= Eukaryotic Initiation Factor 4E Binding Protein 1
ATP	= Adenosine Triphosphate
BM	= Biomarker
Cdk	= Cyclin-dependent Kinase
DLT	= Dose-limiting Toxicity
eIF4E	= Eukaryotic Initiation Factor 4E
ERK	= Extracellular Signal-Regulated Kinase
FDG	= Fluorodeoxyglucose
FOXO	= Forkhead Box O
GPCRs	= G Protein-Coupled Receptors
GSK3	= Glycogen Synthesis Kinase 3
GTP	= Guanosine Triphosphate
HER	= Human Epidermal Growth Factor Receptor
HIF-1alpha	= Hypoxia-Inducible Factor 1alpha
IGF1	= Insulin-Like Growth Factor 1
IkappaB-alpha	= Inhibitor of KappaB Alpha
IKK	= Inhibitor of KappaB Kinase
IRS1	= Insulin Receptor Substrate 1
LOH	= Loss of Heterozygosity

MAPK	= Mitogen-Activated Protein
mTOR	= Mammalian Target of Rapamycin
mTORC1	= mTOR Complex 1 (also known as mTOR-Raptor Complex)
mTORC2	= mTOR Complex 2 (also known as mTOR-Rictor Complex)
NF-kappaB	= Nuclear Factor KappaB
NSCLC	= Non Small Cell Lung Cancer
PDK1	= Phosphoinositide-Dependent Kinase 1
peIF-4G	= Phosphorylated eIF-4G
PET	= Positron Emission Tomography
PH	= Pleckstrin Homology
PI	= Phosphatidylinositol
PI3K	= Phosphoinositide 3-Kinases
PIP	= Phosphatidylinositol 3-Monophosphate
PIP2	= Phosphatidylinositol 4,5-Bisphosphate
PIP3	= Phosphatidylinositol 3,4,5-Trisphosphate
PKA	= Protein Kinase A
PKB	= Protein Kinase B (also known as AKT)
PKC	= Protein Kinase C
PRAS40	= Proline Rich AKT Substrate 40kDa
pS6	= Phosphorylated S6

PTEN = Phosphatase and TENsin Homolog Deleted on Chromosome Ten

Rheb = Ras Homolog Enriched in Brain

RTK = Receptor Tyrosine Kinase

SH2 = Src Homology 2

S6K = S6 Kinases

TKI = Tyrosine Kinase Inhibitors

TSC2 = Tuberous Sclerosis Complex 2

VEGF = Vascular Endothelial Growth Factor

REFERENCES

[1] Cantley LC. The phosphoinositide 3-kinase pathway. Science 2002; 296(5573): 1655-7.

[2] Fruman DA, Meyers RE, Cantley LC. Phosphoinositide kinases. Annu Rev Biochem 1998; 67: 481-507.

[3] Vanhaesebroeck B, Guillermet-Guibert J, Graupera M, Bilanges B. The emerging mechanisms of isoform-specific PI3K signaling. Nat Rev Mol Cell Biol 2010; 11(5): 329-41.

[4] Engelman JA, Luo J, Cantley LC. The evolution of phosphatidylinositol 3-kinases as regulators of growth and metabolism. Nat Rev Genet 2006; 7(8): 606-19.

[5] Zhao L, Vogt PK. Class I PI3K in oncogenic cellular transformation. Oncogene 2008; 27(41): 5486-96.

[6] Hsieh A, Moasser M. Targeting HER proteins in cancer therapy and the role of the non-target HER3. Br J Cancer 2007; 2007(97): 453-7.

[7] Nicholson K, Anderson N. The protein kinase B/AKT signaling pathway in human malignancy. Cell Signal 2002; 14: 381-95.

[8] Toker A, Newton A. Cellular signaling: Pivoting around PDK-1. Cell 2000; 103: 185-8.

[9] Bellacosa A, Chan TO, Ahmed NN, Datta K, Malstrom S, Stokoe D, *et al.* AKT activation by growth factors is a multiple-step process: The role of the PH domain. Oncogene 1998; 17(3): 313-25.

[10] Stokoe D, Stephens LR, Copeland T, Gaffney PR, Reese CB, Painter GF, *et al.* Dual role of phosphatidylinositol-3,4,5-trisphosphate in the activation of protein kinase B. Science 1997; 277(5325): 567-70.

[11] Guertin DA, Stevens DM, Thoreen CC, Burds AA, Kalaany NY, Moffat J, *et al.* Ablation in mice of the mTORC components raptor, rictor, or mLST8 reveals that mTORC2 is required for signaling to AKT-FOXO and PKCalpha, but not S6K1. Dev Cell 2006; 11(6): 859-71.

[12] Jacinto E, Facchinetti V, Liu D, Soto N, Wei S, Jung SY, *et al.* SIN1/MIP1 maintains rictor-mTOR complex integrity and regulates AKT phosphorylation and substrate specificity. Cell 2006; 127(1): 125-37.

[13] Sarbassov DD, Guertin DA, Ali SM, Sabatini DM. Phosphorylation and regulation of AKT/PKB by the rictor-mTOR complex. Science 2005; 307(5712): 1098-101.

[14] Jacinto E, Loewith R, Schmidt A, Lin SF, Ruegg M, Hall A, *et al.* Mammalian TOR complex 2 controls the actin cytoskeleton and is rapamycin insensitive. Nat Cell Biol 2004; 6: 1122-8.

[15] Duronio V. The life of a cell: Apoptosis regulation by the PI3K/PKB pathway. Biochem J 2008; 415(3): 333-44.

[16] Liang J, Zubovitz J, Petrocelli T, Kotchetkov R, Connor MK, Han K, *et al.* PKB/AKT phosphorylates p27, impairs nuclear import of p27 and opposes p27-mediated G1 arrest. Nat Med 2002; 8(10): 1153-60.

[17] Shin I, Rotty J, Wu FY, Arteaga CL. Phosphorylation of p27Kip1 at Thr-157 interferes with its association with importing α during G1 and prevents nuclear re-entry. J Biol Chem 2005; 280(7): 6055-63.

[18] Zhou BP, Liao Y, Xia W, Spohn B, Lee MH, Hung MC. Cytoplasmic localization of p21Cip1/WAF1 by AKT-induced phosphorylation in HER-2/neu-overexpressing cells. Nat Cell Biol 2001; 3(3): 245-52.

[19] Brunet A, Bonni A, Zigmond MJ, Lin MZ, Juo P, Hu LS, *et al.* AKT promotes cell survival by phosphorylating and inhibiting a Forkhead transcription factor. Cell 1999; 96(6): 857-68.

[20] Datta SR, Dudek H, Tao X, Masters S, Fu H, Gotoh Y, *et al.* AKT phosphorylation of BAD couples survival signals to the cell-intrinsic death machinery. Cell 1997; 91(2): 231-41.

[21] Mayo L, Donner D. The PTEN, Mdm2, p53 tumor suppressor oncoprotein network. Trends Biochem Sci 2002; 27: 462-7.

[22] Romashkova J, Makarov S. NF-kappaB is a target of AKT in anti-apoptotic PDGF signaling. Nature 1999; 401: 86-90.

[23] Diehl JA, Cheng M, Roussel MF, Sherr CJ. Glycogen synthase kinase-3β regulates cyclin D1 proteolysis and subcellular localization. Genes Dev 1998; 12(22): 3499-511.

[24] Sekulic A, Hudson C, Homme J, Yin P, Otterness D, Karnitz L, *et al.* A direct linkage between the phosphoinositide 3-kinase-AKT signaling pathway and the mammalian target of rapamycin in mitogen-stimulated and transformed cells. Cancer Res 2000; 60(13): 3504-13.

[25] Inoki K, Li Y, Zhu T, Wu J, Guan K. TSC2 is phosphorylated and inhibited by AKT and suppresses mTOR signaling. Nat Cell Biol 2002; 4(9): 648-57.

[26] Hara K, Maruki Y, Long X, Yoshino K, Oshiro N, Hidayat S, *et al.* Raptor, a binding partner of target of rapamycin (TOR), mediates TOR action. Cell 2002; 110(2): 177-89.

[27] Burnett P, Barrow R, Cohen N, Snyder S, Sabatini DM. RAFT1 phosphorylation of the translational regulators p70 S6 kinase and 4E-BP1. Proc Natl Acad Sci USA 1998; :95(4): 1432-7.

[28] Fonseca B, Smith E, Lee V, MacKintosh C, Proud C. PRAS40 is a target for mammalian target of rapamycin complex 1 and is required for signaling downstream of this complex. J Biol Chem 2007; 282: 24514-24.

[29] Oshiro N, Takahashi R, Yoshino K, Tanimura K, Nakashima A, Eguchi S, *et al.* The proline-rich AKT substrate of 40 kDa (PRAS40) is a physiological substrate of mammalian target of rapamycin complex 1. J Biol Chem 2007; 282(28): 20329-39.

[30] Skinner HD, Zheng JZ, Fang J, Agani F, Jiang BH. Vascular endothelial growth factor transcriptional activation is mediated by hypoxia-inducible factor 1alpha, HDM2, and p70S6K1 in response to phosphatidylinositol 3-kinase/AKT signaling. J Biol Chem 2004; 279(44): 45643-51.

[31] Luo J, Sobkiw CL, Hirshman MF, Logsdon MN, Li TQ, Goodyear LJ, *et al.* Loss of class IA PI3K signaling in muscle leads to impaired muscle growth, insulin response, and hyperlipidemia. Cell Metab 2006; 3(5): 355-66.

[32] Jia S, Liu Z, Zhang S, Liu P, Zhang L, Lee SH, *et al.* Essential roles of PI(3)K-p110β in cell growth, metabolism and tumorigenesis. Nature 2008; 454(7205): 776-9.

[33] Knight ZA, Gonzalez B, Feldman ME, Zunder ER, Goldenberg DD, Williams O, *et al.* A pharmacological map of the PI3-K family defines a role for p110alpha in insulin signaling. Cell 2006; 125(4): 733-47.

[34] Foukas LC, Claret M, Pearce W, Okkenhaug K, Meek S, Peskett E, *et al.* Critical role for the p110α phosphoinositide-3-OH kinase in growth and metabolic regulation. Nature 2006; 441(7091): 366-70.

[35] Maehama T, Dixon JE. The Tumor Suppressor, PTEN/MMAC1, Dephosphorylates the lipid second messenger, phosphatidylinositol 3,4,5-trisphosphate. J Biol Chem 1998; 273(22): 13375-8.

[36] Di Cristofano A, Pesce B, Cordon-Cardo C, Pandolfi PP. PTEN is essential for embryonic development and tumor suppression. Nat Genet 1998; 19(4): 348-55.

[37] Salmena L, Carracedo A, Pandolfi PP. Tenets of PTEN tumor suppression. Cell 2008; 133(3): 403-14.

[38] Harrington LS, Findlay GM, Gray A, Tolkacheva T, Wigfield S, Rebholz H, *et al.* The TSC1-2 tumor suppressor controls insulin-PI3K signaling via regulation of IRS proteins. J Cell Biol 2004; 166(2): 213-23.

[39] Peterson TR, Laplante M, Thoreen CC, Sancak Y, Kang SA, Kuehl WM, *et al.* DEPTOR is an mTOR inhibitor frequently overexpressed in multiple myeloma cells and required for their survival. Cell 2009; 137(5): 873-86.

[40] Trotman LC, Pandolfi PP. PTEN and p53: Who will get the upper hand? Cancer Cell 2003; 3(2): 97-9.

[41] Cully M, You H, Levine AJ, Mak TW. Beyond PTEN mutations: The PI3K pathway as an integrator of multiple inputs during tumorigenesis. Nat Rev Cancer 2006; 6(3): 184-92.

[42] Shaw RJ, Cantley LC. Ras, PI(3)K and mTOR signaling controls tumor cell growth. Nature 2006; 441(7092): 424-30.

[43] Ma L, Chen Z, Erdjument-Bromage H, Tempst P, Pandolfi PP. Phosphorylation and functional inactivation of TSC2 by Erk implications for tuberous sclerosis and cancer pathogenesis. Cell 2005; 121(2): 179-93.

[44] Carracedo A, Ma L, Teruya-Feldstein J, Rojo F, Salmena L, Alimonti A, *et al.* Inhibition of mTORC1 leads to MAPK pathway activation through a PI3K-dependent feedback loop in human cancer. J Clin Invest 2008; 118(9): 3065-74.

[45] Eng C. PTEN: One gene, many syndromes. Hum Mutat 2003; 22(3): 183-98.

[46] Manning BD, Logsdon MN, Lipovsky AI, Abbott D, Kwiatkowski DJ, Cantley LC. Feedback inhibition of AKT signaling limits the growth of tumors lacking Tsc2. Genes Dev 2005; 19(15): 1773-8.

[47] Samuels Y, Wang Z, Bardelli A, Silliman N, Ptak J, Szabo S, *et al.* High Frequency of Mutations of the PIK3CA Gene in Human Cancers. Science 2004; 304(5670): 554.

[48] Campbell IG, Russell SE, Choong DYH, Montgomery KG, Ciavarella ML, Hooi CSF, *et al*. Mutation of the PIK3CA gene in ovarian and breast cancer. Cancer Res 2004; 64(21): 7678-81.

[49] Kang S, Seo SS, Chang HJ, Yoo CW, Park SY, Dong SM. Mutual exclusiveness between PIK3CA and KRAS mutations in endometrial carcinoma. Int J Gynecol Cancer 2008; 18(6): 1339-43.

[50] Massion PP, Kuo WL, Stokoe D, Olshen AB, Treseler PA, Chin K, *et al*. Genomic copy number analysis of non-small cell lung cancer using array comparative genomic hybridization: Implications of the phosphatidylinositol 3-kinase pathway. Cancer Res 2002; 62(13): 3636-40.

[51] Lee JW, Soung YH, Kim SY, Lee HW, Park WS, Nam SW, *et al*. PIK3CA gene is frequently mutated in breast carcinomas and hepatocellular carcinomas. Oncogene 2005; 24(8): 1477-80.

[52] Garcia Pedrero JM, Garcia Carracedo D, Muñoz Pinto C, Herrero Zapatero A, Rodrigo JP, Suarez Nieto C, *et al*. Frequent genetic and biochemical alterations of the PI 3-K/AKT/PTEN pathway in head and neck squamous cell carcinoma. Int J Cancer 2005; 114(2): 242-8.

[53] Stemke-Hale K, Gonzalez-Angulo AM, Lluch A, Neve RM, Kuo WL, Davies M, *et al*. An integrative genomic and proteomic analysis of PIK3CA, PTEN, and AKT mutations in breast cancer. Cancer Res 2008; 68(15): 6084-91.

[54] Samuels Y, Velculescu VE. Oncogenic mutations of PIK3CA in human cancers. Cell Cycle 2004; 3(10): 1221-4.

[55] Velho S, Oliveira C, Ferreira A, Ferreira AC, Suriano G, Schwartz Jr S, *et al*. The prevalence of PIK3CA mutations in gastric and colon cancer. Eur J Cancer 2005; 41(11): 1649-54.

[56] Santarpia L, Qi Y, Stemke-Hale K, Wang B, Young EJ, Booser DJ, *et al*. Mutation profiling identifies numerous rare drug targets and distinct mutation patterns in different clinical subtypes of breast cancers. Breast Cancer Res Treat 2012; 134(1): 333-43.

[57] Banerji S, Cibulskis K, Rangel-Escareno C, Brown KK, Carter SL, Frederick AM, *et al*. Sequence analysis of mutations and translocations across breast cancer subtypes. Nature 2012; 486(7403): 405-9.

[58] Bell D, Berchuck A, Birrer M, Chien J, Cramer D, Dao F, *et al*. Integrated genomic analyses of ovarian carcinoma. Nature 2011; 474(7353): 609-15.

[59] Shah SP, Roth A, Goya R, Oloumi A, Ha G, Zhao Y, *et al*. The clonal and mutational evolution spectrum of primary triple-negative breast cancers. Nature 2012; 486(7403): 395-9.

[60] De Roock W, Claes B, Bernasconi D, De Schutter J, Biesmans B, Fountzilas G, *et al*. Effects of KRAS, BRAF, NRAS, and PIK3CA mutations on the efficacy of cetuximab plus chemotherapy in chemotherapy-refractory metastatic colorectal cancer: A retrospective consortium analysis. Lancet Oncol 2010; 11(8): 753-62.

[61] Huang CH, Mandelker D, Schmidt-Kittler O, Samuels Y, Velculescu VE, Kinzler KW, *et al*. The structure of a human p110α/p85α complex elucidates the effects of oncogenic PI3Kα mutations. Science 2007; 318(5857): 1744-8.

[62] Miled N, Yan Y, Hon WC, Perisic O, Zvelebil M, Inbar Y, *et al*. Mechanism of two classes of cancer mutations in the phosphoinositide 3-kinase catalytic subunit. Science 2007; 317(5835): 239-42.

[63] Zhao L, Vogt PK. Helical domain and kinase domain mutations in p110α of phosphatidylinositol 3-kinase induce gain of function by different mechanisms. Proc Natl Acad Sci USA 2008; 105(7): 2652-7.

[64] Shayesteh L, Lu Y, Kuo WL, Baldocchi R, Godfrey T, Collins C, *et al.* PIK3CA is implicated as an oncogene in ovarian cancer. Nat Genet 1999; 21(1): 99-102.

[65] Mizoguchi M, Nutt CL, Mohapatra G, Louis DN. Genetic alterations of phosphoinositide 3-kinase subunit genes in human glioblastomas. Brain Pathol 2004; 14(4): 372-7.

[66] Philp AJ, Campbell IG, Leet C, Vincan E, Rockman SP, Whitehead RH, *et al.* The phosphatidylinositol 3′-kinase p85α gene is an oncogene in human ovarian and colon tumors. Cancer Res 2001; 61(20): 7426-9.

[67] Shekar SC, Wu H, Fu Z, Yip SC, Nagajyothi, Cahill SM, *et al.* Mechanism of constitutive phosphoinositide 3-kinase activation by oncogenic mutants of the p85 regulatory subunit. J Biol Chem 2005; 280(30): 27850-5.

[68] Ikenoue T, Kanai F, Hikiba Y, Obata T, Tanaka Y, Imamura J, *et al.* Functional analysis of PIK3CA gene mutations in human colorectal cancer. Cancer Res 2005; 65(11): 4562-7.

[69] Bénistant C, Chapuis H, Roche S. A specific function for phosphatidylinositol 3-kinase α (p85α-p110α) in cell survival and for phosphatidylinositol 3-kinase β (p85α-p110β) in *de novo* DNA synthesis of human colon carcinoma cells. Oncogene 2000; 19(44): 5083-90.

[70] Knobbe CB, Reifenberger G. Genetic alterations and aberrant expression of genes related to the phosphatidyl-inositol-3′ kinase/protein kinase B (AKT) signal transduction pathway in glioblastomas. Brain Pathol 2003; 13(4): 507-18.

[71] An HJ, Cho NH, Yang HS, Kwak KB, Kim NK, Oh DY, *et al.* Targeted RNA interference of phosphatidylinositol 3-kinase p110-beta induces apoptosis and proliferation arrest in endometrial carcinoma cells. J Pathol 2007; 212(2): 161-9.

[72] Kang S, Denley A, Vanhaesebroeck B, Vogt PK. Oncogenic transformation induced by the p110β, -γ, and -δ isoforms of class I phosphoinositide 3-kinase. Proc Natl Acad Sci USA 2006; 103(5): 1289-94.

[73] Hickey FB, Cotter TG. BCR-ABL regulates phosphatidylinositol 3-kinase-p110gamma transcription and activation and is required for proliferation and drug resistance. J Biol Chem 2006; 281(5): 2441-50.

[74] Sujobert P, Bardet V, Cornillet-Lefebvre P, Hayflick JS, Prie N, Verdier F, *et al.* Essential role for the p110delta isoform in phosphoinositide 3-kinase activation and cell proliferation in acute myeloid leukemia. Blood 2005; 106(3): 1063-6.

[75] Tamburini J, Green AS, Bardet V, Chapuis N, Park S, Willems L, *et al.* Protein synthesis is resistant to rapamycin and constitutes a promising therapeutic target in acute myeloid leukemia. Blood 2009; 114(8): 1618-27.

[76] Shoji K, Oda K, Nakagawa S, Hosokawa S, Nagae G, Uehara Y, *et al.* The oncogenic mutation in the pleckstrin homology domain of AKT1 in endometrial carcinomas. Br J Cancer 2009; 101(1): 145-8.

[77] Carpten JD, Faber AL, Horn C, Donoho GP, Briggs SL, Robbins CM, *et al.* A transforming mutation in the pleckstrin homology domain of AKT1 in cancer. Nature 2007; 448(7152): 439-44.

[78] Dutt A, Salvesen HB, Greulich H, Sellers WR, Beroukhim R, Meyerson M. Somatic mutations are present in all members of the AKT family in endometrial carcinoma. Br J Cancer 2009; 101(7): 1218-9; 20-1.

[79] Cheng JQ, Godwin AK, Bellacosa A, Taguchi T, Franke TF, Hamilton TC, *et al.* AKT2, a putative oncogene encoding a member of a subfamily of protein-serine/threonine kinases, is amplified in human ovarian carcinomas. Proc Natl Acad Sci USA 1992; 89(19): 9267-71.

[80] Soung YH, Lee JW, Nam SW, Lee JY, Yoo NJ, Lee SH. Mutational analysis of AKT1, AKT2 and AKT3 genes in common human carcinomas. Oncology 2006; 70(4): 285-9.

[81] Davies MA, Stemke-Hale K, Tellez C, Calderone TL, Deng W, Prieto VG, *et al.* A novel AKT3 mutation in melanoma tumors and cell lines. Br J Cancer 2008; 99(8): 1265-8.

[82] Bellacosa A, de Feo D, Godwin AK, Bell DW, Cheng JQ, Altomare DA, *et al.* Molecular alterations of the AKT2 oncogene in ovarian and breast carcinomas. Int J Cancer 1995; 64(4): 280-5.

[83] Nakatani K, Thompson DA, Barthel A, Sakaue H, Liu W, Weigel RJ, *et al.* Up-regulation of AKT3 in estrogen receptor-deficient breast cancers and androgen-independent prostate cancer lines. J Biol Chem 1999; 274(31): 21528-32.

[84] Ruggeri BA, Huang L, Wood M, Cheng JQ, Testa JR. Amplification and overexpression of the AKT2 oncogene in a subset of human pancreatic ductal adenocarcinomas. Mol Carcinogen 1998; 21(2): 81-6.

[85] Sato T, Nakashima A, Guo L, Coffman K, Tamanoi F. Single amino-acid changes that confer constitutive activation of mTOR are discovered in human cancer. Oncogene 2010; 29(18): 2746-52.

[86] García JM, Silva J, Peña C, Garcia V, Rodriguez R, Cruz MA, *et al.* Promoter methylation of the PTEN gene is a common molecular change in breast cancer. Gene Chromosome Canc 2004; 41(2): 117-24.

[87] Goel A, Arnold CN, Niedzwiecki D, Carethers JM, Dowell JM, Wasserman L, *et al.* Frequent inactivation of PTEN by promoter hypermethylation in microsatellite instability-high sporadic colorectal cancers. Cancer Res 2004; 64(9): 3014-21.

[88] Li J, Yen C, Liaw D, Podsypanina K, Bose S, Wang SI, *et al.* PTEN, a putative protein tyrosine phosphatase gene mutated in human brain, breast, and prostate cancer. Science 1997; 275(5308): 1943-7.

[89] Feilotter HE, Coulon V, McVeigh JL, Boag AH, Dorion-Bonnet F, Duboue B, *et al.* Analysis of the 10q23 chromosomal region and the PTEN gene in human sporadic breast carcinoma. Br J Cancer 1999; 79(5-6): 718-23.

[90] Cairns P, Okami K, Halachmi S, Halachmi N, Esteller M, Herman JG, *et al.* Frequent inactivation of PTEN/MMAC1 in primary prostate cancer. Cancer Res 1997; 57(22): 4997-5000.

[91] Reifenberger J, Wolter M, Bostrom J, Buschges R, Schulte KW, Megahed M, *et al.* Allelic losses on chromosome arm 10q and mutation of the PTEN (MMAC1) tumor suppressor gene in primary and metastatic malignant melanomas. Virchows Archiv : Int J Pathol 2000; 436(5): 487-93.

[92] Birck A, Ahrenkiel V, Zeuthen J, Hou-Jensen K, Guldberg P. Mutation and allelic loss of the PTEN/MMAC1 gene in primary and metastatic melanoma biopsies. J Invest Dermatol 2000; 114(2): 277-80.

[93] Byun DS, Cho K, Ryu BK, Lee MG, Park JI, Chae KS, *et al.* Frequent monoallelic deletion of PTEN and its reciprocal associatioin with PIK3CA amplification in gastric carcinoma. Int J Cancer 2003; 104(3): 318-27.

[94] Bilbao C, Rodriguez G, Ramirez R, Falcon O, Leon L, Chirino R, *et al.* The relationship between microsatellite instability and PTEN gene mutations in endometrial cancer. Int J Canc 2006; 119(3): 563-70.

[95] Guldberg P, thor Straten P, Birck A, Ahrenkiel V, Kirkin AF, Zeuthen J. Disruption of the MMAC1/PTEN gene by deletion or mutation is a frequent event in malignant melanoma. Cancer Res 1997; 57(17): 3660-3.

[96] Rhei E, Kang L, Bogomolniy F, Federici MG, Borgen PI, Boyd J. Mutation analysis of the putative tumor suppressor gene PTEN/MMAC1 in primary breast carcinomas. Cancer Res 1997; 57(17): 3657-9.

[97] Tashiro H, Blazes MS, Wu R, Cho KR, Bose S, Wang SI, *et al.* Mutations in PTEN are frequent in endometrial carcinoma but rare in other common gynecological malignancies. Cancer Res 1997; 57(18): 3935-40.

[98] Wang SI, Puc J, Li J, Bruce JN, Cairns P, Sidransky D, *et al.* Somatic mutations of PTEN in glioblastoma multiforme. Cancer Res. 1997; 57(19): 4183-6.

[99] Bose S, Wang SI, Terry MB, Hibshoosh H, Parsons R. Allelic loss of chromosome 10q23 is associated with tumor progression in breast carcinomas. Oncogene 1998; 17(1): 123-7.

[100] McMenamin ME, Soung P, Perera S, Kaplan I, Loda M, Sellers WR. Loss of PTEN expression in paraffin-embedded primary prostate cancer correlates with high Gleason score and advanced stage. Cancer Res 1999; 59(17): 4291-6.

[101] Risinger JI, Hayes K, Maxwell GL, Carney ME, Dodge RK, Barrett JC, *et al.* PTEN mutation in endometrial cancers is associated with favorable clinical and pathologic characteristics. Clin Cancer Res 1998; 4(12): 3005-10.

[102] Rasheed BK, Stenzel TT, McLendon RE, Parsons R, Friedman AH, Friedman HS, *et al.* PTEN gene mutations are seen in high-grade but not in low-grade gliomas. Cancer Res 1997; 57(19): 4187-90.

[103] Smith JS, Tachibana I, Passe SM, Huntley BK, Borell TJ, Iturria N, *et al.* PTEN mutation, EGFR amplification, and outcome in patients with anaplastic astrocytoma and glioblastoma multiforme. J Natl Cancer Inst 2001; 93(16): 1246-56.

[104] Goel VK, Lazar AJ, Warneke CL, Redston MS, Haluska FG. Examination of mutations in BRAF, NRAS, and PTEN in primary cutaneous melanoma. J Invest Dermatol 2006; 126(1): 154-60.

[105] Mikhail M, Velazquez E, Shapiro R, Berman R, Pavlick A, Sorhaindo L, *et al.* PTEN expression in melanoma: Relationship with patient survival, Bcl-2 expression, and proliferation. Clin Cancer Res 2005; 11(14): 5153-7.

[106] Depowski PL, Rosenthal SI, Ross JS. Loss of expression of the PTEN gene protein product is associated with poor outcome in breast cancer. Mod Pathol 2001; 14(7): 672-6.

[107] Ikeda T, Yoshinaga K, Suzuki A, Sakurada A, Ohmori H, Horii A. Anticorresponding mutations of the KRAS and PTEN genes in human endometrial cancer. Oncol Rep 2000; 7(3): 567-70.

[108] To MD, Perez-Losada J, Mao JH, Balmain A. Crosstalk between Pten and Ras signaling pathways in tumor development. Cell Cycle 2005; 4(9): 1185-8.

[109] Kurose K, Gilley K, Matsumoto S, Watson PH, Zhou XP, Eng C. Frequent somatic mutations in PTEN and TP53 are mutually exclusive in the stroma of breast carcinomas. Nat Genet 2002; 32(3): 355-7.

[110] Hollestelle A, Elstrodt F, Nagel JH, Kallemeijn WW, Schutte M. Phosphatidylinositol-3-OH kinase or RAS pathway mutations in human breast cancer cell lines. Mol Cancer Res 2007; 5(2): 195-201.

[111] Perez-Tenorio G, Alkhori L, Olsson B, Waltersson MA, Nordenskjold B, Rutqvist LE, *et al.* PIK3CA mutations and PTEN loss correlate with similar prognostic factors and are not mutually exclusive in breast cancer. Clin Cancer Res 2007; 13(12): 3577-84.

[112] Wee S, Wiederschain D, Maira S-M, Loo A, Miller C, deBeaumont R, *et al.* PTEN-deficient cancers depend on PIK3CB. Proc Natl Acad Sci USA 2008; 105(35): 13057-62.

[113] Oda K, Okada J, Timmerman L, Rodriguez-Viciana P, Stokoe D, Shoji K, *et al.* PIK3CA cooperates with other phosphatidylinositol 3'-kinase pathway mutations to effect oncogenic transformation. Cancer Res 2008; 68(19): 8127-36.

[114] Jia S, Roberts TM, Zhao JJ. Should individual PI3 kinase isoforms be targeted in cancer? Curr Opin Cell Biol 2009; 21(2): 199-208.

[115] Engelman JA, Chen L, Tan X, Crosby K, Guimaraes AR, Upadhyay R, *et al.* Effective use of PI3K and MEK inhibitors to treat mutant Kras G12D and PIK3CA H1047R murine lung cancers. Nat Med 2008; 14(12): 1351-6.

[116] Ihle NT, Lemos R, Wipf P, Yacoub A, Mitchell C, Siwak D, *et al.* Mutations in the phosphatidylinositol-3-Kinase pathway predict for antitumor activity of the inhibitor PX-866 whereas oncogenic Ras is a dominant predictor for resistance. Cancer Res 2009; 69(1): 143-50.

[117] Maira SM, Stauffer F, Brueggen J, Furet P, Schnell C, Fritsch C, *et al.* Identification and characterization of NVP-BEZ235, a new orally available dual phosphatidylinositol 3-kinase/mammalian target of rapamycin inhibitor with potent *in vivo* antitumor activity. Mol Cancer Ther 2008; 7(7): 1851-63.

[118] Serra V, Markman B, Scaltriti M, Eichhorn PJA, Valero V, Guzman M, *et al.* NVP-BEZ235, a dual PI3K/mTOR inhibitor, prevents PI3K signaling and inhibits the growth of cancer cells with activating PI3K mutations. Cancer Res 2008; 68(19): 8022-30.

[119] She QB, Chandarlapaty S, Ye Q, Lobo J, Haskell KM, Leander KR, *et al.* Breast tumor cells with PI3K mutation or HER2 amplification are selectively addicted to AKT signaling. PLoS One 2008; 3(8): e3065.

[120] Tanaka H, Yoshida M, Tanimura H, Fujii T, Sakata K, Tachibana Y, *et al.* The selective class I PI3K inhibitor CH5132799 targets human cancers harboring oncogenic PIK3CA mutations. Clin Cancer Res 2011; 17(10): 3272-81.

[121] Janku F, Wheler JJ, Westin SN, Moulder SL, Naing A, Tsimberidou AM, *et al.* PI3K/AKT/mTOR inhibitors in patients with breast and gynecologic malignancies harboring PIK3CA mutations. J Clin Oncol 2012; 30(8): 777-82.

[122] Weigelt B, Warne PH, Downward J. PIK3CA mutation, but not PTEN loss of function, determines the sensitivity of breast cancer cells to mTOR inhibitory drugs. Oncogene 2011; 30(29): 3222-33.

[123] Jessen K, Kessler L, Kucharski J, Guo X, Staunton J, Janes M, *et al.* Editors. A potent and selective PI3K inhibitor, INK1117, targets human cancers harboring oncogenic PIK3CA mutations [abstract]. AACR-NCI-EORTC: 23rd Molecular Targets and Cancer Therapeutics. San Francisco, USA (2011).

[124] Huang A, Fritsch C, Wilson C, Reddy A, Liu M, Lehar J, *et al.* Editors. Single agent activity of PIK3CA inhibitor BYL719 in a broad cancer cell line panel [abstract]. American Association for Cancer Research - 103rd Annual Meeting. Chicago, USA (2012).

[125] Dan S, Sugita H, Seki M, Mukai Y, Yamazaki K, Ishikawa Y, *et al.* editors. Efficacy of PI3K inhibitors to cancer cells with PIK3CA mutation or loss of PTEN expression. AACR-NCI-EORTC - 21st International Conference: Molecular Targets and Cancer Therapeutics. Boston, USA (2009).

[126] Liu N, Haegebarth A, Bull C, Schatz C, Wiehr S, Hauff P, *et al.* Editors. BAY 80-6946, a highly potent and efficacious class I PI3K inhibitor, induces complete tumor regression or tumor stasis in rat xenograft tumor models with PIK3CA mutant or PTEN deletion. American Association for Cancer Research-102nd Annual Meeting. Orlando, USA (2011).

[127] Vilar E, Mukherjee B, Kuick R, Raskin L, Misek DE, Taylor JM, *et al.* Gene expression patterns in mismatch repair-deficient colorectal cancers highlight the potential therapeutic role of inhibitors of the phosphatidylinositol 3-kinase-AKT-mammalian target of rapamycin pathway. Clin Cancer Res 2009; 15(8): 2829-39.
[128] Nagata Y, Lan KH, Zhou X, Tan M, Esteva FJ, Sahin AA, *et al.* PTEN activation contributes to tumor inhibition by trastuzumab, and loss of PTEN predicts trastuzumab resistance in patients. Cancer Cell 2004; 6(2): 117-27.
[129] Berns K, Horlings HM, Hennessy BT, Madiredjo M, Hijmans EM, Beelen K, *et al.* A functional genetic approach identifies the PI3K pathway as a major determinant of trastuzumab resistance in breast cancer. Cancer Cell 2007; 12(4): 395-402.
[130] Junttila TT, Akita RW, ParsonsK, Fields C, Lewis Phillips GD, Friedman LS, *et al.* Ligand-independent HER2/HER3/PI3K complex is disrupted by trastuzumab and is effectively inhibited by the PI3K inhibitor GDC-0941. Cancer Cell 2009; 15(5): 429-40.
[131] Eichhorn PJA, Gili M, Scaltriti M, Serra V, Guzman M, Nijkamp W, *et al.* Phosphatidylinositol 3-kinase hyperactivation results in lapatinib resistance that is reversed by the mTOR/phosphatidylinositol 3-kinase inhibitor NVP-BEZ235. Cancer Res 2008; 68(22): 9221-30.
[132] Jhawer M, Goel S, Wilson AJ, Montagna C, Ling YH, Byun DS, *et al.* PIK3CA mutation/PTEN expression status predicts response of colon cancer cells to the epidermal growth factor receptor inhibitor cetuximab. Cancer Res 2008; 68(6): 1953-61.
[133] Brognard J, Clark AS, Ni Y, Dennis PA. AKT/protein kinase B is constitutively active in non-small cell lung cancer cells and promotes cellular survival and resistance to chemotherapy and radiation. Cancer Res 2001; 61(10): 3986-97.
[134] Jiang Z, Pore N, Cerniglia GJ, Mick R, Georgescu MM, Bernhard EJ, *et al.* Phosphatase and tensin homologue deficiency in glioblastoma confers resistance to radiation and temozolomide that is reversed by the protease inhibitor nelfinavir. Cancer Res 2007; 67(9): 4467-73.
[135] Leuraud P, Taillandier L, Medioni J, Aguirre-Cruz L, Criniere E, Marie Y, *et al.* Distinct responses of xenografted gliomas to different alkylating agents are related to histology and genetic alterations. Cancer Res 2004; 64(13): 4648-53.
[136] Nakamura JL, Karlsson A, Arvold ND, Gottschalk AR, Pieper RO, Stokoe D, *et al.* PKB/AKT mediates radiosensitization by the signaling inhibitor LY294002 in human malignant gliomas. J Neurooncol 2005; 71(3): 215-22.
[137] Kim SH, Juhnn YS, Song YS. AKT involvement in paclitaxel chemoresistance of human ovarian cancer cells. Ann NY Acad Sci 2007; 1095: 82-9.
[138] Westfall SD, Skinner MK. Inhibition of phosphatidylinositol 3-kinase sensitizes ovarian cancer cells to carboplatin and allows adjunct chemotherapy treatment. Mol Cancer Ther 2005; 4(11): 1764-71.
[139] Krystal GW, Sulanke G, Litz J. Inhibition of phosphatidylinositol 3-kinase-AKT signaling blocks growth, promotes apoptosis, and enhances sensitivity of small cell lung cancer cells to chemotherapy. Mol Cancer Ther 2002; 1(11): 913-22.
[140] Clark AS, West K, Streicher S, Dennis PA. Constitutive and inducible AKT activity promotes resistance to chemotherapy, trastuzumab, or tamoxifen in breast cancer cells. Mol Cancer Ther 2002; 1(9): 707-17.
[141] Nahta R, Yu D, Hung MC, Hortobagyi GN, Esteva FJ. Mechanisms of disease: Understanding resistance to HER2-targeted therapy in human breast cancer. Nat Clin Pract Oncol 2006; 3(5): 269-80.

[142] Shoman N, Klassen S, McFadden A, Bickis MG, Torlakovic E, Chibbar R. Reduced PTEN expression predicts relapse in patients with breast carcinoma treated by tamoxifen. Mod Pathol 2005; 18(2): 250-9.

[143] Smith A, Blois J, Yuan H, Aikawa E, Ellson C, Figueiredo JL, *et al.* The antiproliferative cytostatic effects of a self-activating viridin prodrug. Mol Cancer Ther 2009; 8(6): 1666-75.

[144] Courtney KD, Corcoran RB, Engelman JA. The PI3K pathway as drug target in human cancer. J Clin Oncol 2010; 28(6): 1075-83.

[145] Engelman JA, Settleman J. Acquired resistance to tyrosine kinase inhibitors during cancer therapy. Curr Opin Genet Dev 2008; 18(1): 73-9.

[146] Baselga J. Novel agents in the era of targeted therapy: What have we learned and how has our practice changed? 33rd ESMO Congress. Stockholm, Sweden, 2008; vii281.

[147] Andersen JN, Sathyanarayanan S, Di Bacco A, Chi A, Zhang T, Chen AH, *et al.* Pathway-based identification of biomarkers for targeted therapeutics: Personalized oncology with PI3K pathway inhibitors. Sci Transl Med 2010; 2(43): 43ra55.

[148] Tabernero J, Rojo F, Calvo E, Burris H, Judson I, Hazell K, *et al.* Dose-and schedule-dependent inhibition of the mammalian target of rapamycin pathway with everolimus: A Phase I tumor pharmacodynamic study in patients with advanced solid tumors. J Clin Oncol 2008; 26(10): 1603-10.

[149] Shapiro G, Kwak E, Baselga J, Rodon J, Scheffold C, Laird AD, *et al.* Editors. Phase I dose-escalation study of XL147, a PI3K inhibitor administered orally to patients with solid tumors. American Society of Clinical Oncology. 45th Annual Meeting. Orlando, USA (2009).

[150] LoRusso P, Markman B, Tabernero J, Shazer R, Nguyen L, Heath E, *et al.* Editors. A Phase I dose-escalation study of the safety, pharmacokinetics (PK), and pharmacodynamics of XL765, a PI3K/TORC1/TORC2 inhibitor administered orally to patients (pts) with advanced solid tumors. American Society of Clinical Oncology. 45th Annual Meeting. Orlando, USA (2009).

[151] Diehl F, Schmidt K, Choti MA, Romans K, Goodman S, Li M, *et al.* Circulating mutant DNA to assess tumor dynamics. Nat Med 2007; 14(9): 985-90.

[152] Yao JC, Shah MH, Ito T, Bohas CL, Wolin EM, Van Cutsem E, *et al.* Everolimus for advanced pancreatic neuroendocrine tumors. N Engl J Med 2011; 364(6): 514-23.

[153] Hudes G, Carducci M, Tomczak P, Dutcher J, Figlin R, Kapoor A, *et al.* Temsirolimus, interferon alfa, or both for advanced renal-cell carcinoma. N Engl J Med 2007; 356(22): 2271-81.

[154] Motzer RJ, Escudier B, Oudard S, Hutson TE, Porta C, Bracarda S, *et al.* Efficacy of everolimus in advanced renal cell carcinoma: A double-blind, randomised, placebo-controlled Phase III trial. Lancet 2008; 372(9637): 449-56.

[155] Ellard SL, Clemons M, Gelmon KA, Norris B, Kennecke H, Chia S, *et al.* Randomized Phase II study comparing two schedules of everolimus in patients with recurrent/metastatic breast cancer: NCIC Clinical Trials Group IND. 163. J Clin Oncol 2009; 27(27): 4536-41.

[156] Baselga J, Campone M, Piccart M, Burris III HA, Rugo HS, Sahmoud T, *et al.* Everolimus in postmenopausal hormone-receptor-positive advanced breast cancer. N Engl J Med 2011; 366(6): 520-9.

[157] Jerusalem G, Fasolo A, Dieras V, Cardoso F, Bergh J, Vittori L, *et al.* Phase I trial of oral mTOR inhibitor everolimus in combination with trastuzumab and vinorelbine in pre-treated

patients with HER2-overexpressing metastatic breast cancer. Breast Cancer Res Treat 2011; 125(2): 447-55.

[158] Andre F, Campone M, O'Regan R, Manlius C, Massacesi C, Sahmoud T, *et al.* Phase I study of everolimus plus weekly paclitaxel and trastuzumab in patients with metastatic breast cancer pretreated with trastuzumab. J Clin Oncol 2010; 28(34): 5110-5.

[159] Slomovitz BM, Lu KH, Johnston T, Coleman RL, Munsell M, Broaddus RR, *et al.* A Phase 2 study of the oral mammalian target of rapamycin inhibitor, everolimus, in patients with recurrent endometrial carcinoma. Cancer 2010; 116(23): 5415-9.

[160] O'Reilly KE, Rojo F, She QB, Solit D, Mills GB, Smith D, *et al.* mTOR inhibition induces upstream receptor tyrosine kinase signaling and activates AKT. Cancer Res 2006; 66(3): 1500-8.

[161] Stein R. Prospects for phosphoinositide 3-kinase inhibition as a cancer treatment. Endocr-Relat Cancer 2001; 8(3): 237-48.

[162] Marone R, Cmiljanovic V, Giese B, Wymann MP. Targeting phosphoinositide 3-kinase-moving towards therapy. BBA-Proteins Proteom 2008; 1784(1): 159-85.

[163] Kong D, Yamori T. Advances in development of phosphatidylinositol 3-kinase inhibitors. Cur Med Chem 2009; 16(22): 2839-54.

[164] Maira SM, Stauffer F, Schnell C, García-Echeverría C. PI3K inhibitors for cancer treatment: Where do we stand? Biochem Soc Trans 2009; 37(1): 265.

[165] Knight Z, Shokat K. Chemically targeting the PI3K family. Biochem Soc Trans 2007; 35(Pt 2): 245.

[166] Walker EH, Perisic O, Ried C, Stephens L, Williams RL. Structural insights into phosphoinositide 3-kinase catalysis and signaling. Nature 1999; 402(6759): 313-20.

[167] Walker EH, Pacold ME, Perisic O, Stephens L, Hawkins PT, Wymann MP, *et al.* Structural determinants of phosphoinositide 3-kinase inhibition by wortmannin, LY294002, quercetin, myricetin, and staurosporine. Mol Cell 2000; 6(4): 909-19.

[168] Amzel LM, Huang CH, Mandelker D, Lengauer C, Gabelli SB, Vogelstein B. Structural comparisons of class I phosphoinositide 3-kinases. Nat Rev Cancer 2008; 8(9): 665-9.

[169] Sabbah DA, Simms NA, Brattain MG, Vennerstrom JL, Zhong H. Biological evaluation and docking studies of recently identified inhibitors of phosphoinositide-3-kinases. Bioorg Med Chem Lett 2012; 22(2): 876-80.

[170] Fuchikami K, Togame H, Sagara A, Satoh T, Gantner F, Bacon KB, *et al.* A versatile high-throughput screen for inhibitors of lipid kinase activity: Development of an immobilized phospholipid plate assay for phosphoinositide 3-kinase γ. J Biomol Screen 2002; 7(5): 441-50.

[171] ClinicalTrials.gov A serviceof the US. Available at: http://clinicaltrials.gov (Accessed on July 27, 2012)

[172] Chiorean EG, Mahadevan D, Harris WB, Von Hoff DD, Younger AE, Rensvold DM, *et al.* Editors. Phase I evaluation of SF1126, a vascular targeted PI3K inhibitor, administered twice weekly IV in patients with refractory solid tumors. American Society of Clinical Oncology. 45th Annual Meeting. Orlando, USA (2009).

[173] Mahadevan D, Chiorean EG, Harris W, Von Hoff DD, Younger A, Rensvold DM, *et al.* Editors. Phase I study of the multikinase prodrug SF1126 in solid tumors and B-cell malignancies. American Society of Clinical Oncology. 47th Annual Meeting. Chicago, USA (2011).

[174] Burris H, Rodon J, Sharma S, Tabernero J, Infante JR, Silva A, *et al.* Editors. First-in-human Phase I study of the oral PI3K inhibitor BEZ235 in patients (pts) with advanced

solid tumors. American Society of Clinical Oncology. 46th Annual Meeting. Chicago, USA (2010).

[175] Rodon J, Infante J, Burris H, Tabernero JM. Editors. A Dose-Escalation Study with a Special Drug Delivery System (SDS) of BEZ235, a Novel Dual PI3K/mTOR Inhibitor, in Patients with Metastatic/Advanced Solid Tumors. *2010 San Antonio Breast Cancer Symposium*. San Antonio, USA (2010).

[176] Peyton JD, Rodon Ahnert J, Burris H, Britten C, Chen LC, Tabernero J, *et al*. Editors. A dose-escalation study with the novel formulation of the oral pan-class I PI3K inhibitor BEZ235, solid dispersion system (SDS) sachet, in patients with advanced solid tumors. American Society of Clinical Oncology. 47th Annual Meeting. Chicago, USA (2011).

[177] Krop IE, Saura C, Rodon Ahnert J, Becerra C, Britten CD, Isakoff SJ, *et al*. Editors. A Phase I/IB dose-escalation study of BEZ235 in combination with trastuzumab in patients with PI3-kinase or PTEN altered HER2+ metastatic breast cancer [abstract]. American Society of Clinical Oncology. *47th Annual Meeting Proceeding*. Chicago, USA (2012).

[178] Arkenau H-T, Jones SF, Kurkjian C, Infante JR, Pant S, Burris HA, *et al*. Editors. The PI3K/mTOR inhibitor BEZ235 given twice daily for the treatment of patients (pts) with advanced solid tumors. Americal Society of Clinical Oncology. 48th Annual Meeting; Chicago, USA (2012).

[179] Salkeni MA, Beg MS, Olowokure OO, Fathallah H, Thomas H, Mercer CA, *et al*. Editors. A dose escalation, single arm, Phase Ib/II combination study of BEZ235 with everolimus to determine the safety, pharmacodynamics, and pharmacokinetics in subjects with advanced solid malignancies including glioblastoma multiforme. American Society of Clinical Oncology. 48th Annual Meeting. Chicago, USA (2012).

[180] Markman B, Tabernero J, Krop I, Shapiro GI, Siu L, Chen LC, *et al*. Phase I safety, pharmacokinetic, and pharmacodynamic study of the oral phosphatidylinositol-3-kinase and mTOR inhibitor BGT226 in patients with advanced solid tumors. Ann Oncol 2012; 23(9): 2399-408.

[181] Papadopoulos K, Markman B, Tabernero J, Patnaik A, Heath E, DeCillis A, *et al*. Editors. A Phase I dose-escalation study of the safety, pharmacokinetics (PK), and pharmacodynamics (PD) of a novel PI3K inhibitor, XL765, administered orally to patients (pts) with advanced solid tumors. American Society of Clinical Oncology. 45th Annual Meeting. Chicago, USA (2008).

[182] Markman B, LoRusso P, Patnaik A, Heath E, Laird A, van Leeuwen B, *et al*. Editors. A Phase I dose-escalation study of the safety, pharmacokinetics and pharmacodynamics of XL765, a novel inhibitor of PI3K and mTOR, administered orally to patients with solid tumors. *24th EORTC-NCI-AACR Symposium on Molecular Targets and Cancer Therapeutics*. Geneva, Switzerland, 2008.

[183] Papadopoulos KP, Abrisqueta P, Chambers G, Rasco D, Patnaik A, Tabernero J, *et al*. Editors. A Phase I Dose Expansion Cohort Study of the Safety, Pharmacokinetics and Pharmacodynamics of SAR245409 (S09), An Orally Administered PI3K/mTOR Inhibitor, in Patients with Lymphoma. American Society of Hematology. 53rd Annual Meeting Abstracts. San Diego, USA (2011).

[184] Brana I, Lorusso P, Baselga J, Heath EI, Patnaik A, Gendreau S, *et al*. Editors. A Phase I dose-escalation study of the safety, pharmacokinetics (PK), and pharmacodynamics of XL765 (SAR245409), a PI3K/TORC1/TORC2 inhibitor administered orally to patients

(pts) with advanced malignancies. American Society of Clinical Oncology. 46th Annual Meeting. Chicago, USA (2010).

[185] Janne PA, Felip E, Cedres S, Cohen SJ, Engelman JA, Lucca J, *et al.* Editors. A Phase 1 safety and pharmacokinetic (PK) study of PI3K/TORC1/TORC2 inhibitor, XL765 (SAR245409), in combination with erlotinib in patients (pts) with advanced solid tumors. *25th AACR-NCI-EORTC International Conference on Molecular Targets and Cancer Therapeutics Boston*. USA, 2009.

[186] Cohen RB, Janne PA, Engelman JA, Martinez P, Nishida Y, Gendreau S, *et al.* Editors. A Phase I safety and pharmacokinetic (PK) study of PI3K/TORC1/TORC2 inhibitor XL765 (SAR245409) in combination with erlotinib (E) in patients (pts) with advanced solid tumors. American Society of Clinical Oncology. 46th Annual Meeting. Chicago, USA (2010).

[187] Wen PY, Omuro AM, Batchelor TT, Lai A, Mellinghoff IK, Nghiemphu L, *et al.* Editors. A Phase 1 safety and pharmacokinetic study of XL765 (SAR245409), a novel PI3K/TORC1/TORC2 inhibitor, in combination with temozolomide (TMZ) in patients (pts) with malignant glioma. *25th AACR-NCI-EORTC International Conference on Molecular Targets and Cancer Therapeutics.* Boston, USA (2009).

[188] Nghiemphu PL, Omuro AM, Cloughesy T, Mellinghoff IK, Norden AD, Nguyen LT, *et al.* Editors. A Phase I safety and pharmacokinetic study of XL765 (SAR245409), a novel PI3K/TORC1/TORC2 inhibitor, in combination with temozolomide (TMZ) in patients (pts) with newly diagnosed malignant glioma. American Society of Clinical Oncology. 46th Annual Meeting. Chicago, USA (2010).

[189] Baselga J, Tolaney S, Hart L, Gomez P, Gartner E, DeCillis A, *et al.* Editors. A Phase 1/2 Dose-Escalation Study of SAR245408 (S08) or SAR245409 (S09) in Combination with Letrozole (L) in Subjects with Hormone Receptor-Positive and HER2-Negative (HR+/HER2-) Breast Cancer (BC) Refractory to a Nonsteroidal Aromatase Inhibitor (AI). *2011 San Antonio Breast Cancer Symposium*. San Antonio, USA (2011).

[190] Bendell JC, Wagner AJ, Dolly S, Morgan JA, Papadatos-Pastos D, Ware J, *et al.* Editors. A first-in-human Phase I study to evaluate the dual PI3K/MTOR inhibitor GDC-0980 administered QD in patients with advanced solid tumors or Non-Hodgkin's lymphoma (NHL). *35th ESMO Congress*. Milan, Italy (2010).

[191] Dolly S, Wagner AJ, Bendell JC, Yan Y, Ware JA, Mazina KE, *et al.* Editors. A first-in-human, Phase 1 study to evaluate the dual PI3K/mTOR inhibitor GDC-0980 administered QD in patients with advanced solid tumors or non-Hodgkin's lymphoma. American Society of Clinical Oncology. 46th Annual Meeting. Chicago, USA (2010).

[192] Jin JY, Ware J, Malhi V, Upadhyay S, Wu J, Yan Y, *et al.* Population pharmacokinetics and pharmacody-namics of the dual PI3K/mTOR inhibitor GDC-0980 in Phase I patients with advanced solid tumors. Clin Pharmacol Ther 2011; 89: S81.

[193] Wagner AJ, Burris IHA, De Bono JS, Jayson GC, Bendell JC, Gomez-Roca C, *et al.* Pharmacokinetics and pharmacodynamic biomarkers for the dual PI3K/mTOR inhibitor GDC-0980: Initial Phase I evaluation. Mol Cancer Ther 2009; 8(12): B137.

[194] Wagner AJ, Jayson GC, Gomez-Roca C, Zee YK, Morgan JA, Yan Y, *et al.* A Phase I study evaluating the pharmacokinetics (PK) and pharmacodynamic (PD) activity of the dual PI3K/mTor inhibitor GDC-0980 administered QW. Eur J Cancer Suppl 2010; 8 (7): 123-4.

[195] Wagner AJ, Bendell JC, Dolly S, Morgan JA, Ware JA, Fredrickson J, *et al.* Editors. A first-in-human Phase I study to evaluate GDC-0980, an oral PI3K/mTOR inhibitor, administered QD in patients with advanced solid tumors. American Society of Clinical Oncology. 48th Annual Meeting. Chicago, USA (2011).

[196] Hollebecque A, Clamp A, Horsley L, Morgan JA, Bahleda R, George S, *et al.* Editors. A Phase I study evaluating the pharmacokinetics (PK) and pharmacodynamic (PD) activity of the dual PI3K/mTOR inhibitor GDC-0980 administered once weekly (QW). *AACR-NCI-EORTC - 23rd International Conference: Molecular Targets and Cancer Therapeutics*. San Francisco, USA (2011).

[197] Funke RP, Zhu J, Meng RD, Yan Y, Musib LC, Talluto CC, *et al.* Editors. A Phase Ib/II study testing the safety and efficacy of combined inhibition of the AKT/PI3K and AR signaling pathways in castration-resistant prostate cancer: GDC-0068 or GDC-0980 with abiraterone acetate versus abiraterone acetate. American Society of Clinical Oncology. 48th Annual Meeting. Chicago, USA (2012).

[198] Britten C, Adjei A, Millham R, Houk B, Wainberg Z, Guthrie T, *et al.* 383 First-in-human study of PF-04691502, a small molecule oral dual inhibitor of PI3K and mTOR in patients with advanced cancer: Preliminary report on safety and pharmacokinetics. Eur J Cancer Suppl 2010; 8(7): 121-2.

[199] LoRusso P, Britten C, Millham R, Borzillo G, Houk B, Wainberg Z, *et al.* Editors. First-in-patient study of PF-04691502, a small molecule intravenous dual inhibitor of PI3K and mTOR in patients with advanced cancer: Update on safety, efficacy, and pharmacology. *AACR-NCI-EORTC - 23rd International Conference: Molecular Targets and Cancer Therapeutics*. San Francisco, USA (2011).

[200] Finn R, Crown J, Boer K, Lang I, Parikh R, Breazna A, *et al.* Editors. Phase II Randomized Study of Pre-operative PF-04691502 plus letrozole compared with letrozole (L) in patients with estrogen receptor-positive, HER-2 negative early breast cancer (BC). *4th IMPAKT Breast Cancer Conference*. Brussels, Belgium (2012).

[201] Shapiro GI, Molina J, Bendell J, Brana I, Spicer J, Kwak E, *et al.* First-in-human study of PF-05212384, a small molecule intravenous dual inhibitor of PI3K and mTOR in patients with advanced cancer: Preliminary report on safety and pharmacokinetics. Eur J Cancer Suppl 2010; 8 (7): 123.

[202] Tabernero J, Bell-McGuinn K, Bendell J, Molina J, Kwak E, Millham R, *et al.* Editors. First-in-patient study of PF-05212384, a small molecule intravenous dual inhibitor of PI3K and mTOR in patients with advanced cancer: Update on safety, efficacy, and pharmacology. *AACR-NCI-EORTC - 23rd International Conference: Molecular Cancer Therapeutics*. San Francisco, USA (2011).

[203] Flaherty KT, Puzanov I, Kim KB, Ribas A, McArthur GA, Sosman JA, *et al.* Inhibition of Mutated, Activated BRAF in Metastatic Melanoma. N Engl J Med 2010; 363(9): 809-19.

[204] Munster PN, Van Der Noll R, Voest EE, Dees EC, Tan AR, Specht JM, *et al.* Editors. Phase I first-in-human study of the PI3 kinase inhibitor GSK2126458 (GSK458) in patients with advanced solid tumors (study P3K112826). American Society of Clinical Oncology. 47th Annual Meeting. Chicago, USA (2011).

[205] Grilley-Olson JE, Bedard P, Fasolo A, Blackman SC, Cartee L, Baker-Neblett KL, *et al.* Editors. A Phase I study of the MEK inhibitor GSK1120212 (GSK212) in combination with PI3K/mTOR inhibitor GSK2126458 (GSK458) in patients with advanced solid

tumors. *23rd AACR-NCI-EORTC Molecular Targets and Cancer*. San Francisco, USA (2011).

[206] Bendell JC, Rodon J, Burris HA, De Jonge M, Verweij J, Birle D, *et al*. Phase I, dose-escalation study of BKM120, an oral pan-class I PI3K inhibitor, in patients with advanced solid tumors. J Clin Oncol 2012; 30(3): 282-90.

[207] Baselga J, De Jonge MJ, Rodon J, Burris HA, Birle DC, De Buck SS, *et al*. Editors. A first-in-human Phase I study of BKM120, an oral pan-class I PI3K inhibitor, in patients (pts) with advanced solid tumors. American Society of Clinical Oncology. 46th Annual Meeting. Chicago, USA (2010).

[208] Grana B, Burris HA, Rodon Ahnert J, Abdul Razak AR, De Jonge MJ, Eskens F, *et al*. editors. Oral PI3 kinase inhibitor BKM120 monotherapy in patients (pts) with advanced solid tumors: An update on safety and efficacy. American Society of Clinical Oncology. 47th Annual Meeting. Chicago, USA (2011).

[209] Saura C, Burris H, Arteaga CL, Mayer I, Germa C, Fretault N, *et al*. Phase I safety experience with the oral pan-class I PI3K inhibitor BKM120 in patients with metastatic breast cancer (MBC). Eur J Cancer 2012; 48: S96.

[210] Rodon Ahnert J, Bendell J, Abdul Razak AR, Homji NF, Trandafir L, Quadt C, *et al*. Editors. Safety Profile and Clinical Activity of Single-Agent BKM120, a Pan-Class I PI3K Inhibitor, for the Treatment of Patients with Metastatic Breast Carcinoma. *San Antonio Breast Cancer Symposium*. San Antonio, TX, 2010.

[211] Saura C, Bendell J, Jerusalem G, Graña-Suarez B, Su S, Ru QC, *et al*. Editors. Phase I/II Study of BKM120 in Combination with Trastuzumab in Patients with HER2 Overexpressing Metastatic Breast Cancer Resistant to Trastuzumab-Containing Therapy. *San Antonio Breast Cancer Conference*. San Antonio, TX, 2011.

[212] Bedard P, Tabernero J, Kurzrock R, Britten CD, Stathis A, Perez-Garcia JM, *et al*. Editors. A Phase lb, open-label, multicenter, dose-escalation study of the oral pan-PI3K inhibitor BKM120 in combination with the oral MEK1/2 inhibitor GSK1120212 in patients (pts) with selected advanced solid tumors. American Society Clinical Oncology Annual Meeting. Chicago, USA (2012).

[213] Mayer IA, Abramson VG, Balko JM, Isakoff SJ, Kuba MG, Sanders M, *et al*. Editors. SU2C Phase Ib study of pan-PI3K inhibitor BKM120 with letrozole in ER+/HER2-metastatic breast cancer (MBC). American Society of Clinical Oncology. 48th Annual Meeting. Chicago, USA (2012).

[214] Nagaraj G, Ma CX, Luo J, Ellis MJ. Editors. A Phase I study of BKM120, a novel oral selective phosphatidylinositol-3-kinase (PI3K) inhibitor, in combination with fulvestrant in postmenopausal women with estrogen receptor positive metastatic breast cancer. American Society of Clinical Oncology. 48th Annual Meeting. Chicago, USA (2012).

[215] Kantor A, Daud A, Munster PN, Ea R, Algazi AP. Editors. A Phase I/II trial of BKM120 combined with vemurafenib (PLX4032) in BRAFV600E/k mutant advanced melanoma. American Society of Clinical Oncology. 48th Annual Meeting. Chicago, USA (2012).

[216] Edelman G, Bedell C, Shapiro G, Pandya SS, Kwak EL, Scheffold C, *et al*. Editors. A Phase I dose-escalation study of XL147 (SAR245408), a PI3K inhibitor administered orally to patients (pts) with advanced malignancies [abstract]. American Society of Clinical Oncology- 46th Annual Meeting. Chicago, USA (2010).

[217] Brown JR, Davids MS, Rodon J, Abrisqueta P, DeCillis AP, Rockich K, *et al*. Editors. Phase I Trial of SAR245408 (S08), a Pan-Phosphatidylinositol 3 Kinase (PI3K) Inhibitor,

in Patients with Chronic Lymphocytic Leukemia (CLL) and Lymphoma. American Society of Hematology. 53rd Annual Meeting. San Diego, USA (2011).

[218] Faulkner N, LoRusso PM, Guthrie T, Soria JC, Bahleda R, Bendell JC, *et al.* A Phase 1 safety and pharmacokinetic (PK) study of the PI3K inhibitor XL147 (SAR245408) in combination with erlotinib in patients with advanced solid tumors. Mol Cancer Ther 2009; 8(12 Suppl): C197.

[219] Moldovan C, Soria J, LoRusso P, Guthrie T, Song C, Nguyen LT, *et al.* Editors. A Phase I safety and pharmacokinetic (PK) study of the PI3K inhibitor XL147 (SAR245408) in combination with erlotinib in patients (pts) with advanced solid tumors. American Society of Clinical Oncology. 46th Annual Meeting. Chicago, USA (2010).

[220] Traynor AM, Kurzrock R, Bailey HH, Attia S, Scheffold C, Van Leeuwen B, *et al.* Editors. A Phase I safety and pharmacokinetic (PK) study of the PI3K inhibitor XL147 (SAR245408) in combination with paclitaxel (P) and carboplatin (C) in patients (pts) with advanced solid tumors. American Society of Clinical Oncology. 46th Annual Meeting. Chicago, USA (2010).

[221] Tolaney S, Burris H, Gartner E, Mayer G, Saura C, Maurer M, *et al.* Editors. A Phase 1/2 Study of SAR245408 (S08) in Combination with Trastuzumab (T) or Paclitaxel (P) and T in Patients with HER2+ Metastatic Breast Cancer (MBC) Who Progressed on a Previous T-Based Regimen. *2011 San Antonio Breast Cancer Conference*. San Antonio, USA (2011).

[222] Jimeno A, Hong DS, Hecker S, Clement R, Kurzrock R, Pestano LA, *et al.* Editors. Phase I trial of PX-866, a novel phosphoinositide-3-kinase (PI-3K) inhibitor. American Society of Clinical Oncology. 45th Annual Meeting. Orlando, USA (2009).

[223] Jimeno A, Herbst RS, Falchook GS, Messersmith WA, Hecker S, Peterson S, *et al.* Editors. Final results from a Phase I, dose-escalation study of PX-866, an irreversible, pan-isoform inhibitor of PI3 kinase. American Society of Clinical Oncology. 46th Annual Meeting. Chicago, USA (2010).

[224] Jimeno A, Herbst RS, Falchook GS, Messersmith WA, Camidge DR, Peterson SR, *et al.* A Phase 1 study of continuous dosing with PX-866, an irreversible, pan-isoform inhibitor of PI3 kinase. Eur J Cancer Suppl 2010; 8 (7): 116.

[225] Hong DS, Bowles DW, Falchook GS, Messersmith WA, George GC, O'Bryant CL, *et al.* A multicenter Phase I trial of PX-866, an oral irreversible phosphatidylinositol 3-kinase inhibitor, in patients with advanced solid tumors. Clin Cancer Res 2012; 18(15): 4173-82.

[226] Jimeno A, Senzer N, Wee Ma W, Rudin C, Bowles D, Vo A, *et al.* Results from the Phase 1 portion of a Phase 1/2 study of the irreversible PI-3K inhibitor PX-866 and docetaxel. Mol Cancer Ther 2011; 1.

[227] Jimeno A, Senzer NN, Rudin CM, Ma WW, Halmos B, Schnadig ID, *et al.* Editors. PX-866 and docetaxel in patients with advanced solid tumors. American Society of Clinical Oncology. 46th Annual Meeting. Chicago, USA (2012).

[228] Pitz MW, MacNeil MV, Macdonald DR, Kakumanu AS, Thiessen B, Tsao MS, *et al.* Editors. Phase II study of PX-866 in recurrent glioblastoma. American Society of Clinical Oncology. 48th Annual Meeting. Chicago, USA (2012).

[229] Von Hoff DD, Lorusso P, Tibes R, Shapiro G, Weiss GJ, Ware JA, *et al.* Editors. A first-in-human Phase i study to evaluate the pan-PI3K inhibitor GDC-0941 administered QD or BID in patients with advanced solid tumors. American Society of Clinical Oncology. 46th Annual Meeting. Chicago, USA (2010).

[230] Von Hoff DD, LoRusso P, Demetri GD, Weiss GJ, Shapiro G, Ramanathan RK, *et al.* Editors. A Phase I dose-escalation study to evaluate GDC-0941, a pan-PI3K inhibitor, administered QD or BID in patients with advanced or metastatic solid tumors. American Society of Clinical Oncology. 47th Annual Meeting. Chicago, USA (2011).

[231] Baird RD, Kristeleit RS, Sarker D, Olmos D, Sandhu SK, Yan Y, *et al.* Editors. A Phase I study evaluating the pharmacokinetics (PK) and pharmacodynamics (PD) of the oral panphosphoinositide-3 kinase (PI3K) inhibitor GDC-0941. American Society of Clinical Oncology. 46th Annual Meeting. Chicago, USA (2010).

[232] Sarker D, Kristeleit R, Mazina KE, Ware JA, Yan Y, Dresser M, *et al.* Editors. A Phase I study evaluating the pharmacokinetics (PK) and pharmacodynamics (PD) of the oral pan-phosphoinositide-3 kinase (PI3K) inhibitor GDC-0941. American Society of Clinical Oncology - 45th Annual Meeting. Orlando, USA (2009).

[233] Moreno Garcia V, Baird RD, Shah KJ, Basu B, Tunariu N, Blanco M, *et al.* Editors. A Phase I study evaluating GDC-0941, an oral phosphoinositide-3 kinase (PI3K) inhibitor, in patients with advanced solid tumors or multiple myeloma. American Society of Clinical Oncology. 47th Annual Meeting. Chicago, USA (2011).

[234] Besse B, Soria J, Gomez-Roca C, Ware JA, Adjei AA, Dy GK, *et al.* Editors. A Phase Ib study to evaluate the PI3-kinase inhibitor GDC-0941 with paclitaxel (P) and carboplatin (C), with and without bevacizumab (BEV), in patients with advanced non-small cell lung cancer (NSCLC). American Society of Clinical Oncology. 47th Annual Meeting. Chicago, USA (2011).

[235] Krop I, Wolff A, Winer E, Miller K, Park B, Ware J, *et al.* A Phase Ib Study Evaluating Safety, Tolerability, Pharmacokinetics (PK), and Activity of the Phosphoinositide-3 Kinase (PI3K) Inhibitor GDC-0941 in Combination with Trastuzumab-MCC-DM1 (T-DM1) in Patients with Advanced HER2-Positive Breast Cancer. American Association for Cancer Research - 102nd Annual Meeting. Orlando, USA (2011).

[236] Schoffski P, De Benedictis E, Gendreau S, Gianni L, Krop I, Levy G, *et al.* A Phase Ib, open-label, dose-escalation study of the safety and pharmacology of the PI3-kinase inhibitor GDC-0941 in combination with paclitaxel and bevacizumab in patients with locally recurrent or metastatic breast cancer. *34th Annual CTRC-AACR San Antonio Breast Cancer Symposium.* San Antonio, USA (2012)

[237] Shapiro G, LoRusso P, Kwak EL, Cleary JM, Musib L, Jones C, *et al.* Clinical combination of the MEK inhibitor GDC-0973 and the PI3K inhibitor GDC-0941: A first-in-human Phase Ib study testing daily and intermittent dosing schedules in patients with advanced solid tumors. American Society of Clinical Oncology - 47th Annual Meeting. Chicago, USA (2011).

[238] Bendell J, LoRusso P, Kwak E, Pandya S, Musib L, Jones C, *et al.* Editors. Clinical combination of the MEK inhibitor GDC-0973 and the PI3K inhibitor GDC-0941: A first-in-human Phase Ib study in patients with advanced solid tumors. America Association for Cancer Research. 102nd Annual Meeting. Orlando, USA (2011).

[239] LoRusso P, Shapiro G, Pandya SS, Kwak EL, Jones C, Belvin M, *et al.* Editors. A first-in-human Phase Ib study to evaluate the MEK inhibitor GDC-0973, combined with the pan-PI3K inhibitor GDC-0941, in patients with advanced solid tumors. American Society of Clinical Oncology. 48th Annual Meeting. Chicago, USA (2012).

[240] Result Summaries: GSK1059615. Available at: http://www.gsk-clinicalstudyregister.com/result_comp_list.jsp?Phase=Phase+1&studyType=All&population=All&marketing=All&compound=GSK1059615 (Accessed on July 26, 2012).

[241] Lotze MT, Appleman LJ, Ramanathan RK, Tolcher AW, Beeram M, Papadopoulos KP, *et al.* Editors. Phase I study of intravenous PI3K inhibitor BAY 80-6946: Activity in patients (pts) with advanced solid tumors and non-Hodgkin lymphoma treated in MTD expansion cohorts. Americal Society of Clinical Oncology. 48th Annual Meeting. Chicago, USA (2012).
[242] Patnaik A, Appleman LJ, Mountz JM, Ramanathan RK, Beeram M, Tolcher AW, *et al.* Editors. A first-in-human Phase I study of intravenous PI3K inhibitor BAY 80-6946 in patients with advanced solid tumors: Results of dose-escalation Phase. American Society of Clinical Oncology. 47th Annual Meeting. Chicago, USA (2011).
[243] Omlin AG, Spicer JF, Sarker D, Pinato DJ, Agarwal R, Cassier PA, *et al.* Editors. A pharmacokinetic (PK) pharmacodynamic (PD) driven first-in-human study of the oral class I PI3K inhibitor CH5132799, in patients with advanced solid tumors. American Society of Clinical Oncology. 48th Annual Meeting. Chicago, USA (2012).
[244] Juric D, Rodon J, Gonzalez-Angulo AM, Burris HA, Bendell J, Berlin JD, *et al.* Editors. BYL719, a next generation PI3K alpha specific inhibitor: Preliminary safety, PK, and efficacy results from the first-in-human study [abstract]. American Association for Cancer Research. 103rd Annual Meeting. Chicago, USA (2012).
[245] urman RR, Byrd JC, Flinn IW, Coutre SE, Benson DM, Brown JR, *et al.* Editors. Interim results from a Phase I study of CAL-101, a selective oral inhibitor of phosphatidylinositol 3-kinase p110d isoform, in patients with relapsed or refractory hematologic malignancies. American Society of Clinical Oncology. 46th Annual Meeting. Chicago, USA (2010).
[246] Coutre SE, Byrd JC, Furman RR, Brown JR, Benson DM, Wagner-Johnston ND, *et al.* Editors. Phase I study of CAL-101, an isoform-selective inhibitor of phosphatidylinositol 3-kinase P110d, in patients with previously treated chronic lymphocytic leukemia [abstract]. American Society of Clinical Oncology. 47th Annual Meeting. Chicago, USA (2011).
[247] Flinn IW, Byrd JC, Furman RR, Brown JR, Lin TS, Bello C, *et al.* editors. Preliminary evidence of clinical activity in a Phase I study of CAL-101, a selective inhibitor of the p1108 isoform of phosphatidylinositol 3-kinase (P13K), in patients with select hematologic malignancies. American Society of Clinical Oncology. 45th Annual Meeting. Orlando, USA (2009).
[248] Kahl B, Byrd JC, Flinn IW, Wagner-Johnston N, Spurgeon S, Benson Jr. DM, *et al.* Editors. Clinical Safety and Activity In a Phase 1 Study of CAL-101, An Isoform-Selective Inhibitor of Phosphatidylinositol 3-Kinase P110{delta}, In Patients with Relapsed or Refractory Non-Hodgkin Lymphoma. American Society of Hematology. 52nd Annual Meeting Abstracts. Orlando, USA (2010).
[249] Sharman J, de Vos S, Leonard JP, Furman RR, Coutre SE, Flinn IW, *et al.* Editors. A Phase 1 Study of the Selective Phosphatidylinositol 3-Kinase-Delta (PI3K{delta}) Inhibitor, CAL-101 (GS-1101), in Combination with Rituximab and/or Bendamustine in Patients with Relapsed or Refractory Chronic Lymphocytic Leukemia (CLL). American Society of Hematology. 53rd Annual Meeting. San Diego, CA (2011).
[250] Flinn IW, Schreeder MT, Coutre SE, Leonard J, Wagner-Johnston ND, De Vos S, *et al.* Editors. A Phase I study of CAL-101, an isoform-selective inhibitor of phosphatidylinositol 3-kinase P110 {delta}, in combination with anti-CD20 monoclonal antibody therapy and/or bendamustine in patients with previously treated B-cell malignancies. American Society of Clinical Oncology. 47th Annual Meeting. Chicago, USA (2011).

[251] de Vos S, Schreeder MT, Flinn IW, Coutre SE, Leonard JP, Wagner-Johnston ND, *et al.* Editors. A Phase 1 Study of the Selective Phosphatidylinositol 3-Kinase-Delta (PI3K{delta}) Inhibitor, Cal-101 (GS-1101), in Combination with Rituximab and/or Bendamustine in Patients with Previously Treated, Indolent Non-Hodgkin Lymphoma (iNHL). American Society of Hematology. 53rd Annual Meeting. San Diego, USA (2011).

[252] Furman RR, Barrientos JC, Sharman JP, De Vos S, Leonard J, Coutre SE, *et al.* Editors. A Phase I/II study of the selective phosphatidylinositol 3-kinase-delta (PI3K{delta}) inhibitor, GS-1101 (CAL-101), with ofatumumab in patients with previously treated chronic lymphocytic leukemia (CLL). Americal Society of Clinical Oncology. 48th Annual Meeting. Chicago, USA (2012).

[253] Tolcher AW, Yap TA, Fearen I, Taylor A, Carpenter C, Brunetto AT, *et al.* Editors. A Phase I study of MK-2206, an oral potent allosteric AKT inhibitor (AKTi), in patients (pts) with advanced solid tumor (ST). American Society of Clinical Oncology. 45th Annual Meeting. Orlando, USA (2009).

[254] Yap TA, Yan L, Patnaik A, Fearen I, Olmos D, Papadopoulos K, *et al.* Editors. First-in-man clinical trial of the oral pan-AKT inhibitor MK-2206 in patients with advanced solid tumors. American Society of Clinical Oncology. 47th Annual Meeting. Chicago, USA (2011).

[255] Biondo A, Yap TA, Yan L, Patnaik A, Fearen I, Baird RD, *et al.* Editors. Phase I clinical trial of an allosteric AKT inhibitor, MK-2206, using a once weekly (QW) dose regimen in patients with advanced solid tumors. American Society of Clinical Oncology. 47th Annual Meeting. Chicago, USA (2011).

[256] Yap TA, Papadopoulos K, Fearen I, Carpenter C, Delgado L, Taylor A, *et al.* First-in-man, first-in-class Phase I study of two schedules of MK-2206, a novel oral AKT inhibitor, in patients (pts) with advanced solid tumors including ovarian and castration resistant prostate cancer (CRPC). Mol Cancer Ther 2009; 8(12): B135.

[257] Yap TA, Yan L, Patnaik A, Olmos D, Fearen I, Baird RD, *et al.* Editors. Final results of a translational Phase I study assessing a QOD schedule of the potent AKT inhibitor MK-2206 incorporating predictive, pharmacodynamic (PD), and functional imaging biomarkers. American Society of Clinical Oncology. 47th Annual Meeting. Chicago, USA (2011).

[258] Knowling M, Blackstein M, Tozer R, Bramwell V, Dancey J, Dore N, *et al.* A Phase II study of perifosine (D-21226) in patients with previously untreated metastatic or locally advanced soft tissue sarcoma: A National Cancer Institute of Canada Clinical Trials Group trial. Invest New Drugs 2006; 24(5): 435-9.

[259] Argiris A, Cohen E, Karrison T, Esparaz B, Mauer A, Ansari R, *et al.* A Phase II trial of perifosine, an oral alkylphospholipid, in recurrent or metastatic head and neck cancer. Cancer Biol Ther 2006; 5(7): 766-70.

[260] Molife LR, Minton S, Vitfell-Pedersen J, Chen E, Sullivan D, Yan L, *et al.* A Phase I study of the potent AKT inhibitor MK-2206 in combination with carboplatin and paclitaxel, docetaxel or erlotinib in patients with advanced solid tumors. *2011 European Multidisciplinary Cancer Congress*. Stockholm, Sweden (2011).

[261] Han HS, Swanton C, Janjigian YY, Sutherland SC, Chandarlapaty S, Lehman R, *et al.* A Phase I study of the AKT inhibitor (MK-2206) with concurrent trastuzumab and lapatinib in patients with HER2-positive solid tumors. American Society of Clinical Oncology - 47th Annual Meeting, Chicago. Chicago, USA (2011).

[262] Khan KH, Yan L, Mezynski J, Patnaik A, Moreno V, Papadopoulos KP, *et al.* A Phase I dose escalation study of oral MK-2206 (allosteric AKT inhibitor) with oral selumetinib (AZD6244; ARRY-142866) (MEK 1/2 inhibitor) in patients with advanced or metastatic solid tumors. American Society of Clinical Oncology - 48th Annual Meeting. Chicago, USA (2012).

[263] Tolcher AW, Baird RD, Patnaik A, Moreno Garcia V, Papadopoulos KP, Garrett CR, *et al.* A Phase I dose-escalation study of oral MK-2206 (allosteric AKT inhibitor) with oral selumetinib (AZD6244; MEK inhibitor) in patients with advanced or metastatic solid tumors. American Society of Clinical Oncology - 47th Annual Meeting. Chicago, USA (2011).

[264] Brana I, Gray JE, Haluska P, Berger R, Golan T, Jones ME, *et al.* Editors. Rational molecularly targeted combinations: A parallel-arm Phase I trial of the humanized anti-IGF-1R antibody dalotuzumab (D) in combination with the allosteric AKT inhibitor MK-2206 or the gamma secretase inhibitor MK-0752, in patients with advanced solid tumors. American Society of Clinical Oncology. 48th Annual Meeting. Chicago, USA (2012).

[265] Kalinsky K, Sparano J, Kim M, Crew K, Maurer M, Taback B, *et al.* Pre-surgical evaluation of the AKT inhibitor MK-2206 in patients with operable invasive breast Cancer: New York Cancer Consortium Trial P8740. American Association for Cancer Research - 103rd Annual Meeting. Chicago, IL (2012).

[266] Speranza G, Kinders RJ, Khin S, Weil MK, Do KT, Horneffer Y, *et al.* Pharmacodynamic biomarker-driven trial of MK-2206, an AKT inhibitor, with AZD6244 (selumetinib), a MEK inhibitor, in patients with advanced colorectal carcinoma (CRC). Americal Society of Clinical Oncology - 48th Annual Meeting. Chicago, USA (2012).

[267] Burris HA, Siu LL, Infante JR, Wheler JJ, Kurkjian C, Opalinska J, *et al.* Safety, pharmacokinetics (PK), pharmacodynamics (PD), and clinical activity of the oral AKT inhibitor GSK2141795 (GSK795) in a Phase I first-in-human study. American Society of Clinical Oncology - 47th Annual Meeting. Chicago, USA (2011).

[268] Gungor H, Stronach E, Curry E, Saleem A, Agarwal R, Blagden S, *et al.* Mutation and protein expression biomarkers correlate with response to AKT inhibition in a Phase I trial of the oral pan AKT inhibitor GSK2141795 (GSK795) in patients (pts) with platinum resistant ovarian cancer. Eur J Cancer 2011; 47: 12-3.

[269] Kurzrock R, Patnaik A, Rosenstein L, Fu S, Papadopoulos KP, Smith DA, *et al.* Editors. Phase I dose-escalation of the oral MEK1/2 inhibitor GSK1120212 (GSK212) dosed in combination with the oral AKT inhibitor GSK2141795 (GSK795). American Society of Clinical Oncology. 47th Annual Meeting. Chicago, USA (2011).

[270] Tabernero J, Saura C, Roda Perez D, Dienstmann R, Rosello S, Prudkin L, *et al.* Editors. First-in-human Phase I study evaluating the safety, pharmacokinetics (PK), and intratumor pharmacodynamics (PD) of the novel, oral, ATP-competitive AKT inhibitor GDC-0068. American Society of Clinical Oncology. 47th Annual Meeting. Chicago, USA (2011).

[271] S Saura C, Jones S, Mateo J, Hollebecque A, Cleary JM, Roda Perez D, *et al.* Editors. A Phase Ib study of the AKT inhibitor GDC-0068 with docetaxel (D) or mFOLFOX-6 (F) in patients (pts) with advanced solid tumors. American Society of Clinical Oncology. 48th Annual Meeting. Chicago, USA (2012).

[272] Calvo E, Benhadji KA, Azaro A, Duran I, Argiles G, Boni V, *et al.* Editors. First-in-human Phase I study of LY2780301, an oral P70S6K/AKT inhibitor, in patients with refractory

solid tumors. American Society of Clinical Oncology. 48th Annual Meeting. Chicago, USA (2012).

[273] Infante JR, Tabernero J, Burris HA, Macarulla T, Martin M, Liu Y, *et al.* A Phase I, open label, dose escalation study of an oral mammalian target of rapamycin inhibitor INK128 administered once daily in patients with advanced malignancies. American Association for Cancer Research - 103rd Annual Meeting. Chicago, IL (2012).

[274] Tabernero J, Cervantes A, Gordon MS, Chiorean EG, Burris HA, Macarulla T, *et al.* A Phase I, open label, dose escalation study of oral mammalian target of rapamycin inhibitor INK128 administered by intermittent dosing regimens in patients with advanced malignancies. American Association for Cancer Research - 103rd Annual Meeting. Chicago, IL (2012).

[275] Naing A, Aghajanian C, Raymond E, Kurzrock R, Blanco M, Oelmann E, *et al.* First results from a Phase I trial of AZD8055, a dual mTORC1 and mTORC2 inhibitor. *AACR-NCI-EORTC - 27th International Conference on Molecular Targets and Cancer Therapeutics.* San Francisco, USA (2011).

[276] Tan DS, Dumez H, Olmos D, Sandhu SK, Hoeben A, Stephens AW, *et al.* Editors. First-in-human Phase I study exploring three schedules of OSI-027, a novel small molecule TORC1/TORC2 inhibitor, in patients with advanced solid tumors and lymphoma. American Society of Clinical Oncology. 46th Annual Meeting. Chicago, USA (2010).

[277] Banerji U, Dean EJ, Gonzalez M, Greystoke AP, Basu B, Krebs M, *et al.* Editors. First-in-human Phase I trial of the dual mTORC1 and mTORC2 inhibitor AZD2014 in solid tumors. American Society of Clinical Oncology. 48th Annual Meeting. Chicago, USA (2012).

[278] Shih KC, Bendell JC, Reinert A, Jones S, Kelley RK, Infante JR, *et al.* Editors. Phase I trial of an oral TORC1/TORC2 inhibitor (CC-223) in advanced solid and hematologic cancers. American Society of Clinical Oncology. 48th Annual Meeting. Chicago, USA (2012).

[279] Garlich JR, De P, Dey N, Jing DS, Peng X, Miller A, *et al.* A vascular targeted pan phosphoinositide 3-kinase inhibitor prodrug, SF1126, with antitumor and antiangiogenic activity. Cancer Res 2008; 68(1): 206-15.

[280] Garlich J, Qi W, Becker M, Stejskal A, Mahadevan D. Editors. Translational studies of the novel prodrug PI3K/mTOR/PIM1 inhibitor SF1126 in DLBCL. American Association for Cancer Research. 102nd Annual Meeting. Orlando, USA (2011).

[281] Maira SM, Stauffer F, Brueggen J, Furet P, Schnell C, Fritsch C, *et al.* Identification and characterization of NVP-BEZ235, a new orally available dual phosphatidylinositol 3-kinase/mammalian target of rapamycin inhibitor with potent *in vivo* antitumor activity. Mol Cancer Ther 2008; 7(7): 1851-63.

[282] Schnell CR, Stauffer F, Allegrini PR, O'Reilly T, McSheehy PM, Dartois C, *et al.* Effects of the dual phosphatidylinositol 3-kinase/mammalian target of rapamycin inhibitor NVP-BEZ235 on the tumor vasculature: Implications for clinical imaging. Cancer Res 2008; 68(16): 6598-607.

[283] Brachmann SM, Hofmann I, Schnell C, Fritsch C, Wee S, Lane H, *et al.* Specific apoptosis induction by the dual PI3K/mTor inhibitor NVP-BEZ235 in HER2 amplified and PIK3CA mutant breast cancer cells. Proc Natl Acad Sci USA. 2009; 106(52): 22299-304.

[284] Eichhorn PJ, Gili M, Scaltriti M, Serra V, Guzman M, Nijkamp W, *et al.* Phosphatidylinositol 3-kinase hyperactivation results in lapatinib resistance that is reversed

by the mTOR/phosphatidylinositol 3-kinase inhibitor NVP-BEZ235. Cancer Res 2008; 68(22): 9221-30.

[285] Markman B, Serra V, Scaltriti M, Valero V, Guzman M, Garcia-Echevarria C, *et al.* Editors. Pharmacodynamic (PD) endpoints and cellular proliferation effects of NVP-BEZ235, a dual PI3K/mTOR inhibitor, in breast cancer cells and xenografts with wild-type (WT) and activating PI3K mutations. American Society of Clinical Oncology. 44th Annual Meeting. Chicago, USA (2008).

[286] Serra V, Markman B, Scaltriti M, Eichhorn PJ, Valero V, Guzman M, *et al.* NVP-BEZ235, a dual PI3K/mTOR inhibitor, prevents PI3K signaling and inhibits the growth of cancer cells with activating PI3K mutations. Cancer Res 2008; 68(19): 8022-30.

[287] Dubrovska A, Kim S, Salamone RJ, Walker JR, Maira SM, Garcia-Echeverria C, *et al.* The role of PTEN/AKT/PI3K signaling in the maintenance and viability of prostate cancer stem-like cell populations. Proc Natl Acad Sci USA 2009; 106(1): 268-73.

[288] Oishi T, Itamochi H, Kudoh A, Nonaka M, Sato S, Naniwa J, *et al.* Editors. NVP-BEZ235, a dual PI3K/ mTOR inhibitor, suppress tumorigenicity of ovarian clear cell carcinoma cells. American Association for Cancer Research. 103rd Annual Meeting. Chicago, USA (2012).

[289] Kwan SY, Fung A, Izaguirre D, Zu Z, Tsang-Lee Y, Mok S, *et al.* Editors. Sensitivity of ovarian clear cell carcinoma cells to PI3K inhibitors. American Association for Cancer Research. 102nd Annual Meeting. Orlando, USA (2011).

[290] Montero JC, Chen X, Ocana A, Pandiella A. Predominance of mTORC1 over mTORC2 in the regulation of proliferation of ovarian cancer cells: Therapeutic implications. Mol Cancer Ther 2012; 11(6): 1342-52.

[291] Shoji K, Oda K, Nakagawa S, Ikeda Y, Kuramoto H, Nishida M, *et al.* Editors. Activity of dual PI3K/mTOR inhibitor, NVP-BEZ235, and mTOR inhibitor, RAD001 (everolimus), in endometrial cancer cell lines. American Society of Clinical Oncology. 46th Annual Meeting. Chicago, USA (2010).

[292] Yang S, Xiao X, Meng X, Leslie KK. Combination therapy with mTOR and PI3 kinase inhibitors is broadly synergistic in a wide variety of endometrial cancer cells. American Association for Cancer Research. 102nd Annual Meeting. Orlando, USA (2011).

[293] Muller A, Bachmann E, Linnig M, Khillimberger K, Galle PR, Mohler M. Selective PI3K inhibition in wild type and PIK3CA mutated human gastrointestinal cancer. Jahrestagung der Deutschen, Österreichischen und Schweizerischen Gesellschaften für Hämatologie und Onkologie Basel, Switzerland (2011).

[294] Cao P, Maira SM, Garcia-Echeverria C, Hedley DW. Activity of a novel, dual PI3-kinase/mTor inhibitor NVP-BEZ235 against primary human pancreatic cancers grown as orthotopic xenografts. Br J Cancer 2009; 100(8): 1267-76.

[295] Cho DC, Cohen MB, Panka DJ, Collins M, Ghebremichael M, Atkins MB, *et al.* The efficacy of the novel dual PI3-kinase/mTOR inhibitor NVP-BEZ235 compared with rapamycin in renal cell carcinoma. Clin Cancer Res 2010; 16(14): 3628-38.

[296] Engelman JA, Chen L, Tan X, Crosby K, Guimaraes AR, Upadhyay R, *et al.* Effective use of PI3K and MEK inhibitors to treat mutant Kras G12D and PIK3CA H1047R murine lung cancers. Nat Med 2008; 14(12): 1351-6.

[297] Gong HC, Wang S, Mayer G, Chen G, Leesman G, Singh S, *et al.* Signatures of drug sensitivity in nonsmall cell lung cancer. Int J Proteom 2011; 2011: Article ID 215496.

[298] Walsh KJ, Fan S, Patel A, Jacobs CL, Smith J, Liu Q, *et al.* Editors. Hedgehog pathway inhibition is a novel therapeutic approach in lymphomas and its efficacy is inversely related to PI3 kinase inhibition. American Society of Hematology. 52nd Annual Meeting. Orlando, USA (2010).

[299] Buglio D, Lemoine M, Neelapu SS, Vega F, Berry D, Younes A. NVP-BEZ235, a dual inhibitor of phosphoinositol-3-kinase (PI3K) and Mammalian Target of Rapamycin (mTOR), is a potent inhibitor of lymphoma cell growth and survival. American Society of Hematolog. 52nd Annual Meeting. Orlando, USA (2011).

[300] Wong J, Welschinger R, Baraz R, Weiss J, Bradstock K, Bendall LJ. Comparision of dual PI-3K/mTOR inhibitors with mtor inhibitors using a pre-clinical model of acute lymphoblastic leukemia. American Society Hematology. 52nd Annual Meeting; Orlando, USA (2010).

[301] Badura S, Tesanovic T, Pfeifer H, Hohnloser C, Serve H, Ruthardt M, *et al.* Editors. Inhibition of the PI3K/AKT/mTOR pathway overcomes resistance to ABL-directed TKI in long-term cultured acute lymphoblastic leukemia (ALL) cells. Jahrestagung der Deutschen, Österreichischen und Schweizerischen Gesellschaften für Hämatologie und Onkologie; Basel, Switzerland (2011).

[302] Liu H, Diaz-Flores E, Poire X, Odenike O, Koval G, Malnassy G, *et al.* Editors. Combination of a MEK inhibitor, AZD6244, and dual PI3K/MTOR inhibitor, NVP-BEZ235: An effective therapeutic strategy for acute myeloid leukemia. American Society of Hematology. 52nd Annual Meeting. Orlando, USA (2010).

[303] Chapuis N, Tamburini J, Green AS, Vignon C, Bardet V, Neyret A, *et al.* Dual inhibition of PI3K and mTORC1/2 signaling by NVP-BEZ235 as a new therapeutic strategy for acute myeloid leukemia. Clin Cancer Res 2010; 16(22): 5424-35.

[304] Chiarini F, Grimaldi C, Ricci F, Tazzari PL, Evangelisti C, Ognibene A, *et al.* Activity of the novel dual phosphatidylinositol 3-kinase/mammalian target of rapamycin inhibitor NVP-BEZ235 against T-cell acute lymphoblastic leukemia. Cancer Res 2010; 70(20): 8097-107.

[305] Guenther A, Burger R, Klapper W, Staudinger M, Richter K, Ahrens T, *et al.* Editors. Inhibitors of mtor and PI3K synergistically block plasmacytoma cell growth. American Society of Hematology. 53rd Annual Meeting. San Diego, USA (2011).

[306] De PKR, Sun Y, Dey N, Leyland-Jones B. Preclinical efficacy of the novel dual PI3K/mTOR inhibitor, BEZ235 compared with RAD001 in HER2+ breast tumors. American Association for Cancer Research. 102nd Annual Meeting. Orlando, USA (2011).

[307] Chakrabarty A, Rexer BN, Wang SE, Cook RS, Engelman JA, Arteaga CL. H1047R phosphatidylinositol 3-kinase mutant enhances HER2-mediated transformation by heregulin production and activation of HER3. Oncogene 2010; 29(37): 5193-203.

[308] Wang L, Zhang Q, Zhang J, Sun S, Guo H, Jia Z, *et al.* PI3K pathway activation results in low efficacy of both trastuzumab and lapatinib. BMC Cancer 2011; 11: 248.

[309] Crowder RJ, Phommaly C, Tao Y, Hoog J, Luo J, Perou CM, *et al.* PIK3CA and PIK3CB inhibition produce synthetic lethality when combined with estrogen deprivation in estrogen receptor-positive breast cancer. Cancer Res 2009; 69(9): 3955-62.

[310] Baumann P, Schneider L, Mandl-Weber S, Oduncu F, Schmidmaier R. Simultaneous targeting of PI3K and mTOR with NVP-BGT226 is highly effective in multiple myeloma. Anti-Cancer Drugs 2012; 23(1): 131-8.

[311] Wong J, Welschinger R, Baraz R, Bradstock KF, Bendall LJ. Application of dual PI-3K/mTOR inhibitors is not always superior to inhibition of mTOR alone. American Society of Hematology. 52nd Annual Meeting. Orlando, USA (2011).

[312] Chang KY, Tsai SY, Wu CM, Yen CJ, Chuang BF, Chang JY. Novel phosphoinositide 3-kinase/mTOR dual inhibitor, NVP-BGT226, displays potent growth-inhibitory activity against human head and neck cancer cells *in vitro* and *in vivo*. Clin Cancer Res 2011; 17(22): 7116-26.

[313] Sanchez CG, Ma CX, Crowder RJ, Guintoli T, Phommaly C, Gao F, *et al.* Preclinical modeling of combined phosphatidylinositol-3-kinase inhibition with endocrine therapy for estrogen receptor-positive breast cancer. Breast Cancer Res 2011; 13(2): R21.

[314] Glienke W, Hausmann E, Bergmann L. Activity of NVP-BGT226 in human pancreatic cancer cell lines. Jahrestagung der Deutschen, Österreichischen und Schweizerischen Gesellschaften für Hämatologie und Onkologie. Berlin, Germany (2010).

[315] Glienke W, Maute L, Wicht J, Bergmann L. The dual PI3K/mTOR inhibitor NVP-BGT226 induces cell cycle arrest and regulates Survivin gene expression in human pancreatic cancer cell lines. Tumor Biol 2012; 33(3): 757-65.

[316] Patnaik A, Lorusso P, Tabernero J. Biomarker development for XL765, a potent and selective oral dual inhibitor of PI3K and mTOR currently being administered to patients in a Phase I clinical trial (abstract B265). *AACR-NCI-EORTC - 23rd International Conference on Molecular Targets and Cancer Therapeutics*. San Francisco, USA, 2007.

[317] Wallin JJ, Edgar KA, Guan J, Berry M, Prior WW, Lee L, *et al.* GDC-0980 is a novel class I PI3K/mTOR kinase inhibitor with robust activity in cancer models driven by the PI3K pathway. Mol Cancer Ther 2011; 10(12): 2426-36.

[318] Yuan J, Mehta PP, Yin MJ, Sun S, Zou A, Chen J, *et al.* PF-04691502, a potent and selective oral inhibitor of PI3K and mTOR kinases with antitumor activity. Mol Cancer Ther 2011; 10(11): 2189-99.

[319] Mallon R, Feldberg LR, Lucas J, Chaudhary I, Dehnhardt C, Delos Santos E, *et al.* Antitumor efficacy of PKI-587, a highly potent dual PI3K/mTOR kinase inhibitor. Clin Cancer Res 2011; 17(10): 3193-203.

[320] Mayer IA, Abramson VG, Balko JM, Isakoff SJ, Kuba MG, Sanders M, *et al.* SU2C Phase Ib study of pan-PI3K inhibitor BKM120 with letrozole in ER+/HER2- metastatic breast cancer (MBC) [abstract]. American Society of Clinical Oncology. 48th Annual Meeting. Chicago, USA (2012).

[321] Ihle NT, Williams R, Chow S, Chew W, Berggren MI, Paine-Mrrieta G, *et al.* Molecular pharmacology and antitumor activity of PX-866, a novel inhibitor of phosphoinositide-3-kinase signaling. Mol Cancer Ther 2004; 3(7): 763-72.

[322] Ihle NT, Paine-Murrieta G, Berggren MI, Baker A, Tate WR, Wipf P, *et al.* The phosphatidylinositol-3-kinase inhibitor PX-866 overcomes resistance to the epidermal growth factor receptor inhibitor gefitinib in A-549 human non-small cell lung cancer xenografts. Mol Cancer Ther 2005; 4(9): 1349-57.

[323] Senzer N, Bowles D, Cohen RB, Vo A, Klucher K, Peterson S, *et al.* Results from the Phase 1 portion of a Phase 1/2 study of the irreversible PI-3K inhibitor PX-866 and cetuximab. *AACR-NCI-EORTC - 27th International Conference on Molecular Targets and Cancer Therapeutics.* San Francisco, USA, 2011

[324] Folkes AJ, Ahmadi K, Alderton WK, Alix S, Baker SJ, Box G, *et al.* The identification of 2-(1H-indazol-4-yl)-6-(4-methanesulfonyl-piperazin-1- ylmethyl)-4-morpholin-4-yl-thieno[3,2-d]pyrimidine (GDC-0941) as a potent, selective, orally bioavailable inhibitor of class I PI3 kinase for the treatment of cancer. J Med Chem 2008; 51(18): 5522-32.

[325] Raynaud FI, Eccles S, Clarke PA, Hayes A, Nutley B, Alix S, *et al.* Pharmacologic characterization of a potent inhibitor of class I phosphatidylinositide 3-kinases. Cancer Res 2007; 67(12): 5840-50.
[326] Sampath D, Cao T, Oeh J, Barck KH, Reslan HB, Wyatt S, *et al.* PI3K inhibition is necessary and sufficient to induce an antiangiogenic response *in vivo* based on suppression of tumor vascular structure. *EORTC-NCI-AACR - 22nd Symposium on Molecular targets and Cancer Therapeutics*. Berlin, Germany, 2010.
[327] Liu N, Rowley B, Schneider C, Bull C, Kaekoenen S, Hentemann M, *et al.* BAY 80-6946, a highly selective and potent pan class I PI3K inhibitor induces tumor apoptosis *in vitro* and tumor regression *in vivo* in a sub-set of tumor models. American Association for Cancer Research - 102nd Annual Meeting. Orlando, USA (2011).
[328] Y Yaguchi SI, Fukui Y, Koshimizu I, Yoshimi H, Matsuno T, Gouda H, *et al.* Antitumor activity of ZSTK474, a new phosphatidylinositol 3-kinase inhibitor. J Natl Cancer Inst 2006; 98(8): 545-56.
[329] Kong D, Yamori T. ZSTK474 is an ATP-competitive inhibitor of class I phosphatidylinositol 3 kinase isoforms. Cancer Sci 2007; 98(10): 1638-42.
[330] Fritsch CM, Schnell C, Chatenay-Rivauday C, Guthy DA, Pover AD, Wartmann M, *et al.* NVP-BYL719, a novel PI3Kalpha selective inhibitor with all the characteristics required for clinical development as an anti-cancer agent [abstract]. American Association for Cancer Research. 103rd Annual Meeting. Chicago, USA (2012).
[331] Rivero RA, Hardwicke MA. Identification of GSK2636771, a potent and selective, orally bioavailable inhibitor of phosphatidylinositol 3-kinase-beta (PI3K{alpha}) for the treatment of PTEN deficient tumors [abstract]. American Association for Cancer Research. 103rd Annual Meeting. Chicago, IL (2012).
[332] Blackman SC, Gainer SD, Suttle BB, Skordos KW, Greshock JD, Motwani M, *et al.* A Phase I/IIa, first time in human, open-label dose-escalation study of GSK2636771 in subjects with advanced solid tumors with PTEN deficiency. American Association for Cancer Research. 103rd Annual Meeting. Chicago, USA (2012).
[333] Billottet C, Grandage VL, Gale RE, Quattropani A, Rommel C, Vanhaesebroeck B, *et al.* A selective inhibitor of the p110 isoform of PI 3-kinase inhibits AML cell proliferation and survival and increases the cytotoxic effects of VP16. Oncogene 2006; 25(50): 6648-59.
[334] Tamburini J, Chapuis N, Bardet V, Park S, Sujobert P, Willems L, *et al.* Mammalian target of rapamycin (mTOR) inhibition activates phosphatidylinositol 3-kinase/AKT by up-regulating insulin-like growth factor-1 receptor signaling in acute myeloid leukemia: Rationale for therapeutic inhibition of both pathways. Blood 2008; 111(1): 379-82.
[335] Lannutti BJ, Meadows SA, Herman SEM, Kashishian A, Steiner B, Johnson AJ, *et al.* CAL-101, a p110δ selective phosphatidylinositol-3-kinase inhibitor for the treatment of B-cell malignancies, inhibits PI3K signaling and cellular viability. Blood 2011; 117(2): 591-4.
[336] Herman SEM, Gordon AL, Wagner AJ, Heerema NA, Zhao W, Flynn JM, *et al.* Phosphatidylinositol 3-kinase- inhibitor CAL-101 shows promising preclinical activity in chronic lymphocytic leukemia by antagonizing intrinsic and extrinsic cellular survival signals. Blood 2010; 116(12): 2078-88.
[337] Meadows SA, Kashishian A, Johnson D, Ulrich RG, Miller LL, Lannutti BJ. CAL-101 (GS-1101), a Specific Inhibitor of Phosphatidylinositol-3-Kinase-Delta (PI3K{delta}), Disrupts Signals From the Microenvironment, Induces Apoptosis, and Enhances the Antitumor Activity of Everolimus (RAD001), An Inhibitor of Mammalian Target of

Rapamycin (mTOR), in Mantle Cell Lymphoma (MCL). American Society of Hematology. 53rd Annual Meeting. San Diego, USA (2011).

[338] Meadows SA, Kashishian A, Johnson D. CAL-101 a Potent selective inhibitor of the p110{delta} Isoform of Phosphatidylinositol 3-kinase Attenuates pathway signaling induces apoptosis and overcomes signals from the microenvironment in cellular models of Hodgkin lymphoma. American Society of Hematology. 52nd Annual Meeting. Orlando, USA (2010).

[339] Ikeda H, Hideshima T, Fulciniti M, Perrone G, Miura N, Yasui H, *et al.* PI3K/p110 is a novel therapeutic target in multiple myeloma. Blood 2010; 116(9): 1460-8.

[340] Hoellenriegel J, Meadows SA, Sivina M, Wierda WG, Kantarjian H, Keating MJ, *et al.* The phosphoinositide 3′-kinase delta inhibitor, CAL-101, inhibits B-cell receptor signaling and chemokine networks in chronic lymphocytic leukemia. Blood 2011; 118(13): 3603-12.

[341] Davids MS, Lannutti BJ, Brown JR, Letai AG. BH3 profiling demonstrates that CAL-101 restores apoptotic priming in stroma-exposed chronic lymphocytic leukemia cells. *XIV International Workshop on Chronic Lymphocytic Leukemia*. Houston, USA (2011).

[342] Furman RR, Byrd JC, Brown JR, Coutre SE, Benson DM, Jr., Wagner-Johnston ND, *et al.* CAL-101, An Isoform-Selective Inhibitor of Phosphatidylinositol 3-Kinase P110{delta}, Demonstrates Clinical Activity and Pharmacodynamic Effects In Patients with Relapsed or Refractory Chronic Lymphocytic Leukemia. American Society of Hematology. 52nd Annual Meeting. Orlando, USA (2010).

[343] Flinn IW, Byrd JC, Furman RR, Brown JR, Benson DM, Coutre SE, *et al.* Evidence of Clinical Activity in a Phase 1 Study of CAL-101, An Oral P110{Delta} Isoform-Selective Inhibitor of Phosphatidylinositol 3-Kinase, in Patients with Relapsed or Refractory B-Cell Malignancies. American Society of Hematology. 51st Annual Meeting. New Orleans, USA (2009).

[344] Hallek M, Cheson BD, Catovsky D, Caligaris-Cappio F, Dighiero G, Döhner H, *et al.* Guidelines for the diagnosis and treatment of chronic lymphocytic leukemia: A report from the International Workshop on Chronic Lymphocytic Leukemia updating the National Cancer Institute-Working Group 1996 guidelines. Blood 2008; 111(12): 5446-56.

[345] Liu L, Sun B-C, Pistillo J, Payton M, Wang L, Archibeque I, *et al.* Phosphatidylinsoitol-3 Kinase Delta (PI3K{delta}) Inhibitor AMG 319 Combined with Vincristine Enhances G2/M Arrest and Apoptotic Death in Neoplastic B Cells. *American Society of Hematology - 53rd Annual Meeting*, San Diego, USA (2011).

[346] Sinclair A, Metz D, Cushing T, Liu L, Brake R, Starnes C, *et al.* Phosphatidylinositol-3 Kinase Delta (PI3K{delta}) Inhibitor AMG 319 Is a Potent, Selective and Orally Bioavailable Small Molecule Inhibitor That Suppresses PI3K-Mediated Signaling and Viability in Neoplastic B Cells. American Society of Hematology. 53rd Annual Meeting. San Diego, USA (2011).

[347] Lindsley CW. The AKT/PKB family of protein kinases: A review of small molecule inhibitors and progress towards target validation: A 2009 update. Curr Top Med Chem 2010; 10(4): 458-77.

[348] Gonzalez E, McGraw TE. The AKT kinases: Isoform specificity in metabolism and cancer. Cell Cycle 2009; 8(16): 2502-8.

[349] Garcia-Echeverria C, Sellers WR. Drug discovery approaches targeting the PI3K/AKT pathway in cancer. Oncogene 2008; 27(41): 5511-26.

[350] Vasudevan KM, Barbie DA, Davies MA, Rabinovsky R, McNear CJ, Kim JJ, *et al.* AKT-independent signaling downstream of oncogenic PIK3CA mutations in human cancer. Cancer Cell 2009; 16(1): 21-32.
[351] Meuillet EJ, Zuohe S, Lemos R, Ihle N, Kingston J, Watkins R, *et al.* Molecular pharmacology and antitumor activity of PHT-427, a novel AKT/phosphatidylinositide-dependent protein kinase 1 pleckstrin homology domain inhibitor. Mol Cancer Ther 2010; 9(3): 706-17.
[352] Hennessy BT, Lu Y, Poradosu E, Yu Q, Yu S, Hall H, *et al.* Pharmacodynamic markers of perifosine efficacy. Clin Cancer Res 2007; 13(24): 7421-31.
[353] Van Ummersen L, Binger K, Volkman J, Marnocha R, Tutsch K, Kolesar J, *et al.* A Phase I trial of perifosine (NSC 639966) on a loading dose/maintenance dose schedule in patients with advanced cancer. Clin Cancer Res 2004; 10(22): 7450-6.
[354] Posadas EM, Gulley J, Arlen PM, Trout A, Parnes HL, Wright J, *et al.* A Phase II study of perifosine in androgen independent prostate cancer. Cancer Biol Ther 2005; 4(10): 1133-7.
[355] Hedley D, Moore MJ, Hirte H, Siu L, Vincent M, Jonker D, *et al.* A Phase II trial of perifosine as second line therapy for advanced pancreatic cancer. A study of the Princess Margaret Hospital [PMH] Phase II Consortium. American Society of Clinical Oncology - 41th Annual Meeting. Orlando, USA (2005).
[356] Ernst DS, Eisenhauer E, Wainman N, Davis M, Lohmann R, Baetz T, *et al.* Phase II study of perifosine in previously untreated patients with metastatic melanoma. Invest New Drugs 2005; 23(6): 569-75.
[357] Marsh Rde W, Rocha Lima CM, Levy DE, Mitchell EP, Rowland KM, Jr., Benson AB. A Phase II trial of perifosine in locally advanced, unresectable, or metastatic pancreatic adenocarcinoma. Am J Clin Oncol 2007; 30(1): 26-31.
[358] Chee KG, Longmate J, Quinn DI, Chatta G, Pinski J, Twardowski P, *et al.* The AKT inhibitor perifosine in biochemically recurrent prostate cancer: A Phase II California/Pittsburgh cancer consortium trial. Clin Genitourinary Cancer 2007; 5(7): 433-7.
[359] Conley AP, Araujo D, Ludwig J, Ravi V, Samuels BL, Choi H, *et al.* A randomized Phase II study of perifosine (P) plus imatinib for patients with imatinib-resistant gastrointestinal stromal tumor (GIST). American Society of Clinical Oncology - 45th Annual Meeting. Orlando, USA (2009).
[360] Cho DC, Hutson TE, Samlowski W, Sportelli P, Somer B, Richards P, *et al.* Two Phase 2 trials of the novel AKT inhibitor perifosine in patients with advanced renal cell carcinoma after progression on vascular endothelial growth factor-targeted therapy. Cancer 2012; 118(24): 6055-62.
[361] Bendell JC, Nemunaitis J, Vukelja SJ, Hagenstad C, Campos LT, Hermann RC, *et al.* Randomized placebo-controlled Phase II trial of perifosine plus capecitabine as second- or third-line therapy in patients with metastatic colorectal cancer. J Clin Oncol 2011; 29(33): 4394-400.
[362] Bendell JC, Ervin TJ, Senzer NN, Richards DA, Firdaus I, Lockhart AC, *et al.* Results of the X-PECT study: A Phase III randomized double-blind, placebo-controlled study of perifosine plus capecitabine (P-CAP) versus placebo plus capecitabine (CAP) in patients (pts) with refractory metastatic colorectal cancer (mCRC). American Society of Clinical Oncology - 48th Annual Meeting. Chicago, USA (2012).
[363] Ghobrial IM, Roccaro A, Hong F, Weller E, Rubin N, Leduc R, *et al.* Clinical and translational studies of a Phase II trial of the novel oral AKT inhibitor perifosine in relapsed

or relapsed/refractory Waldenstrom's macroglobulinemia. Clin Cancer Res 2010; 16(3): 1033-41.

[364] Ghobrial IM, Leleu X, Rubin N, Xie W, Hong F, Chuma S, *et al.* Final Results of a Phase II Trial of the Novel Oral AKT Inhibitor Perifosine in Relapsed and/or Refractory Waldenstrom Macroglobulinemia (WM). American Society of Hematology - 50th Annual Meeting. San Francisco, USA (2008).

[365] Richardson PG, Wolf J, Jakubowiak A, Zonder J, Lonial S, Irwin D, *et al.* Perifosine plus bortezomib and dexamethasone in patients with relapsed/refractory multiple myeloma previously treated with bortezomib: results of a multicenter Phase I/II trial. J Clin Oncol 2011; 29(32): 4243-9.

[366] Jakubowiak AJ, Richardson PG, Zimmerman T, Alsina M, Kaufman JL, Kandarpa M, *et al.* Perifosine plus lenalidomide and dexamethasone in relapsed and relapsed/refractory multiple myeloma: A Phase I Multiple Myeloma Research Consortium study. Br J Haematol 2012; 158(4): 472-80.

[367] Yang L, Dan HC, Sun M, Liu Q, Sun XM, Feldman RI, *et al.* AKT/protein kinase B signaling inhibitor-2, a selective small molecule inhibitor of AKT signaling with antitumor activity in cancer cells overexpressing AKT. Cancer Res 2004; 64(13): 4394-9.

[368] Feun LG, Savaraj N, Bodey GP, Lu K, Yap BS, Ajani JA, *et al.* Phase I study of tricyclic nucleoside phosphate using a five-day continuous infusion schedule. Cancer Res 1984; 44(8): 3608-12.

[369] Schilcher RB, Haas CD, Samson MK, Young JD, Baker LH. Phase I evaluation and clinical pharmacology of tricyclic nucleoside 5'-phosphate using a weekly intravenous regimen. Cancer Res 1986; 46(6): 3147-51.

[370] Feun LG, Blessing JA, Barrett RJ, Hanjani P. A Phase II trial of tricyclic nucleoside phosphate in patients with advanced squamous cell carcinoma of the cervix. A Gynecologic Oncology Group Study. Am J Clin Oncol 1993; 16(6): 506-8.

[371] Hoffman K, Holmes FA, Fraschini G, Esparza L, Frye D, Raber MN, *et al.* Phase I-II study: Triciribine (tricyclic nucleoside phosphate) for metastatic breast cancer. Cancer Chemother Pharmacol 1996; 37(3): 254-8.

[372] Phillips CL, Fouladi M, Perentesis JP, Leary S, McGovern RM, Reid JM, *et al.* A Phase I trial of MK 2206 in children with refractory solid tumors: A Children's Oncology Group study. American Society of Clinical Oncology - 48th Annual Meeting. Chicago, USA (2012).

[373] Heerding DA, Rhodes N, Leber JD, Clark TJ, Keenan RM, Lafrance LV, *et al.* Identification of 4-(2-(4-amino-1,2,5-oxadiazol-3-yl)-1-ethyl-7-{[(3S)-3-piperidinylmethyl]oxy}-1H- imidazo[4,5-c]pyridin-4-yl)-2-methyl-3-butyn-2-ol (GSK690693), a novel inhibitor of AKT kinase. J Med Chem 2008; 51(18): 5663-79.

[374] Gungor H, Saleem A, Agarwal R, Blagden SP, Michael A, Stronach EA, *et al.* Pharmacokinetic (PK)/pharmacodynamic (PD) analysis of escalating repeat doses of the AKT inhibitor GSK2141795 (GSK795) in patients (pts) with ovarian cancer. American Society of Clinical Oncology - 47th Annual Meeting. Chicago. USA (2011).

[375] Spencer A, Yoon SS, Harrison SJ, Morris S, Smith D, Freedman SJ, *et al.* Novel AKT inhibitor GSK2110183 shows favorable safety, pharmacokinetics, and clinical activity in multiple myeloma. preliminary results from a Phase i first-time-in-human study. American Society of Hematology - 53rd Annual Meeting. San Diego, USA (2011).

[376] Lin K. GDC-0068: A novel, selective, ATP-competitive inhibitor of AKT. American Association for Cancer Research - 102nd Annual Meeting. Orlando, USA (2011)

[377] Marshall J, Posey J, Hwang J, Malik S, Shen R, Kazempour K, *et al.* A Phase I trial of RX-0201 (AKT anti-sense) in patients with an advanced cancer. American Society of Clinical Oncology - 43th Annual Meeting. Chicago, USA (2007).

[378] Jessen K, Wang S, Kessler L, Guo X, Kucharski J, Staunton J, *et al.* INK128 is a potent and selective TORC1/2 inhibitor with broad oral antitumor activity. *AACR-NCI-EORTC - 25th International Conference on Molecular Targets and Cancer Therapeutic.* Boston, USA, 2009

[379] Kessler L, Jessen K, Janes M, Staunton J, Kucharski J, Guo X, *et al.* INK128, a TORC1/2 kinase inhibitor, enhances the efficacy of cytotoxic therapies in endometrial tumor models. American Association for Cancer Research - 103rd Annual Meeting. Chicago, IL (2012)

[380] Kessler L, Wang S, Guo X, Kucharski J, Staunton J, Lan L, *et al.* INK128, an orally active TORC1/2 kinase inhibitor, shows broad antitumor activity and enhances efficacy of cytotoxic as well as targeted agents. American Association for Cancer Research - 102nd Annual Meeting. Orlando (2011)

[381] Leyland-Jones B, Wu H, Sun Y, Rommel C, Yi L, De P, *et al.* Preclinical activity of INK128, a TORC1/2 inhibitor, in triple negative breast cancer: A combination of PARP inhibitor with PI3K-mTOR pathway-targeted inhibitor. American Association for Cancer Research - 103rd Annual Meeting. Chicago, IL (2012)

[382] Wang S, Jessen K, Kessler L, Kucharski J, Lan L, Guo X, *et al.* INK128, a novel TORC1/2 inhibitor with potent oral antitumor activity in preclinical models of renal cancer. American Association for Cancer Research - 102nd Annual Meeting. Orlando, USA (2011)

[383] Banerji U, Aghajanian C, Raymond E, Kurzrock R, Blanco-Codesido M, Oelmann E, *et al.* First results from a Phase I trial of AZD8055, a dual mTORC1 and mTORC2 inhibitor. American Society of Clinical Oncology - 47th Annual Meeting, Chicago, USA (2011).

[384] Gokhale PC, Bhagwat SV, Crew AP, Cooke A, Mantis C, Workman JE, *et al.* OSI-027, a selective dual mTORC1/TORC2 kinase inhibitor displays broad spectrum anti-tumor activity in preclinical models of human cancer. American Association for Cancer Research - 101st Annual Meeting. Washington DC, USA (2010)

[385] Guichard SM, Howard Z, Heathcote D, Roth M, Hughes G, Curwen J, *et al.* AZD2014, a dual mTORC1 and mTORC2 inhibitor is differentiated from allosteric inhibitors of mTORC1 in ER+ breast cancer. American Association for Cancer Research - 103rd Annual Meeting, Chicago, IL (2012)

[386] Stewart A, Thavasu P, Heaton S, Banerjee S, Kaye SB, Banerji U. The combination of the dual mTORC1/mTORC2 inhibitor AZD2014 and paclitaxel in human ovarian cancer models. American Association for Cancer Research - 103rd Annual Meeting. Chicago, IL (2012)

[387] Castro, A.C., Evans, C.A., Lescarbeau, A., Liu, T., Snyder, D.A., Tremblay, M.R., Ren, P., Liu, Y., Li, L., Chan, K. Heterocyclic compounds and uses thereof. US20130029984 (**2013**).

[388] Nagarathnam, D., Vakkalanka, S.K., Muthuppalaniappan, M., Babu, G., Bhavar, P.K. Novel compounds as modulator of protein kinases. WO2012151525 (**2012**).

[389] Pastor Fernandez, J., Martinez Donzalez, S., Lorenzo Garcia, M., Blanco-Aparicio, C., Palacios Doiztua, I., Cebria Gomez, A., Quinones Sanchez, H., Fominaya Gutierrez, J. Imidazopyrazines derivates as kinase inhibitors. EP2524918 (**2012**).

[390] Pastor Fernandez, J., Martinez Gonzalez, S., Alvarez Escobar, R.M., Rodriguez Aristegui, S., Gonzalez Cantalapiedra, E., Hernandez Higueras, A.I., Varela Busto, C. Fused Imidazo [3,2 - D] Pyrazines as P13 Kinase Inhibitors. US20130029967 (**2013**).

[391] Kumar, S., Joshi, K.S., Deore, V., Bhonde, M.R., Yewalkar, N.N., Padgaonkar, A.A., Kulkarni-Almeida, A.A., Rathos, M.J., Parikh, S., Dagia, N.M. Pyridyl derivatives, their preparation and use. US8314103 (**2012**).

[392] Ren, P., Liu, Y. Reactive mTOR and PI3 kinase inhibitor and uses thereof. WO2012154608 (**2012**).

[393] Ren, P., Liu, Y. Reactive PI3K kinase inhibitors and uses thereof. WO2012154610 (**2012**).

[394] Ren, P., Liu, Y., Jessen, K., Guo, X., Rommel, C., Wilson, T.E. Combination of kanase inhibitors and use thereof. WO2012148540 (**2012**).

[395] Mitchell, I., Blake, J. Dihydrothienopyrimidines as AKT protein kinase inhibitors. US20120329808 (**2012**).

[396] Bencsik, J., Blake, J. Hydroxylated pyrimidyl cyclopentane as AKT protein kinase inhibitor. EP2240455 (**2012**).

[397] Seefeld, M.A., Rouse, M.B. Inhibitors of AKT activity. US8338434 (**2012**).

[398] Banka, A., Bencsik, J., Blake, J., Hentemann, M.F., Kallan, N.C., Liang, J., Mitchell, I.S., Schlachter, S.T., Wallace, E.M., Xu, R., Tang, T.P. Cyclopenta[D]pyrimidines as AKT protein kinase inhibitors. US8329709 (**2012**).

[399] Mitchell, I., Blake, J., Xu, R., Kallan, N.C., Xiao, D., Spencer, K.L., Bencsik, J.R. Dihydrofuro Pyrimidines as AKT protein kinase inhibitors. US8329701 (**2012**)

[400] Banka, A., Blake, J.F., Bencsik, J.R., Fong, K.C., Hentemann, M.F., Sammond, D.M., Miitchell, I.S., Xu, R., Wallace, E.M., Tang, T. Pyrimidyl cyclopentanes as AKT protein kinase inhibitors. US8324221 (**2012**).

[401] Brollo, M., Carry, J.C., Certal, V., Didier, E., Doerflinger, G., El Ahmad, Y., Filoche-Romme, B., Halley, F., Karlsson, K.A., Schio, L., Thompson, F.Novel pyrimidine derivates, preparation thereof, and pharmaceutical use thereof as AKT (PKB) phosphorylation inhibitors. WO2012089633 (**2012**).

[402] Carry, J.-C., Certal, V., Halley, F., Karlsson, A., Schio, L., Thomson, F. Novel (6-oxo-1,6-dihydropyrimidin-2-yl) amide derivates, preparation thereof and pharmaceutical use thereof as AKT (PKB) Phosphorylation inhibitors. US20120270867 (**2012**).

[403] Akinsanmi, L., Kincaid, J. Compounds useful as AKT/PKB modulators and uses thereof. WO2012158197 (**2012**).

[404] O'Neil, J., Benita, Y., Marine, S., Haines, B. Compositions and methods for treating cancer. US20120289481 (**2012**).

[405] Davies, T.G., Boyle, R.G., Collins, I., Garrett, M.D. Pharmaceutical compounds. US8343953 (**2013**).

[406] Hidalgo M, Bruckheimer E, Rajeshkumar NV, Garrido-Laguna I, De Oliveira E, Rubio-Viqueira B, *et al.* A pilot clinical study of treatment guided by personalized tumorgrafts in patients with advanced cancer. Mol Cancer Ther 2011; 10(18): 1311-6.

[407] Liu P, Cheng H, Santiago S, Raeder M, Zhang F, Isabella A, *et al.* Oncogenic PIK3CA-driven mammary tumors frequently recur *via* PI3K pathway-dependent and PI3K pathway-independent mechanisms. Nat Med 2011; 17(9): 1116-21.

[408] Brana I, Siu LL. Clinical development of phosphatidylinositol 3-kinase inhibitors for cancer treatment. BMC Med 2012; 10: 161.

[409] Yamasaki F, Johansen MJ, Zhang D, Krishnamurthy S, Felix E, Bartholomeusz C, *et al.* Acquired resistance to erlotinib in A-431 epidermoid cancer cells requires down-regulation of MMAC1/PTEN and up-regulation of phosphorylated AKT. Cancer Res 2007; 67(12): 5779-88.

[410] Guix M, Faber AC, Wang SE, Olivares MG, Song Y, Qu S, *et al.* Acquired resistance to EGFR tyrosine kinase inhibitors in cancer cells is mediated by loss of IGF-binding proteins. J Clin Invest 2008; 118(7): 2609-19.

[411] Sequist LV, Waltman BA, Dias-Santagata D, Digumarthy S, Turke AB, Fidias P, *et al.* Genotypic and histological evolution of lung cancers acquiring resistance to EGFR inhibitors. Sci Trans Med 2011; 3(75): 75ra26.

[412] Chakrabarty A, Bhola NE, Sutton C, Ghosh R, Kuba MG, Dave B, *et al.* Trastuzumab-resistant cells rely on a HER2-PI3K-FoxO-survivin axis and are sensitive to PI3K inhibitors. Cancer Res 2013; 73(3): 1190-200.

[413] Dave B, Migliaccio I, Gutierrez MC, Wu MF, Chamness GC, Wong H, *et al.* Loss of phosphatase and tensin homolog or phosphoinositol-3 kinase activation and response to trastuzumab or lapatinib in human epidermal growth factor receptor 2-overexpressing locally advanced breast cancers. J Clin Oncol 2011; 29(2): 166-73.

[414] Yamnik RL, Holz MK. mTOR/S6K1 and MAPK/RSK signaling pathways coordinately regulate estrogen receptor α serine 167 phosphorylation. FEBS Lett 2010; 584(1): 124-8.

[415] Yamnik RL, Digilova A, Davis DC, Brodt ZN, Murphy CJ, Holz MK. S6 kinase 1 regulates estrogen receptor α in control of breast cancer cell proliferation. J Biol Chem 2009; 284(10): 6361-9.

[416] Tabernero J, Rojo F, Calvo E, Burris H, Judson I, Hazell K, *et al.* Dose- and schedule-dependent inhibition of the mammalian target of rapamycin pathway with everolimus: A Phase I tumor pharmacodynamic study in patients with advanced solid tumors. J Clin Oncol 2008; 26(10): 1603-10.

[417] Shi Y, Yan H, Frost P, Gera J, Lichtenstein A. Mammalian target of rapamycin inhibitors activate the AKT kinase in multiple myeloma cells by up-regulating the insulin-like growth factor receptor/insulin receptor substrate-1/phosphatidylinositol 3-kinase cascade. Mol Cancer Ther 2005; 4(10): 1533-40.

[418] Di Cosimo S, Bendell JC, Cervantes-Ruiperez A, Roda D, Prudkin L, Stein MN, *et al.* A Phase I study of the oral mTOR inhibitor ridaforolimus (RIDA) in combination with the IGF-1R antibody dalotozumab (DALO) in patients (pts) with advanced solid tumors. American Society of Clinical Oncology. 46th Annual Meeting. Chicago, USA (2010).

[419] Ibrahim YH, García-García C, Serra V, He L, Torres-Lockhart K, Prat A, *et al.* PI3K inhibition impairs BRCA1/2 expression and sensitizes BRCA-proficient triple-negative breast cancer to PARP inhibition. Cancer Discov 2012; 2(11): 1036-47.

[420] Juvekar A, Burga LN, Hu H, Lunsford EP, Ibrahim YH, Balmañà J, *et al.* Combining a PI3K inhibitor with a PARP inhibitor provides an effective therapy for BRCA1-related breast cancer. Cancer Discov 2012; 2(11): 1048-63.

Send Orders of Reprints at reprints@benthamscience.net
Topics in Anti-Cancer Research, Vol. 2, **2013, 197-230** **197**

CHAPTER 5

Cell Cycle and Energy Metabolism in Tumor Cells: Strategies for Drug Therapy

Nivea D. Amoêdo, Tatiana El-Bacha Porto, Mariana F. Rodrigues and Franklin D. Rumjanek*

Universidade Federal do Rio de Janeiro, Instituto de Bioquímica Médica, Centro de Ciências da Saúde, Cidade Universitária, Ilha do Fundão Rio de Janeiro CEP 21941-590, RJ, Brazil

Abstract: Recent results obtained from research on the intermediary metabolism of tumor cells have uncovered the biochemical reprogramming that takes place upon malignant transformation. Many features have been highlighted that are currently being exploited for specific chemotherapy. Many more will become available shortly as a consequence of the recognition of potentially useful targets for treatment. General interest in this area can be gauged by the number of recent patents that have been deposited, or are in the process of application. Because the metabolic subversion that is a hallmark of cancer cells involves disruption of its homeostasis, the regulatory pathways dealt with in this chapter were broadly divided into those that encompass the main stages of the cell cycle and its various regulatory mechanisms and those that involve the aerobic glycolysis typical of cancer cells. It becomes apparent that both, the cell cycle and the intermediary metabolism are interconnected and rely on reactions many of which are dependent on kinases and phosphatases. Kinases and phosphatases are responsive to cellular redox signaling and may have a key role in determining whether cells progress towards malignant transformation as a result of continuous oxidative stress. The data discussed here underline aspects of the signaling pathways that lend themselves to specific inhibition by natural and synthetic compounds. The mitochondria and its role in programmed cell death is briefly commented, but special emphasis is placed on biochemical regulation at the level of chromatin structure, particularly the reactions that involve acetylation and deacetylation of histones. Within this context, inhibitors that act on histone deacetylases are discussed as promising alternatives to available treatments.

Keywords: Acetylation, aminopeptidases, angiogenesis, ATP, CDKs, chromossomes, CKIs, homeostasis, hypoxia, kinases, lactate, metabolomics, mitochondria, oncogenes, phosphatases, pyruvate kinase, ROS, sumoylation, ubiquitin.

***Address correspondence to Franklin D. Rumjanek:** Bloco E, Sala 22 Instituto de Bioquímica Médica CCS-Universidade Federal do Rio de Janeiro, Ilha do Fundão, Rio de Janeiro, Brazil CEP 21941-590; Tel: (5521) 25609625; E-mail: franklin@bioqmed.ufrj.br

Atta-ur Rahman and Khurshid Zaman (Eds)

INTRODUCTION

Whether sporadic or hereditary, most if not all types of cancer ultimately derive from single cells that have undergone irreversible biochemical reprogramming. The phenotypes acquired by the clones of transformed cells are such that the intrinsic pathways normally acting as safeguards for the tissue and the organism become subverted and/or abrogated. External and internal factors contribute to this abnormal situation. External factors include environmental variations that usually involve the interaction of carcinogens, physical or chemical, with the cell genomes (nuclear and mitochondrial). Internal factors on the other hand result from defects introduced by the cell machinery normally participating in the regulation of gene expression, which includes the cell cycle and the intermediary metabolism.

Biochemical reprogramming associated to cancer seems to rely heavily on altered properties of oncogenic kinases that normally act as growth signals. These growth factors can then affect the cell cycle machinery in many ways and subvert the sequential activation of cyclin-dependent kinases (CDKs). Kinases and phosphatases can also interfere with the metabolic pathways that support cell proliferation. The metabolic reprogramming that accompanies malignant transformation also involves reactions occurring within the mitochondria. Protein phosphorylation and dephosphorylation by tyrosine kinases and phosphatases, a recurrent regulatory theme in cell signaling, are themselves regulated by reactive oxygen species (ROS), especially hydrogen peroxide produced by the mitochondrial respiratory chain. H_2O_2 and other types of ROS are thus emerging as key regulatory elements and highlight the intertwined relation between mitochondria and the cell cycle, Fig (**1**).

In this chapter, we will present a brief description of the events leading to deregulation of cell proliferation and how the aberrant metabolic profiles typical of cancer cells can contribute to this state of affairs. It is hoped that such depictions will highlight causal relationships and that these in turn could suggest further strategies for control and treatment.

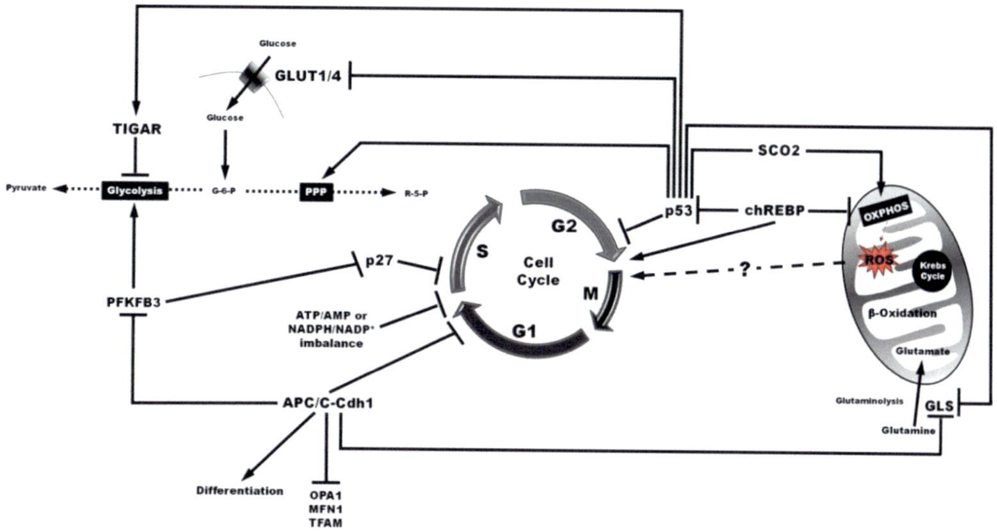

Figure 1: Schematic representation of some molecules and pathways linking metabolism and cell cycle progression. To maintain the proliferative state of tumor cells a tight interaction between cell cycle and energy metabolism is required. The ubiquitin ligase complex APC/CCdh1 mediates de degradation of both 6-phosphfructo-2-kinase/fructose-2,6-bisphosphatase isoform 3 (PFKB3). Glutaminase 1 (GLS1) also arrests cell cycle. PFKB3, a crucial allosteric regulator of PFK is a member of the glycolytic pathway. When PFKB3 is inhibited, glycolysis is interrupted. PFKB3 inhibits p27, another regulator of cell cycle. ATP/AMP and NADPH/NADP$^+$ balance are sensors of cell proliferation. The carbohydrate responsive element binding protein (ChREBP) regulates p53 and consequently cell cycle, mitochondrial function and the glycolytic flux. Although ROS may induce cell proliferation the mechanism is poorly understood. *TIGAR* (TP53-induced glycolysis and apoptosis regulator), SCO2 (synthesis of cytochrome c oxidase), GLUT1/4 (Glucose transporter 1/4), G-6-P (Glucose-6-phosphate), PPP (pentose phosphate pathway), R-5-P (Ribulose-5-phosphate).

Cell Cycle and Cyclin-Dependent Kinases

Uncontrolled cell proliferation is perhaps the most obvious feature of cancer cells. Since regulation of the cell cycle is largely dependent on the binding of specific cyclins to kinases, it is worth dissecting this mechanism in more detail. In the cell cycle there are checkpoints and go-ahead signals. The checkpoints are transition stages consisting of control systems that act as barriers along the cell cycle. There are three major checkpoints: the start checkpoint that determines whether a quiescent cell will enter a round of duplication, the G_2/M checkpoint which allows a cell to undergo metaphase and the metaphase-anaphase checkpoint after which sister chromatid separation, mitosis and cytokinesis occur. The control systems consist in fact of several reactions that collectively reflect biochemical mechanisms of cellular surveillance, that is, made up of many sensor reactions. Many of these sensor reactions involve protein phosphorylation. The end result is information that effectively tells the cell that it could proceed to the next stage in the cycle. When abnormalities occur, for example, in DNA synthesis, or chromosome assembly and segregation, cell-cycle arrest is induced so that the repair systems may come into action. Depending on the degree of damage, the defective cells themselves could be eliminated by a series of events whose outcome is either senescence or apoptosis. Why has protein phosphorylation become a recurrent device used by the cell for many regulatory reactions? The most outstanding influence of the epigenetically added phosphate groups may stem from the negative charges that are introduced into the polymer. In neutral pH each phosphate group contains two negative charges and thus the phosphoryl oxygens can establish hydrogen bonds that attract a cluster of positively charged amino acid side chains. This usually produces dramatic changes in the protein conformation and consequently modulates its functions. Apart from phosphate mediated intra-chain conformational changes, the adducts can promote the attraction of positively charged amino acids from other protein subunits. Thus, the introduction of phosphate groups contributes as well to the formation of docking sites for other proteins and ligands in general. This feature confers plasticity to the complex and generally favors the establishment of self-regulating networks. Furthermore, the covalent modification of enzymes by phosphate can be conveniently reversed by phosphatases. Both reactions, phosphorylation and dephosphorylation are energetically favorable because the kinase mediated addition of the gamma phosphate group of ATP or its removal by hydrolysis catalyzed by phosphatases is equivalent in fact to the net hydrolysis of ATP. It can be appreciated, therefore, that profound conformational differences can be achieved without too much investment in terms of energy, a feature that is definitely selectable from the evolutionary point of view.

Many of the compounds that are currently being clinically evaluated as anticancer drugs show broad anti-kinase properties which target the CDKs among others. Because these kinases play important roles in many regulatory events in the cell, much effort has been directed at characterizing phosphoproteins structurally and functionally. As a result of the general interest, the human kinome became available in 2002 [1] as a spinoff of the human genome sequencing project. This screening revealed the occurrence of more than 500 protein kinases that could potentially become drug targets for the treatment of a broad collection of diseases, particularly cancer. These include members of the cell division cycle 25 (Cdc25). By dephosphorylating Cdks, Cdc25 phosphatases render them active and, therefore promote progression along the cell cycle [2]. Indeed, Cdc25 phosphatases are considered to be classical proto-oncogenes since it has been found that they are overexpressed in several types of cancer. Interestingly, besides their action on Cdks, Cdc25 B, one of the three Cdc25 homologues has the ability to interact with several other key homeostatic proteins such as steroid receptors, c-AMP response element binding protein and the histone acetyl transferase co-activating binding proteins p300/CBP. Adding to this, the kinases are also amenable to regulation by specific inhibitors. A case in point is protein p21 that binds to G1-SCDK and S-CDK complexes and acts by blocking the cell cycle during passage from G1 to S when anomalies relating to DNA damage occur. Apart from DNA damage, protein p21 mediated cell cycle arrest can also be induced by glucose restriction. When cells are starved of glucose, the inhibition of expression of the glucose transcription factor carbohydrate responsive element binding protein (ChREBP) occurs. Because ChREBP is essential for cell proliferation, its suppression, accompanied, or triggered by p53 activation was found to lead to cell cycle arrest in colorectal cancer cells. If p53 loses its function through mutation, a frequent event in many types of cancer there is no cell cycle arrest. Again, ChREBP involvement on cell proliferation stresses the strong link between cell metabolism and regulation of the cell cycle [3-9] Fig (**1**).

Another connection between the cell cycle and the energy metabolism of neoplastic and non-neoplastic cells is provided by the E3 ubiquitin ligase APC/C-Cdh1 and the $SCF^{ßTrCP}$ complexes. They are known to degrade cell cycle proteins so that its over expression negatively affects the progression of the cell cycle leading on to inhibition of cell proliferation. Concomitantly, APC/C-Cdh1 and $SCF^{ßTrCP}$ are known to inhibit glycolysis and glutaminolysis by targeting 6-phosphofructo-2-kinase/fructose-2,6-bisphosphatase, isoform 3 (PFKFB3) and glutaminase 1 (GLS1), respectively. Because PFKFB3 and GLS1 are key regulatory enzymes in glycolysis and glutaminolysis, it is thought that suppression of expression the APC and $SCF^{ßTrCP}$ systems may be at the heart of the high glucose and glutamine consumption in cancer cells [10-12]. Figure **1** summarizes the main connections between metabolism and the cell cycle.

The key role that kinases and protein phosphorylation have on cell homeostasis can be best appreciated by detailing the emblematic Mdm2-$p14^{ARF}$-p53 regulatory axis [13]. Phosphorylated p53 normally drives cells into cell-cycle arrest, senescence or apoptosis. However, p53 function can be prevented by protein Mdm2 which binds to its dephosphorylated form promotes its ubiquitylation and subsequent degradation in the cytoplasmic proteasomes. Importantly, the interaction between Mdm2 and p53 in the nucleus is conformation-based and is tightly regulated at multiple levels, one of which is site-specific phosphorylation. It is known, for example that phosphorylation of Mdm2 at Thr-216 weakens its interaction with p53. Mdm2 itself is inactivated by protein $p14^{ARF}$ which binds to Mdm 2 and promotes its degradation within the nucleolus. Incidentally, because Mdm2 is overproduced in many tumors, it also constitutes another potential target for chemotherapy.

The importance of the kinome project and cancer can be gauged by the concentrated effort, mainly by pharmaceutical companies, to develop kinase inhibitors. This is reflected by the number of patent applications, which so far is in the order of tens of thousands. Moreover, kinases can be easily inhibited by small organic molecules, a fact that has contributed to the existence of more than 200 inhibitors undergoing clinical trials [14].

Several major groups of CDKs have been described, among which the cyclin-dependent kinases have attracted much interest [15, 16]. These enzymes consist of a catalytic unit, the Cdk proper and a regulatory unit consisting of the cyclins. Functionally, the Cdks differ from the receptor tyrosine kinases present on the cell surface in that they phosphorylate the aminoacids serine and threonine. The CDKs that have been studied in more detail within the context of the cell cycle are CDK1, CDK2, CDK4 and CDK6. CDK7, 8 and 9 are involved in regulation of transcription. It must be reminded that these protein kinases are catalytically inactive when in a free state, i.e., dissociated from the cyclins. Enzymatic activity is only achieved when a complex is formed between the catalytic subunit and cyclin proteins. The cyclins that form heterodimers with the catalytic moiety of the kinases are cyclin A1, A2, B1, B2, B3, D1, D2, D3, E1 and E2. Apart from these, G1-cyclins are accessory to CDKs of late G1 phase and are important for entry into the S-phase. Different combinations of CDKs and the cyclins produce the holoenzymes that can then phosphorylate other downstream protein substrates that will act as effectors of the transitions observed along the cell cycle. To complicate matters further *in vitro* experiments have shown that binding of different cyclins to the same CDK can change the substrate specificity [17].

Rather than the CDKs themselves, it is the intracellular cyclin concentration that oscillates. The variations in cyclin concentration result from regulation at the transcriptional, translational and degradation levels. CDKs proteolysis is accomplished in proteasomes after ubiquitylation of the protein complex. However, detailed knowledge of the CDKs protein substrates is still fragmentary. Only now as a result of approaches involving combinatorial analysis using large scale screening (microarrays, etc.), some of the putative protein substrates are beginning to be characterized. Their functional characterization, however, is an ongoing endeavor. Without the complete set of data it will hard to understand how the entry of cells into the S-phase, which depends on the activation of CDK2 by cyclin E and cyclin A, does not propel the cells into a different stage of the cycle such as mitosis. Or, for that matter, why entry into mitosis mediated by the corresponding CDKs does not initiate DNA synthesis [18]. One clue for the orderly and sequential progress along the cycle is the rapid elimination of cyclins as a result of the action of ubiquitin ligases. By attaching polyubiquitin chains to the cyclins the ligases mark them for proteolytic degradation, an action that hinders reversibility of the process. Proteolytic degradation is countered by small ubiquitin-like modifier proteins (SUMO) that compete with ubiquitin for certain substrates and thus act antagonistically as natural modulators of ubiquitins. Sumoylation increases protein stability, and thus SUMO could be an important player in tumorigenesis, by extending the cellular half-life of certain growth transcription factors that would otherwise be tagged for degradation via proteasomes. Although, SUMO constitutes a potential target in cancer therapy [19], a proteasome inhibitor, Bortezomib, has already been extensively used for the treatment of individuals with multiple myeloma. In this case, the idea was to promote the general degradation of oncogenic proteins assuming that these would outnumber the proapoptotic factors. This situation illustrates how anticancer strategies could take advantage of either branch of modulatory systems [20].

There are different classes of cyclins that are functionally allocated to each of the stages of the cell cycle. These classes are called, therefore, G_1, S and M cyclins. G1/S cyclins are involved in the entry of a cell into the cycle itself, S-cyclins participate in chromosome duplication and hence, DNA synthesis. Finally M-cyclins initiate mitosis at the G_2/M stage. The CDKs bind to G1-cyclins, G1/S-cyclins, S-cyclins and M-cyclins, respectively. A description of the steps involved in the S-phase illustrates how CDK mediated protein phosphorylation plays a key role in the cell cycle and how the CDKs themselves can be specifically inhibited by other regulatory proteins in connection with the sensor reactions already alluded to. This can be illustrated by considering the detection of DNA damage such as the occurrence of single strand cleavages. Protein kinases ATR (Ataxia telangiectasia and Rad3 related protein) and ATM (Ataxia telangiectasia mutated protein) become activated by conformational changes in DNA. As a result, the transcription factor protein p53 stimulates the expression of protein p21 which in turn inhibits the kinase activity of cyclinE-Cdk2 complex. The inhibition of this CDK by p21 blocks the phosphorylation of the retinoblastoma protein (pRb) thus ablating transcription factor E2F. E2F itself is further regulated by the so called pocket proteins that when hypophosphorylated, form repressor complexes that cause their silencing [21]. Consequently, the cell cycle remains arrested in G1. In mice models, pocket proteins p107 and p130 have been shown to function as tumor suppressors. Furthermore, it was found that the viral oncoprotein E7 believed to be one of the main agents involved in formation of head and neck cancer, was able to inactivate the repressive action of heterodimer pRb/p107 thus suggesting that the mechanism whereby virus E7 exert its oncogenic properties involves the silencing of E2F and consequently progression past the G1 stage [22]. In highly proliferative tumors E2F1 was found to be up regulated, which in turn led to increased *de novo* lipid synthesis [23]. Incidentally, the degree of phosphorylation of pRb is central to many events pertaining to the cell cycle. Recently, a specific inhibitor of CDK1/cyclin B1 activity, RO-3306 was shown to reversible down-regulate the expression of protein p21, the anti-apoptotic protein

Bcl2 and surviving, thus making it a candidate for cancer therapy [4]. In the cell cycle, only after DNA damage is corrected by the repair system the blockage induced by high levels of p21 will be reversed and it will proceed to the S-phase. Similar sensor reactions take place at the other checkpoints, thus underscoring the central role of protein phosphorylation in cell homeostasis. For example, when cells proliferate the kinase cyclin D-CDK4/6 is expressed in response to mitogenic signals and thus it acts as a mitogenic sensor. It must be emphasized, however, that the CDKs represent only one aspect of the overall regulatory network. It can be appreciated that each of the main elements briefly described above is itself subjected to regulation at various levels with the result that a network is formed that includes hundreds of proteins.

Are there observable changes in the overall pattern of CDKs in cancer cells? There is general agreement that of all the CDKs characterized so far, Cdk4 and Cdk6 alterations seem to be the most common manifestation in several types of tumors [24, 25]. As mentioned before, CDK deregulation actually implies in cyclin variation (*de novo* synthesis and degradation), since ultimately it is the fluctuation of these proteins that promote CDK activity. Down regulation of CDKs can be achieved by lowering local cyclin concentration. As mentioned before a regulatory switch could be formed either by direct inhibition of the complex by the so called CDK inhibitors (CKIs) and by phosphatases that remove the activating phosphate residues from the cyclin-CDK comple. CKIs are small peptides that constitute two major families. The INK4 family that downregulates Cdk4 and 6 and the Cip/kip inhibitor family which is composed by potent inhibitors of CDK2 [10]. The p21 protein involved in DNA repair is one of the members of the family, which aggregate as well p27 and p57. In the case of p27 besides its clear inhibitory effect on CDK2, it also downregulates CDK4/cyclinD, although in the latter case, it appears that the inhibition is dependent on the degree of phosphorylation of the inhibitor itself [15]. Interestingly, the degree phosphorylation of the Cip/Kip inhibitor family introduces yet another level of regulation. When phosphorylated through the Akt/PKB pathway after mitogen activation, p21 and p27 cannot enter the nucleus and exert their canonical inhibitory effects on several cyclin-CDK complexes. Thus, besides direct modulation of activators and inhibitors, the interplay between kinases and phosphatases also affects the intracellular traffic and localization of the individual factors.

Apart from the increased concentration of cognate cyclins, hyperactivity of CDKs could result from structural alterations that prevent them from binding CKIs or from alterations in the CKIs themselves. In theory, uncontrolled cell proliferation could occur as a result of overexpression of the CDKs. However, as mentioned before, it is known that during the cell cycle the catalytic moiety of CDKs are expressed at more or less constant rates which do not seem to change significantly during cell transformation. On the other hand, the levels of cyclins whose fluctuations normally regulate the cell division cycles have been shown to be altered in cancer. This will be further discussed below.

An example of the former situation is found in some melanoma patients, in which a missense mutation Arg24Cys present in CDK4 blocks the binding of INK4 inhibitors. Likewise, suppression of p21 and p27 promotes overexpression of E-cyclins and this in turn produces cell proliferation. Suppression mediated by p21 and p27 affects cell proliferation mainly by way of CDK2. CDK1 mediated cell proliferation may also be involved since this complex has been shown to be a ligand to these two inhibitors. Analysis of some human tumours has evidenced p21 and p27 suppression [26]. Upregulation of CDKs as a function of p21 and p27 silencing has been associated to gene hypermethylation of those genes. As for the overexpression or amplification of the CDKs, chromosomal translocations affecting CDK4 and CDK6 genes have been implicated in many types of cancer such as sarcoma, glioma, breast tumors, lymphoma and melanoma [25].

In practically, all types of cancer, the progression of G1 to S is altered due to deregulation of the D1/CDK4 complex. More notably, it is the cyclin moiety of the CDK complex which varies abnormally during neoplasia. Whereas most cyclins fluctuate according to internal control loops, D-cyclins stand out in terms of their unique responsiveness to extracellular mitogenic stimulation. Mitogens act through activation of receptor tyrosine kinase and the downstream signaling cascades that ultimately induce upregulation of cyclin D1 transcription, as well as increased translation and reduced post-translational proteolysis. Therefore, this cyclin has been definitely implicated as a culprit in cell transformation. Drugs targeting this cyclin would be of clinical interest, but so far no such direct inhibitors have been found. Alternatively, approaches aiming at controlling cyclin D1 levels by means of stimulation of its proteolytic degradation are under way [27]. However, controlling cyclin D1 production cannot be regarded as a panacea. A recent meta-analysis involving 2731 patients with non-small-cell lung cancer, revealed that there was no correlation between cyclin D1 expression and survival [24].

From the above, it can be concluded that the cyclical CDK activity can be controlled in many different ways. Whatever regulatory loop is being considered, the outcome of the event will depend ultimately on the active bimolecular complex kinase-cyclins. Consequently, it is not surprising that considerable attention has been directed at the development of drugs that could abrogate cell proliferation by way of inhibition of CDK activity. Indeed, several compounds are already being used clinically, many of which target the ATP binding sites of the kinases. Although, the ATP binding site is similar for all protein kinases, the compounds derive specificity by binding to the so called pockets lying adjacent to the ATP site. These pockets are formed by side chains in the kinase structure that display aliphatic and aromatic hydrophobic groups and that are amenable to different types of hydrogen bonding with the inhibitors. With these binding sites in mind, the inhibitors can be designed so that they will, in some cases, bind to the active or inactive forms of the protein kinases, depending on how each fits within the regulatory pathway. With this strategy, it becomes possible to engineer drugs that differentiate the individual kinases and thus attack specific disorders. The protein kinase inhibitors are not only employed for cancer treatment, but a large proportion of the available ones have been employed for that purpose.

Within the next few years the list of compounds will no doubt be substantially enlarged since at the moment there is a plethora of drugs undergoing clinical trials (Table **1**). An example is flavopiridol, a drug that inhibits CDKs in general, but displays lower K_i values for CDK9-cyclin T. This CDK participates in the elongation of mRNA and therefore it affects several pathways that generate transcription factors sharing different regulatory roles in the cell. Although, CDK9-cyclin is not directly involved in the cell cycle, its inhibition by flavopiridol induces a decrease in mRNA elongation of several short lived factors such as cytokines, cell-cycle regulators and kinases in general [28]. Apart from flavopiridol and other compounds which are based on natural substances various other synthetic molecules have been described as CDK inhibitors that are now being tested in clinical trials [5].

Table 1: Drugs that affect CDKs and the cell cycle [25].

CDK Inhibitor in Clinical Trial	**Clinical Indications**	**Know Targets**
Alvocidib (Flavopiridol)	Phase II clinical trials as a CDK9 inhibitor for a number of cancers, with promising results for the treatment of B-cell chronic lymphocytic leukaemia (CLL)	Broad-specificity CDK inhibitor with a distinct preference for CDK9
PD0332991	Phase II clinical trials for multiple myeloma	Potent and selective CDK4 and CDK6 inhibitor
AT-7519	Phase I clinical trials for advanced or metastatic tumours	CDK1, CDK2, CDK4, CDK5, GSK3β inhibitor
P276-00	Phase I/II clinical trials for neoplasms, Phase II for advanced malignant melanoma positive for cyclin D1 expression and treatment of recurrent and/or locally advanced head and neck Cancer	Specific Cdk4-D1, Cdk1-B and Cdk9-T inhibitor
P1446A-05	Phase I clinical study for advanced refractory malignancies	CDK4 inhibitor
PD-0332991	Phase I clinical trials for Neoplasms, Lymphoma Non-Hodgkin	CDK4, CDK6 inhibitor
R547	Phase I/II clinical trials for advanced solid tumors	CDK1, CDK2, CDK4, CDK7 inhibitor
SNS-032	Phase I clinical trials for Advanced B-Lymphoid Malignancies and Advanced Solid Tumors	CDK1, CDK2, CDK4, CDK7,CDK9, GSK3β inhibitor
SCH 727965	Phase I clinical trials for advanced cancer	CDK1, CDK2, CDK5, CDK9 inhibitor

Despite the central roles that CDKs play in the cell cycle, the first clinical trials employing CDK inhibitors have been disappointing. Many explanations have been put forward. For example, drugs such as flavopiridol may be acting on pathways other than those directly linked to the CDKs and might be specific only for certain tumors. CDK targets currently undergoing clinical trials include CDK1, CDK2, CDK4, CDK5, CDK6, CDK7, CDK8 and CDK9, most of them indicated for cases of advanced cancer [25]. In addition, due to the high functional redundancy that exists in cells, tumors continue to be viable even if single kinases become specifically inhibited. In other words, an efficient therapy might require the concomitant inhibition by various kinases that form salvage pathways without compromising normal cells, a very difficult task indeed. Another common observation is the development of resistance to the kinase inhibitors. The selective appearance of mutations that hinder drug binding to the target site has been reported in many trials [29]. Another set of inhibitors that is being considered as therapeutic options target not the CDKs directly, but the phosphatases. The Cdc25 family of phosphatases that participate in the transitions between the cell cycle phases is an example. By dephosphorylating CDKs, Cdc25 phosphatases render them active and hence display oncogenic properties in some cancers. Therefore, specific inhibitors against these enzymes have been developed and are currently being tested. These have been recently reviewed by Lavecchia *et al.* [2].

A recent trend towards cell cycle arrest and induction of apoptosis and necrosis has centered on the synthesis of peptides that mimic CDK inhibitors. These are synthetic peptides ranging from 8-34 aminoacid residues peptides that can be designed to bind specifically to cyclins or to CDKs and thus reproduce the effect of the naturally occurring proteins p21, p16 and p27. In many cases of cancer, these proteins have lost their ability to regulate CDKs. The importance of CDK inhibitor proteins can be appreciated by the observation that inactivation of INK4a is one of the most frequent genetic traits in tumorigenesis. Whilst therapy with peptides show great promise, there are technical problems involving the delivery of these synthetic peptides, and so far most of the experiments conducted have been carried out with cell lines [30].

The plasticity and interconnectivity exhibited by the cell homeostatic pathways have suggested alternative strategies for cancer treatment. Recently, metformin (dimethylbiguanide) a drug that has been employed as a first line pharmacologic treatment of type II diabetes is now being considered as an anti-tumorigenic agent in endometrial cancer and as an adjuvant in the treatment of breast cancer. Metformin may derive its beneficial effects on cancer by an indirect route that involves the intermediary metabolism. It is known that metformin activates AMP-activated protein kinase (AMPK) in several tissues. This kinase complex only allows cell division in situations where the energy level is compatible with proliferation, thus turning it into an energy sensor switch. When the cells are depleted of ATP, AMPK stimulates catabolism at the same time it blocks anabolic reactions. AMPK becomes active by a phosphorylation reaction catalyzed by the kinase LKB1, which is itself a tumor suppressor factor (see Fig. (**1**)). Because metformin activates AMPK it is thought that the drug's antineoplastic effect results from a parallel increase in the levels of LKB1. Incidentally, many types of cancer show a loss of LKB1 function [31-33]. The role of AMPK as an energy sensor and tumor suppressor has also been exploited for the development of new compounds which might activate this kinase. Two inventions have been recently patented dealing with this topic (WO2011029855; Glaxosmithkline LLC, 2011; WO2011163319, Cash AB, 2011) [34, 35]. Recently, AMPK has been shown to be an important effector of tumor cell survival by acting as a regulator of cellular NADPH availability [36]. These results add support to the all-important notion that besides the pro-tumorigenic stimulus for cell proliferation mediated by deregulated mitogens, it is the redox equilibrium in tumor cells that can dictate whether they will be viable or not.

An altogether different approach employed specific inhibitors of methionine aminopeptidases (MetAPs) which are now being tested as anti-cancer agents. The MetAPs that in normal cells catalyze the removal of initiator *N*-terminal methionine residues from nascent proteins, have been found to be overexpressed in various types of cancers. Overexpression of MetAPs and indeed other cognate genes would be expected by considering that the higher proliferative rates typical of tumor cells would be accompanied by higher rates of protein synthesis. Clinical trials are now being carried out with synthetic inhibitor compounds such as fumagillin analogs and natural inhibitors of aminopeptidases such as 2-hydroxy-3-aminoamide and the fused ketide amino acid derivatives, bengamides, isolated from sponges. All these compounds induce cell arrest at both, G1 and G2/M phases and had significant effects inhibiting tumor growth in mouse tumor models [37].

The G2/M phase of the cell cycle has also become a potential target for pharmacological interference in cancer treatment. In many types of cancer, one of the most visible alterations of transformed cells is the occurrence of structurally abnormal chromosomes. These could result from irregular microtubule nucleation at the centrosomes and hence lead to aberrant mitotic spindle formation. This in turn is directly subordinated to the Wnt-ß-catenin signaling pathway, which has been recently shown to be important components of the centrosomes. ß-catenin which is essential for centrosomal separation accumulates at the G2/M as a result of phosphorylation of low density lipoprotein receptor-related protein 6 (LRP6) by CDK14/cyclin Y complex [3]. Thus, in highly proliferating cells progression to mitosis could in theory be blocked by inhibitors affecting CDK14/cyclin complex formation or its function. Indeed, in certain cancers such as breast and prostate, expression of Wnt is increased which in turn leads to stabilization and accumulation of ß-catenin in the nucleus. In this context, it is accepted that Wnt hyper activation is in fact a hallmark of many types of cancer stem cells and this growth factor might be determinant in metastasis as well, particularly in colorectal tumors. Wnt itself is amenable to regulation by miRNAs. These are noncoding RNAs that bind to the UTRs of mRNA targets and repress their translation. Recently, it has been found that members of the family miRNA-34 (miRNA-34a-5p, miRNA-34b-5p and miRNA-34c-5p) are able to suppress the Wnt signaling pathway by interacting with genes encoding proteins downstream of Wnt [38]. Furthermore, it is known that in several types of cancer, deletions occur in chromosomal locations where putatively miR-34 family is synthesized. Therefore, stimulation of miRNA-34 production may well represent an additional strategy for anti-cancer intervention.

Tumor Cell Energy Requirements

With all its mechanistic subtleties, the cell cycle is costly in terms of energy. The human genome contains many genes that encode for proteins in charge of cellular processes, intracellular signaling, DNA replication, metabolism, transcription and translation. The energy situation clearly stands out when one considers that one of the more apparent characteristics of the tumor cells, is their limitless replication. In rapidly growing tumors, constant anabolism must be accompanied by upregulated pathways that ultimately accelerate the rate of ATP synthesis for all processes involved. Indeed, in order to support cell growth and proliferation, cancer cells must suffer metabolic reprogramming, which results in distinct bioenergetic phenotypes [39-41]. Hence, the energy metabolism of a malignant cell represents a promising target for cancer treatment.

The classic bioenergetic phenotype of cancer cells was described by Otto Warburg, over 90 years ago, in which an enhanced glycolysis with concomitant production of lactate is observed, even in the presence of high oxygen tension [42]. This so called Warburg phenomenon, also termed aerobic glycolysis, actually forms the basis of a widely used diagnostic tool for cancer that relies on the visualization of tumors as a result of enhanced glucose uptake revealed by positron emission tomography. In addition, a method using a glucose nanosensor to measure the rate of glucose consumption in highly proliferative cells both *in vivo* and *in vitro* has been developed (WO2012002963 Centro de Estudios Cientificos de Valdivia, 2012) [43]. Another invention that took advantage of the increased utilization of glucose by cancer cells was the conjugation of 2-deoxyglucose to anti-cancer drugs. 2-deoxyglucose is a glucose analogue that is taken up but not metabolized by the cells. As a result, a more efficient delivery of the drug should produce a better response to treatment (US7943586 The Trustees of the University of Pennsylvania, 2011) [44].

After the pioneering studies of Warburg, a great deal of information was generated and nowadays it is known that several other elements take part in the general metabolic reprogramming observed in the tumor cell. In this regard, in addition to the highly glycolytic "classic Warburg" phenotype, there are some tumors that present an active and even enhanced oxidative phosphorylation [45, 46]. It is important to stress at this point that the increased rate of glucose utilization (and enhanced glycolysis) presented by several types of tumors does not imply that cancer cells rely exclusively or even predominantly on glycolytic derived ATP to supply its energy needs [47-49]. Accordingly, ATP synthesis by the mitochondria seems to be an important feature of many types of cancer [45, 46].

Irrespectively of the physiological status of the mitochondria of tumor cells, a common feature is an increased glucose utilization required as a source of energy for bulk macromolecule synthesis [40, 50]. The fluctuation in oxygen tension experienced by many tumors may limit nutrient oxidation and ATP synthesis by oxidative phosphorylation and, therefore, glucose utilization assumes an important role under these unfavorable conditions [51]. The degradation of glucose molecules generates several intermediates that are used for biosynthetic purposes, e.g., glucose-6-phosphate for glycogen and ribose-5-phosphate synthesis; dihydroxyacetone phosphate for triacylglycerol synthesis and pyruvate for alanine synthesis [52]. Maintenance of high levels of NADPH relies not only on the inhibition of its consumption, for example during fatty acid biosynthesis, but also on alternative pathways for its production. Glucose molecules are also channeled by cancer cells to the pentose phosphate pathway, which produces NADPH (for antioxidative defense and fatty acid synthesis) and ribose-5-phosphate for purine/pirimidines synthesis [52]. In addition, the increased flux through the glycolytic pathway generates high amounts of lactate, which creates an acid environment and facilitate tumor invasion [53]. This aspect of the tumor cell shows that the increased glucose utilization by tumor cells has far reaching consequences that collectively illustrate a situation of selective adaptation. Metabolic reprogramming of cancer cells involve a gain-of-function of oncogenic factors, such as HIF-1 and PI3k/Akt/mTor axis and/or a loss-of-function of tumor suppressors, such as p53 [40, 47]. When the balance between glycolysis and oxidative phosphorylation is altered, activation of the Hypoxia-Inducible Factor-1 (HIF-1) takes place. This in turn can affect the expression of hundreds of other genes that interfere with several steps of the cell cycle and metabolic reprogramming of cancer cells. This regulation includes an enhanced conversion of glucose to pyruvate and lactate and mitochondrial dysfunction resulting in the reduction and/or suppression of oxidative phosphorylation and decreased mitochondrial biogenesis [39-40]. HIF-1 also is accessory for angiogenesis, the production of reactive oxygen species and the general regulation of intracellular Ca^{++} homeostasis [54]. Since p53 activity is associated with decreased glycolytic and increased oxidative phosphorylation activities, the loss-of-function of this tumor suppressor protein, typical of many types of cancer, also contributes to the observed increase in utilization of the carbons from glucose by tumor cells [40] (Fig (**2**)).

The identification of metabolic targets linked to the modulation of glucose utilization provides useful information that can be used in the treatment of cancer [40]. Indeed, several small molecules have been used to modulate target enzymes/proteins which occupy central roles in cancer metabolism. One important strategy for efficient targeting would be to decrease glucose/substrate supply by way of HIF-1 alfa modulation. Two methods based on the inhibition of HIF-1 expression by locked nucleic acid oligonucleotides (US7939507 Enzol Pharmaceuticals, Inc., 2011) [55] or prevention of HIF-1 activation by nitrosylation (US20110054023 Duke University, 2011) [56] have been developed which might inhibit angiogenesis and halt tumor proliferation. Targeting PI3k/akt/mTor axis would also affect the metabolic reprogramming of cancer cells and potentially regulate tumor growth. In this sense, small molecule antagonists of phosphatidyl inositol-3,4,5-triphosphate, which is the main product of PI3k and which regulates Akt activation, have also been patent protected (WO2011022028 Tufts University, 2011) [57].

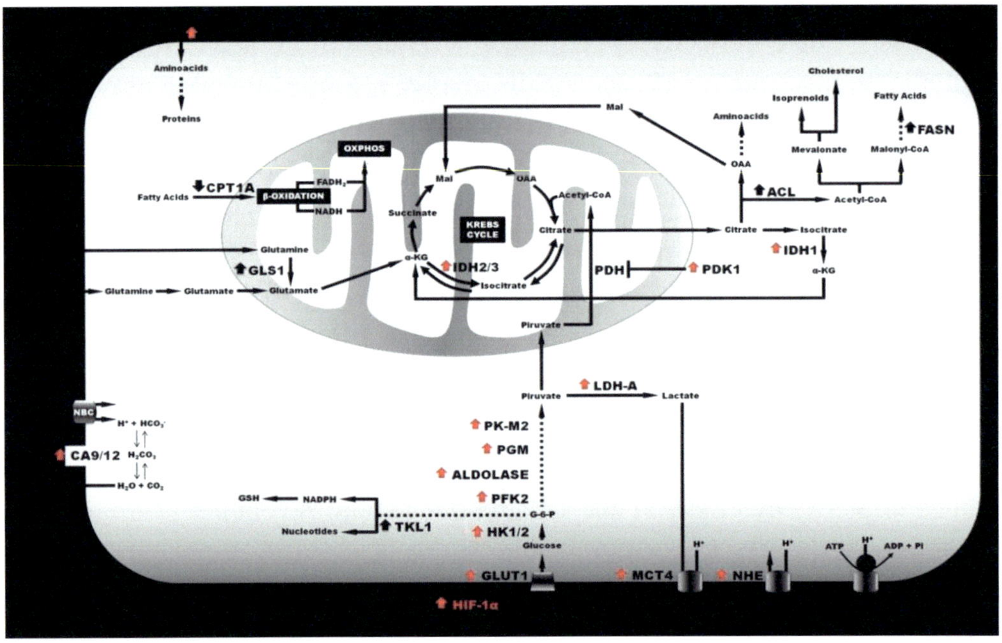

Figure 2: Energy metabolism in tumor cells. The tumorigenesis is accompanied by metabolic reprogramming. Activation of HIF-1α (hypoxia-inducible factor) is one of the main events promoting alterations in selected metabolic pathways. Red arrows represent alterations caused by the activation of HIF-1. LAT1 (large neutral amino acid transporter), CPT1A (carnitine palmitoyltransferase 1A), GLS1 (glutaminase 1), CA9 and CA12, carbonic anhydrases 9 and 12; CPT, carnitine palmitoyltransferase; GLUT, glucose transporter, GSH (glutathione), HK (hexokinase), OXPHOS (oxidative phosphorylation), LDHA (lactate dehydrogenase) isoform A, MCT (monocarboxylate transporter), PDH (pyruvate dehydrogenase), PDK (pyruvate dehydrogenase kinase) PFK (phosphofructokinase), PGM (phosphoglycerate mutase), PKM2 (pyruvate kinase isoform M2), TLK (transketolase), ACL (ATP citrate lyase), IDH2/3 (isocitrate dehydrogenase isoform 2 and 3), FASN (fatty acid synthase).

As mentioned above, increased production of lactate seems to facilitate tumor invasion. Lactate dehydrogenase is the enzyme that catalyzes the reversible conversion of pyruvate from glycolysis to lactate. Different methods for inhibiting lactate dehydrogenase have been patented (US20120003156 The Johns Hopkins University, 2012) [58] and could be important for the treatment of cancer. Therefore, blockage of pyruvate conversion to lactate could be important to maintain pH in the surrounding micro environment and also would make the former more available for oxidation.

In addition to the modulation of glucose metabolism, there has been a great deal of interest in compounds which modulate mitochondrial function and have a profound effect as promoters of apoptosis [48, 59]. This has become particularly noticeable by examination of tumor cell metabolic profile that led to the discovery of tumor-specific alterations on mitochondrial biogenesis-related genes [39, 60]. Thus, mitochondrial shape and size [61], accumulation of mutations in mitochondrial DNA [62], respiratory chain complexes activities [63], truncation of the Kreb's cycle via modulation of ATP citrate lyase [38], increased expression of mitochondria-bound hexokinase [50] and inhibition of pyruvate dehydrogenase complex [64, 65] are all potential targets for intervention.

The following section contains data from recent studies involving compounds that exploit aberrant metabolism and that could be used as anti-cancer drugs.

Bromopyruvate

There are several fundamental proteins that assist malignant tumors in scavenging and metabolizing glucose at an abnormal rate [40]. For instance, an increase in hexokinase (HK) activity, the enzyme that catalyzes the first step of the glycolytic pathway in which glucose is phosphorylated to glucose-6-phosphate via phosphate transfer from ATP, appears to be a typical phenotype of malignant tumor growth and proliferation [50, 66]. It has been demonstrated that many malignant tumors over-express type II (and possibly type I) HK, an isoform of the enzyme which is preferentially bound to mitochondria through interaction with the voltage-dependent anion channel (VDAC), a protein located on the outer mitochondrial membrane [67]. This scenario facilitate the utilization of mitochondrial generated ATP via the mitochondrial adenine nucleotide translocator (ANT) by HK, committing glucose to glycolysis and other biosynthetic pathways that use it as a precursor. This occurs because HK binding to mitochondria binding also decreases its inhibition by glucose-6-phosphate [50, 67, 68]. Apart from the metabolic advantages conferred by the increased expression of type II HK in malignant tumors, overexpression seems to be central in protecting cells from apoptotic stimuli [69]. In this context, studies on the interaction between HK and mitochondria and mitochondrial-bound proteins prompted the search for potential molecular targets that could lead to inhibition of tumor proliferation. It has been shown that the pyruvate/lactate analogue, 3-bromopyruvate (3-BrPA), an alkylating agent which is able to react with thiol and hydroxy groups of several enzymes [70-72], inhibits both, glycolysis and oxidative phosphorylation and, therefore, cellular ATP production [50,73, 74]. The beneficial aspects of 3-BrPA as an inhibitor of cancer cell proliferation and tumor growth has generated a patent based on the inhibition of ATP production that has been recently deposited [75, 76]. Some analogues of 3-bromopyruvate have also been patent protected such as 3-halopyruvate (US20100221220) [77] and were shown to be effective in the treatment of liver tumors. It has been shown that 3-BrPA treatment eradicated hepatocellular carcinoma implanted in rats possibly due to inhibition of type II HK and mitochondrial function [73]. Such a result emphasizes the important role of HK-mitochondria interaction for tumor survival. 3-BrPA was also shown to decrease the viability of a human hepatocarcinoma cell line by significantly decreasing the rate of glucose utilization (by inhibiting glyceraldehyde-3-phosphate dehydrogenase and phosphoglycerate kinase activities) and oxidative phosphorylation (via succinate dehydrogenase inhibition) [74]. These studies support the idea that the selective modulation of energy-related pathways in cancer cells is a very promising strategy to control the rate of cellular proliferation and tumor development. A recent report has suggested that the anti-tumor activity of 3-BrPA in a human mammary cell line, apart from its effect on energy homeostasis, involved the inhibition of histone deacetylases and, consequently, regulation of cell proliferation [78] and below. In addition to 3-bromopyruvate, compounds which affect ATP availability have also been considered as anti-cancer drugs. Two main systems are involved in the synthesis of ATP in mitochondria: Oxidative phosphorylation, which comprises the respiratory complexes and the phosphorylation system, which is a functional unit consisting of ANT, phosphate carrier and ATP synthase. ATP is synthesized in the mitochondrial matrix and ANT exchanges ADP for ATP in an electrogenic antiport across the inner mitochondrial membrane. Therefore, ANT is a potential target for anti-cancer treatment since any alteration in ANT expression/activity, would result in decreased availability of ATP and its accumulation in mitochondria. Indeed, a method for treating breast cancer by using ANT small interfering RNA or ANT short hairpin RNA has been recently patent protected (US20110207798 Bioinfra Inc., 2011) [79].

Pyruvate Kinase Inhibitors

Regulation of the glycolytic pathway occurs at several levels involving the allosteric and covalent modulation of glycolytic enzymes. In this regard, the enzymes that catalyze thermodynamically favorable and, virtually irreversible reactions of the glycolytic pathways, represent prime metabolic targets in cancer cells. Pyruvate kinase, the enzyme which catalyzes the conversion of phosphoenolpyruvate to pyruvate and ATP, belongs to this category. Like mitochondrial-bound HK isoforms, the expression pattern of PK isoforms is altered in many cancers [40], as reflected by overexpression of the embryonic isoform of PK. Overexpression confers metabolic advantages to tumor cells [40]. Indeed, a patent was deposited recently in which novel inhibitors of PK, which chemically modify this enzyme's structure, were effective in inhibiting the proliferation of breast and glioma cell lines [80]. Modulators that allosterically inhibit PK catalytic activity were also patented [81].

Dichloroacetate

Given that a shift from oxidative to glycolytic metabolism represents an important aspect of carcinogenesis, compounds that revert or re-program energy metabolism of cancer cells, e.g., by stimulating glucose oxidation and modulating mitochondrial function, are also very promising for cancer treatment [40, 48]. In this regard, dichloroacetate (DCA) is a compound that inhibits pyruvate dehydrogenase kinase (PDK) and consequently reverts the inhibition of pyruvate dehydrogenase. Such an action of DCA favors pyruvate (and indirectly glucose) oxidation to Acetyl CoA. It has been shown that DCA decreases mitochondrial membrane potential, increases mitochondrial generation of H_2O_2 and activates mitochondrial K^+ channels, all of which contribute to apoptosis induction and to a decrease in tumor proliferation and growth [64]. Interestingly, it was observed that the molecular inhibition of PDK isoform 2 by siRNA mimics DCA effects in non-small cell lung cancer, glioblastoma and mammary carcinoma cell lines [64]. A patent describing this strategy in cancer treatment using dichloroacetate was recently deposited [82]. The patent claims are that the treatment of non-small cell lung cancer, glioblastoma and mammary carcinoma cell lines with DCA resulted in a modulation of mitochondrial function measured by an increase in cytochrome *c* release and mitochondrial depolarization, which ultimately turn cells more prone to apoptotic death.

Acetylation and Deacetylation in Tumorigenesis

In eukaryotic cells, the DNA is packaged into chromatin, a highly organized and dynamic protein-DNA complex. The fundamental subunits of this structure are the nucleosomes, octamers formed by four core histones, i.e., an H3/H4 tetramer and two H2A/H2B dimers, enfolded by DNA. Chromatin structures can exhibit alteration between compacted and relaxed conformations and these states are related to acetylation and deacetylation processes. Histones acetyl transferases (HATs) add acetyl groups to lysine residues, while histones deacetylases (HDACs) remove the acetyl groups. These enzymes have been linked to gene expression activation and repression, respectively. In general, hyperacetylation is associated with increased transcriptional activity, whereas hypoacetylation is associated with repression of gene expression.

Besides histone proteins, the HDACs/HATs have many other non-histone protein substrates, such as transcriptional factors-p53, retinoblastoma protein- Rb; chaperones (HSP90); cytoskeleton-actin, α-tubulin, BAX, HMGB1, metabolic enzymes (pyruvate kinase; acetyl-CoA synthase) and steroid receptors among others. For this reason, these enzymes are involved in control of a broad spectrum of biological functions. Among them are growth arrest, DNA repair, cellular bioenergetics, cell death pathways (apoptosis, and autophagy), mitosis, generation of reactive oxygen species, senescence and angiogenesis [83-85].

High expression and activity of HDAC was associated with progressions and poor prognosis of different tumors [84]. Considering the involvement of HDACs in the multiple cellular functions mentioned above they have clearly become potential targets within the context of therapy in cancer.

Histone Deacetylase Inhibitors

A wide range of HDAC inhibitors (HDACi) with different chemical structures have been identified. These inhibitors, obtained from natural or synthetic sources, are usually grouped into five classes including, hydroxamic acid and derived compounds, benzamides, cyclic peptides, short chain fatty acids and ketones. In spite of their structural differences, these HDACis have a similar spectrum of anti-tumoral activity, but different efficacy depending on cell type, concentration of the inhibitor and time of incubation with the corresponding drug.

The mechanisms of action of this class of drugs are still uncertain. However, it is known that HDACis regulate gene transcription (about 2 - 10% of genes) through inhibition of HDAC, leading to alterations at the level of target proteins acetylation and deacetylation. This action may cause transcriptional and post-translational modifications. For example, a tumor suppressor can be reactivated and restore the control of cell cycle and thus lead to tumor cell apoptosis. A well documented example is the transcriptional induction of $p21^{WAF1/CIP1}$ by HDACi, which inhibits the CyclinD/CDK4 complex formation and G1 arrest [61]. Besides $p21^{WAF1/CIP1}$, other genes related to cell cycle control are up or down regulated by HDACis: genes related to apoptosis (BAX, BCL2), transcriptional factors (NFKB, STAT3, c-MYC, GATA-2), growth factors (erb-1, erb-2), angiogenesis (VEGF) and chaperones (HSP90, HSP70) [86-89]. These effects of HDAC have been observed in solid and hematological disperse tumors, which present different levels of response to the drugs. Sensitivity also depends on the degree of tumor differentiation, replicative status and metastasis.

Several different HDACis are being evaluated in clinical trials for the cancer treatment after Food and Drug Administration (FDA) approval of Suberoylanilide Hydroxamic Acid (SAHA) in 2006 for the treatment of advanced cutaneous T-cell Lymphoma [90]. Additionally, an increase in patent applications claiming novel HDCAis as potential drug candidates has been observed [91]. In the last year, several patents were deposited and, in general, they described news compounds with HDACi activity (US20120035257, US20120041001) [92, 93], HDACi in combination with others drugs such as cell cycle modulators or tyrosine kinase inhibitors. Also there are methods for determining HDAC resistance (US2011005316) [94] and methods for identifying patients responsive to these inhibitors.

HDAC is display pleiotropic effects in different tumors, inducing growth arrest, differentiation and apoptosis. Interestingly, some reports show that HDAC is have lower inhibitory activity on normal cells when compared to transformed ones [95]. It is believed that the difference in sensitivity is due, among other things, to the higher ability of normal cells to counteract the high levels of reactive oxygen species generated by HDAC treatment. In normal fibroblasts, for example, increased levels of thioredoxin a natural ROS scavenger, was detected upon HDAC treatment, in contrast to transformed fibroblasts. For these reasons, the HDAC have been regarded as potential therapeutic agents for cancer treatment. Currently, there is a massive search for novel compounds exhibiting HDAC properties, mainly because of their far reaching effects at the chromatin level. In some cases, such as sodium butyrate, a natural end product of the cell metabolism, the side effects are not as severe as those obtained with other classes of drugs.

HDAC Inhibitors and Mitochondria

As discussed above, the mechanism of action of HDAC may be related to alterations on the acetylation status of transcriptional factors and consequent regulation of gene expression. However, it is not understood why tumor cells are more sensitive to these drugs than normal cells. Clearly, thioredoxin levels alone cannot explain the observed effects. The answers may be connected to the peculiarities of mitochondrial metabolism in cancer, for example those that involve Ca^{2+} uptake by mitochondria. Although to date there are no available data, it has been suggested that the different phenotype of cancer cells regarding Ca^{2+} uptake may be directly correlated to functional alterations of the Ca^{2+} pump itself [96]. As a result of a repressed mitochondrial respiration, the electron transport complexes remain in the reduced state, a situation that favors the production of ROS. Due to the close vicinity to the source of ROS and the lack of the protective histones, in the long run the mitochondrial DNA itself becomes damaged by the oxidative stress and this in turn produces mutations that ultimately contribute to malfunction of the respiratory chain [97]. The vicious circle thus established creates one of the hallmarks of cancer cells, namely, phenotypes characterized by mitochondrial DNA mutations. It is still debatable, however, whether mitDNA mutations are a cause or consequence of malignant transformation. In this context, the role that ROS play on cell metabolism remains somewhat ambiguous [8]. On one hand, superoxide anion, hydrogen peroxide, hydroxyl radical, organic peroxides and reactive nitrogen species generated under hypoxic conditions can contribute towards lipid peroxidation and protein modifications that increase the risk of mutagenesis and are associated to many degenerative diseases. On the other hand, the oxidative stress appears to constitute a normal control in situations such as cell proliferation, differentiation and migration. Viewed like that ROS in general and H_2O_2 in particular take part as elements in untransformed cell signaling and are known to be produced in cells stimulated by various growth factors. H_2O_2 can modify the activity of protein tyrosine kinases which in turn, as mentioned before, can regulate a series of vital cellular events. Phosphatases are also affected by H_2O_2 and thus introduce a balance in the modulation that depends on reactions involving protein phosphorylation and dephosphorylation. For example, tyrosine phosphatase activity is reversibly inhibited in cells that have been stimulated with PDGF, EGF, insulin and various B cell receptor ligands. Likewise, cells stimulated with TNF-α produce H_2O_2 that inactivate mitogen-activated protein kinase phosphatases. As a consequence, other effectors such as c-Jun become activated and promote specific cellular responses. It appears, therefore, that the overall effect that oxidative stress has on cells is a matter of degree. Plausibly, when antioxidant enzymes such as catalase, glutathione peroxidase and peroxiredoxin fail to degrade the excess of ROS produced in the mitochondria, a situation conducive to carcinogenesis becomes established. Cancer cells are in fact exquisitely sensitive to ROS and it is well established that they can effectively lead to inhibition of cell growth and cell death. In this scenario malignant transformation would be produced by DNA strand breaks and point mutations directly affecting proto-oncogenes and tumor suppressor genes. In this respect, it has been shown that ROS can increase the expression of DNA methyltransferases that silence several genes including cyclin-dependent kinase inhibitor-2, BRCA1 and importantly, the retinoblastoma protein, the controlling hub in the cell cycle.

Whatever the situation, the viability of tumor cells depends heavily on a constant energy supply. A variety of compounds targeting energy metabolism, specially at the level of the mitochondria, have been identified. Recently, attention has been directed at several known compounds, such as tamoxifen, resveratrol and HDACis that have effects on cellular metabolism [98, 99]. Besides their potential chemotherapeutic use, these drugs are now helping to dissect details of the metabolic reprogramming that accompanies cell transformation.

Little is known about HDACi effects on the glycolytic and oxidative pathways. Studies of mitochondria of rat liver treated with the short chain fatty acid derivate Valproate (VPA) have shown that this HDACi inhibits fatty acid β-oxidation and in general depresses cell oxidative metabolism leading to a decrease in both, the rate of oxygen consumption coupled to ATP synthesis and cytochrome oxidase activity. VPA induces an increase in acyl-CoA/Coenzyme A ratio in the mitochondrial matrix, which may also be associated to lower acetyl-CoA concentration. These effects can be related to the conversion of VPA to Coenzyme A derivatives, i.e. valproyl-CoA [100-102] The metabolic effects of VPA might be exacerbated by a decrease in PDH complex activity, which also promotes a decrease in acetyl-CoA concentration, thus contributing to the energy collapse of cancer cells. Colorectal adeno carcinomas cells (HT29) treated with sodium butyrate (NaB), another short chain fatty acid class HDACi, inhibited glucose uptake and oxidation, as well as ribose synthesis and increased *de novo* fatty acid synthesis along with activation of the pentose phosphate pathway. Another group showed that theses cells metabolize NaB without increasing the oxygen consumption-synthesis ATP coupled [103]. However MIA cells, butyrate-resistant pancreatic adenocarcinoma, did not display any changes in their metabolic profile after treatment. These metabolic changes can be correlated to the induction of differentiation processes by butyrate and consequently with its growth inhibitory effects [104]. In myeloma cells the HDACis VPA and SAHA, decrease fatty acid oxidation and acetyl-CoA levels. In addition, these inhibitors induced a decrease on glucose uptake and hexokinase activity leading to metabolic reprogramming and apoptosis in tumor cells [105]. In neuroblastoma cells, TSA and VPA are upregulated PGC1α and GLUT 4. These alterations were important to increase mitochondrial function [106].

We have shown that the sodium butyrate and trichostatin A (TSA), both of them deacetylase inhibitors, decreased the glycolytic flux and induced a shift of towards a more oxidative metabolism in H460 cells. Interestingly, panobinostat (LBH589), a pan-deacetylase inhibitor that has been extensively used in clinical trials for various types of cancer was found to down regulate, among other factors, glucose transporter GLUT1 in Hodgkin lymphoma cell lines [107]. Although, our own results with sodium butyrate agree with the inhibition of GLUT1 expression, we found in addition that GLUT3 expression was significantly increased by the HDACi. Metabolomic analysis showed that NaB altered the glycolytic metabolite profile of intact H460 cells. Concomitantly, we detected an activation of the pentose phosphate pathway. These results showed alterations in the energetic metabolism of H460 cells after treatment with 10 mM NaB for 24 hours [108].

Recently, different papers have showed that most enzymes from energy metabolism are acetylated. This pos-translational modification can up regulate or down regulate activity of specific enzymes from glycolysis and oxidative pathways (overview in [109]) Regulation of intermediary metabolism by protein acetylation, 2010). In this scenario, the HDACs NAD-dependent from family Sirt have emerged as important proteins because they can regulate either cytoplasmic or mitochondrial proteins involved in cellular bioenergetics. Hallows and collaborators showed that Sirt1 deacetylated phosphoglycerate mutase-1, a glycolytic enzyme and decreased its activity [110]. Another report showed that Sirt 3, a mitochondrial HDAC, increased ATP levels in the cell and complex I activity from electron transport system [111]. In this context, it is noteworthy the publication of one patent related to inhibition of HDAC from class III, in other words, Sirt family (US20110104177) [112].

CURRENT & FUTURE DEVELOPMENTS

Recent results have shown that several pathways of the intermediary metabolism are subverted when cells transform into tumors. Indeed, current strategies for chemotherapy have taken advantage of some features of the metabolic reprogramming that takes place in tumor cells with a view to adopting a more selective approach to cancer treatment. Because there are common nodes between the energy metabolism and factors that control the cell cycle many of these strategies will certainly focus on those pathways that will produce maximum disruption of cancer cells. For example, drugs that concomitantly stimulate ROS production and promote methylation-dependent gene silencing. Among likely target candidates for such drug interference are the cyclin-dependent kinase inhibitor-2 and the retinoblastoma protein. In this context, much attention is being directed at the effect that pulse treatment with ROS has on replicative senescence, a process that besides the Rb protein does involve checkpoint proteins such as p53, p21 and p16.

ACKNOWLEDGEMENTS

The authors wish to acknowledge the financial support of CNPq, FAPERJ, FAF and INCT/CNPq-Cancer.

CONFLICT OF INTEREST

Regarding the present chapter, the authors wish to declare that to their knowledge no conflict of interest exist regarding either the present paper, the supporting agencies and the patents cited in the text.

DISCLOSURE

The chapter submitted for Patent eBook Series "Topics in Anti-Cancer Research", Volume 2 is an update of our article "Cell Cycle and Energy Metabolism in Tumor Cells: Strategies for Drug Therapy", published in the journal 'Recent Patents on Anti-Cancer Drug Discovery', Volume 6, Number 1, January, 2011, Page 15 to 25 with additional text and references.

REFERENCES

[1] Manning G, Whyte DB, Martinez R, Hunter T, Sudarsanam S. The protein kinase complement of the human genome. Science 2002; 298(5600): 1912-34.

[2] Lavecchia A, Di Giovanni C, Novellino E. CDC25A and B dual-specificity phosphatase inhibitors: Potential agents for cancer therapy. Curr Med Chem 2009; 16(15): 1831-49.

[3] Davidson G, Niehrs C. Emerging links between CDK cell cycle regulators and Wnt signaling. Trends Cell Biol 2010; 20(8): 453-60.

[4] Kojima K, Shimanuki M, Shikami M, Andreeff M, Nakakuma H. Cyclin-dependent kinase 1 inhibitor RO-3306 enhances p53-mediated Bax activation and mitochondrial apoptosis in AML. Cancer Sci 2009; 100(6): 1128-36.

[5] Krystof V, Uldrijan S. Cyclin-dependent kinase inhibitors as anticancer drugs. Curr Drug Targets 2010; 11(3): 291-302.
[6] Mason EF, Rathmell JC. Cell metabolism: An essential link between cell growth and apoptosis. Biochim Biophys Acta 2011; 1813(4): 645-54.
[7] Ralph SJ, Rodriguez-Enriquez S, Neuzil J, Saavedra E, Moreno-Sanchez R. The causes of cancer revisited: "Mitochondrial malignancy" and ROS-induced oncogenic transformation - why mitochondria are targets for cancer therapy. Mol Aspects Med 2010; 31(2): 145-70.
[8] Reuter S, Gupta SC, Chaturvedi MM, Aggarwal BB. Oxidative stress, inflammation, and cancer: How are they linked? Free Radic Biol Med 2010; 49(11): 1603-16.
[9] Tong X, Zhao F, Mancuso A, Gruber JJ, Thompson CB. The glucose-responsive transcription factor ChREBP contributes to glucose-dependent anabolic synthesis and cell proliferation. Proc Natl Acad Sci USA 2009; 106(51): 21660-5.
[10] Duan S, Pagano M. Linking metabolism and cell cycle progression via the APC/CCdh1 and SCFbetaTrCP ubiquitin ligases. Proc Natl Acad Sci USA 2011; 108(52): 20857-8.
[11] Almeida A, Bolanos JP, Moncada S. E3 ubiquitin ligase APC/C-Cdh1 accounts for the Warburg effect by linking glycolysis to cell proliferation. Proc Natl Acad Sci USA 2010; 107(2): 738-41.
[12] Colombo SL, Palacios-Callender M, Frakich N, Carcamo S, Kovacs I, Tudzarova S, *et al.* Molecular basis for the differential use of glucose and glutamine in cell proliferation as revealed by synchronized HeLa cells. Proc Natl Acad Sci USA 2011; 108(52): 21069-74.
[13] Sherr CJ. Tumor surveillance via the ARF-p53 pathway. Genes Dev 1998; 12(19): 2984-91.
[14] Akritopoulou-Zanze I, Hajduk PJ. Kinase-targeted libraries: The design and synthesis of novel, potent, and selective kinase inhibitors. Drug Discov Today 2009; 14(5-6): 291-7.
[15] Echalier A, Endicott JA, Noble ME. Recent developments in cyclin-dependent kinase biochemical and structural studies. Biochim Biophys Acta 2010; 1804(3): 511-9.
[16] Hochegger H, Takeda S, Hunt T. Cyclin-dependent kinases and cell-cycle transitions: Does one fit all? Nat Rev Mol Cell Biol 2008; 9(11): 910-6.
[17] Murray AW. Recycling the cell cycle: Cyclins revisited. Cell 2004; 116(2): 221-34.
[18] Errico A, Deshmukh K, Tanaka Y, Pozniakovsky A, Hunt T. Identification of substrates for cyclin dependent kinases. Adv Enzyme Regul 2010; 50(1): 375-99.
[19] Bettermann K, Benesch M, Weis S, Haybaeck J. SUMOylation in carcinogenesis. Cancer Lett 2012; 316(2): 113-25.
[20] Tanaka T, Nakatani T, Kamitani T. Inhibition of NEDD8-conjugation pathway by novel molecules: Potential approaches to anticancer therapy. Mol Oncol 2012; 6(3): 267-75.
[21] Kurimchak A, Grana X. PP2A holoenzymes negatively and positively regulate cell cycle progression by dephosphorylating pocket proteins and multiple CDK substrates. Gene 2012; 499(1): 1-7.
[22] Shin MK, Pitot HC, Lambert PF. Pocket proteins suppress head and neck cancer. Cancer Res 2012; 72(5): 1280-9.
[23] Bhatia B, Hsieh M, Kenney AM, Nahle Z. Mitogenic Sonic hedgehog signaling drives E2F1-dependent lipogenesis in progenitor cells and medulloblastoma. Oncogene 2011; 30(4): 410-22.
[24] Hayward NK. Genetics of melanoma predisposition. Oncogene 2003; 22(20): 3053-62.
[25] Malumbres M, Barbacid M. Cell cycle, CDKs and cancer: A changing paradigm. Nat Rev Cancer 2009; 9(3): 153-66.

[26] Blain SW. Switching cyclin D-Cdk4 kinase activity on and off. Cell Cycle 2008; 7(7): 892-8.
[27] Kim JK, Diehl JA. Nuclear cyclin D1: An oncogenic driver in human cancer. J Cell Physiol 2009; 220(2): 292-6.
[28] Johnson LN. The regulation of protein phosphorylation. Biochem Soc Trans 2009; 37(Pt 4): 627-41.
[29] Knight ZA, Lin H, Shokat KM. Targeting the cancer kinome through polypharmacology. Nat Rev Cancer 2010; 10(2): 130-7.
[30] Raucher D, Moktan S, Massodi I, Bidwell GL, 3rd. Therapeutic peptides for cancer therapy. Part II - cell cycle inhibitory peptides and apoptosis-inducing peptides. Expert Opin Drug Deliv 2009; 6(10): 1049-64.
[31] Cantrell LA, Zhou C, Mendivil A, Malloy KM, Gehrig PA, Bae-Jump VL. Metformin is a potent inhibitor of endometrial cancer cell proliferation-implications for a novel treatment strategy. Gynecol Oncol 2010; 116(1): 92-8.
[32] Grenader T, Goldberg A, Shavit L. Metformin as an addition to conventional chemotherapy in breast cancer. J Clin Oncol 2009; 27(35): e259.
[33] Memmott RM, Dennis PA. LKB1 and mammalian target of rapamycin as predictive factors for the anticancer efficacy of metformin. J Clin Oncol 2009; 27(34): e226.
[34] Mirguet, O. Pyrrolo-pyridine derivatives as activators of AMPK. WO2011029855 (**2011**).
[35] Cash, A.B. Activation of AMP-protein activated kinase by oxaloacetate compounds. WO2011163319 (**2011**).
[36] Jeon SM, Chandel NS, Hay N. AMPK regulates NADPH homeostasis to promote tumour cell survival during energy stress. Nature 2012; 485(7400): 661-5.
[37] Yin SQ, Wang JJ, Zhang CM, Liu ZP. The development of MetAP-2 inhibitors in cancer treatment. Curr Med Chem 2012; 19(7): 1021-35.
[38] Cha YH, Kim NH, Park C, Lee I, Kim HS, Yook JI. miRNA-34 intrinsically links p53 tumor suppressor and Wnt signaling. Cell Cycle 2012; 11(7): 1273-81.
[39] Bellance N, Lestienne P, Rossignol R. Mitochondria: From bioenergetics to the metabolic regulation of carcinogenesis. Front Biosci 2009; 14: 4015-34.
[40] Kroemer G, Pouyssegur J. Tumor cell metabolism: Cancer's Achilles' heel. Cancer Cell 2008; 13(6): 472-82.
[41] Wu M, Neilson A, Swift AL, Moran R, Tamagnine J, Parslow D, *et al.* Multiparameter metabolic analysis reveals a close link between attenuated mitochondrial bioenergetic function and enhanced glycolysis dependency in human tumor cells. Am J Physiol Cell Physiol 2007; 292(1): C125-36.
[42] Warburg O. On respiratory impairment in cancer cells. Science 1956; 124(3215): 269-70.
[43] Barros Olmedo, L.F., Bittner Hofmann, C.X. Method to measure the metabolic rate or rate of glucose consumption of cells or tissues with high spatiotemporal resolution using a glucose nanosensor. WO2012002963 (**2012**).
[44] Zheng, G., Glickson, J.D., Chance, B. Antineoplastic agents targeted via glut transporters. US7943586 (**2011**).
[45] Guppy M, Leedman P, Zu X, Russell V. Contribution by different fuels and metabolic pathways to the total ATP turnover of proliferating MCF-7 breast cancer cells. Biochem J 2002; 364(Pt 1): 309-15.
[46] Zu XL, Guppy M. Cancer metabolism: Facts, fantasy, and fiction. Biochem Biophys Res Commun 2004; 313(3): 459-65.

[47] Costello LC, Franklin RB. Tumor cell metabolism: The marriage of molecular genetics and proteomics with cellular intermediary metabolism; proceed with caution! Mol Cancer 2006; 5: 59.

[48] Ralph SJ, Low P, Dong L, Lawen A, Neuzil J. Mitocans: Mitochondrial targeted anti-cancer drugs as improved therapies and related patent documents. Recent Pat Anticancer Drug Discov 2006; 1(3): 327-46.

[49] Takai N, Kawamata N, Gui D, Said JW, Miyakawa I, Koeffler HP. Human ovarian carcinoma cells: Histone deacetylase inhibitors exhibit antiproliferative activity and potently induce apoptosis. Cancer 2004; 101(12): 2760-70.

[50] Mathupala SP, Ko YH, Pedersen PL. Hexokinase-2 bound to mitochondria: Cancer's stygian link to the "Warburg Effect" and a pivotal target for effective therapy. Semin Cancer Biol 2009; 19(1): 17-24.

[51] Pouyssegur J, Dayan F, Mazure NM. Hypoxia signaling in cancer and approaches to enforce tumour regression. Nature 2006; 441(7092): 437-43.

[52] Gatenby RA, Gillies RJ. Why do cancers have high aerobic glycolysis? Nat Rev Cancer 2004; 4(11): 891-9.

[53] Swietach P, Vaughan-Jones RD, Harris AL. Regulation of tumor pH and the role of carbonic anhydrase 9. Cancer Metastasis Rev 2007; 26(2): 299-310.

[54] Taylor CT, Pouyssegur J. Oxygen, hypoxia, and stress. Ann NY Acad Sci 2007; 1113: 87-94.

[55] Westergaard, M., Thrue, C.A., Rasmussen, F.W., Hansen, H.F., Potent LNA oligonucleotides for the inhibition of HIF-1a expression. US7939507 (**2011**).

[56] Dewhirst, M.W., Cao, Y. Inhibition of HIF-1 activation for anti-tumor and anti-inflammatory responses. US20110054023 (**2011**).

[57] Degterev, A., Reibark, M., Wagner, G., Yuan, J. Small molecule antagonists of phosphatidylinositol-3, 4, 5 triphosphate (PIP3) and uses thereof. WO2011022028 (**2011**).

[58] Dang, C.V., Le, Q.H., Dinavahi, R. Methods for treating neoplasia by inhibiting lactate dehydrogenase and/or nicotinamide phosphoribosyltransferase. US20120003156 (**2012**).

[59] Ralph SJ, Neuzil J. Mitochondria as targets for cancer therapy. Mol Nutr Food Res 2009; 53(1): 9-28.

[60] Bellance N, Benard G, Furt F, Begueret H, Smolkova K, Passerieux E, *et al.* Bioenergetics of lung tumors: Alteration of mitochondrial biogenesis and respiratory capacity. Int J Biochem Cell Biol 2009; 41(12): 2566-77.

[61] Arismendi-Morillo G. Electron microscopy morphology of the mitochondrial network in human cancer. Int J Biochem Cell Biol 2009; 41(10): 2062-8.

[62] Ishikawa K, Takenaga K, Akimoto M, Koshikawa N, Yamaguchi A, Imanishi H, *et al.* ROS-generating mitochondrial DNA mutations can regulate tumor cell metastasis. Science 2008; 320(5876): 661-4.

[63] Simonnet H, Alazard N, Pfeiffer K, Gallou C, Beroud C, Demont J, *et al.* Low mitochondrial respiratory chain content correlates with tumor aggressiveness in renal cell carcinoma. Carcinogenesis 2002; 23(5): 759-68.

[64] Bonnet S, Archer SL, Allalunis-Turner J, Haromy A, Beaulieu C, Thompson R, *et al.* A mitochondria-K^+ channel axis is suppressed in cancer and its normalization promotes apoptosis and inhibits cancer growth. Cancer Cell 2007; 11(1): 37-51.

[65] Kim JW, Tchernyshyov I, Semenza GL, Dang CV. HIF-1-mediated expression of pyruvate dehydrogenase kinase: A metabolic switch required for cellular adaptation to hypoxia. Cell Metab 2006; 3(3): 177-85.

[66] Bustamante E, Morris HP, Pedersen PL. Energy metabolism of tumor cells. Requirement for a form of hexokinase with a propensity for mitochondrial binding. J Biol Chem 1981; 256(16): 8699-704.
[67] Pastorino JG, Hoek JB. Regulation of hexokinase binding to VDAC. J Bioenerg Biomembr 2008; 40(3): 171-82.
[68] Mathupala SP, Ko YH, Pedersen PL. Hexokinase II: Cancer's double-edged sword acting as both facilitator and gatekeeper of malignancy when bound to mitochondria. Oncogene 2006; 25(34): 4777-86.
[69] Gottlob K, Majewski N, Kennedy S, Kandel E, Robey RB, Hay N. Inhibition of early apoptotic events by Akt/PKB is dependent on the first committed step of glycolysis and mitochondrial hexokinase. Genes Dev 2001; 15(11): 1406-18.
[70] Chang GG, Hsu RY. Mechanism of pigeon liver malic enzyme: Kinetics, specificity, and half-site stoichiometry of the alkylation of a cysteinyl residue by the substrate-inhibitor bromopyruvate. Biochemistry 1977; 16(2): 311-20.
[71] Korotchkina LG, Showkat Ali M, Patel MS. Involvement of alpha-cysteine-62 and beta-tryptophan-135 in human pyruvate dehydrogenase catalysis. Arch Biochem Biophys 1999; 369(2): 277-87.
[72] Tunnicliff G, Ngo TT. Mechanism of inactivation of brain glutamic decarboxylase by 3-bromopyruvate. Int J Biochem 1978; 9(4): 249-52.
[73] Ko YH, Smith BL, Wang Y, Pomper MG, Rini DA, Torbenson MS, *et al.* Advanced cancers: Eradication in all cases using 3-bromopyruvate therapy to deplete ATP. Biochem Biophys Res Commun 2004; 324(1): 269-75.
[74] Pereira da Silva AP, El-Bacha T, Kyaw N, dos Santos RS, da-Silva WS, Almeida FC, *et al.* Inhibition of energy-producing pathways of HepG2 cells by 3-bromopyruvate. Biochem J 2009; 417(3): 717-26.
[75] Ko, Y.H., Geschwind, J.-F.H., Pedersen, P.L. Therapeutics for cancer using 3-bromopyruvate and other selective inhibitors of ATP production. US7547673 (**2009**).
[76] Geschwind, J.-H., Vali, M. Therapeutics for cancer using 3-bromopyruvate and other selective inhibitors of ATP production. US20100203110 (**2010**).
[77] Ko, Y.H. Therapeutics for cancer using 3-bromopyruvate and other selective inhibitors of ATP production. US20100221220 (**2010**).
[78] Thangaraju M, Karunakaran SK, Itagaki S, Gopal E, Elangovan S, Prasad PD, *et al.* Transport by SLC5A8 with subsequent inhibition of histone deacetylase 1 (HDAC1) and HDAC3 underlies the antitumor activity of 3-bromopyruvate. Cancer 2009; 115(20): 4655-66.
[79] Kim, C.W., Jang, J.Y., Method for treating breast cancer using adenine nucleotide translocator 2 (ANT2) siRNA or ANT2 shRNA. US20110207798 (**2011**).
[80] Smith, B.R., Chang, T.-H., Leyland-Jones, B. Novel inhibitors of pyruvate kinase as therapeutic agents for cancer. US20080311183 (**2008**).
[81] Abraham, D.J., Wang, C., Danso-Danquah, R., Burnett, J.C., Joshi, G.S., Hoffman, S.J. Allosteric inhibitors of pyruvate kinase. US6534501 (**2003**).
[82] Michelakis, M., Archer, S. Method of treating cancer using dichloroacetate. US20090118370 (**2009**).
[83] Gu W, Roeder RG. Activation of p53 sequence-specific DNA binding by acetylation of the p53 C-terminal domain. Cell 1997; 90(4): 595-606.

[84] Witt O, Deubzer HE, Milde T, Oehme I. HDAC family: What are the cancer relevant targets? Cancer Lett 2009; 277(1): 8-21.

[85] Xie H, Bandhakavi S, Roe MR, Griffin TJ. Preparative peptide isoelectric focusing as a tool for improving the identification of lysine-acetylated peptides from complex mixtures. J Proteome Res 2007; 6(5): 2019-26.

[86] Aoyagi S, Archer TK. Modulating molecular chaperone Hsp90 functions through reversible acetylation. Trends Cell Biol 2005; 15(11): 565-7.

[87] Quivy V, Van Lint C. Regulation at multiple levels of NF-kappaB-mediated transactivation by protein acetylation. Biochem Pharmacol 2004; 68(6): 1221-9.

[88] Roy S, Packman K, Jeffrey R, Tenniswood M. Histone deacetylase inhibitors differentially stabilize acetylated p53 and induce cell cycle arrest or apoptosis in prostate cancer cells. Cell Death Differ 2005; 12(5): 482-91.

[89] Yu X, Guo ZS, Marcu MG, Neckers L, Nguyen DM, Chen GA, *et al.* Modulation of p53, ErbB1, ErbB2, and Raf-1 expression in lung cancer cells by depsipeptide FR901228. J Natl Cancer Inst 2002; 94(7): 504-13.

[90] FDA approval and New Drug Application (NDA) documents for ZolinzaTM (SAHA, vorinostat).

[91] Wang H, Dymock BW. New patented histone deacetylase inhibitors. Expert Opin Ther Pat 2009; 19(12): 1727-57.

[92] Lan-Hargest, H.-Y., Kaufman, R.J., Wiech, N.L. Histone deacetylase inhibitors. US20120035257 (**2012**).

[93] Van Emelen, K., Verdonck, M.G.C., Van Brandt, S.F.A., Backx, L.J.J. Carbonylamino-derivatives as novel inhibitors of histone deacetylase. US20120041001 (**2012**).

[94] Buggy, J.J., Balasubramanian, S. Methods for determining cancer resistance to histone deacetylase inhibitors. US20110053164 (**2011**).

[95] Ungerstedt JS, Sowa Y, Xu WS, Shao Y, Dokmanovic M, Perez G, *et al.* Role of thioredoxin in the response of normal and transformed cells to histone deacetylase inhibitors. Proc Natl Acad Sci USA 2005; 102(3): 673-8.

[96] Wojtczak L, Teplova VV, Bogucka K, Czyz A, Makowska A, Wieckowski MR, *et al.* Effect of glucose and deoxyglucose on the redistribution of calcium in ehrlich ascites tumour and Zajdela hepatoma cells and its consequences for mitochondrial energetics. Further arguments for the role of Ca^{2+} in the mechanism of the crabtree effect. Eur J Biochem 1999; 263(2): 495-501.

[97] Gogvadze V, Orrenius S, Zhivotovsky B. Mitochondria in cancer cells: What is so special about them? Trends Cell Biol 2008; 18(4): 165-73.

[98] Kallio A, Zheng A, Dahllund J, Heiskanen KM, Harkonen P. Role of mitochondria in tamoxifen-induced rapid death of MCF-7 breast cancer cells. Apoptosis 2005; 10(6): 1395-410.

[99] Tinhofer I, Bernhard D, Senfter M, Anether G, Loeffler M, Kroemer G, *et al.* Resveratrol, a tumor-suppressive compound from grapes, induces apoptosis via a novel mitochondrial pathway controlled by Bcl-2. FASEB J 2001; 15(9): 1613-5.

[100] Ponchaut S, van Hoof F, Veitch K. Cytochrome aa3 depletion is the cause of the deficient mitochondrial respiration induced by chronic valproate administration. Biochem Pharmacol 1992; 43(3): 644-7.

[101] Silva MF, Ruiter JP, L IJ, Jakobs C, Duran M, de Almeida IT, *et al.* Differential effect of valproate and its Delta2- and Delta4-unsaturated metabolites, on the beta-oxidation rate of long-chain and medium-chain fatty acids. Chem Biol Interact 2001; 137(3): 203-12.

[102] Turnbull DM, Bone AJ, Bartlett K, Koundakjian PP, Sherratt HS. The effects of valproate on intermediary metabolism in isolated rat hepatocytes and intact rats. Biochem Pharmacol 1983; 32(12): 1887-92.

[103] Leschelle X, Delpal S, Goubern M, Blottiere HM, Blachier F. Butyrate metabolism upstream and downstream acetyl-CoA synthesis and growth control of human colon carcinoma cells. Eur J Biochem 2000; 267(21): 6435-42.

[104] Boren J, Lee WN, Bassilian S, Centelles JJ, Lim S, Ahmed S, *et al.* The stable isotope-based dynamic metabolic profile of butyrate-induced HT29 cell differentiation. J Biol Chem 2003; 278(31): 28395-402.

[105] Wardell SE, Ilkayeva OR, Wieman HL, Frigo DE, Rathmell JC, Newgard CB, *et al.* Glucose metabolism as a target of histone deacetylase inhibitors. Mol Endocrinol 2009; 23(3): 388-401.

[106] Cowell RM, Talati P, Blake KR, Meador-Woodruff JH, Russell JW. Identification of novel targets for PGC-1alpha and histone deacetylase inhibitors in neuroblastoma cells. Biochem Biophys Res Commun 2009; 379(2): 578-82.

[107] Lemoine M, Derenzini E, Buglio D, Medeiros LJ, Davis RE, Zhang J, *et al.* The pan-deacetylase inhibitor panobinostat induces cell death and synergizes with everolimus in Hodgkin lymphoma cell lines. Blood 2012; 119(17): 4017-25.

[108] Amoedo ND, Rodrigues MF, Pezzuto P, Galina A, da Costa RM, de Almeida FC, *et al.* Energy metabolism in H460 lung cancer cells: Effects of histone deacetylase inhibitors. PLoS One 2011; 6(7): e22264.

[109] Guan KL, Xiong Y. Regulation of intermediary metabolism by protein acetylation. Trends Biochem Sci 2011; 36(2): 108-16.

[110] Hallows WC, Yu W, Denu JM. Regulation of glycolytic enzyme phosphoglycerate mutase-1 by Sirt1 protein-mediated deacetylation. J Biol Chem 2012; 287(6): 3850-8.

[111] Ahn BH, Kim HS, Song S, Lee IH, Liu J, Vassilopoulos A, *et al.* A role for the mitochondrial deacetylase Sirt3 in regulating energy homeostasis. Proc Natl Acad Sci USA 2008; 105(38): 14447-52.

[112] Baylin, S., Pruitt, K. Histone deacetylase inhibitors, combination therapies and methods of use. US20110104177 (**2011**).

Topics in Anti-Cancer Research, Vol. 2, 2013, 231-256

CHAPTER 6

V-ATPase Inhibitors in Cancer Therapy: Targeting Intraorganellar Acidification

Agustín Hernández*, **Gloria Serrano-Bueno, Rosana Herrera-Palau, José R. Pérez-Castiñeira and Aurelio Serrano**

Instituto de Bioquímica Vegetal y Fotosíntesis, CSIC-Universidad de Sevilla, Avda. Américo Vespucio 49, 41092 Seville, Spain

Abstract: Vacuolar-type ATPases are multicomponent proton pumps involved in the acidification of single membrane intracellular compartments such as endosomes and lysosomes. They couple the hydrolysis of ATP to the translocation of one or two protons across the membrane. Acidification of the lumen of single membrane organelles is a necessary factor for the correct traffic of membranes and cargo to and from the different internal compartments of a cell. V-ATPases are also involved in the regulation of pH at the cytosol and, possibly, extracellular milieu. The inhibition of V-ATPases has been shown to induce apoptosis as well as cell cycle arrest in tumor cells; therefore, chemicals that behave as inhibitors of this kind of proton pumps have been proposed as putative treatment agents against cancer and many have been patented as such. The compounds filed in patents fall into five major types: plecomacrolides, benzolactone enamides, archazolids, chondropsins and indoles. All these have proved to be apoptosis inducers in cell culture and many are able to reduce xenograft tumor growth in murine models. The present chapter will summarize their general structure, origin and mechanisms of action and put them in relation to the patents registered so far for the treatment of cancer.

Keywords: Acidification, apicularen, apoptosis, archazolid, bafilomycin, cell cycle arrest, cell death, chondropsin, concanamycin, endosome, hidrazide, indole, lobatamide, lysosome, macrolide, organelle, palmerolide, salicylihalamide, V-ATPase, Warburg-effect.

INTRODUCTION

Transport of cargo and membranes from the endoplasmic reticulum to their final destinations is vital for eukaryotic cells. The major players in this flux of vesicles

***Address correspondence to Agustín Hernández:** IBVF, CSIC-Universidad de Sevilla, Avda. Americo Vespucio 49, 41092 Seville, Spain; Tel: +34 954 489500; Fax +34 954 460065; E-mail: agustin.hernandez@csic.es

Atta-ur Rahman and Khurshid Zaman (Eds)

and proteins are the endoplasmic reticulum (ER, the site where both proteins and lipids are synthesized), the Golgi apparatus, early and late endosomes, other single-membrane vesicular organelles derived from these, such as peroxysomes and exocytic vesicles, and the lysosome. The latter, along with the plasma membrane, can roughly be considered as terminal destinations. Nevertheless, membrane and cargo can flow both ways; for example, from ER to the lysosome (anterograde) or from the plasma membrane to the ER (retrograde). The detailed mechanisms and players involved in fission, fusion and transport of vesicles are an active field of research. However, one of the requirements known for a correct function of the endo/exocytic pathway is the presence of an electrochemical gradient across the membranes of these organelles, mostly in the form of a proton gradient [1, 2]. The extent of this gradient is different in each compartment, as shown in Fig. (**1**). While ER remains at near-neutral pH and shows no remarkable difference with respect to the cytosol, lysosomes can hold a 3-pH unit transmembrane gradient [2]. Other compartments show pH values somewhere in between these two extremes. As a rule of thumb, the extent of lumenal acidification for vesicular organelles is greater the farther they are from the ER and the closer they are to a terminal destination (plasma membrane or lysosome). Indeed, the idea that these pH gradients are only a part of the vesicle transport mechanism is an oversimplification. The acidification of the vesicular lumina is also necessary for the numerous functions of these organelles; for example, glycosylation of proteins in the Golgi apparatus is impaired if the pH gradient is abolished in this organelle [3, 4]. The generation of these positive-inside proton gradients is carried out by a class of proton pumping ATPases, usually called Vacuolar ATPases (V-ATPases), in concert with counter ion conductance driven by channels and other transporters. It is also balanced by the intrinsic proton permeability of the membrane and the activity of proton-consuming transporters such as H^+ antiporters [2]. V-ATPases were first described in vacuoles (the plant and fungal equivalent of the animal lysosome), but later they were found across the range of single-membrane organelles in all eukaryotic organisms. Mitochondria and chloroplasts do not bear this kind of proton pumps but the closely related F_0F_1 type. At any rate, V-ATPases are not only found at the endo/exocytic system, but they also exist to accomplish physiologically important functions at the plasma membrane of certain mammalian cell types, such as those at the *vas deferens* and osteocytes [5, 6]. Diseases like osteoporosis and osteopetrosis owe a great deal to plasma membrane V-ATPase dysfunction [7, 8]. In cancer they have been suggested to influence metastatic potential by providing an acidic extracellular environment that would ease protease action on the extracellular matrix [9]. Although, it is a promising hypothesis that deserves future attention, the actual importance of V-ATPase-mediated extracellular acidification, as opposed to improvement of other intracellular organelle functions, has not been sufficiently addressed yet. Conversely, their effect on drug resistance and proliferation through acidification of endocellular compartments and changes in cytosolic pH homoeostasis seems, comparatively, well established. We will thus concentrate on V-ATPases and their inhibitors as modulators of lumenal and cytosolic pH in cancer.

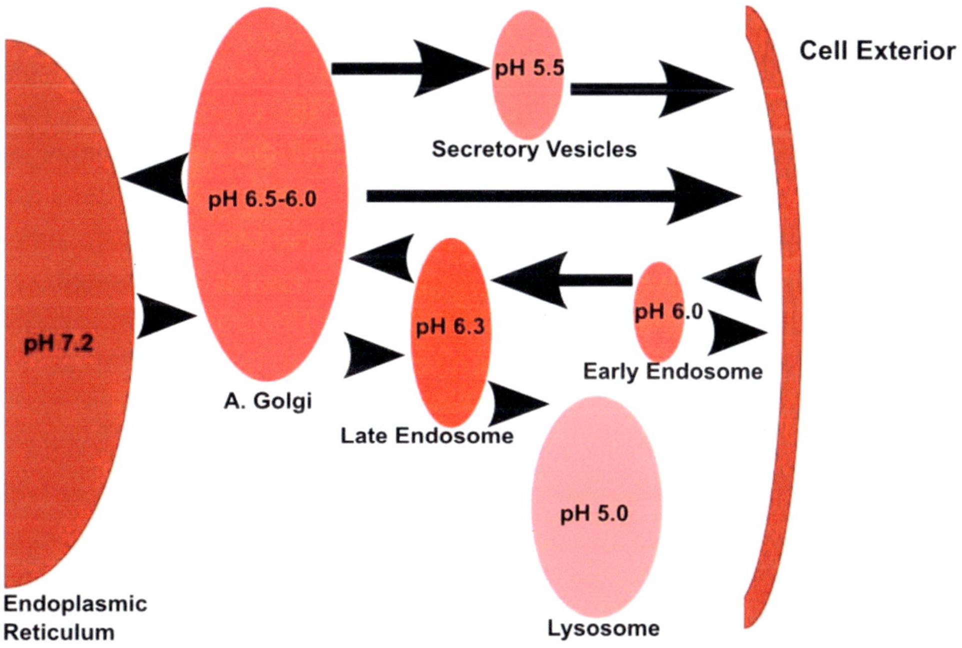

Figure 1: Traffic between intracellular compartments and their internal characteristic pH values. Vesicle flux between single membrane organelles is shown by arrows.

V-ATPASE STRUCTURE AND TRANSPORT MECHANISM

V-type ATPases are very complex biochemical machines, they are multimeric proteins consisting of two main domains (V_0 and V_1). A general model is depicted in Fig. (**2**). From extensive experimentation on the yeast enzyme, it is now known that the membrane-embedded domain (V_0) is composed of 9 polypeptides: single copies of a, c', c'' d and e, and four copies of c. The hydrophilic domain, named V_1 by similarity to the F_1 domain in F_0F_1 ATPases, is composed of eight different polypeptides (named always using capital letters, A to H) Fig. (**2**). The stoichiometry of these polypeptides is three for A, B, E and G and one for C, D, H, and F. In mammals, another c subunit substitutes for subunit c' and an additional regulatory subunit (Ac45) is present. However, these differences do not alter significantly the catalytic mechanism or the general model for the mammalian enzyme. Proton pumping is achieved by a rotary mechanism similar to that observed in the closely related F_0F_1 proton pump in mitochondria. Subunits A harbour catalytic domains that, by hydrolysing ATP, provide torque to the V_1 domain that is transmitted to the V_0 domain by stalk subunits D, F and subunit d at the V_0 domain. This induces the rotation of the membrane ring complex composed of subunits c_4, c', c'' while subunit a and the A_3B_3 complex remain static. The current line of thought proposes that this movement provides a path for proton transport through two hemi-channels that would be present in subunit a. One proton from the cytosol enters the first hemi-channel and it is complexed to a protonable glutamate residue on subunits c, c' or c''. The cation remains associated to its ring subunit until sector V_0 makes a new full turn; the stability of the cation-protein interaction is enhanced due to its direct contact with a non-polar environment such as the lipid milieu [10]. When a protonated proteolipid in the rotor reaches again subunit a, the protonated residue enters in contact with the second polar hemi-channel and the cation is released into the lumen. Subunits B, albeit carrying ATP binding sites, are not capable of hydrolysis and are considered regulatory [10].

In vivo modulation of V-ATPase activity can be achieved by several mechanisms. V_1 domains can exist both as soluble cytosolic complexes and bound to V_0 domains. Since neither free V_0 nor V_1 domains are capable of proton transport or

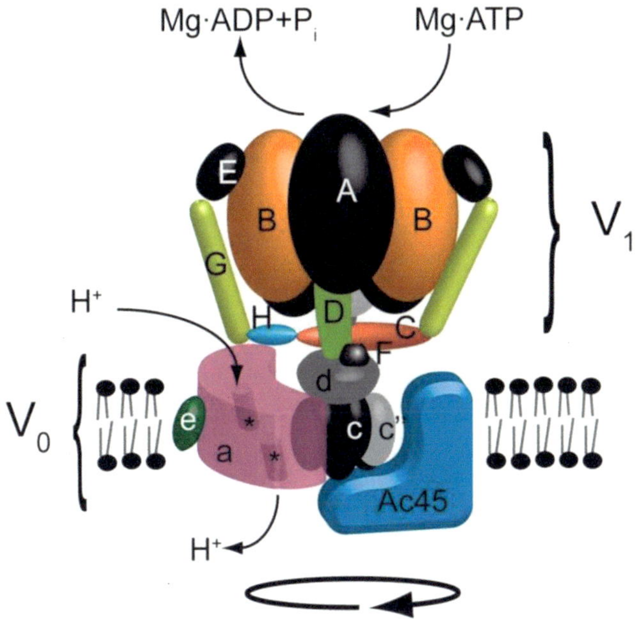

Figure 2: Subunit structure of V-ATPases. Subunits A to F constitute the hydrophilic V_1 domain; subunits a to e comprise the V_0 membrane-embedded domain.

ATP hydrolysis, respectively, assembly and disassembly of V_1 from V_0 is believed to be a mechanism providing fast regulation of pump activity, especially in situations of dynamic glucose availability [1, 11]. Modulation of H^+/ATP transport stoichiometry is another mechanism of regulation. Subunit a holds both hemi-channels on its *C*-terminus and can produce V-ATPases with varying stoichiometry, depending on the integration of different isoforms of this polypeptide into the mature protein complex. For example, in yeast, V-ATPases bearing isoform Stv1p show a stoichiometry of 1 proton per hydrolysed ATP, whereas if the same enzyme carries isoform Vph1p that parameter increases up to 2 H^+/ATP [10]. Also, other subunits may, in theory, alter the ratio of transported protons per ATP as seen in mutagenesis studies over subunits A, C or D [12]. In mouse and humans, there are four genes coding for subunit a. In addition to this, at least three transcript variants for A1 have been found in humans. However, although it seems plausible that a similar mechanism of variable stoichiometry applies in mammals, this has not been demonstrated so far. Phosphorylation of the holoenzyme has also been reported. In insect cells, it was first described that C subunit was phosphorylated by protein kinase A and that this was instrumental for correct V_1/V_0 assembly [13]. Shortly after, yeast Dbf2p protein kinase was shown to phosphorylate both A and B subunits, moreover *dbf2Δ* deletion strains were unable to acidify their vacuoles [14]. In mammals, phosphorylation of epididymides V-ATPase by PKA has also been observed [15]. Yet another mechanism of transport regulation is the control of the number of ATPase pumps resident in an organelle. This regulation has been clearly observed for the plasma-membrane resident V-ATPase, the abundance of which is affected by the rate of sequestration into recycling endosomes [12]. Indeed, changes in exo/endocytic flux dynamics could provide a possible explanation to the increased number of V-ATPases found at the plasma membrane of malignant tumor cells. However, to date, no indications exist as to whether a similar mechanism is at work in other membranes.

IMPORTANCE OF V-ATPASES FOR A CANCER CELL

A tumor cell's fast pace of growth is supported by an accelerated metabolism. The latter fuels the synthesis of new cellular components, such as proteins or lipids, that need to be transported to their final destinations. In this context, the importance of V-ATPases for tumor cell can easily be understood. Despite this, V-ATPases do not seem to be greatly overexpressed in neoplastic cells, as opposed to many other proteins in rapidly dividing cells, such as growth factor signalling or cell cycle-related proteins [16, 17]. The subunit/gene complexity of these proton pumps probably makes the overexpression of all of them in a coordinated way a phenomenon very unlikely to occur. However, increased expression of several isoforms has been reported, for example, it has been shown that ATP6V1C1 human gene (encoding subunit C) is overexpressed in oral squamous carcinoma cells and that this may promote a greater degree of V_1V_0 assembly than in normal tissue [18]. Similarly, different subunit genes have been found to be overexpressed in drug-resistant cell lines, including ATP6L (ATP6V0C, subunit c) in the case of cisplatin resistance [19]. Moreover, it has been demonstrated that overexpression of proteolipid c leads to increased invasiveness in stable transfectants [20]. One of the consequences of all this is that tumor cells depend more heavily on the activity of V-ATPases than normal cells. This is exemplified by the well known capability of V-ATPase inhibitors to induce apoptosis in tumor cells [21, 22]. It has been proposed that the acidic environment within endosomes helps dissociation of ligands from their receptors, thereby facilitating the recycling of the latter back to the plasma membrane [23]. Alternatively, inhibition of the V-ATPase would lead to endo/exocytic malfunction that, in turn, should cause receptors for growth factors such as EGFR to remain associated to their ligands in endosomes, thus preventing their degradation [24]. In addition, alkalinization of intracellular vesicular compartments would lead to protein missorting. In yeast models, plasma membrane proteins have been observed to mislocalize in V-ATPase mutants [25]. In mammals, glycosyltransferases at the Golgi apparatus have been proven to be sensitive to the lumenal ion composition. In particular, these enzymes are rapidly missorted to endosomes if the pH value within the Golgi is affected by merely 0.4 units [3, 4]. This same phenomenon has been observed for secreted proteins such as chromogranin A [26] and viral VSV-G [27], although, in the latter case, it might also be connected to the already mentioned redistribution of glycosyltransferases.

Tumor cells live in a harsh microenvironment. Hypoxic conditions and rapid growth rates make these cells rely on glycolysis and lactic acid fermentation, rather than on respiration, to obtain the energy they need; this is the so-called Warburg Effect [28]. This anaerobic metabolism has the downturn of producing great amounts of protons that need to be neutralized from the cytosol. At the same time, deficient perfusion of solid tumors leads to low extracellular pH that can contribute to select cells able to thrive in such an environment because they can efficiently drive away protons from their cytoplasms [29-31]. These cells could be more effective at sequestering cytosolic protons into intracellular vesicular compartments or could be expelling them back to the intercellular milieu. In all of these cases, V-ATPases play an important role. It has been proven that V-ATPases are present at the plasma membrane of tumor cells and that their abundance correlates with proliferation and metastatic potential [9, 32, 33]. However, it is still unclear whether many of the phenotypes observed in these cells are caused by V-ATPases at the plasma membrane or due to concomitant increased endo/exocytic rates. Cathepsins, matrix metalloproteases and other proteases involved in metastasis, have been invoked as the beneficiaries of increased plasma membrane proton extrusion and acidification of the extracellular medium since they need an acidic environment to loosen the extracellular protein matrix. However, bearing in mind that there are several other factors involved, it is still difficult to ascertain to which extent plasma membrane V-ATPases contribute to extracellular acidification. Moreover, many of these proteases are intracellular in normal cells but in neoplastic ones they become overexpressed and secreted [34]. This differential location can greatly be influenced by enhanced activity of endocellular V-ATPases which would make transit of the overproduced proteases more speedy and become secreted as a side effect. At any rate, more work is needed to shed light into the influence of plasma membrane V-ATPases on extracellular acidification. Under the mentioned growth conditions, internal pH homoeostasis is of paramount importance: on the one hand, protons are rapidly produced in glycolysis-lactic acid fermentation and, on the other, they also tend to invade the cytosol from the acidic extracellular medium. In this context, a robust V-ATPase activity, either at the plasma membrane or at intracellular compartments can represent a clear proliferative advantage by transporting protons away from the cytosol. Moreover, it is known that acidic conditions at the cytosol promote apoptosis while a mildly alkaline pH at the cytoplasm is a requisite for proliferation [35]. At the same time, a neutral to mildly alkaline cytosol and the establishment of well formed pH gradients across intracellular vesicular compartments such as the lysosome are vital for drug resistance since many drugs are lysosomotropic cations. This means that alkaline cytosols provide a barrier against drug diffusion across the plasma membrane and, once inside, drugs tend to get sequestered in the lumen of acidic intracellular compartments [36-38]. Remarkably, tumor cells able to maintain greater pH gradients in these compartments are more drug-resistant than normal ones [39-40].

INHIBITORS OF V-ATPASES

Due to the great importance of V-ATPases in many physiological and pathological situations, including cancer, there has been an active search for specific inhibitors that could be used both in the clinic and in research. As a result, nowadays there is a large amount of different inhibitors against V-ATPases that fall into different categories, although they tend to share some common characteristics. For a more comprehensive list, the reader could consider reading [41]. On the whole, with the exception of the indoles and azaindoles, all inhibitors may be considered as polyketides, i.e. large structures that are putatively synthesized in a manner akin to the first steps of fatty acid synthesis (Claisen condensation of propionyl or acetyl residues). Furthermore, many fall in the category of macrolides (structures with large lactone rings). This complexity in the structures has made the search for simpler easier-to-synthesize compounds an active field of research, with little success so far.

The effect of treatment of tumor cells with V-ATPase inhibitors has mostly been analysed using the classical macrolide inhibitors bafilomycin A and concanamycin A; however, most of the effects observed have been confirmed with other types of inhibitors. As expected, inhibition of proton transport by V-ATPases results in alkalinization of intracellular vesicular compartments and acidification of the cytosol [38, 42-44]. In B cell lymphoma lines, this process has been observed to be concomitant to an increase in reactive oxygen species that, in turn, induced cell death [43]. Under these conditions, sequestration of hydrogen peroxide with *N*-acetylcysteine inhibited cell death but inhibition of caspase activity was ineffective. Although, antisense experiments directed against c proteolipids in Hela cells reported necrosis [45], in all reports where details of the cell death ensued from inhibition of V-ATPases have been investigated, apoptosis is the only mechanism described so far [22, 46-49]. Noticeably, not all types of compounds have been studied as to their mode of cell death induction. Thus, there exist no data yet for archazolids and indoles, and very few in the case of benzolactone enamides. Nevertheless, with the exceptions noted above, the intrinsic pathway of apoptosis is involved in this process through mitochondrial depolarization and liberation of cytochrome c to the cytosol [22, 43, 50, 51]. Furthermore, caspases are central for V-ATPase inhibitor-induced apoptosis [22, 51, 52], although it has been reported that bafilomycin A induces caspase-independent cell death in B-cell tumor lines [43]. On the other hand, in EGFR overexpressing cancer cell lines, the extrinsic pathway of apoptosis has also been reported to play a decisive role through Fas/FasL in concanamycin B-induced cell death [21].

Cell cycle arrest is also a common outcome of V-ATPase inhibition. Cells tend to arrest in G1 due to increased expression of the G1/M transition inhibitor p21 [42, 46, 53, 54], although the exact mechanisms to this end are still somewhat obscure.

In HT-29 colon cancer cells, it was observed that p53 was stabilized as a response to intracellular compartment alkalinization but p21 induction was partially p53 independent [42]. Alternatively, it has been proposed that G1 arrest may be related to inhibition of the degradation of hypoxia-inducible factor 1α (HIF-1α) [54]. However, the link between HIF-1α degradation and V-ATPase inhibition has not been put forward. HIF-1α is a transcription factor responsible for the induction of p21 under conditions of hypoxia and is kept at low levels in normal oxygenic conditions by degradation via the proteasome [55].

In vivo testing has produced promising results, albeit few reports have been published so far. The proof of concept that reduction of V-ATPase activity can be effective against cancer *in vivo* may have come from RNAi studies. Silencing of ATP6L (the gene encoding membrane bound c subunit) was found to severely inhibit proliferation and metastatic potential of HCCLM3 xenografts into the livers of BalB/c (nu^+/nu^+) mice, even though the silencing only reached a mere 60% [32]. On their turn, V-ATPase inhibitors have also shown *in vivo* antitumoral activity, for example, omeprazole was seen effective against B-cell lymphoma proliferation in murine models [43]. NiK-12192, an indole, has recently been reported to inhibit growth and metastatic potential of non-small cell lung cancer H460 xenografts in mice, although it was not effective against artificially established metastasis [56]. Another line of thought is based on the importance of V-ATPases for the sequestration of chemotherapeutic drugs into intracellular compartments, leading to drug-resistance. This has prompted studies on the ability of chemical inhibitors to enhance drug sensitivity. Thus, NiK-12192 reportedly produced the cytoplasmic redistribution of camptothecins in treated cells and the potentiation of topotecan antitumoral effects in HT29 topotecan resistant tumor xenografts [56]. In a murine model of breast cancer, FR202126 has also been shown to inhibit metastasis growth in the bone but not the invasion and the proliferation of metastatic cells. This was mostly due to the antiosteolytic effect of this compound [57]. Probably for this reason, this new kind of compounds that show promising differential specificity towards different V-ATPases [58] has not been patented specifically as antitumoral drugs, but are just proposed as putative coadjuvant treatments. Omeprazole, on its turn, has shown effectiveness against tumoral progression in a murine lymphoma model in combination with drugs such as cisplatin [38].

Plecomacrolides: Bafilomycins, Concanamycins, Iejimalides and Palmerolides

Bafilomycin A was the first reported specific inhibitor of V-ATPases [59], closely followed by concanamycin A [60]. Both compounds are very similar, consisting of large macrocyclic lactone rings, which place them in the macrolide group, being generally referred to as plecomacrolides. In nature, they can be isolated from several species of *Streptomyces* bacteria when grown as a mycelium [61]. General structures of bafilomycin A and concanamycin A are shown in Fig. (**3**). It took more than ten years to ascertain the binding site of these compounds on the V-ATPase complex, although it was clear that they bound somewhere within the V_0 domain. Indeed, early suspicions of binding to subunit a [62] have been confirmed recently [63], thus explaining some details of their effect. However, it is now well established that the major inhibitory mechanism of plecomacrolides is another: these compounds bind to the c proteolipid subunit at a site near or the same where DCCD (*N,N'*-dicyclohexylcarbodiimide) binds, thereby impairing the transport of protons through this peptide [64]. An important consequence of this is that bafilomycins and concanamycins are not selective against V-ATPases from different origins, since proteolipid c is the most conserved subunit in V-ATPases. Their IC_{50s} are in the low nanomolar range, which makes this type of compounds extremely potent and useful in research to distinguish between different families of ATPases in a cell. For example, P-type ATPases are only inhibited by plecomacrolides in the micromolar range and the closely related F_0F_1 ATPases from mitochondria are not inhibited at all.

Apart from their effect on the proton conductance through V_0, there are other possibilities to explain the anticancer capability of plecomacrolides. For example, it has been proposed that bafilomycin A induces the expression of hypoxia-inducible factor 1α (HSF-1α) and, concomitantly, p21 [54] leading to cell cycle arrest. Similar results have been reported for the bafilomycin analog hygrolidin [53]. Moreover, both concanamycin A and bafilomycin A_1 have been shown to induce the production of nitric oxide in RAW 264.7 leukemia cells which, in turn, activated c-Jun *N*-terminal kinase and NF-κB leading to apoptosis [65]. These effects might be related to a different mode of action recently reported for bafilomycin A: in mitochondria isolated from rat liver, sub-micromolar concentrations of this compound were found to transport potassium into the mitochondrial lumen leading to swelling and depolarization in a manner resembling that observed for valinomycin; this phenomenon was independent of any effects on the F_0F_1 ATPase [66].

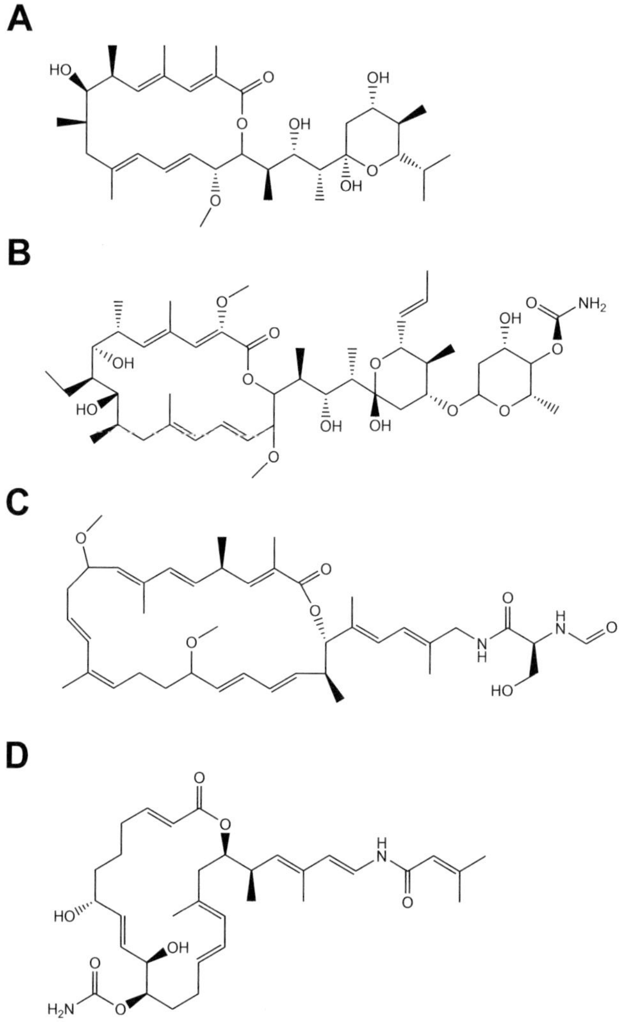

Figure 3: Structure of some plecomacrolides. A, Bafilomycin A; B, Concanamycin A; C, Iejimalide B; D, Palmerolide A.

Total synthesis of bafilomycin A was achieved as early as 1997 [67] and that of concanamycin (concanamycin F) in 2001 [68]. Prior to that, their first putative use in cancer chemotherapy had already been filed [69]; since then, several other derivatives and uses have been patented. The importance of intracellular compartment acidification is recognised as central for the anticancer mechanism of plecomacrolides [70] and for the usefulness of these compounds to overcome drug resistance [71]. On the other hand, plecomacrolides tend to be unstable in alkaline conditions, which has driven the search for more stable derivatives [72].

Iejimalides Fig. (**3C**) are a class of compounds very similar to bafilomycins and concanamycins with a 24 carbon lactone ring. They were first isolated from the tunicate *Eudistoma cf. rigida* but named after the Japanese name of the island where the specimens were first collected (Ie Jima) [73]. Both iejimalide A and B have been fully synthesized and have been proposed to have microtubule depolarizing activity [74-76] in addition to their effect on V-ATPases [77]. Although all these compounds were known to inhibit tumor cell proliferation since they were first isolated [73], only one of these compounds, iejimalide B, has been proven to induce apoptosis in a tumor cell line (LNCaP); noticeably, it was also shown that it only induced cell cycle arrest in p53 defective lines [78]. No patents on iejimalides seem to have been filed thus far.

Palmerolide A Fig. (**3D**) is a more recent but similar case to iejimalides, it was first isolated from a tunicate (*Synoicum adareanum*) and shown to inhibit tumor cell proliferation via V-ATPase inhibition [79]. Its total synthesis and that of some derivatives has already been achieved [80, 81]. The interest this compound has raised resulted in two very recent patents [82, 83].

Apoptolidin is a peculiar plecomacrolide: its mechanism of action was described as inhibition of the mitochondrial F_0F_1 ATPase [84], but the actual mechanism has been suggested to be similar to that of bafilomycins and concanamycins in subsequent patent filings [85]. However, no data support this hypothesis in peer-reviewed journals to date.

Benzolactone Enamides: Salicylihalimides, Lobatamides and Apicularens

Following the discovery of plecomacrolides, a series of compounds with strong inhibitory potency against V-ATPases were described within a short period during the late 1990s. The first of these (salicylihalimide) was obtained from sponges of the genus *Haliclona sp.* [86], lobatamides where first obtained from the tunicate *Aplidium lobatum* (hence its name) [87] and apicularens from mixobacteria of the genus *Chondromyces* [88]. The apparent wide range of organisms used as sources may be misleading, since it is plausible that they are actually synthesized by symbiotic microorganisms [89]. All these compounds share a benzolactone enamide core and show a cytotoxic profile similar to that of plecomacrolides in NCI's 60-Cell screens [89]. Their IC_{50}s also lie within the nanomolar range [61, 90]. Structures for representative compounds of this class are depicted in Fig. (**4**).

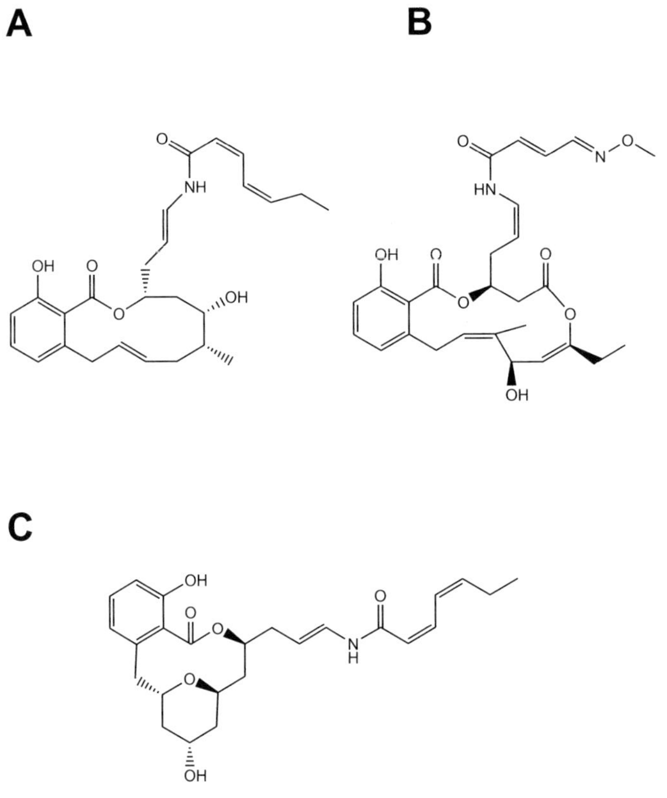

Figure 4: Examples of benzolactone enamides. A, Salicylihalimide A; B, Lobatamide A; C, Apicularen A.

Benzolactone enamides have raised a great interest due to their selectivity towards animal V-ATPases, as opposed to fungal proton pumps (no studies on plant enzymes have been published so far) [89, 91]. The reason for this selectivity is still unknown, but it is probably related to their different modes of inhibition. In studies using brain and tobacco hornworm V-ATPase, it was shown that salicylihalimide A bound the V_0 domain and that this binding could not be inhibited by the addition of bafilomycin or concanamycin derivatives [64, 90]. This was later confirmed for lobatamide [91]. However, a clear picture on the actual subunit and binding site for this type of compounds still has to emerge.

Total synthesis of benzolactone enamides was reported within a few years of their discovery. Thus, salicylihalimide A synthesis was published in the year 2000 [92], followed by lobatamide C [93] and apicularen A [94]. Apart from these representatives, this class of compounds has rendered many other chemicals that have not been discussed here, such as the cruentarens or the oximidines, that share a similar structure and mode of action. These have been reviewed in more detail elsewhere [61, 95]. Patents have not lagged behind and the application of salicylihalimides and apicularens was filed as early as 2003 [96] and extended later in successive applications [96]. At times, the potential use of V-ATPase inhibitors -irrespective of their class- has been filed, for example, a patent comprising the use of plecomacrolides or benzolactone enamides as sensitizers towards irradiation [70]. Actually, lobatamides, together with other benzolactone enamides, have recently received some attention [97]. The last type of these compounds to be registered has been the palmerolides, with a patent application in 2008 [83].

Other Compounds: Chondropsins, Archazolids and Indoles

The search for new V-ATPase inhibitors has rendered new classes of compounds: chondropsins, archazolids and indoles (and their derivatives, the azaindoles). Most of them have been obtained from natural sources but indoles have been chemically synthesized.

Chondropsins are complex macrolides comprising 33-37 members in a large lactone ring and long polyketide extensions Fig. (**5A**). They show potent death inducing capability and were first isolated from marine sponges of the genera *Chondropsis* and *Siliquariaspongia* [98, 99]. Later, they were described as V-ATPase inhibitors on the basis of their profile on NCI-60 tests and *in vitro* assays [100]. Surprisingly, these compounds preferentially inhibit fungal V-ATPases, with IC_{50}s in the sub-micromolar range, rather than mammalian V-ATPases, which typically show IC_{50}s in the low micromolar range. Despite this, chondropsins seem to share a similar mode of inhibition with plecomacrolides such as bafilomycins, since mutations affecting bafilomycin sensitivity in the *Neurospora crassa* enzyme also affect chondropsin inhibition [100].

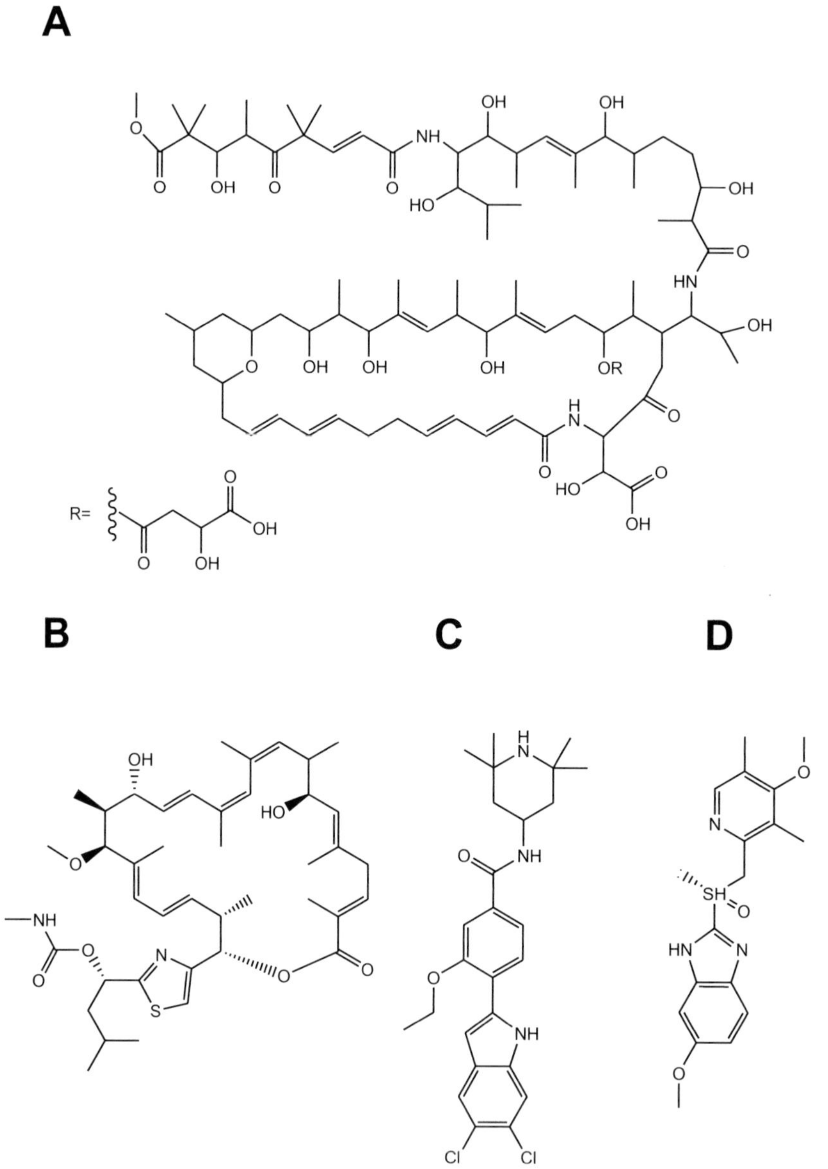

Figure 5: Other diverse V-ATPase inhibitors. A, Chondropsin A; B, Archazolid A; C, NiK12192 (indole); D, (R)-Omeprazole.

Archazolids are compounds structurally related to the plecomacrolides that also comprise a thiazole ring in a side chain Fig. (**5B**). First isolated from the mixobacterium *Archangium gephyra* [101], archazolid A was shown to inhibit V-ATPases from the tobacco hornworm *Manduca sexta* (IC_{50} = 20nM) and acidification of intracellular compartments in mammalian cells [91]. Their mode of action seems to be the inhibition of the holoenzyme rotation by binding to subunit c, since archazolid A competes with plecomacrolide concanolide A for the binding to the V_0 domain [91]. In order to assess the important residues in the molecule derivatives of archazolides have been produced. Substitutions at carbon 7 in these compounds (marked with an asterisk on Fig. (**5B**)) severely affected their effectiveness in mammalian cell assays with comparatively minor effects on their inhibitory capacity in *in vitro* assays; the ultimate reasons for this are still unknown.

Ten years after the discovery of bafilomycin, Farina and co-workers applied the information obtained by then in structural studies to produce simpler compounds that were able to inhibit V-ATPases while easy to synthesize [102, 103]. These compounds are characterized by an indole core with electron-withdrawing residues (usually chloro) at positions 5 and 6, and an amino substituent after a three- to four-carbon atom spacer. Similarly to plecomacrolides, this kind of inhibitors also bind subunit c [104, 105]. Also, like bafilomycins and concanamycins, it was thought for some time that binding to subunit a could also be part of its mechanism of action, but this hypothesis is now abandoned [106]. It was an attractive hypothesis because binding to this subunit could help to explain their unique preferential inhibition of osteoclast ATPases *vs*. other mammalian V-ATPases [102, 103, 107].

A special case is that of omeprazole and similar derivatives such as lanzoprazole, or pantoprazole, commonly known as PPI (proton pump inhibitors). These compounds are imidazole derivatives that present a tricoordinated sulfur atom in a pyramidal structure (Fig. (**5D**)) thus, these molecules can coexist in both S and R enantiomeric forms. They are normally used as inhibitors of the gastric H^+/K^+-ATPase, a P-type ATPase, hence its denomination as PPI. Its mode of action on this enzyme is related to its reactivity with a cysteine residue at the active site of the ATPase. At high concentrations they seem to inhibit V-ATPases and increase tumor cell sensitivity towards other chemotherapeutic agents used against cancer [38]. This has prompted the filing of a patent for their use as antitumoral agents [108].

The synthesis and registration of all these compounds have fared different paths. No reports on the total synthesis of chondropsins are known to the authors to date and, presumably, the isolation of these compounds from scarce natural sources is very difficult. Regardless of this, their use, either alone or in conjunction with irradiation, has been registered [109, 110]. Archazolids are still in a preliminary stage and neither total synthesis nor putative uses have been reported. Indoles, on their part, are fully synthetic molecules and, due to their apparent selectivity against osteoclast V-ATPases, they were first registered as putative treatment agents against osteoporosis [111]. It has been recently shown that they can also inhibit metastasis initiation and bone invasion in animal models [56, 57], probably, this has fuelled the registration of this kind of compounds as anticancer agents [111].

Since the first version of this chapter was written, a new class of compounds has been described and patented as useful V-ATPase inhibitors: the hidrazides. So far, their only known example is KM91104 (3,4-dihydroxy-*N'*-2-(hydroxybenzylidene)benzohydrazide) [112]. The novelty of this compound relies on its ability to disturb also the newly described interaction between subunits A and B, in particular, a3 and B2 [113]. As it is easily understandable from its mode of action, this compound or derivatives show potential as small molecules with the sorely needed specificity to discriminate between V-ATPase isoforms.

CURRENT & FUTURE DEVELOPMENTS

So far, no cancer clinical trials with V-ATPase inhibitors are known. This is probably due to the difficulty in obtaining them in sufficient amounts and also because of their high toxicity [41, 58]. The latter stems from the high potency but lack of selectivity towards different tissues that most inhibitors show to date [58]. Indoles could be considered an exception, but they are not likely to be specific enough due to the small differences in affinity displayed by the different variants of this type of molecules. In this sense, inhibition of V-ATPases in pancreas has been suggested to be linked to the risk of induced glucose intolerance [114]. This is probably the most important issue to overcome before any compound inhibiting intracellular compartment acidification can reach the market. To this end, studies on different derivatives are paramount, specially those involving compounds already showing some kind of specificity. No doubt that these studies must come accompanied by structural studies on the mode of inhibition and binding site of these inhibitors. A fruitful approach can also be the simplification of compounds, as it was done with plecomacrolides rendering indoles and azaindoles. This can be specially important for compounds such as the chondropsins, which can be cumbersome to synthesize and difficult to obtain from natural sources. The search for new classes of compounds can also yield interesting results, as it is proven from the fact that several classes of totally unrelated compounds and tens of derivatives are already available since the discovery of bafilomycin A in 1988. With the availability of high throughput screening techniques, it can be expected that new compounds will come up soon. Noteworthy in this respect is the discovery of hidrazides, which may be the first of a series of compounds identified on the basis of their interactions with specific V-ATPase subunits. As it is, the interest in these compounds remains high as judged by preclinical tests and the fair amount of patents issued.

ACKNOWLEDGEMENTS

The authors thank the Andalusian Regional Government and the Spanish Ministry of Science and Innovation for their support to PAIDI group BIO-261 through grants P07-CVI-3082 and BFU2010-15622, all of them partially funded by the EU FEDER program. PAIDI group BIO-261 belongs to the CeiA3 and Andalucia TECH Campuses of International Excellence. Also, thanks are due to Ms. I. Jiménez for her invaluable technical assistance.

CONFLICT OF INTEREST

The authors confirm that this chapter content has no conflict of interest.

DISCLOSURE

The chapter submitted for Patent eBook Series “Topics in Anti-Cancer Research”, Volume 2 is an update of our article “Intraorganellar Acidification by V-ATPases:

A Target in Cell Proliferation and Cancer Therapy", published in the journal "Recent Patents on Anti-Cancer Drug Discovery", Volume 5, Number 2, June Issue 2010, Page 88 to 98 with modified title, additional text and recent references.

REFERENCES

[1] Kane PM. The where, when, and how of organelle acidification by the yeast vacuolar H^+-ATPase. Microbiol Mol Biol Rev 2006; 70: 177-91.

[2] Weisz OA. Acidification and protein traffic. Int Rev Cytol 2003; 226: 259-319.

[3] Rivinoja A, Hassinen A, Kokkonen N, Kauppila A, Kellokumpu S. Elevated Golgi pH impairs terminal *N*-glycosylation by inducing mislocalization of Golgi glycosyltransferases. J Cell Physiol 2009; 220: 144-54.

[4] Axelsson MA, Karlsson NG, Steel DM, Ouwendijk J, Nilsson T, Hansson GC. Neutralization of pH in the Golgi apparatus causes redistribution of glycosyltransferases and changes in the *O*-glycosylation of mucins. Glycobiology 2001; 11: 633-44.

[5] Brown D, Breton S. H(+)V-ATPase-dependent luminal acidification in the kidney collecting duct and the epididymis/vas deferens: Vesicle recycling and transcytotic pathways. J Exp Biol 2000; 203: 137-45.

[6] Kaunitz JD, Yamaguchi DT. TNAP, TrAP, ecto-purinergic signaling, and bone remodeling. J Cell Biochem 2008; 105: 655-62.

[7] Frattini A, Orchard PJ, Sobacchi C, Giliani S, Abinun M, Mattsson JP, *et al*. Defects in TCIRG1 subunit of the vacuolar proton pump are responsible for a subset of human autosomal recessive osteopetrosis. Nat Genet 2000; 25: 343-6.

[8] Hinton A, Bond S, Forgac M. V-ATPase functions in normal and disease processes. Eur J Physiol 2009; 457: 589-98.

[9] Sennoune SR, Bakunts K, Martínez GM, Chua-Tuan JL, Kebir Y, Attaya MN, *et al*. Vacuolar H^+-ATPase in human breast cancer cells with distinct metastatic potential: Distribution and functional activity. Am J Physiol Cell Physiol 2004; 286: C1443-52.

[10] Forgac M. Vacuolar ATPases: Rotary proton pumps in physiology and pathophysiology. Nat Rev Mol Cell Biol 2007; 8: 917-29.

[11] Sautin YY, Lu M, Gaugler A, Zhang L, Gluck SL. Phosphatidylinositol 3-kinase-mediated effects of glucose on vacuolar H^+-ATPase assembly, translocation, and acidification of intracellular compartments in renal epithelial cells. Mol Cell Biol 2005; 25: 575-89.

[12] Breton S, Brown D. New insights into the regulation of V-ATPase-dependent proton secretion. Am J Physiol Renal Physiol 2007; 292: F1-10.

[13] Voss M, Vitavska O, Walz B, Wieczorek H, Baumann O. Stimulus-induced phosphorylation of vacuolar H(+)-ATPase by protein kinase A. J Biol Chem 2007; 282: 33735-42.

[14] Makrantoni V, Dennison P, Stark MJR, Coote PJ. A novel role for the yeast protein kinase Dbf2p in vacuolar H^+-ATPase function and sorbic acid stress tolerance. Microbiology 2007; 153: 4016-26.

[15] Hallows KR, Alzamora R, Li H, Gong F, Smolak C, Neumann D, *et al*. AMP-activated protein kinase inhibits alkaline pH- and PKA-induced apical vacuolar H^+-ATPase accumulation in epididymal clear cells. Am J Physiol Cell Physiol 2009; 296: C672-81.

[16] Butt AJ, Caldon CE, McNeil CM, Swarbrick A, Musgrove EA, Sutherland RL. Cell cycle machinery: Links with genesis and treatment of breast cancer. Adv Exp Med Biol 2008; 630: 189-205.

[17] Hernández A, López-Lluch G, Bernal JA, Navas P, Pintor-Toro JA. Dicoumarol down-regulates human PTTG1/Securin mRNA expression through inhibition of Hsp90. Mol Cancer Ther 2008; 7: 474-82.

[18] Otero-Rey EMA, Somoza-Martín M, Barros-Angueira F, García-García A. Intracellular pH regulation in oral squamous cell carcinoma is mediated by increased V-ATPase activity via over-expression of the ATP6V1C1 gene. Oral Oncol 2008; 44: 193-9.

[19] Torigoe T, Izumi H, Ishiguchi H, Uramoto H, Murakami T, Ise T, *et al.* Enhanced expression of the human vacuolar H^+-ATPase c subunit gene (ATP6L) in response to anticancer agents. J Biol Chem 2002; 277: 36534-43.

[20] Kubota S, Seyama Y. Overexpression of vacuolar ATPase 16-kDa subunit in 10T1/2 fibroblasts enhances invasion with concomitant induction of matrix metalloproteinase-2. Biochem Biophys Res Commun 2000; 278: 390-4.

[21] Yoshimoto Y, Imoto M. Induction of EGF-dependent apoptosis by vacuolar-type H(+)-ATPase inhibitors in A431 cells overexpressing the EGF receptor. Exp Cell Res 2002; 279: 118-27.

[22] Aiko K, Tsujisawa T, Koseki T, Hashimoto S, Morimoto Y, Amagasa T, *et al.* Involvement of cytochrome c and caspases in apoptotic cell death of human submandibular gland ductal cells induced by concanamycin A. Cell Signal 2002; 14: 717-22.

[23] van Weert AW, Dunn KW, Gueze HJ, Maxfield FR, Stoorvogel W. Transport from late endosomes to lysosomes, but not sorting of integral membrane proteins in endosomes, depends on the vacuolar proton pump. J Cell Biol 1995; 130: 821-34.

[24] Alwan HAJ, van Zoelen EJJ, van Leeuwen JEM. Ligand-induced lysosomal epidermal growth factor receptor (EGFR) degradation is preceded by proteasome-dependent EGFR de-ubiquitination. J Biol Chem 2003; 278: 35781-90.

[25] Perzov N, Nelson H, Nelson N. Altered distribution of the yeast plasma membrane H^+-ATPase as a feature of vacuolar H^+-ATPase null mutants. J Biol Chem 2000; 275: 40088-95.

[26] Taupenot L, Harper KL, O'Connor DT. Role of H^+-ATPase-mediated acidification in sorting and release of the regulated secretory protein chromogranin A: Evidence for a vesiculogenic function. J Biol Chem 2005; 280: 3885-97.

[27] Seog D-H. SS33410, an inhibitor of V-ATPase, blocks intracellular protein transport of the VSV-G protein in the Golgi compartment. Biosci Biotechnol Biochem 2003; 67: 2591-7.

[28] Vander Heiden MG, Cantley LC, Thompson CB. Understanding the Warburg effect: The metabolic requirements of cell proliferation. Science 2009; 324: 1029-33.

[29] Fais S, De Milito A, You H, Qin W. Targeting vacuolar H^+-ATPases as a new strategy against cancer. Cancer Res 2007; 67: 10627-30.

[30] Iessi E, Marino ML, Lozupone F, Fais S, De Milito A. Tumor acidity and malignancy: Novel aspects in the design of anti-tumor therapy. Cancer Ther 2008; 6: 55-66.

[31] Swietach P, Vaughan-Jones RD, Harris AL. Regulation of tumor pH and the role of carbonic anhydrase 9. Cancer Metast Rev 2007; 26: 299-310.

[32] Lu X, Qin W, Li J, Tan N, Pan D, Zhang H, *et al.* The growth and metastasis of human hepatocellular carcinoma xenografts are inhibited by small interfering RNA targeting to the subunit ATP6L of proton pump. Cancer Res 2005; 65: 6843-9.

[33] Sennoune SR, Luo D, Martínez-Zaguilán R. Plasmalemmal vacuolar-type H^+-ATPase in cancer biology. Cell Biochem Biophys 2004; 40: 185-206.

[34] Joyce JA, Hanahan D. Multiple roles for cysteine cathepsins in cancer. Cell Cycle 2004; 3: 1516-9.

[35] Lagadic-Gossmann D, Huc L, Lecureur V. Alterations of intracellular pH homeostasis in apoptosis: Origins and roles. Cell Death Differ 2004; 11: 953-61.

[36] Simon S, Roy D, Schindler M. Intracellular pH and the control of multidrug resistance. Proc Natl Acad Sci USA 1994; 91: 1128-32.

[37] Chen VY, Rosania GR. The great multidrug-resistance paradox. ACS Chem Biol 2006; 1: 271-3.

[38] Luciani F, Spada M, De Milito A, Molinari A, Rivoltini L, Montinaro A, *et al.* Effect of proton pump inhibitor pretreatment on resistance of solid tumors to cytotoxic drugs. J Nat Cancer Inst 2004; 96: 1702-13.

[39] Millot C, Millot J-M, Morjani H, Desplaces A, Manfait M. Characterization of acidic vesicles in multidrug-resistant and sensitive cancer cells by acridine orange staining and confocal microspectrofluorometry. J Histochem Cytochem 1997; 45: 1255-64.

[40] Weylandt KH, Nebrig M, Jansen-Rosseck N, Amey JS, Carmena D, Wiedenmann B, *et al.* ClC-3 expression enhances etoposide resistance by increasing acidification of the late endocytic compartment. Mol Cancer Ther 2007; 6: 979-86.

[41] Beutler JA, McKee TC. Novel marine and microbial natural product inhibitors of vacuolar ATPase. Curr Med Chem 2003; 10: 787-96.

[42] Castillo-Avila W, Abal M, Robine S, Pérez-Tomás R. Non-apoptotic concentrations of prodigiosin (H^+/Cl^- symporter) inhibit the acidification of lysosomes and induce cell cycle blockage in colon cancer cells. Life Sciences 2005; 78: 121-7.

[43] De Milito A, Iessi E, Logozzi M, Lozupone F, Spada M, Marino ML, *et al.* Proton pump inhibitors induce apoptosis of human B-cell tumors through a caspase-independent mechanism involving reactive oxygen species. Cancer Res 2007; 67: 5408-17.

[44] Liao C, Hu B, Arno MJ, Panaretou B. Genomic screening *in vivo* reveals the role played by vacuolar H^+ ATPase and cytosolic acidification in sensitivity to DNA-damaging agents such as cisplatin. Mol Pharmacol 2007; 71: 416-25.

[45] Zhan H, Yokoyama K, Otani H, Tanigaki K, Shirota N, Takano S, *et al.* Different roles of proteolipids and 70-kDa subunits of V-ATPase in growth and death of cultured human cells. Genes Cells 2003; 8: 501-13.

[46] Chevallier C, Laprévote O, Bignon J, Debitus C, Guénard D, Sévenet T. Isolation of cytotoxic chondropsins, macrolide lactams from the New-Caledonian marine sponge *Psammoclemma* sp. and electrospray ion trap multiple stage MS study of these macrolides. Nat Prod Res 2004; 18: 479-84.

[47] Hong J, Yokomakura A, Nakano Y, Ishihara K, Kaneda M, Onodera M, *et al.* Inhibition of vacuolar-type (H^+)-ATPase by the cytostatic macrolide apicularen A and its role in apicularen A-induced apoptosis in RAW 264.7 cells. FEBS Lett 2006; 580: 2723-30.

[48] Morimura T, Fujita K, Akita M, Nagashima M, Satomi A. The proton pump inhibitor inhibits cell growth and induces apoptosis in human hepatoblastoma. Pediatr Surg Int 2008; 24: 1087-94.

[49] Xu J, Feng HT, Wang C, Yip KHM, Pavlos N, Papadimitriou JM, *et al.* Effects of Bafilomycin A1: An inhibitor of vacuolar H (+)-ATPases on endocytosis and apoptosis in RAW cells and RAW cell-derived osteoclasts. J Cell Biochem 2003; 88: 1256-64.

[50] Huang X, Masselli A, Frisch SM, Hunton IC, Jiang Y, Wang JYJ. Blockade of tumor necrosis factor-induced bid cleavage by caspase-resistant Rb. J Biol Chem 2007; 282: 29401-13.

[51] Sasazawa Y, Futamura Y, Tashiro E, Imoto M. Vacuolar H(+)-ATPase inhibitors overcome Bcl-xL-mediated chemoresistance through restoration of a caspase-independent apoptotic pathway. Cancer Sci 2009; 100: 1460-7.

[52] Hong J, Yamaki K, Ishihara K, Ahn JW, Zee O, Ohuchi K. Induction of apoptosis of RAW 264.7 cells by the cytostatic macrolide apicularen A. J Pharm Pharmacol 2003; 55: 1299-306.

[53] Kawada M, Usami I, Ohba S, Someno T, Kim J, Hayakawa Y, *et al.* Hygrolidin induces p21 expression and abrogates cell cycle progression at G1 and S phases. Biochem Biophys Res Commun 2002; 298: 178-83.

[54] Lim J-H, Park J-W, Kim M-S, Park S-K, Johnson RS, Chun Y-S. Bafilomycin induces the p21-mediated growth inhibition of cancer cells under hypoxic conditions by expressing hypoxia-inducible factor-1alpha. Mol Pharmacol 2006; 70: 1856-65.

[55] Koshiji M, Huang LE. Dynamic balancing of the dual nature of HIF-1alpha for cell survival. Cell Cycle 2004; 3: 853-4.

[56] Supino R, Petrangolini G, Pratesi G, Tortoreto M, Favini E, Bo LD, *et al.* Antimetastatic effect of a small-molecule vacuolar H^+-ATPase inhibitor in *in vitro* and *in vivo* preclinical studies. J Pharmacol Exp Ther 2008; 324: 15-22.

[57] Niikura K. Effect of a V-ATPase inhibitor, FR202126, in syngeneic mouse model of experimental bone metastasis. Cancer Chemother Pharmacol 2007; 60: 555-62.

[58] Niikura K. Vacuolar ATPase as a drug discovery target. Drug News Perspect 2006; 19: 139-44.

[59] Bowman EJ, Siebers A, Altendorf K. Bafilomycins: A class of inhibitors of membrane ATPases from microorganisms, animal cells, and plant cells. Proc Natl Acad Sci USA 1988; 85: 7972-6.

[60] Dröse S, Bindseil KU, Bowman EJ, Siebers A, Zeeck A, Altendorf K. Inhibitory effect of modified bafilomycins and concanamycins on P- and V-type adenosinetriphosphatases. Biochemistry 1993; 32: 3902-6.

[61] Huss M, Wieczorek H. Inhibitors of V-ATPases: Old and new players. J Exp Biol 2009; 212: 341-6.

[62] Zhang J, Feng Y, Forgac M. Proton conduction and bafilomycin binding by the V_0 domain of the coated vesicle V-ATPase. J Biol Chem 1994; 269: 23518-23.

[63] Wang Y, Inoue T, Forgac M. Subunit of the yeast V-ATPase participates in binding of bafilomycin. J Biol Chem 2005; 280: 40481-8.

[64] Huss M, Ingenhorst G, Konig S, Gassel M, Drose S, Zeeck A, *et al.* Concanamycin A, the Specific Inhibitor of V-ATPases, Binds to the Vo Subunit c. J Biol Chem 2002; 277: 40544-8.

[65] Hong J, Nakano Y, Yokomakura A, Ishihara K, Kim S, Kang Y-S, *et al.* Nitric oxide production by the vacuolar-type (H^+)-ATPase inhibitors bafilomycin A1 and concanamycin A and its possible role in apoptosis in RAW 264.7 cells. J Pharmacol Exp Ther 2006; 319: 672-81.

[66] Teplova VV, Tonshin AA, Grigoriev PA, Saris N-EL, Salkinoja-Salonen MS. Bafilomycin A1 is a potassium ionophore that impairs mitochondrial functions. J Bioenerg Biomembr 2007; 39: 321-9.

[67] Toshima K, Jyojima T, Yamaguchi H, Noguchi Y, Yoshida T, Murase H, *et al.* Total Synthesis of bafilomycin A(1). J Org Chem 1997; 62: 3271-84.

[68] Toshima K, Jyojima T, Miyamoto N, Katohno M, Nakata M, Matsumura S. The first total synthesis of concanamycin f (concanolide a). J Org Chem 2001; 66: 1708-15.

[69] Holt, T.G., Monaghan, R.L. Methods of achieving antileukemia activity using 16-membered-macrolide-type compounds. US5306716 (**1994**).

[70] Paglin, S., Yahalom, J., Hollister, T., Delohery, T. Inhibition of vacuolar proton ATPase activity and/or the modulation of acidic organelle function sensitizes cells to radiation, chemotherapy and biological agents. US6982252 (**2006**).

[71] Khosla, C., Salomon, A. Screening method for cancer therapeutics and stable antitumor drug. US6974664 (**2005**).

[72] Khosla, C., Fujie, A. Stable antitumor drug. US6548485 (**2003**).

[73] Kobayashi J, Cheng J, Ohta T, Nakamura H, Nozoe S, Hirata Y, *et al.* Iejimalides A and B, novel 24-membered macrolides with potent antileukemic activity from the Okinawan tunicate *Eudistoma cf. rigida*. J Org Chem 1988; 53: 6147-50.

[74] Fürstner A, Nevado C, Tremblay M, Chevrier C, Teplý F, Aïssa C, *et al.* Total synthesis of iejimalide B. Angewandte Chemie 2006; 45: 5837-42.

[75] Fürstner A, Nevado C, Waser M, Tremblay M, Chevrier C, Teplý F, *et al.* Total synthesis of iejimalide A-D and assessment of the remarkable actin-depolymerizing capacity of these polyene macrolides. J Am Chem Soc 2007; 129: 9150-61.

[76] Schweitzer D, Kane JJ, Strand D, McHenry P, Tenniswood M, Helquist P. Total synthesis of iejimalide B. An application of the Shiina macrolactonization. Org Lett 2007; 9: 4619-22.

[77] Kazami S, Muroi M, Kawatani M, Kubota T, Usui T, Kobayashi JI, *et al.* Iejimalides show anti-osteoclast activity via V-ATPase inhibition. Biosci Biotech Biochem 2006; 70: 1364-70.

[78] Wang W-LW, McHenry P, Jeffrey R, Schweitzer D, Helquist P, Tenniswood M. Effects of Iejimalide B, a marine macrolide, on growth and apoptosis in prostate cancer cell lines. J Cell Biochem 2008; 105: 998-1007.

[79] Diyabalanage T, Amsler CD, McClintock JB, Baker BJ. Palmerolide A, a cytotoxic macrolide from the antarctic tunicate *Synoicum adareanum*. J Am Chem Soc 2006; 128: 5630-1.

[80] Jiang X, Liu B, Lebreton S, Brabander JKD. Total synthesis and structure revision of the marine metabolite palmerolide A. J Am Chem Soc 2007; 129: 6386-7.

[81] Nicolaou KC, Leung GYC, Dethe DH, Guduru R, Sun Y-P, Lim CS, *et al.* Chemical synthesis and biological evaluation of palmerolide A analogues. J Am Chem Soc 2008; 130: 10019-23.

[82] Baker, B.J., Diyabalanage, T., McClintock, J.B., Amsler, C.D. Cytotoxin compound and method of isolation. US20050187286 (**2005**).

[83] De Brabander, J.K., Jiang, X., Liu, B. Palmerolides: Methods of preparation and derivatives thereof. US20080249162 (**2008**).

[84] Salomon AR, Voehringer DW, Herzenberg LA, Khosla C. Apoptolidin, a selective cytotoxic agent, is an inhibitor of F_0F_1-ATPase. Chem Biol 2001; 8: 71-80.

[85] Wender, P.A., Jankowski, O.D., Tabet, E.A. Apoptolidin analogs and derivatives for inducing apoptosis in transformed cells. US20060101 (**2006**).

[86] Erickson K, Beutler J, Cardellina J, Boyd M. Salicylihalamides A and B, novel cytotoxic macrolides from the marine sponge *Haliclona* sp. J Org Chem 1997; 62: 8188-92.
[87] Galinis DL, McKee TC, Pannell LK, Cardellina JH, Boyd MR. Lobatamides A and B, novel cytotoxic macrolides from the tunicate *Aplidium lobatum*. J Org Chem 1997; 62: 8968-9.
[88] Kunze B, Jansen R, Sasse F, Höfle G, Reichenbach H. Apicularens A and B, new cytostatic macrolides from Chondromyces species (myxobacteria): Production, physico-chemical and biological properties. J Antibiot 1998; 51: 1075-80.
[89] Boyd MR, Farina C, Belfiore P, Gagliardi S, Kim JW, Hayakawa Y, *et al*. Discovery of a novel antitumor benzolactone enamide class that selectively inhibits mammalian vacuolar-type (H^+)-atpases. J Pharmacol Exp Ther 2001; 297: 114-20.
[90] Xie X-S, Padron D, Liao X, Wang J, Roth MG, De Brabander JK. Salicylihalamide A inhibits the V_0 sector of the V-ATPase through a mechanism distinct from bafilomycin A1. J Biol Chem 2004; 279: 19755-63.
[91] Huss M, Sasse F, Kunze B, Jansen R, Steinmetz H, Ingenhorst G, *et al*. Archazolid and apicularen: Novel specific V-ATPase inhibitors. BMC Biochem 2005; 6: 13.
[92] Wu Y, Seguil OR, De Brabander JK. Synthesis and initial structure--activity relationships of modified salicylihalamides. Org Lett 2000; 2: 4241-4.
[93] Shen R, Lin CT, Porco JA. Total synthesis and stereochemical assignment of the salicylate antitumor macrolide lobatamide C(1). J Am Chem Soc 2002; 124: 5650-1.
[94] Lewis A, Stefanuti I, Swain SA, Smith SA, Taylor RJ. A formal total synthesis of (+)-apicularen A: Base-induced conversion of apicularen-derived intermediates into salicylihalamide-like products. Org Biomol Chem 2003; 1: 104-16.
[95] Yet L. Chemistry and biology of salicylihalamide A and related compounds. Chem Rev 2003; 103: 4283-306.
[96] De Brabander, J.K., Wu, Y. Synthetic salicylihalamides, apicularens and derivatives thereof. US6617348 (**2003**), US6734209 (**2004**) & US6936723 (**2005**).
[97] Boyd, M.R. Vacuolar-type (H^+)-ATPase-inhibiting compounds, compositions and uses thereof. US20080275108 (**2008**).
[98] Cantrell CL, Gustafson KR, Cecere MR, Pannell LK, Boyd MR. Chondropsins A and B: Novel tumor cell growth-inhibitory macrolide lactams from the marine sponge chondropsis sp. J Am Chem Soc 2000; 122: 8825-9.
[99] Rashid MA, Cantrell CL, Gustafson KR, Boyd MR. Chondropsin D, a new 37-membered-ring macrolide lactam from the marine sponge Chondropsis species. J Nat Prod 2001; 64: 1341-4.
[100] Bowman EJ, Gustafson KR, Bowman BJ, Boyd MR. Identification of a new chondropsin class of antitumor compound that selectively inhibits V-ATPases. J Biol Chem 2003; 278: 44147-52.
[101] Sasse F, Steinmetz H, Höfle G, Reichenbach H. Archazolids, new cytotoxic macrolactones from *Archangium gephyra* (Myxobacteria). Production, isolation, physico-chemical and biological properties. J Antibiot 2003; 56: 520-5.
[102] Gagliardi S, Nadler G, Consolandi E, Parini C, Morvan M, Legave MN, *et al*. 5-(5,6-Dichloro-2-indolyl)-2-methoxy-2,4-pentadienamides: Novel and selective inhibitors of the vacuolar H^+-ATPase of osteoclasts with bone antiresorptive activity. J Med Chem 1998; 41: 1568-73.

[103] Nadler G, Morvan M, Delimoge I, Belfiore P, Zocchetti A, James I, *et al.* (2Z,4E)-5-(5,6-dichloro-2-indolyl)-2-methoxy-*N*-(1,2,2,6,6-pentamethylpiperidin-4-yl)-2,4-entadienamide, a novel, potent and selective inhibitor of the osteoclast V-ATPase. Bioorg Med Chem Lett 1998; 8: 3621-6.

[104] Whyteside G, Meek PJ, Ball SK, Dixon N, Finbow ME, Kee TP, *et al.* Concanamycin and indolyl pentadieneamide inhibitors of the vacuolar H^+-ATPase bind with high affinity to the purified proteolipid subunit of the membrane domain. Biochemistry 2005; 44: 15024-31.

[105] Páli T, Dixon N, Kee TP, Marsh D. Incorporation of the V-ATPase inhibitors concanamycin and indole pentadiene in lipid membranes. Spin-label EPR studies. Biochim Biophys Acta 2004; 1663: 14-8.

[106] Hesselink RW, Fedorov A, Hemminga MA, Prieto M. Membrane-bound peptides from V-ATPase subunit a do not interact with an indole-type inhibitor. J Pept Sci 2008; 14: 383-8.

[107] Farina C, Gagliardi S, Nadler G, Morvan M, Parini C, Belfiore P, *et al.* Novel bone antiresorptive agents that selectively inhibit the osteoclast V-H^+-ATPase. Farmaco 2001; 56: 113-6.

[108] Fais, S., Luciani, F. Novel uses for proton pump inhibitors. US20080160106 (**2008**).

[109] Boyd, M.R., Gustafson, K.R., Cantrell, C.L. Biologically active macrolides, compositions, and uses thereof. US7144918 (**2006**).

[110] Boyd, M.R., Gustafson, K.R. Chondropsin-class antitumor V-ATPase inhibitor compounds, compositions and methods of use thereof. US7205334 (**2007**) & US7521475 (**2009**).

[111] Farina, C., Gagliardi, S., Misiano, P., Celestini, P., Zunino, F. Indole and azaindole derivatives with antitumor action. US0248672 (**2007**).

[112] Kartner, N., Manolson, M.F. Compounds, compositions and treatments for V-ATPase related diseases. US20110189306 (**2011**).

[113] Kartner N, Yao Y, Li K, Crasto GJ, Datti A, Manolson MF. Inhibition of osteoclast bone resorption by disrupting vacuolar H^+-ATPase a3-B2 subunit interaction. J Biol Chem 2010; 285: 37476-90.

[114] Hettiarachchi KD, Zimmet PZ, Myers MA. The effects of repeated exposure to sub-toxic doses of plecomacrolide antibiotics on the endocrine pancreas. Food Chem Tox 2006; 44: 1966-77.

Send Orders of Reprints at reprints@benthamscience.net
Topics in Anti-Cancer Research, 2013, 257-278

CHAPTER 7

Insights into the Role of Fc Gamma Receptors (FcγRs) Genetic Variations in Monoclonal Antibody-Based Anti-cancer Therapy

Fabio Concetti[1] and Valerio Napolioni[1,*]

[1]*School of Biosciences and Biotechnologies, University of Camerino, Camerino, Italy*

Abstract: Recently, the field of oncology has witnessed the introduction of several effective chemotherapeutic agents. Still, not all cancers respond to the use of conventional chemotherapy and thus combination therapy is an emerging weapon in the battle against cancer. There is emerging evidence in support of the use of Monoclonal antibodies (MoAbs) in cancer therapy. The mechanisms behind their efficacy are multi-faceted; they can kill tumor cells through antibody-dependent cell-mediated cytotoxicity (ADCC), complement-dependent cytotoxicity (CDC), and apoptosis as well as target ligands or growth factor receptors favoring tumor growth. The interaction of the Fc domains of antibodies with the Fcγ (gamma) receptors is an essential prerequisite for biological response to antibodies, including ADCC. This interaction is strongly regulated and is largely dependent upon receptor conformation and number. It is accepted that germ-line single nucleotide polymorphisms (SNPs) and copy number variations (CNVs) have the potential to predict the outcome of therapy. The possibility of predicting patients response to monoclonal antibody therapy is of particular importance, as response rates are moderate, with the risk of serious side effects all at a high financial cost. This patent chapter provides an insight into the role of Fcγ receptors (FcγRs) genetic variation in Monoclonal Antibody-based anti-cancer therapy.

Keywords: ADCC, Alemtuzumab, Bevacizumab, cancer, Cetuximab, chemotherapeutic agents, copy number variations, drug responses, drug toxicity, engineered antibodies, Fc gamma receptors, genetic polymorphism, monoclonal antibody-based therapy, Ofatumumab, oncology, personalized medicine, pharmacogenomics, single nucleotide polymorphism, Rituximab, Trastuzumab.

INTRODUCTION

Pharmacogenomics is a branch of pharmacology dedicated to understanding the

***Address correspondence to Valerio Napolioni:** School of Biosciences and Biotechnologies, University of Camerino, Via Gentile III da Varano, 62032 Camerino, Italy; Tel: 39 0737 403293; Fax: 39 0737 402727; E.mail: valerio.napolioni@unicam.it

Atta-ur Rahman and Khurshid Zaman (Eds)

hereditary basis for drug responses that are idiosyncratic in nature. In oncology, pharmacogenomics is currently used to predict cancer susceptibility, tumor progression and recurrence, patient survival, and response to and toxicity associated with traditional chemotherapy treatments [1-3].

The use of monoclonal antibodies (MoAbs) shows promise in cancer therapy. MoAbs can induce tumor cell death directly through antibody-dependent cell-mediated cytotoxicity (ADCC), complement-dependent cytotoxicity (CDC), and apoptosis in- or directly by binding and “inactivating” ligands or growth factor receptors normally favoring tumor growth. ADCC is mediated by Fcγ receptors (FcγRs), where individual FcγRs exert unique effector functions as well as they are expressed on unique effector cell types [4, 5].

Since FcγRs display genetic polymorphisms affecting their expression as well as their functional properties, the preferential interaction of particular anti-cancer MoAbs with specific FcγRs alleles (natural variations within the genetic locus) translates into distinct biological effects as well as genetic variations in the Fc region (GM allotypes) of IgG molecules [6]. In this chapter, we will focus on the pharmacogenomics of Fcγ receptors in MoAbs-based anti-cancer therapy.

HUMANIZED AND ENGINEERED MONOCLONAL ANTIBODIES AND THEIR USE IN ANTI-CANCER THERAPY

The most common strategy in cancer immunotherapy involves the use of antibodies, or antibody fragments, that either directly target antigen-expressing cells, or act by blocking soluble factors that support tumorigenesis, tumor vascularization, metastasis, etc. Antibodies, or antibody fragments themselves may have direct or indirect cytotoxic effects. Direct effects include the induction of apoptosis, the blocking of growth factor receptors, the blocking of ligands and anti-idiotype antibody formation. Indirect effects include ADCC and CDC.

The first experiments with antibodies in anti-cancer therapy performed with murine MoAbs were plagued by low efficacy due to weak binding between human Fc receptors and the Fc murine domain of the antibody as well as induction of an immune response against the mouse MoAb recognized as non-self by the human immune system [7]. These drawbacks have been circumvented by the recent generation of chimeric, humanized and fully human antibodies through recombinant DNA technique, as well as their improved engineering. The fusion between human Fc domains of the antibody with the murine variable region (chimeric antibodies) has yielded a remarkable decrease of immune rejections of the antibodies as well as their stronger and more specific binding to human Fc receptors [8]. One encouraging approach in the field of antibody engineering is represented by the manipulation of Fc region: a new patent reported the procedure to obtain, through the modification of one or more specific amino acid in the Fc region, a greater affinity for FcγRIIIA and/or FcγRIIA. This invention could be particularly useful in cancer treatment and/or prevention through the employment of therapeutic antibodies with enhanced ADCC mediated by FcγRs [9]. Several technical obstacles prevented the large scale production of fully human antibodies, but there are ongoing efforts to overcome these problems providing hope for the future. Another promising aspect in improving antibody-based therapies is represented by the manipulation of glycosylation of MoAb variations. Indeed, the last generation of antibodies with no- or low-fucose demonstrate a very promising increase in binding to activating FcγRIIIA, triggering a stronger ADCC compared to highly-fucosylated MoAbs [10]; recently, the structural basis underlying the reason of this enhanced ADCC is becoming clearer [11]. Notably, FcγRIIA mediates processes associated with cell activation, including phagocytosis of IgG-opsonized particles, whereas co-engagement of the inhibitory FcγRIIB down-regulates such signaling [12]. Thus, activation/inhibitory ratios of Fc receptors likely set the threshold for effector responses including ADCC and CDC.

Fcγ RECEPTORS GENOMICS AND VARIATION

Fcγ receptors are a heterogeneous family of molecules expressed on most immune cell types. They are composed of a ligand-binding α-chain sometimes associated with the homodimeric, cell-signaling common γ-chain. These molecules bind the Fc region of IgG antibodies; this association is critical in immunity because receptors represent the link between humoral and cellular response. Other receptors bind different classes of Ig: FcεRI and FcεRII bind IgE, FcαR bind IgA and Fcα/μR bind IgA and IgM. The neonatal Fc receptor (FcRn) plays a crucial role in the placental transfer of IgG from the mother to her fetus or through the milk. However, the main function of this receptor is to regulate the homeostasis of serum IgGs and albumin through their binding, in order to prevent a premature catabolism of these molecules. In this way FcRn continues to play an important immunological role throughout adult life, possibly also affecting MoAbs-based anti-cancer therapy. All Fc receptors, excepting FcεRII, belong to the Ig super family. IgG is the most abundant immunoglobulin in the serum (75% of total) whereas IgA is the most abundant form in the human body (as total mass). They are both synthesized and secreted by plasma cells. IgGs are divided in four subclasses: IgG1, IgG2, IgG3 and IgG4. The main function of IgGs is to protect the organism against pathogens by complement activation, agglutination and immobilization, and opsonization for phagocytosis; IgGs are also involved in ADCC.

Fcγ receptors display coordinated and opposing roles in the immune system depending on the domains composition of their cytoplasmic region and/or their associated chains. A key regulatory domain is the Immunoreceptor Tyrosine-based Activation Motif (ITAM) located in the cytoplasmic region (or in the associated signal transducing unit) of activating Fcγ receptors. Following IgG binding and subsequent aggregation, these receptors can initiate the inflammatory, cytolytic and phagocytic activities of immune effector cells where they are expressed. Conversely, at the cytoplasmic tail of inhibitory receptors, there is an Immunoreceptor Tyrosine-based Inhibitory Motif (ITIM). These receptors negatively regulate antigen-specific proliferation and differentiation of B cells, IgE-triggered mediator release by mast cells, or internalization of IgG-immune complexes by macrophages. The level of and type of cellular response is determined by the relative expression of activating and inhibitory receptors. Indeed many cell types express both classes of receptors whose ratio is influenced by cytokines.

The human Fcγ receptors are encoded by eight distinct genes grouped in three highly homologous classes: FcγRI, FcγRII and FcγRIII. Thanks to alternative splicing the total number of protein products is at least 10 [5, 13]. The high homology among these genes suggests that the evolution of this cluster is likely the result of gene duplications and recombination events. The precise orientation and relative position of the cluster's genes has been clarified by Su *et al.* [14] as reported in Fig. (**1**).

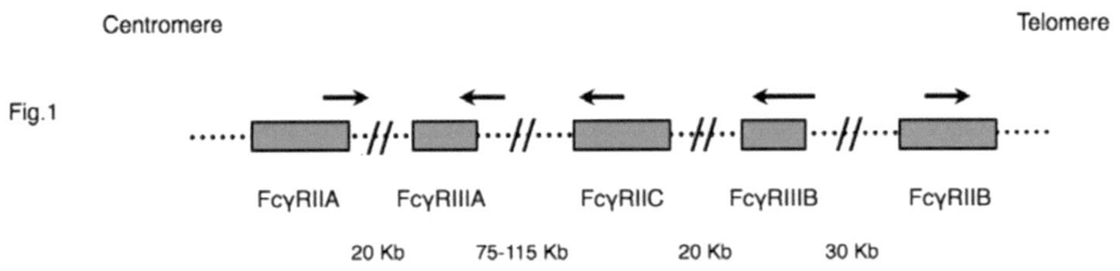

Figure 1: Genomic organization and relative distances among genes of classic low-affinity Fc receptors cluster.

FcγRI are high affinity receptors ($K_d = 10^{-8}$M for momomeric IgG) while FcγRII and FcγRIII exhibit low affinity for monomeric IgG (K_d from 10^{-5} to 10^{-7}M) and they bind mainly IgG in immune complexes. Main features of FcγRs are summarized in Table **1**.

Table 1: Main features of Fcγ receptors.

Receptor Family	**Human Genes**	**Chromosomal Locus**	**Signaling Unit**	**Immune Cells in which Receptors are Expressed**
FcγRI (CD64)	*FCGR1A*	1q21.2-q21.3	α + γ (ITAM)	Dendritic cells, macrophages, monocytes, neutrophils
	FCGR1B	1p11.2	Not Known	
	FCGR1C	1q21.1	Not Known	
FcγRII (CD32)	*FCGR2A*	1q23	α (ITAM)	Dendritic cells, macrophages, monocytes, neutrophils
	FCGR2B	1q23	α (ITIM)	B lymphocytes, dendritic cells, macrophages, monocytes, neutrophils, mast cells
	FCGR2C	1q23.3	α (ITAM)	NK cells
FcγRIII (CD16)	*FCGR3A*	1q23	α + γ,β,ζ (ITAM)	Dendritic cells, macrophages, monocytes, NK cells, mast cells
	FCGR3B	1q23	(? lipid rafts)	Neutrophils

Three genes belong to the FcγRI (CD64) family, namely *FCGR1A*, *FCGR1B* and *FCGR1C*. A rare mutation at codon 92 in the first extracellular domain (EC1) of *FCGR1A* leads to a stop codon, nevertheless individuals carrying this mutation appear clinically well [15].

Also the family FcγRII (CD32) has three genes encoding for FcγRIIA, B and C, respectively. Extracellular domains of these receptors are very similar, whereas the cytoplasmic domain of the B receptor, which carries a distinctive inhibitory signaling motif (ITIM), diverges from the A and C domains. Three isoforms of B gene are known: FcγRIIb1, b2 and b3 differing by only a few amino acids and arising from alternative splicing. The C gene has a FcγRIIB-like extracellular domain and a FcγRIIA-like cytoplasmic domain; this is probably due to an unequal crossover event occurring during evolution between *FCGR2A* and *FCGR2B* genes [16]. *FCGR2C* is expressed on NK cells [17, 18]. However, *FCGR2C* is not expressed by a large proportion of individuals due to a *FCGR2C* c.169C >T (p.Gln57*) polymorphism changing a glutamine to a stop codon and causes premature truncation of the protein abolishing its expression [19]. Moreover, an important SNP in the coding region of *FCGR2A*, the most widely expressed human FcγR, leads to a structural polymorphism at residue 131 [20]: the histidine (H) to arginine (R) change confers a lower affinity for IgG_2 and it has been associated to several autoimmune diseases [21] and to a higher risk for serious infections [22]. This polymorphism also displays an east-west geographic gradient of allele frequencies [23].

Another big source for inter-individual differences is the gene copy number variation (CNV). Thanks to human genome project, thousands of common CNVs have been identified [24, 25]. Their role in disease susceptibility is largely unknown, but there is increasing evidence that altered copy numbers of dosage sensitive genes may be responsible for a variety of diseases. The gene cluster of Fcγ receptors exhibits a great variation in copy numbers. Both the *FCGR3A* and the *FCGR3B* genes showed variation in copy number; CNV in *FCGR3B* is directly linked to similar variation in the *FCGR2C* gene number which is strongly associated with idiopathic thrombocytopenic purpura [26].

The FcγRIII (CD16) family possesses only two genes encoding for FcγRIIIA, with medium affinity for ligand (K_d from 1 to 2 x 10^{-7}M), and FcγRIIIB with low affinity for ligand ($K_d > 10^{-7}$M). *FCGR3A* gene displays a well known A to C change (*rs396991*) leading to a valine→ phenylalanine substitution at amino acid 158 [27, 28]; this amino acid change affects the binding of monomeric IgG_1 and IgG_3 and it is characterized by a stronger binding for homozygote V158 compared to homozygote F158. *FCGR3B* displays two common haplotypes, NA1 and NA2 [29] arising from the precise grouping of 5 different SNPs which consists of four non-synonymous and one synonymous mutation (i.e., substitution of the codon of one exon with a new one that codes for the same amino acid such that the polypeptide sequence is not modified) within the membrane distal Ig-like domain of the receptor. Furthermore, *FCGR3B* exhibits numerous other allotypes in addition to NA1 and NA2, such as SH antigen (a A78D amino acid change), which, whilst at lower frequency, may be functionally important and should be characterized [30]. Similarly to *FCGR2C*, also FcγRIII family displays CNVs associated with human diseases. Findings suggest that low *FCGR3B* copy number, and in particular complete *FCGR3B* deficiency, has a key role in the development of systemic lupus erythematosus and rheumatoid arthritis [31, 32]. *FCGR3B* deletion is a result of independent non-allelic homologous recombination events with a frequency of approximately 0.1% [33]. Notably, pathogen diversity, in particular helminthes diversity, has played a critical role in shaping the functional variation at these genes both between mammalian species and between human populations [33]. Moreover, the East Asian populations have a higher frequency of *FCGR3B* duplication compared to Europeans [34]. A recent meta-analysis showed that *FCGR3B* deletion is a risk factor for non-organ-specific autoimmunity [35]. Main allelic variants of genes are summarized in Table **2** [36-38].

Table 2: Main allelic variants of Fcγ receptors and their physiological effects.

Receptor Family	Human Genes	Variants	Effects	Reference
FcγRI (CD64)	*FCGR1A*	R92X	X92: Undetectable expression of FcγRIA on phagocyte	[15]
FcγRII (CD32)	*FCGR2A*	R131H	H131: Higher affinity for IgG2	[20]
	FCGR2B	I232T	T232: lower affinity for lipid rafts/decreased inhibitory activity	[36]
	FCGR2C	CNV	Supposable higher number of receptors related to higher number of copies of the gene with altered balance of activating and inhibitory FcγRs	[26]
FcγRIII (CD16)	*FCGR3A*	V158F CNV	V158: Higher affinity for IgG1 and IgG3, binds IgG4 Supposable higher number of receptors related to higher number of copies of the gene with altered balance of activating and inhibitory FcγRs	[27] [28]
	FCGR3B	NA 1/2 CNV	NA 1: Higher affinity for IgG1 and IgG3 Supposable higher number of receptors related to higher number of copies of the gene with altered balance of activating and inhibitory FcγRs	[29] [37]

Fcγ RECEPTORS AND MONOCLONAL ANTIBODY-BASED THERAPY

Alemtuzumab

The anti-CD52 antibody "Alemtuzumab", also known as "MoAb CD52" or "Campath™" is a humanized MoAb directed against CD52, a protein with unknown functions expressed on the surface of T and B-lymphocytes, monocytes and eosinophils [38]. This antibody was initially developed for its ability to prevent graft-versus-host disease (GVHD). In 2001 it was approved for the treatment of the B-cell chronic lymphocytic leukemia (CLL) [39]. Alemtuzumab is also active against T cell pro-lymphocytic leukemia and adult T cell leukemia and lymphoma, but it is currently not approved for the treatment of these diseases [40].

It is increasingly apparent that post-translational modifications of antibodies play an important role in modulating receptor binding. Human IgG has only one conserved glycosylation site located within the Cγ2 domain (Asn297): the carbohydrate composition of the glycan linked to this asparagine has a strong impact on the binding ability of IgGs to FcγRs and thereby on the FcγRs effector functions. Interestingly, therapeutic antibodies which have been engineered to be no- or low-fucose antibodies display an increased binding to FcγRIIIA and trigger a stronger ADCC in comparison with highly-fucosylated MoAb [41]. In this context, fucose-free Alemtuzumab displays a higher affinity for FcγRIIIA compared to the fucosylated form. However, both Alemtuzumab types show similar affinity for FcγRI and FcγRII [42]. It has been demonstrated that human FcγRs polymorphisms have a remarkable effect on patient response to the therapeutically treatment with MoAb [43]. It also has been reported that antibodies without fucose show a slight increase in their binding to *FCGR2A* R131 variant [44]. It is conceivable that higher copy number of *FCGR3A* could affect the response to Alemtuzumab.

Bevacizumab

The anti-VEGF (vascular endothelial growth factor) antibody "Bevacizumab", also known as "rhuMAb VEGF" or "Avastin™" is a chimeric anti-VEGF MoAb [45]. It consists of mutated human IgG1 framework regions and antigen-binding complementary-determining regions from the murine anti-hVEGF MoAb A.4.6.1 which blocks binding of human VEGF to its receptors. Bevacizumab is currently being investigated clinically for use in treating various cancers (approved in 2004 for treatment of lung and colorectal cancers); although some early stage trials have shown promising results [46, 47], arterial thromboembolism has been reported in colorectal cancer (CRC) patients.

Using FcγRIIA transgenic (hFcR) mice, Meyer *et al.* [48] provided compelling evidence that Bevacizumab-immune complexes (Bevacizumab + VEGF), which induce *in vitro* (via FcγRIIA) platelet aggregation and granule release, cause thrombocytopenia and thrombosis *in vivo*. Notably, Bevacizumab-immune complexes were shown to be thrombotic in hFcR mice in the presence of heparin. This activity required the heparin-binding domain of VEGF. Heparin promoted Bevacizumab-immune complexes deposition on to platelets in a mechanism similar to that observed with antibodies from patients with heparin-induced thrombocytopenia [48]. In light of this evidence, *FCGR2A* genetic polymorphisms should be studied to address whether they will affect the occurrence of arterial thromboembolism in CRC patients.

Cetuximab

The anti-EGFR antibody "Cetuximab", also known as "IMC-C225"(pre-clinical name) or "Erbitux™" is a chimeric MoAb that targets the extra-cellular domain of epidermal growth factor receptor (EGFR), blocking ligand binding to the receptor. Based on a randomized Phase II clinical trial, Cetuximab was approved in the US in 2004 for use in combination with irinotecan, or as monotherapy in EGFR-positive irinotecan-refractory metastatic CRC. However, Cetuximab has an objective response rate (ORS) of only 9% when used as a single agent, along with side effects of diarrhea, skin rash and infusion reactions [49, 50].

There are no biomarkers that reliably predict responses to Cetuximab, but examination of the correlation between patient response and *KRAS* mutations shows promise. *KRAS* encodes a small G protein that links ligand-dependent receptor activation to intracellular pathways of the EGFR signaling cascade. Mutations at key sites within the gene, commonly at codons 12 and 13, cause constitutive activation of KRAS-associated signaling. Growing evidence indicates that tumor *KRAS* mutations are associated to Cetuximab inefficacy [50-54] and the monoclonal anti-EGFR IgG_2 antibody Panitumumab [55], most likely because blockade of the surface receptor is inadequate on cells with downstream activated transduction pathway.

Cetuximab may also exert anti-tumor effects through ADCC. ADCC is influenced by *FCGR2A* H131R and *FCGR3A* V158F polymorphisms that are clinically relevant in follicular lymphoma and metastatic breast cancer treated with Rituximab and Trastuzumab, respectively [43, 56]. Recently, Bibeau *et al.* [57] reported an association of *FCGR* polymorphisms and *KRAS* mutation with the outcome of irinotecan-refractory metastatic CRC patients treated with Cetuximab plus irinotecan. They found patients with *FCGR2A* 131H/H and/or *FCGR3A* 158V/V genotypes had longer progression-free survival (PFS) than 131R and 158F carriers (5.5 vs. 3.0 months; P = 0.005). The difference remained significant for *KRAS* mutated patients. By multivariate analysis, *KRAS* mutation and *FCGR* combined status were independent risk factors for PFS. Overall, the combined *FCGR2A*/*FCGR3A* polymorphisms may be considered relevant prognostic factors for disease progression in metastatic CRC patients treated with Cetuximab plus irinotecan [58]. The reliability of *FCGR2A* polymorphisms as predictive markers of Cetuximab efficacy in EFGR downstream-mutated metastatic CRC was also confirmed in a recent study reporting a higher disease control rate for *FCGR2A* 131H/H genotype compared to the other genotypes (67% vs. 33%, p = 0.017) [59]. A recent study conducted on patients with advanced CRC demonstrated a significant influence of *FCGR3A* F158V polymorphism on survival, both in the whole population as well as in patients with a wild-type *KRAS* tumor, with *FCGR3A* 158V/V patients presenting a dramatically shorter survival [60]. A shorter disease free survival time was also observed for CRC patients with V/V phenotype after treatment with chemotherapy, Bevacizumab and Cetuximab [61]. This correlation study was performed in a large cohort of wild-type *KRAS* cancer patients demonstrating no additional benefit of Cetuximab to conventional treatment [62].

Despite the small sample study, the finding that *FCGR3A* F158V polymorphism was a significant independent predictor of the overall survival of wild-type *KRAS* cancer patients suggests a possible employment of this polymorphism as an additional marker for predicting Cetuximab efficacy, time to progression and overall survival. However, an opposite trend was observed towards a higher response rate and a longer overall survival in CRC patients bearing the *FCGR3A*

158V allele in a recent study performed on patients receiving Cetuximab in combination with irinotecan and tegafur-uracil plus folinic acid [63].

Rituximab

The anti-CD20 antibody "Rituximab", also known as "IDEC-C2B8" (pre-clinical name) or "Rituxan™" is a chimeric MoAb directed against the CD20 antigen expressed on B cells. The first therapeutic trials were reported in 1993, but 4 years elapsed before the Food and Drug Administration approved Rituximab for its use in oncology (it was approved for treatment of lymphoma in 1997). One year later, in 1998, the French Drug Agency followed suit [64]. More recently (2004), Rituximab has been approved for the maintenance treatment of autoimmune diseases and the prevention of graft rejection [65, 66].

Rituximab mediates its anti-tumor activity by multiple mechanisms that include CDC, ADCC and induction of apoptosis following CD20 cross-linking [67, 68]. The inhibitory FcγRIIb on target B cells promotes internalization of rituximab from the surface of certain B-cell malignancies, and is largely responsible for the observed heterogeneity across a range of B-cell malignancies. Internalization correlated strongly with FcγRIIb expression on normal and malignant B cells, and resulted in reduced macrophage phagocytosis of mAb-coated targets [69].

Rituximab sensitizes drug-resistant B Non-Hodgkin's lymphoma (NHL) cell lines to the apoptotic effects of various chemotherapeutic drugs via the selective down-regulation of Bcl-$_{XL}$ expression. Down-regulation of Bcl-xL expression resulted from the inhibition of both Raf/MEK/ERK1/2 and NF-κB survival pathways [70-72]. However, a subgroup of patients did not respond, and in patients with initial response early relapses occur, indicating rituximab resistance. This indicates a clear unmet need to explore alternative antibodies, non-cross resistant to Rituximab, such as Ofatumumab (HuMax-CD20; Genmab, Copenhagen, Denmark), which is a fully human CD20 mAb with a potential low incidence of human-antihuman antibody formation.

Ofatumumab targets a novel epitope of the CD20 molecule on B cells and releases very slowly from the target compared to Rituximab. Ofatumumab induces significant complement-dependent cell lysis *in vitro*, particularly in cells with low

CD20 expression. The FDA recently approved Ofatumumab for treatment of CLL refractory to fludarabine and Alemtuzumab [73]. Although, Ofatumumab has demonstrated a higher potency and a longer duration of efficacy than Rituximab in several preclinical model studies, and even kills Rituximab refractory B cells [74], the identification of factors predicting Rituximab response would allow Rituximab to be reserved for those patients who are most likely to benefit.

Polymorphisms of activating FcγRIIIA (CD16) and FcγRIIA (CD32a) have been found to influence Rituximab response, most likely due to the relative efficiency of different FcγR variants in performing ADCC. The inhibitory FcγRIIB (CD32b) has an opposing effect on effector cells.

Diffuse large B-cell lymphoma (DLBCL) is the most common lymphoid neoplasm accounting for approximately 30-40% of all NHLs. Recently, the combination of Rituximab (R) and CHOP (cyclophosphamide, doxorubicin, vincristin, prednisone) has led to a significant improvement of DLBCL patients outcomes, establishing R-CHOP as the new standard treatment [75, 76]. Recent studies reported a lack of association of *FCGR2A* and *FCGR3A* polymorphisms with survival and response to R-CHOP in DLBCL patients [77] and with follicular lymphoma (FL) [78]. However, another recent work showed a correlation between *FCGR3A* polymorphism and event-free survival and PFS on elderly DLBCL patients after R-CHOP treatment, but not with CHOP alone, suggesting the possibility to design new CD20 antibodies for low-responder patients [79]. FL patients carrying *FCGR3A* 158 V/V genotype respond better than F carriers to Rituximab monotherapy [42, 80, 81], but not to R-CHOP [82, 83].

A new patent established that the association between the *FCGR3A* genotype and clinical and molecular responses to therapeutic antibodies can be used to select only human patient homozygous for V/V at position 158 for the treatment of follicular CD20 positive NHL with Rituximab [84]. However, new approaches have also been suggested to use human or humanized chimeric MoAbs (with high ADCC activity) for treating selected groups of weak-responsive patients carrying *FCGR3A*-158F homozygous or *FCGR3A*-158V/F heterozygous genotypes [85]. *FCGR3A* 158 V/V genotype is associated with improved response to Rituximab monotherapy in Waldenstrom's macroglobulinemia [86], but not in CLL [87]. A recent study on Korean DLBCL patients showed that carriers of *FCGR3A* 158 V/V genotype respond better to R-CHOP than F carriers; however, there were no differences in event-free survival and overall survival [88]. In one series, FL patients carrying *FCGR2A* 131H/H genotype responded better to Rituximab monotherapy than heterozygous patients or patients homozygous for arginine [81]. Other studies failed to confirm this association [80, 82, 87-90].

Mantle cell lymphoma (MCL) accounts for 3-10% of all NHLs, with median overall survival not exceeding 3-4 years. Rituximab in combination with the Hyper-CVAD regimen appears the most promising regimen; Galimberti *et al.* [91] evaluated the clinical success of the regimen, as well as the possible role of *FCGR3A* and *FCGR2A* polymorphisms. The overall response rate was 62.5%, with 33% of complete responses after four cycles of R-Hyper-CVAD. Two-year PFS was 78% for 158V/V patients *vs.* 75% for cases carrying phenylalanine ($p = 0.88$). When the *FCGR2A* polymorphism was assessed, the 2-year PFS was 82% for 131H/H patients vs. 75% for those carrying arginine ($p = 0.26$). These results confirm that Rituximab plus Hyper-CVAD is an effective regimen for the induction of prolonged remission in patients with aggressive MCL and suggests that Rituximab effectiveness is independent from *FCGR* polymorphisms.

Trastuzumab

The anti-HER-2/neu antibody "Trastuzumab", also known as "rhuMAb HER2" or "Herceptin™" is a humanized MoAb approved in 1998 for the treatment of breast cancer. It has been shown to bind both activatory (FcγRIIIA; FcγRIIA) and inhibitory (FcγRIIB) antibody receptors. Additionally, several *FCGR* polymorphisms have been identified that may affect the ADCC of natural-killer cells/monocytes. Notably, Arnould *et al.* [92] have shown immune cell infiltration in HER2-positive breast cancer in the neoadjuvant setting following trastuzumab treatment, underlining the impact of ADCC.

FCGR polymorphisms were found to be associated with clinical outcome of patients with breast cancer who received Trastuzumab. Fifty-four patients with HER2/neu-amplified breast cancer receiving Trastuzumab plus taxane for metastatic disease were evaluated for *FCGR3A*-V158F, *FCGR2A*-H131R, and *FCGR2B*-I232T polymorphisms. The *FCGR3A*-158 V/V genotype was significantly correlated with objective response rate and PFS. Additionally, a significant trend in objective response rate and PFS was noticed for the *FCGR2A* 131H/H genotype. The combination of the two favorable genotypes (V/V and/or H/H) was independently associated with better objective response rate and PFS compared to the other combinations. The ADCC analysis showed that peripheral blood mononuclear cells (PBMCs) carrying V/V and/or H/H genotypes had a significantly higher Trastuzumab-mediated cytotoxicity than PBMCs harboring different genotypes. Overall, these data support the hypothesis that FcγR-mediated ADCC plays an important role in the clinical effect of Trastuzumab [56].

Recent data from 15 operable and 35 metastatic HER2-positive breast cancer patient, treated with Trastuzumab, showed that the *FCGR2A*-131 H/H genotype was significantly correlated to the pathologically documented response (pathological response) ($P = 0.015$) and the objective response ($P = 0.043$). The *FCGR3A*-158 V/V genotype was not correlated to the pathological response, but exhibited a trend toward correlation with the objective response. Patients with the *FCGR2A*-131 H/H genotype had also a significant longer PFS in the metastatic setting ($P = 0.034$) [93]. However, different results were obtained in non-metastatic HER2-positive early breast cancer patient; no-correlation was detected between disease free survival and *FCGR2A* polymorphism (131H/H vs. H/R vs. R/R, $P = 0.76$) as well as for *FCGR3A* polymorphism (158V/V vs. V/F vs. F/F, $P = 0.98$) [94].

CURRENT & FUTURE DEVELOPMENTS

It is accepted that germ-line polymorphisms (both SNPs and CNV) have the potential to predict the outcome of therapy. Predicting outcome of MoAb-therapy is especially warranted, as response rates are moderate, with possible serious adverse side effects, at high financial cost. In this chapter, we provided an overview of studies on polymorphisms within FcγReceptors (FCGRs) genetic clusters and their effects on MoAb-based anti-cancer therapy.

These studies highlighted the biological complexity behind the role of FcγRs in determining MoAb therapeutic effectiveness. To summarize, the patient response to MoAb therapy can be affected by differences in the degree of dependency on

ADCC, immunoglobulin subtype among individual MoAbs, and also, likely by inherent molecular differences in various subclasses of disease. Before embracing an approach to predict clinical responses or to modify dosing based on patients FcγR polymorphisms, either in clinical trials or in clinical practice, one must first appreciate the multifaceted nature of this approach. Moreover, FcγR triggering results in more than ADCC or phagocytosis. Recent studies indicated that therapeutic antibodies might lead to activation of tumor-associated macrophages and thereby even promote tumor growth [95].

In vitro binding studies of individual MoAbs to recombinant FcγR may help to define the importance of different polymorphic alleles in the antitumor mechanism of MoAb *in vivo*. An accurate prediction of outcome based on *FCGR* genotype can help identify patients most likely to benefit from a specific form of MoAb (i.e. fucosylated vs. non). Historically, *FCGR2A* polymorphism is particularly important among patients with complement deficiency where phagocytosis is the only intact defense for clearing infections. Thus, one might expect *FCGR2A* genotype to be most critical if the antitumor mechanism is complement-independent.

Identification of the clinically important FcγR for each MoAb will help focus efforts on improving Fc affinities for their specific FcγR. Since FcγR is only one of the many receptors important in ADCC and antigen presenting cell function, a better understanding of genetic polymorphisms in antibody-based therapies may provide insight into how to render this modality even more effective [96]. For this reason, new patents on novel diagnostic methods to predict the responsiveness to therapy in personalized way, based on copy number variations and SNPs on FcγR gene cluster, are promising and welcomed [97].

However, besides the important efforts contributed by pharmacogenomics studies on the role of FcγR natural variations in MoAb anti-cancer therapy, the engineering of antibody molecules [98, 99] will enhance their antitumor activity, leading to improved therapeutic outcomes and reduced doses.

In conclusion, through the use of genetic pre-screening of patients it may be possible to differentiate non-responders from responders. Additionally, as our knowledge increases, there will be the possibility to engineer antibodies with the maximum FcγR binding potential.

CONFLICT OF INTERESTS

None declared.

ACKNOWLEDGEMENTS

We would like to thank Kristina Havas for critical reading of the chapter.

DISCLOSURE

The chapter submitted for Patent eBook Series "Topics in Anti-Cancer Research" Volume 2 is an update of our article "Insights into the Role of Fc Gamma Receptors (FcγRs) Genetic Variations in Monoclonal Antibody-Based Anti-Cancer Therapy", published in the journal 'Recent Patents on Anti-Cancer Drug Discovery' Volume 5, Number 3, November Issue 2010, Page 197 to 204 with additional text and recent references.

REFERENCES

[1] Sarries C, Haura EB, Roig B, Taron M, Abad A, Scagliotti G, *et al.* Pharmacogenomic strategies for developing customized chemotherapy in non-small cell lung cancer. Pharmacogenomics 2002; 3(6): 763-80.

[2] Stoehlmacher J, Goekkurt E, Lenz HJ. Pharmacogenetic aspects in treatment of colorectal cancer-an update. Pharmacogenomics 2003; 4(6): 767-77.

[3] Tan BR, McLeod HL. Pharmacogenetic influences on treatment response and toxicity in colorectal cancer. Semin Oncol 2005; 32(1): 113-9.

[4] Van Sorge NM, van der Pol WL, van de Winkel JG. FcγR polymorphisms: Implications for function, disease susceptibility and immunotherapy. Tissue Antigens 2003; 61(3): 189-202.

[5] Ravetch JV, Bolland S. IgG Fc receptors. Annu Rev Immunol 2001; 19: 275-90.

[6] Namboodiri AM, Pandey JP. Differential inhibition of trastuzumab- and Cetuximab-induced cytotoxicity of cancer cells by immunoglobulin G1 expressing different GM allotypes. Clin Exp Immunol 2011; 166(3): 361-5.

[7] Nissim A, Chernajovsky Y. Historical development of monoclonal antibody therapeutics. Handb Exp Pharmacol 2008; (181): 3-18.

[8] Kipriyanov SM, Le Gall F. Generation and production of engineered antibodies. Mol Biotechnol 2004; 26(1): 39-60.

[9] Stavenhagen, J., Vijh, S., Rankin, C., Gorlatov, S., Huang, L. Identification and engineering of antibodies with variant Fc regions and methods of using same. US7960512 (**2011**).

[10] Yamane-Ohnuki N, Satoh M. Production of therapeutic antibodies with controlled fucosylation. MAbs 2009; 1(3): 230-6.

[11] Mizushima T, Yagi H, Takemoto E, Shibata-Koyama M, Isoda Y, Iida S, *et al.* Structural basis for improved efficacy of therapeutic antibodies on defucosylation of their Fc glycans. Genes Cells 2011; 16(11): 1071-80.

[12] Syam S, Mero P, Pham T, McIntosh CA, Bruhns P, Booth JW. Differential recruitment of activating and inhibitory Fc gamma RII during phagocytosis. J Immunol 2010; 184(6): 2966-73.

[13] Unkeless JC, Scigliano E, Freedman VH. Structure and function of human and murine receptors for IgG. Annu Rev Immunol 1988; 6: 251-81.

[14] Su K,Wu J, Edberg JC, McKenzie SE, Kimberly RP. Genomic organization of classical human low-affinity Fcg receptor genes. Genes Immun 2002; 3 Suppl 1: S51-6

[15] Van de Winkel JGJ, de Wit TP, Ernst LK, Capel PJA, Ceuppens JL. Molecular basis for a familial defect in phagocyte expression of IgG receptor I (CD64). J Immunol 1995; 154(6): 2896-903.

[16] Warmerdam PA, Nabben NM, van de Graaf SA, van de Winkel JG, Capel PJ. The human low affinity immunoglobulin G Fc receptor IIC gene is a result of an unequal crossover event. J Biol Chem 1993; 268(10): 7346-9.

[17] Morel PA, Ernst LK, Metes D. Functional CD32 molecules on human NK cells. Leuk Lymphoma 1999; 35(1-2): 47-56.

[18] Metes D, Ernst LK, Chambers WH, Sulica A, Herberman RB, Morel PA. Expression of functional CD32 molecules on human NK cells is determined by an allelic polymorphism of the FcγRIIC gene. Blood 1998; 91(7): 2369-80.

[19] van der Heijden J, Breunis WB, Geissler J, de Boer M, van den Berg TK, Kuijpers TW. Phenotypic variation in IgG receptors by nonclassical FCGR2C alleles. J Immunol 2012; 188(3): 1318-24.

[20] Warmerdam PA, van de Winkel JG, Vlug A, Westerdal NA, Capel PJ. A single amino acid in the second Ig-like domain of the human Fcγ receptor II is critical in human IgG2 binding. J Immunol 1991; 147(4): 1338-43.

[21] Yun HR, Koh HK, Kim SS, Chung WT, Kim DW, Hong KP, *et al.* FcγRIIa/IIIa polymorphism and its association with clinical manifestations in Korean lupus patients. Lupus 2001; 10(7): 466-72.

[22] Domingo P, Muniz-Diaz E, Baraldes MA, Arilla M, Barquet N, Pericas R, *et al.* Associations between Fc gamma receptor IIA polymorphisms and the risk and prognosis of meningococcal disease. Am J Med 2002; 112(1): 19-25.

[23] Carrington CV, Norman PJ, Vaughan RW, Kondeatis E, Ramdath DD, Hameed K, *et al.* Analysis of Fc gamma receptor II (CD32) polymorphism in populations of African and South Asian ancestry reveals east-west geographic gradients of allele frequencies. Eur J Immuno genet 2003; 30(5): 375-9

[24] Redon R, Ishikawa S, Fitch KR, Feuk L, Perry GH, Andrews TD, *et al.* Global variation in copy number in the human genome. Nature 2006; 444: 444-54.

[25] Conrad DF, Pinto D, Redon R, Feuk L, Gokcumen O, Zhang Y, *et al.* Origins and functional impact of copy number variation in the human genome. Nature 2010; 464(7289): 704-12.

[26] Breunis WB, van Mirre E, Bruin M, Geissler J, de Boer M, Peters M, *et al.* Copy number variation of the activating FCGR2C gene predisposes to idiopathic thrombocytopenic purpura. Blood 2008; 111(3): 1029-38

[27] Thabet MM, Huizinga TW, Marques RB, Stoeken-Rijsbergen G, Bakker AM, Kurreeman FA, *et al.* The contribution of Fcgamma receptor IIIA gene 158V/F polymorphism and copy number variation to the risk of ACPA positive rheumatoid arthritis. Ann Rheum Dis 2009; 68(11): 1775-80

[28] Wu J, Edberg JC, Redecha PB, Bansal V, Guyre PM, Coleman K, *et al.* A novel polymorphism of FcγRIIIa (CD16) alters receptor function and predisposes to autoimmune disease. J Clin Invest 1997; 100(5): 1059-70.
[29] Salmon JE, Edberg JC, Kimberly RP. Fc gamma receptor III on human neutrophils. Allelic variants have functionally distinct capacities. J Clin Invest 1990; 85(4): 1287-95
[30] Flesch BK, Doose S, Siebert R, Ntambi E, Neppert J. FCGR3 variants and expression of human neutrophil antigen-1a, -1b, and -1c in the populations of northern Germany and Uganda. Transfusion 2002; 42(4): 469-75.
[31] Fanciulli M, Norsworthy PJ, Petretto E, Dong R, Harper L, Kamesh L, *et al.* FCGR3B copy number variation is associated with susceptibility to systemic, but not organ-specific, autoimmunity. Nat Genet 2007; 39(6): 721-3.
[32] McKinney C, Fanciulli M, Merriman ME, Phipps-Green A, Alizadeh BZ, Koeleman BP, *et al.* Association of variation in Fcgamma receptor 3B gene copy number with rheumatoid arthritis in Caucasian samples. Ann Rheum Dis 2010; 69(9): 1711-6.
[33] Machado LR, Hardwick RJ, Bowdrey J, Bogle H, Knowles TJ, Sironi M, *et al.* Evolutionary history of copy-number-variable locus for the low-affinity Fcγ receptor: Mutation rate, autoimmune disease, and the legacy of helminth infection. Am J Hum Genet 2012; 90(6): 973-85.
[34] Hollox EJ, Detering JC, Dehnugara T. An integrated approach for measuring copy number variation at the FCGR3 (CD16) locus. Hum Mutat 2009; 30(3): 477-84.
[35] McKinney C, Merriman TR. Meta-analysis confirms a role for deletion in FCGR3B in autoimmune phenotypes. Hum Mol Genet 2012; 21(10): 2370-6.
[36] Kono H, Kyogoku C, Suzuki T, Tsuchiya N, Honda H, Yamamoto K, *et al.* FcgammaRIIB Ile232Thr transmembrane polymorphism associated with human systemic lupus erythematosus decreases affinity to lipid rafts and attenuates inhibitory effects on B cell receptor signaling. Hum Mol Genet 2005; 14(19): 2881-92.
[37] Willcocks LC, Lyons PA, Clatworthy MR, Robinson JI, Yang W, Newland SA, *et al.* Copy number of FCGR3B, which is associated with systemic lupus erythematosus, correlates with protein expression and immune complex uptake. J Exp Med 2008; 205(7): 1573-82.
[38] Gilleece MH, Dexter TM. Effect of Campath-1H antibody on human hematopoietic progenitors *in vitro*. Blood 1993; 82(3): 807-12.
[39] Robak T. Alemtuzumab in the treatment of chronic lymphocytic leukemia. BioDrugs 2005; 19(1): 9-22.
[40] Morris JC, Waldmann TA. Antibody-based therapy of leukaemia. Expert Rev Mol Med 2009; 11: e29.
[41] Abès R, Teillaud JL. Impact of glycosylation on effector functions of therapeutic IgG. Pharmaceuticals 2010; 3(1): 146-157.
[42] Natsume A, In M, Takamura H, Nakagawa T, Shimizu Y, Kitajima K, *et al.* Engineered antibodies of IgG1/IgG3 mixed isotype with enhanced cytotoxic activities. Cancer Res 2008; 68(10): 3863-72.
[43] Cartron G, Dacheux L, Salles G, Solal-Celigny P, Bardos P, Colombat P, *et al.* Therapeutical activity of humanized anti-CD20 monoclonal antibody and polymorphism in IgG Fc receptor FcgammaRIIIa gene. Blood 2002; 99(3): 754-8.
[44] Shields RL, Lai J, Keck R, O'Connell LY, Hong K, Meng YG, *et al.* Lack of fucose on human IgG1 N-linked oligosaccharide improves binding to human Fcgamma RIII and antibody-dependent cellular toxicity. J Biol Chem 2002; 277(30): 26733-40.

[45] Fyfe, G., Holmgren, E., Mass, R.D., Novotny, W. Treatment with anti-VEGF antibodies. US7622115 (**2009**).

[46] Kerbel RS. Clinical trials of antiangiogenic drugs: Opportunities, problems, and assessment of initial results. J Clin Oncol 2001; 19(18 Suppl): 45S-51S.

[47] Kabbinavar F, Hurwitz HI, Fehrenbacher L, Meropol NJ, Novotny WF, Lieberman G, *et al.* Phase II, randomized trial comparing bevacizumab plus fluorouracil (FU)/leucovorin (LV) with FU/LV alone in patients with metastatic colorectal cancer. J Clin Oncol 2003; 21(1): 60-52003; 21: 60-5.

[48] Meyer T, Robles-Carrillo L, Robson T, Langer F, Desai H, Davila M, *et al.* Bevacizumab immune complexes activate platelets and induce thrombosis in FCGR2A transgenic mice. J Thromb Haemost 2009; 7(1): 171-81.

[49] Goel, S., Mariadason, J.M. Method of determining the sensitivity of cancer cells to EGFR inhibitors including Cetuximab, panitumumab and erlotinib. US20090258364 (**2009**).

[50] De Roock W, Piessevaux H, De Schutter J, Janssens M, De Hertogh G, Personeni N, *et al.* KRAS wild-type state predicts survival and is associated to early radiological response in metastatic colorectal cancer treated with Cetuximab. Ann Oncol 2008; 19(3): 508-15.

[51] Di Fiore F, Blanchard F, Charbonnier F, Le Pessot F, Lamy A, Galais MP, *et al.* Clinical relevance of KRAS mutation detection in metastatic colorectal cancer treated by Cetuximab plus chemotherapy. Br J Cancer 2007; 96(8): 1166-9.

[52] Lièvre A, Bachet JB, Boige V, Cayre A, Le Corre D, Buc E, *et al.* KRAS mutations as an independent prognostic factor in patients with advanced colorectal cancer treated with Cetuximab. J Clin Oncol 2008; 26(3): 374-9.

[53] Lièvre A, Bachet JB, Le Corre D, Boige V, Landi B, Emile JF, *et al.* KRAS mutation status is predictive of response to Cetuximab therapy in colorectal cancer. Cancer Res 2006; 66(8): 3992-5.

[54] Cervantes A, Macarulla T, Martinelli E, Rodriguez-Braun E, Ciardiello F, Stroh C, *et al.* Correlation of KRAS status (wild type [wt] vs. mutant [mt]) with efficacy to first-line Cetuximab in a study of Cetuximab single agent followed by Cetuximab + FOLFIRI in patients (pts) with metastatic colorectal cancer (mCRC). American Society of Clinical Oncology - Annual Meeting, (2008).

[55] Van Cutsem E, Peeters M, Siena S, Humblet Y, Hendlisz A, Neyns B, *et al.* Open-label Phase III trial of panitumumab plus best supportive care compared with best supportive care alone in patients with chemotherapy-refractory metastatic colorectal cancer. J Clin Oncol 2007; 25(13): 1658-64.

[56] Musolino A, Naldi N, Bortesi B, Pezzuolo D, Capelletti M, Missale G, *et al.* Immunoglobulin G fragment C receptor polymorphisms and clinical efficacy of trastuzumab-based therapy in patients with HER-2/neu-positive metastatic breast cancer. J Clin Oncol 2008; 26(11): 1789-96.

[57] Bibeau F, Lopez-Crapez E, Di Fiore F, Thezenas S, Ychou M, Blanchard F, *et al.* Impact of Fc{gamma}RIIa-Fc{gamma}RIIIa polymorphisms and KRAS mutations on the clinical outcome of patients with metastatic colorectal cancer treated with Cetuximab plus irinotecan. J Clin Oncol 2009; 27(7): 1122-9.

[58] Lenz, H.-J. Fcgamma polymorphisms for predicting disease and treatment outcome. US20090181016 (**2009**) & US20120094291 (**2012**).

[59] Rodríguez J, Zarate R, Bandres E, Boni V, Hernández A, Sola JJ, *et al.* Fc gamma receptor polymorphisms as predictive markers of Cetuximab efficacy in epidermal growth factor receptor downstream-mutated metastatic colorectal cancer. Eur J Cancer 2012; 48(12): 1774-80.

[60] Dahan L, Norguet E, Etienne-Grimaldi MC, Formento JL, Gasmi M, Nanni I, *et al.* Pharmacogenetic profiling and Cetuximab outcome in patients with advanced colorectal cancer. BMC Cancer 2011; 11: 496.

[61] Pander J, Gelderblom H, Antonini NF, Tol J, van Krieken JH, van der Straaten T, *et al.* Correlation of FCGR3A and EGFR germline polymorphisms with the efficacy of Cetuximab in KRAS wild-type metastatic colorectal cancer. Eur J Cancer 2010; 46(10): 1829-34.

[62] Tol J, Koopman M, Cats A, Rodenburg CJ, Creemers GJ, Schrama JG, *et al.* Chemotherapy, bevacizumab, and Cetuximab in metastatic colorectal cancer. N Engl J Med 2009; 360(6): 563-72.

[63] Etienne-Grimaldi MC, Bennouna J, Formento JL, Douillard JY, Francoual M, Hennebelle I, *et al.* Multifactorial pharmacogenetic analysis in colorectal cancer patients receiving 5-fluorouracil-based therapy together with Cetuximab-irinotecan. Br J Clin Pharmacol 2012; 73(5): 776-85.

[64] Maloney DG, Grillo-López AJ, White CA, Bodkin D, Schilder RJ, Neidhart JA, *et al.* IDEC-C2B8 (rituximab) anti-CD20 monoclonal antibody therapy in patients with relapsed low-grade non-Hodgkin's lymphoma. Blood 1997; 90(6): 2188-95.

[65] Edwards JC, Szczepanski L, Szechinski J, Filipowicz-Sosnowska A, Emery P, Close DR, *et al.* Efficacy of B cell-targeted therapy with rituximab in patients with rheumatoid arthritis. N Engl J Med 2004; 350(25): 2572-81.

[66] Becker YT, Becker BN, Pirsch JD, Sollinger HW. Rituximab as treatment for refractory kidney transplant rejection. Am J Transplant 2004; 4(6): 996-1001.

[67] Shan D, Ledbetter JA, Press OW. Apoptosis of malignant human B cells by ligation of CD20 with monoclonal antibodies. Blood 1998; 91(5): 1644-52.

[68] Jazirehi AR, Bonavida B. Cellular and molecular signal transduction pathways modulated by rituximab (rituxan, anti-CD20 mAb) in non-Hodgkin's lymphoma: Implications in chemosensi- tization and therapeutic intervention. Oncogene 2005; 24(13): 2121-43.

[69] Lim SH, Vaughan AT, Ashton-Key M, Williams EL, Dixon SV, Chan HT, *et al.* Fc gamma receptor IIb on target B cells promotes rituximab internalization and reduces clinical efficacy. Blood 2011; 118(9): 2530-40.

[70] Bonavida, B., Jazirehi, A.R. Molecular signaling pathways triggered by Rituximab: Prognostic, diagnostic, and therapeutic uses. US20070172847 (**2007**).

[71] Jazirehi AR, Vega MI, Chatterjee D, Goodglick L, Bonavida B. Inhibition of the Raf-MEK1/2-ERK1/2 signaling pathway, Bcl-xL down-regulation, and chemosensitization of non-Hodgkin's lymphoma B cells by Rituximab. Cancer Res 2004; 64(19): 7117-26.

[72] Jazirehi AR, Huerta-Yepez S, Cheng G, Bonavida B. Rituximab (chimeric anti-CD20 monoclonal antibody) inhibits the constitutive nuclear factor-{kappa}B signaling pathway in non-Hodgkin's lymphoma B-cell lines: Role in sensitization to chemotherapeutic drug-induced apoptosis. Cancer Res 2005; 65(1): 264-76.

[73] Osterborg A. Ofatumumab, a human anti-CD20 monoclonal antibody. Expert Opin Biol Ther 2010; 10(3): 439-49.

[74] Hagenbeek A, Gadeberg O, Johnson P, Pedersen LM, Walewski J, Hellmann A, *et al.* First clinical use of ofatumumab, a novel fully human anti-CD20 monoclonal antibody in relapsed or refractory follicular lymphoma: Results of a Phase 1/2 trial. Blood 2008; 111(12): 5486-95.

[75] Feugier P, Van Hoof A, Sebban C, Solal-Celigny P, Bouabdallah R, Fermé C, *et al.* Long-term results of the RCHOP study in the treatment of elderly patients with diffuse large B-cell lymphoma: A study by the Groupe d'Etude des Lymphomes de l'Adulte. J Clin Oncol 2005; 23(18): 4117-26.

[76] Pfreundschuh M, Trumper L, Osterborg A, Pettengell R, Trneny M, Imrie K, *et al.* CHOP-like chemotherapy plus rituximab versus CHOP-like chemotherapy alone in young patients with good-prognosis diffuse large-B cell lymphoma: A randomized controlled trial by the MabThera International Trial (MInT) Group. Lancet Oncol 2006; 7(5): 379-91.

[77] Fabisiewicz A, Paszkiewicz-Kozik E, Osowiecki M, Walewski J, Siedlecki JA. FcγRIIA and FcγRIIIA polymorphisms do not influence survival and response to rituximab, cyclophosphamide, doxorubicin, vincristine, and prednisone immunochemotherapy in patients with diffuse large B-cell lymphoma. Leuk Lymphoma 2011; 52(8): 1604-6.

[78] Prochazka V, Papajik T, Gazdova J, Divoka M, Rozmanova S, Faber E, *et al.* FcγRIIIA receptor genotype does not influence an outcome in patients with follicular lymphoma treated with risk-adapted immunochemotherapy. Neoplasma 2011; 58(3): 263-70.

[79] Ahlgrimm M, Pfreundschuh M, Kreuz M, Regitz E, Preuss KD, Bittenbring J. The impact of Fc-γ receptor polymorphisms in elderly patients with diffuse large B-cell lymphoma treated with CHOP with or without rituximab. Blood 2011; 118(17): 4657-62.

[80] Levy, R., Weng, W.K. Methods and compositions for determining responsiveness to antibody therapy. US20060008825 (**2006**).

[81] Weng WK, Levy R. Two immunoglobulin G fragment C receptor polymorphisms independently predict response to rituximab in patients with follicular lymphoma. J Clin Oncol 2003; 21(21): 3940-7.

[82] Boetcher S, Pott C, Ritgen M, Hiddeman W, Unterhalt M, Kneba M. Evidence for FcgRIIIA-independent rituximab effector mechanisms in patients with follicular lymphoma treated with combined immunochemotherapy. American Society of Hematology - Annual Meeting, (2004).

[83] Carlotti E, Palumbo GA, Oldani E, Acerboni S, Di Raimondo F, Cortelazzo S, *et al.* Bone marrow bcl2/IgH+ cells at diagnosis and not FcgRIIIA polymorphism predict response in follicular non-Hodgkin's lymphoma patients treated with sequential CHOP and rituximab. Blood 2005; 106(11): 289A-90A.

[84] Watier, H., Cartron, G., Colombat, P. Methods and compositions to evaluate antibody treatment response. US7858300 (**2010**).

[85] Bourel, D., Jorieux, S., Romeuf, C.D., Klein, P., Gaucher, C., Bihoreau, N., Nony, E. Use of ADCC-optimized antibodies for treating low-responder patients. US7713524 (**2010**).

[86] Treon SP, Hansen M, Branagan AR, Verselis S, Emmanouilides C, Kimby E, *et al.* Polymorphisms in FcgRIIIA (CD16) receptor expression are associated with clinical response to rituximab in Waldenstrom's macroglobulinemia. J Clin Oncol 2005; 23(3): 474-81.

[87] Farag SS, Flinn IW, Modali R, Lehman TA, Young D, Byrd JC. Fc gamma RIIIa and Fc gamma RIIa polymorphisms do not predict response to rituximab in B-cell chronic lymphocytic leukemia. Blood 2004; 103(4): 1472-4.

[88] Kim DH, Jung HD, Kim JG, Lee JJ, Yang DH, Park YH, *et al.* FCGR3A gene polymorphisms may correlate with response to frontline R-CHOP therapy for diffuse large B-cell lymphoma. Blood 2006; 108(8): 2720-5.

[89] Mitroviç Z, Aurer I, Radman I, Ajdukoviç R, Sertiç J, Labar B. FCgammaRIIIA and FCgammaRIIA polymorphisms are not associated with response to rituximab and CHOP in patients with diffuse large B-cell lymphoma. Haematologica 2007; 92(7): 998-9.

[90] Weng WK, Levy R. Genetic polymorphism of the inhibitory IgG Fc receptor FcgammaRIIb is not associated with clinical outcome in patients with follicular lymphoma treated with rituximab. Leuk Lymphoma 2009; 50(5): 723-7.

[91] Galimberti S, Palumbo GA, Caracciolo F, Benedetti E, Pelosini M, Brizzi S, *et al.* The efficacy of rituximab plus Hyper-CVAD regimen in mantle cell lymphoma is independent of FCgammaRIIIa and FCgammaRIIa polymorphisms. J Chemother 2007; 19(3): 315-21.

[92] Arnould L, Gelly M, Penault-Llorca F, Benoit L, Bonnetain F, Migeon C, *et al.* Trastuzumab-based treatment of HER2-positive breast cancer: An antibody-dependent cellular cytotoxicity mechanism? Br J Cancer 2006; 94(2): 259-67.

[93] Tamura K, Shimizu C, Hojo T, Akashi-Tanaka S, Kinoshita T, Yonemori K, *et al.* FcγR2A and 3A polymorphisms predict clinical outcome of trastuzumab in both neoadjuvant and metastatic settings in patients with HER2-positive breast cancer. Ann Oncol 2011; 22(6): 1302-7.

[94] Hurvitz SA, Betting DJ, Stern HM, Quinaux E, Stinson J, Seshagiri S, *et al.* Analysis of Fcγ receptor IIIa and IIa Polymorphisms: Lack of correlation with outcome in trastuzumab-treated breast cancer patients. Clin Cancer Res 2012; 18(12): 3478-86.

[95] Pander J, Heusinkveld M, van der Straaten T, Jordanova ES, Baak-Pablo R, Gelderblom H, *et al.* Activation of tumor-promoting type 2 macrophages by EGFR-targeting antibody Cetuximab. Clin Cancer Res 2011; 17(17): 5668-73. 2008; 26: 1789-96.

[96] Erichsen HC, Chanock SJ. SNPs in cancer research and treatment. Br J Cancer 2004; 90(4): 747-51.

[97] Roos, D., Kuijpers, T.W. Diagnostic methods involving determining gene copy numbers and SNPs in the FcyRII/FcyRIII gene cluster, and probes for use in such methods to detect susceptibility to and treatment efficacy in autoimmune diseases. US7994300 (**2011**).

[98] Lazar, G.A., Dang, W., Desjarlais, J.R., Karki, S.B., Vafa, O., Hayes, R., Arthur, C.J. Optimized Fc variants and methods for their generation. US20090215991 (**2009**) & CN1867583 (**2012**).

[99] Lazar, G.A., Dang, W., Desjarlais, J.R., Karki, S.B., Vafa, O., Hayes, R. Fc variants having decreased affinity for FcyRIIb. US20090010920 (**2009**).

Topics in Anti-Cancer Research, Vol. 2, 2013, 279-298

CHAPTER 8

Angiogenesis: Therapeutic Target in Renal Cell Carcinoma

Manisha Singh[1], Sudip Nanda[2], Santo Longo[3] and Shree G. Sharma[4]

[1]Department of Internal Medicine, University of Arkansas for Medical Sciences, Little Rock, Arkansas, USA; [2]Division of Cardiovascular Medicine, Mayo Clinic, Rochester, Minnesota; [3]Department of Pathology, St. Luke's Hospital, Bethlehem, Pennsylvania; [4]Department of Pathology, University of Arkansas for Medical Sciences, Little Rock, Arkansas, USA

Abstract: Renal cell carcinoma (RCC) is one of the most common cancers in the United States. Recent achievements in translational research have led to significant developments in treatment strategies for this malignancy. RCC is a richly vascular neoplasm. A better understanding of disease biology has helped in the development of anti-angiogenic therapy. Vascular endothelial growth factor (VEGF) is the most important molecular target in the treatment of RCC. Patents have been filed for anti-VEGF and other molecular pathways involved in the pathogenesis of RCC. This chapter provides an overview of angiogenesis in RCC, important anti-angiogenic drugs for treating RCC and some developmental drugs and patents which might shape the treatment of RCC in future.

Keywords: Angiogenesis, antiangiogenic therapy, axitinib, bevacizumab, mTOR, patents, pazopanib, renal cell carcinoma, sorafenib, sunitinib, temsirolimus, VEGF, VHL.

INTRODUCTION

Renal cell carcinoma (RCC) is one of the common cancers in United States. An estimated 64,770 new cases (including renal pelvis) will occur in 2012, which will cause approximately 13,570 deaths [1]. The first and most pursued of targeted therapies is in the area of anti-angiogenesis. Anti-angiogenic therapy is the treatment of choice for patients with recurrent and stage IV RCC. Approved drugs

*__Address correspondence to Shree G Sharma:__ Department of Pathology, University of Arkansas for Medical Sciences, 4301 West Markham # 517, Little Rock, Ar, 72205, USA; Tel: 501-526-6477; Fax: 501-686-5959; E-mail: drshreegopal@gmail.com

Atta-ur Rahman and Khurshid Zaman (Eds)

affecting angiogenesis are sunitinib, bevacizumab, sorafenib, pazopanib, axitinib, temsirolimus and everolimus [2]. Blood vessels are the fundamental structural supply of the nutritional and metabolic needs of cells. From very early embryogenesis, the initiation of blood vessel growth and their development is regulated by a balance of stimulatory and inhibitory factors Fig. (**1**). Sources of these factors include host cells, endothelial cells, and the extracellular matrix. When the balance of these factors favor angiogenesis, special endothelial cells, called "tip cells", begin sprouting new capillary-like vessels. The proliferation of tip cells is followed closely by the growth of "stalk cells." "Stalk cells" form a supportive trunk of the neo-capillary and provide the connection to the main parent vessel [3]. In addition, angiogenesis is a source of hematopoietic stem cells [4].

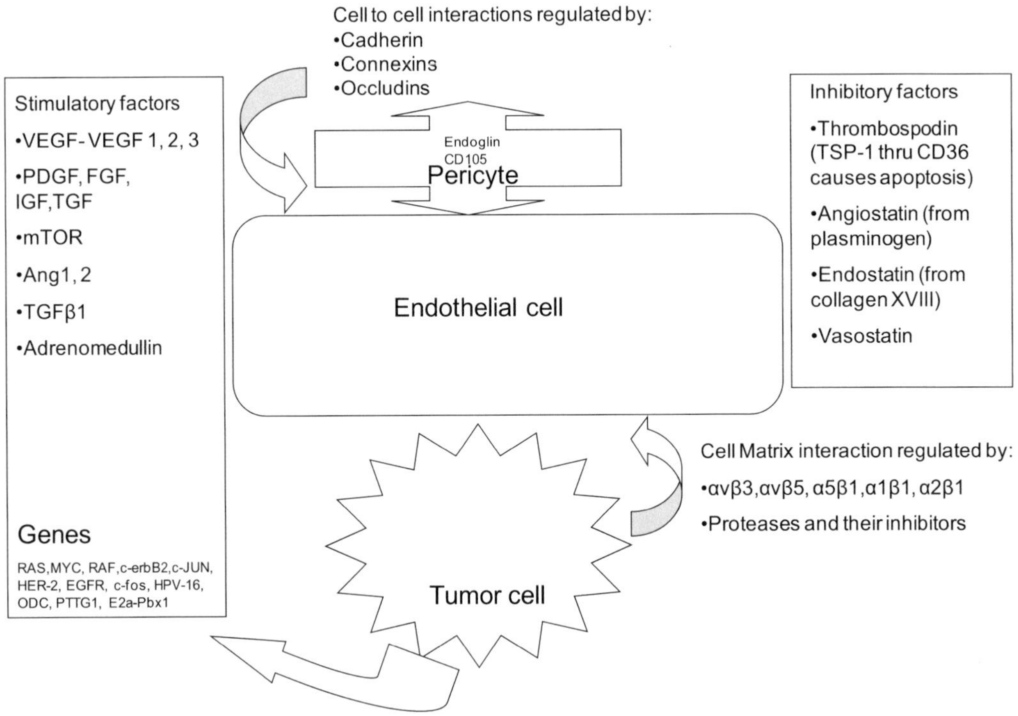

Figure 1: Regulatory factors in angiogenesis.

The study of new vessel formation (angiogenesis) has defined more precise use of some existing terms and has generated some specific neologisms. Both of these language changes require specific understanding. Angiogenesis indicates the formation of new blood vessels from existing blood vessels by the processes of "sprouting," "branching," or "intussusceptions" [5]. Vasculogenesis denotes *de novo* blood vessel formation during fetal life, by endothelial differentiation from totipotential stem cells [6]. Post-natal neo-vessels (capillaries), formed by the proliferation of endothelial cells (EC), are very fragile. Composed only of a single layer of endothelial cells, the walls of these capillaries are leaky and architecturally haphazard. Newly-formed capillaries are subsequently intimately surrounded by smooth muscle cells, designated "mural cells" (MCs) and pericytes. MCs are smooth muscle cells within the walls of larger vessels and the pericytes around smaller vessels. In tandem, the acquisition of MCs and pericytes accomplishes two essential needs. First, the immediate structural stabilization of the neo-capillaries is accomplished. Second, where needed, the addition of MCs and pericytes provide the construction of more complex arteries and veins, called arteriogenesis [7].

The specific selection of endothelial cells for either arterial or venous development occurs very early in the development process. This process is regulated by hemodynamic, genetic, and local tissue factors [3]. The entire process of development of vessels is a continuously dynamic process. New vessels adapt and are modified in response to local signals, provided by the needs of particular organ.

Ultimately, the neo-vessel uniqueness, of each organ, resides in the array of genomic markers expressed by the endothelial cells. These markers are the actual targets for selective anti-angiogenic therapy. In addition, markers can be identified by their structure of origin. The different markers expressed by the arteries (VEGFR2, NRP1, DII4, Notch, ephrin B2, Cx37 and Cx40); veins (VEGFR3, NRP2, COUP-TFII, EphB4, Msr/Apj), and lymphatics (VEGFR3, NRP2, LYVE-1, podoplanin, Prox 1, ephrin-B2/EphB4 and CCL21) are known [8]. The markers expressed by the tumor vasculature are also known and are very unique [9].

It is imperative to students of this subject to envision angiogenesis occurring in two different venues. Chronic disorders with prolonged and sustained angiogenesis (diabetes, psoriasis, rheumatoid arthritis, tumor, and atherosclerosis) are in sharp contrast to a "self-limited" angiogenesis. The latter results from specific identifiable initiators, among which the best known are: wound healing, reproduction, development, and the unique angiogenesis for the metabolic demands of tumor growth. Tumor angiogenesis is an uncontrolled vascular growth driven to nourish cells which are not required for normal function [7].

The intense study of angiogenesis has identified endothelial factors which are the targets of a novel tumor therapy. These factors, their origin, and main action are summarized in Table **1**. The key therapeutic objective is to target markers on the endothelial cells of angiogenic vessels within tumors. Faster than endothelial cells, tumor cells acquire mutations which are prone to develop resistance to therapy. Thus, the more stable angiogenic endothelial cells express unique vascular "zip codes" and certain markers. So unique are these markers that therapeutic agents can distinguish the angiogenic endothelium within tumors, from the rest of the vascular system of the body [10].

Table 1: Summary of factors involved in angiogenesis, cell of origin and functions in brief.

Factor/Receptor	**Cell**	**Function**
VEGF	EC	Differentiation, proliferation & migration of endothelial cells
Notch Pathway	EC, MC	Development of arteries
Ephrin b2/EphB4	EC	Cell specialization (arterial or venous)
PDGFβ/PDGFR-β	EC, MC	Differentiation, proliferation & migration of mural cells
Ang-1/Tie-2	EC	Decreases permeability & stabilizes vessels
Ang-2/Tie2	EC	Induce apoptosis in absence of VEGF and role in lymphangiogenesis
TGF-β1/TGF-BrII	EC, MC	Synthesis of ECM & proteases, formation of mural cell
TGF-β1/ALK1/ALK5	EC	Proliferation & migration of endothelial cells, vessel maturation
Cadherin	EC	Junction inbetween EC and b/w MC and EC
Connexins	EC, MC	Junction inbetween EC and b/w MC and EC
Occludins & Claudins	EC	Formation of tight junction and interaction of EC and MC
Integrins	EC	Suppressing EC apoptosis
Proteases	EC, MC	Cleavage of ECM
Protease inhibitors		Inhibition of ECM cleavage
mTOR	EC, MC	Cell proliferation, angiogenesis

Ref: [7, 75] (Abbreviation: EC- Endothelial cell, MC- Mural cell, ECM- Extracellular matrix)

RCC is one of the best examples of neoplasms which reflect development in translational research. Anti-angiogenic therapy is most successful in the clear cell variant of RCC. In the present chapter, important aspects of angiogenesis in RCC will be discussed along with important current and future anti-angiogenic drugs, including patents.

1. ROLE OF VHL GENE IN RCC

The Von Hippel Lindau (VHL) gene mutation occurs in both the familial and sporadic forms of the RCC. Normally, the VHL protein degrades the Hypoxia Inducible Factor- alpha (HIF- α) by ubiquitination. This leads to its subsequent degradation by the proteasomal pathway. In the absence of normal VHL function, HIF- α accumulates, even in normoxic conditions, forming a dimer with HIF-β. The formation of this dimer causes production or alteration of VEGF, transforming growth factor-α (TGF- α), platelet derived growth factor (PDGF), erythropoietin (EP), fibroblast growth factor (FGF) [11], glycolytic enzyme genes (anaerobic metabolism), i-NOS & HO-1 genes (vasodilatation), and tyrosine hydroxylase gene (increased breathing) Fig. (**2**) [12]. Collectively, all the growth factors lead to tumor proliferation and angiogenesis.

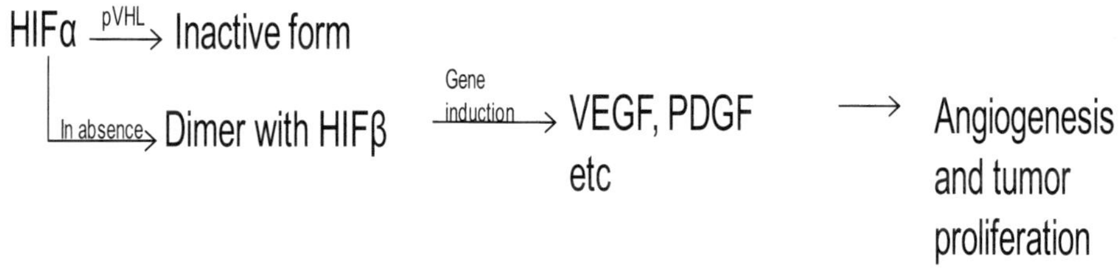

Figure 2: RAS-MAP kinase pathway.

2. ROLE OF VEGF IN RCC

Vascular endothelial growth factor (VEGF) is one of the most important regulators of angiogenesis in RCC. It promotes angiogenesis by promoting endothelial cell proliferation, migration, invasion, and permeability [13]. VEGF also plays a crucial role in the assignment of endothelial cells to an arterial or venous fate [8]. At present, there are seven types of VEGF- VEGF A, VEGF B, VEGF C, VEGF D, VEGF E, VEGF F and placental growth factor (PlGF) [14].

All VEGFs act through three tyrosine kinase receptors (RTK) VEGFR1/Flt-1, VEGFR2/KDR/Flk-1, and VEGFR3/Flt-4. RTK's have a single transmembranal α helix. On the cytosolic side it has the tyrosine kinase. The signaling is via any of the three pathways-i) RAS-MAP kinase pathway; ii) IP3/DAG pathway; 3) PI3-kinase pathway [15].

The RAS signaling pathway is important in the biology of RCC and is the potential target for many anti-angiogenic drugs Fig. (**3**). VEGFR2 is considered to be important in angiogenesis and is one of the prime targets for anti-angiogenic drugs. VEGFR2 receptors are expressed in almost all endothelial cells. VEGF-C and VEGFR3 receptors are predominantly confined to post-embryonic lymphatic channels [8]. VEGF-A and VEGF-B are recognized to be important in renal cell carcinoma [16]. In clear cell carcinomas, the regulation of VEGF can be independent of the VHL mutation, so targeting the receptor can be more effective [16].

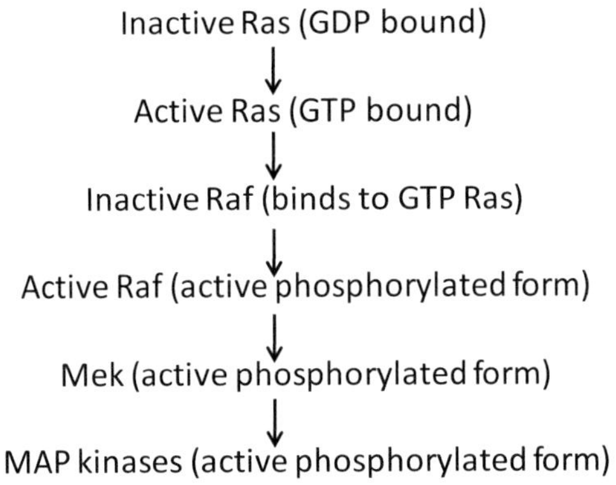

Figure 3: Role of VHL in HIF- α degradation.

3. ROLE OF ANGIOPOIETINS IN RCC

Angiopoietins (Ang) are endothelial growth factors that act via phosphorylation of tyrosine kinase Tie-2 receptors. Ang1 and Ang2 are the most thoroughly studied of the currently four known angiopoietins [17]. Ang1 promotes vascular sprouting. Ang1 also increases the interaction between endothelial cells and adjacent stromal cells, promoting the adhesiveness of the cells [18]. Ang2 promotes the development of immature vessels. Counteracting the role of Ang1, Ang2 loosens the adhesion between the endothelial cells and adjacent stromal cells, in the presence of VEGF [17]. RCC shows increased concentration of Ang2 and increased gene expression of Tie2 [19]. These make them a potential target for anti-angiogenic therapy.

4. ROLE OF INTEGRINS IN RCC

Integrins are the cell surface molecules that provide cell-to-cell adhesion and the adherence of cells to matrix. Integrins up-regulate intracellular signals that promote cell migration and proliferation. Integrins are over-expressed on the tumor cells and the tumor vasculature. Integrin $\alpha v\beta 3$, selectively expressed on vessel endothelium within tumors, serves an important target for treating malignancies [18, 20]. Expression of $\alpha v\beta 3$ integrin on vascular endothelium of renal cell carcinoma is targeted by nanoparticles. Nanoparticles specific for $\alpha v\beta 3$ integrin carrying doxorubicin have shown anti-metastatic effect in the orthotopic models of renal cell carcinoma [21].

5. ROLE OF MATRIX METALLOPROTEINASES IN RCC

Matrix metalloproteinases (MMP) are important in the progression of tumor. MMPs degrade the stroma and basement membrane adjacent to tumors. They also act on growth factor receptors, cytokines, angiogenic factors, and apoptotic ligands [20]. MMP expression is regulated by the effects of tissue inhibitor of matrix metalloproteinase (TIMP). Angiogenesis is promoted when MMP releases VEGF and TGF-β from the stromal cells [20].

6. ROLE OF MAMMALIAN TARGET OF RAPAMYCIN IN RCC

Mammalian target of rapamycin (mTOR) is an intracellular serine/threonine protein kinase system that plays an important role in angiogenesis, cell growth and protein degradation [22]. It receives signals and interacts with multiple pathways to execute its function. It receives signals from protein kinase B which in turn receives signals from phosphoinositide 3-kinase and phosphatase and tensin homolog (PTEN) [23]. RCC shows frequent alterations in the mTOR pathway [24]. Increased mTOR activity leads to silencing of VHL resulting in increased HIFα levels [25], leading to angiogenesis and tumor proliferation as discussed earlier. RCC also shows PTEN mutation which increases mTOR activity. Loss of PTEN and increased mTOR activity are associated with poor prognosis in RCC [24].

7. ROLE OF FIBROBLAST GROWTH FACTOR IN RCC

Fibroblast growth factors (FGFs) play an important role in angiogenesis. Besides acting on endothelial cells FGFs can act on other cell lineages and regulates angiogenesis by facilitating cell-cell interactions [26]. Amongst the FGFs, FGF-2 is considered to play an important role in mediating angiogenesis in RCC [27]. FGF-2 angiogenic response is mediated through VEGF and once VEGF is expressed its angiogenic response appears to be independent of FGF [26]. Angiogenesis is targeted in RCC by antisense oligonucleotides against FGF-2 [27] and monoclonal antibodies that target FGF-2 ligand [27, 28].

CURRENT DRUGS USED IN THERAPY OF RCC

A. Current anti-VEGF drugs

1. Bevacizumab

The first anti-VEGF antibody was the mouse anti-VEGF. Bevacizumab (Avastin) is a monoclonal anti-VEGF antibody developed by Genentech Inc, South San Francisco, CA. It is active against all types of VEGF. Avastin blocks the interaction of VEGF with their respective receptors. Avastin is ninety-three percent (93%) human and seven percent (7%) murine origin, respectively [29]. It is used widely, especially in metastatic renal cell carcinoma. It neutralizes all isoforms of VEGF without affecting the receptor. After showing significant response in preclinical Phase I and Phase II trials, Bevacizumab was introduced in combination with IFN and IL-2 in Phase III trials. With doses of 10 mg/kg every 2 weeks, significant improvements of progression-free survival and overall survival were obtained with the combination of Bevacizumab and IFN α [30, 31]. Hypertension is a frequent side effect of bevacizumab. Other adverse complications in the study included thromboembolism and gastrointestinal perforation [31]. Bevacizumab plus interferon is considered suitable for patients with favorable prognosis and/or indolent disease [32].

2. Sorafenib

Sorafenib (Nexavar; Bayer Pharmaceuticals) is a RTK inhibitor. Besides inhibiting the VEGF receptors it also inhibits the PDGF, c-kit, RET receptors [33] and the Ras-Raf/MEK/ERK signaling pathway [11]. Sorafenib is an oral agent and has shown promising results in clinical trials. It has a half-life of 25-48 hrs and is metabolized in the liver by CYP3A4 and UGT1A9 [11]. The IC_{50} concentration for sorafenib is in the nanomolar range. Escudier *et al.* [33] performed a Phase III trial on 903 patients of renal cell carcinoma who were resistant to other forms of therapy. The cases were randomized to receive either sorafenib (451 patients, 400mg twice daily) or placebo (452 patients). The study demonstrated significant improvement in the progression free survival of the patients on sorafenib, with previous failed therapy. The most commonly reported side effects were diarrhea and minor dermatologic reactions. Adverse cardiovascular events were more frequent in the treated group, compared to the placebo group, but there frequency was low. Therapy was interrupted in 21% of patients, due to adverse events mostly constitutional, gastrointestinal, dermal and pulmonary. Sorafenib may be particularly beneficial in the elderly and the patients with multiple comorbidities.

3. Sunitinib (SU011248)

Sunitinib (Pfizer Inc) is an oral tyrosine kinase inhibitor with a half-life of 40-60 hrs and is metabolized in liver by CYP3A4. The IC_{50} concentration for sunitinib is in the nanomolar range. It is active against VEGF and PDGF receptors and inhibits fibroblast growth factor receptors at higher concentration [34]. In Phase I trials, sunitinib was used to treat solid tumors, refractory to all other therapy [34]. In Phasc II trials sunitinib was used as the second line single agent therapy in cases of metastatic RCC [35]. It blocks the receptors of intracellular signaling and kinase dependent functions. In a Phase III multicenter trial for metastatic RCC, sunitinib performed better as a first line therapeutic agent than IFN-α [36]. In one treatment arm of this study, the dosage schedule of sunitinib (50mg once daily) was 4 weeks on and 2 weeks off. In the other arm, IFN-α 9 million units was given subcutaneously three times weekly. Patients given sunitinib had a longer median progression free survival and higher objective response rate. The adverse effects reported in the study were hypertension, hand foot syndrome, and gastrointestinal symptoms including diarrhea [36]. A trial to determine the efficacy of continuous-dosing of sunitinib was compared to the 4/2 schedule [37]. The trial did not reveal any greater efficacy of continuous sunitinib dosing over the 4/2 schedule. Therefore, the approved 50 mg/d dose on 4/2 schedule is recommended for patients with advanced RCC [37]. Sunitinib is currently recommended for patients of all prognosis groups [32].

4. Axitinib

Given orally, Axitinib (Pfizer Inc.) is an active selective inhibitor of all VEGF receptors. Rixe *et al.* [38] conducted a Phase II clinical trial for metastatic renal cell carcinoma on patients' refractory to cytokine. In a fasting state, 5 mg of Axitinib was given twice daily. These patients had a median time to progression of 15.7 months and a 44.2% objective response rate. The most common side effects were diarrhea, nausea, hypertension, hoarseness and fatigue. A randomized Phase III trial, involving 723 patients, was conducted to compare the efficacy of axitinib (5mg twice a day) over sorafenib (400mg twice a day) [39]. All the patients in this study experienced disease progression despite the use of first line therapy. This study showed significant improvement in progression-free survival with axitinib, which became the recommended treatment option after first line therapy for advanced renal cell carcinoma [39]. Axitinib was approved by FDA in 2012 for treatment of advanced RCC.

5. Pazopanib

Pazopanib (GlaxoSmithKline) was approved by FDA in 2009 for targeted therapy of RCC. It exerts its antiangiogenic effect by inhibiting numerous tyrosine kinases including VEGF and PDGF receptors [40]. It is approved at a dose of 800 mg daily. That maximal dose is decreased to a dose 200mg daily for patients with impaired hepatic function. The adverse events are similar to those of the other tyrosine kinase inhibitors. In Phase III trials, the use of pazopanib significantly improved the progression free survival from 4.2 to 9.2 months as compared to a placebo [41]. Pazopanib is considered as a reasonable option to sunitinib for patients with good and intermediate prognosis [32].

B. Current Drugs Against mTOR Pathway

1. Temsirolimus

Temsirolimus (Wyeth) is an analog of rapamycin and is a specific inhibitor mTOR kinase along with its primary metabolite sirolimus [42]. It requires weekly intravenous administration. Temsirolimus binds to the intracellular protein FKBP-12 to inhibit further signaling in the mTOR pathway. Using temsirolimus, Hudes *et al.* [42] conducted a randomized trial on 626 patients with newly diagnosed metastatic renal cell carcinoma. The patients were divided in three groups: 207 patients received interferon alone; 209 temsirolimus alone; and 210 patients received both interferon and temsirolimus. Improved median overall survival was obtained in the group on temsirolimus alone (10.9 months) compared to the group on interferon alone (7.3 months) and the group on the combination therapy (8.4 months). In this study, using temsirolimus alone, reported adverse side effects were asthenia, rash, anemia, nausea, dyspnea, diarrhea, peripheral edema, hyperlipidemia, and hyperglycemia. The grade 3&4 adverse events were most common in the group with combination therapy. Temsirolimus is under trial for other solid tumors [43]. Temsirolimus most likely benefit the patients of metastatic renal cell carcinoma with ECOG performance status 2 and/or non-clear cell disease [32].

2. Everolimus

Everolimus (Novartis) is an orally active mTOR inhibitor which also binds to the intracellular FKBP-12 protein. Motzer *et al.* [35, 44] conducted a Phase III trial on patients with metastatic RCC. The disease in these patients progressed while on anti-VEGF therapy namely sunitinib, sorafenib, or both. Everolimus improved the median progression-free survival. The adverse effects included rash, stomatitis, diarrhea, hyperglycemia, hypercholesterolemia, hyperlipidemia and non-infectious pneumonitis. Independent of [drug] causality, serious adverse events included infections, dyspnea, and fatigue [44]. Everolimus is considered to be safe and effective in patients who have progressed on VEGF inhibitors [44]. FDA in 2009 approved everolimus for use after progression on sunitinib, sorafenib or both.

CURRENT DRUG RECOMMENDATIONS IN THERAPY OF RCC

It is recommended that sequential therapy should be considered in all patients who can tolerate it.

FUTURE DRUGS IN THERAPY OF RCC

A. Anti-VEGF

VEGF Trap (Sanofi-aventis and Regeneron Pharmaceuticals, USA) is a decoy receptor protein with high affinity for VEGF A and placental growth factor. It is currently in clinical trials for solid tumors, other than RCC [13]. It is developed by fusing the Fc portion of the IgG1 and the extracellular domains of VEGFR-1 and VEGFR-2 [14]. VEGF Trap significantly inhibited the growth of primary and metastatic RCC and improved survival in murine model [45].

IMC-1121b and IMC-18F1(ImClone and Eli Lilly and Company, Indianapolis, USA) are the two antibodies which are developed against the VEGF receptors. IMC-1121b, after successful Phase I trial, is in Phase II trial for advanced RCC [13]. IMC-18F1 has shown activity against breast cancer in xenograft models [13] and preliminary clinical studies have indicated favorable safety profile [46].

Enzastaurin (LY317615) [Eli Lilly and Company, Indianapolis, USA]: Keyes *et al.* [47] studied this drug in human tumor xenografts. Against these xenografts, the drug resulted in decreased plasma concentration of VEGF and decreased intra-tumoral vascular density. Enzastaurin has been tried in Phase I trial for human solid tumors [48].

B. Anti-Angiopoietins

AMG-386 (Amgen, Thousand Oaks, CA, USA): AMG-386 targets angiopoietins. It is a recombinant peptibody and binds angiopoietins 1 and 2. Binding subsequently inhibits Tie-2 dependent action on endothelial cells [49]. The drug is under Phase I trial and Phase II study with some encouraging results [19].

CVX-060 (CovX research LLC, San Diego, CA, USA): CVX-060 is another peptide targeting the angiopoietins. This is a combination of two Ang-2-binding peptides. It has undergone Phase I and will soon undergo a Phase II trial [19].

CVX-241 (CovX research LLC, San Diego, CA, USA): CVX-241 is a fusion protein in this group which in addition to Ang-2 also targets VEGF [19].

C. Anti-Integrins

Volociximab (PDL Biopharma Inc and Biogen Idec Inc): Volociximab is a chimeric monoclonal antibody. It inhibits binding of fibronectin to $\alpha5\beta1$ leading to apoptosis of endothelial cells [50]. Besides RCC it has a touted potential in the treatment of other solid tumors and is currently in Phase I/II trials [51]. In patients with metastatic renal cell carcinoma, volociximab has undergone Phase II multicenter study [50]. Anti-integrins used for advanced malignancies and in Phase 1 trial are Medi 522, EMD 121974, ATN-161, and Vitaxin [52].

D. Nanoparticles

Nanoparticles can be used as vehicles for gene therapy [9], in targeted chemotherapy [53], and to assess angiogenesis by MRI [54]. Nanoparticles containing the antibody against $\alpha v\beta3$ become concentrated in vessels within tumors. In combination with a gene, the complex may prove to be an important model for tumor therapy [9].

E. Matrix metalloproteinase inhibitors

AE-941(AEterna laboratories Inc., Quebec, Canada): It is an orally active agent containing water soluble molecules, which is an extract of cartilage (US Patent No. 5618925) [55]. It inhibits MMP-2, 9 and 12 and competes with VEGF for its receptor. In a Phase II trial, conducted by Batist *et al.* [56] an oral dose of 240ml/day showed a significant improvement in survival of patients with RCC. It has been used in Phase III clinical trials for patients with metastatic RCC that failed immunotherapy [57].

ONO-4817 (ONO pharmaceutical company, Osaka, Japan) is the new synthetic inhibitor of MMP [58]. In the study of Muraishi *et al.* [58], it was given orally in a dose of 50-200 mg/kg/day to the murine model of renal cell carcinoma. The drug successfully inhibited lung metastases, by inhibiting the MMP-2 enzyme.

Several MMP inhibitors are in use for other malignancies, in different Phase trials. To date, they have not been used in RCC. Some of them are Batimastat, Marimastat, Neovastat, AG3340, BAY 12-9566 [52].

PATENTS FOR ANTI VEGF THERAPY

US8053430 Haraldsson *et al.* November 8, 2011

The patent is about a particular formulation of Orellanine and it also includes administration and dosing schedules [59].

US 7989501 Mertins *et al.* August 2, 2011

The patent is about pharmaceutical combination of dimethylsulfonate compounds and it also includes administration and dosing schedules for treating RCC [60].

US 7745156 Terret JA Jun 29, 2010

The patent is about the use of polypeptide CD27L in diagnosis and treatment of epithelial cancers including RCC [61].

US 7727526 Massfelder *et al.* Jun 1, 2010

The patent is about the use of antagonist to parathyroid hormone-related peptide to prepare a pharmaceutical compound which can be used to treat RCC and its metastatic foci [62].

US7375193 Baca *et al.* May20, 2008

The patent is for an anti-VEGF antibody. The anti-VEGF antibody is a heavy chain variable domain consisting of a specific heavy chain CDR amino acid sequence [63].

US7354579 Holash *et al.* April 8, 2008

The patent is for a combination of anti-VEGF and anti-proliferative agent. The VEGF antagonist is VEGFR1R2-Fc.DELTA.C1 (a) [the amino acid sequence of SEQ ID NO: 2]. The anti-proliferative agent is selected from the group of paclitaxel, docetaxel or a derivative, analogue, or mixture of paclitaxel and a platinum-based chemotherapeutic [64].

Other Patents

The patents [65-70] targeting the other pathways with their main mechanisms of action are mentioned in Table **2**.

Table 2: Mechanism of action of patented molecules with potential therapeutic application in renal cell carcinoma.

Target/Agent	Mechanism of Action	Patent No.	Ref
Phosphodiesterase 10	Inhibtion leads to cell death	US6538029	[65]
N-Acetylmuramyl-L-alanyl-D-isogutamin-yl-L-alanine-2-(1,2-dipalmitoyl-sn-g lyc ro-3-hydroxyphosphoryloxy) ethylamide monosodium salt	Decreases size of pulmonary metastasis	US4994440	[66]
Hybridome, 5C5 (CNCM no I-2184) producing monoclonal antibody 5C5	Specifically recognizes RCC	US7074613	[67]
Gene expression profile	Identified genes for targeted therapy	US20050130193	[68]
Hypoxia inducible protein 2 (hig2)	Monoclonal antibody against hig2	US20070059814	[69]
Tumor necrosis factor (TNF)	Anti-TNF antibody	US20070160606	[70]

CURRENT & FUTURE DEVELOPMENTS

In the rapidly expanding field of cancer research, a viable future lies ahead in the study of the molecular biology of angiogenesis. New anti-angiogenesis agents, in the treatment of solid tumors have already been brought to clinical practice [71]. With the widespread use of the anti-angiogenic drugs the complications associated with therapy have also surfaced, the most concerning of them is the increase in the rate of tumor growth and metastasis [72]. Different regimens have been recommended for the effective use of anti-angiogenic therapy, the sequential therapy should be considered in all patients who can tolerate it [32]. Angiogenesis is regulated by multiple pathways, therefore resistance to therapy for one pathway, up regulates the other pathways, resulting in increased angiogenesis [28].

The properties of the vasculature can be explored for effective treatment. The various vessels within each organ are highly specialized. They express unique markers on their endothelial cells, pericytes and in extracellular matrices [9]. The development of phage peptide libraries have helped to identify sequences unique to tumor vasculature. The adhesion receptors $\alpha_v\beta_3$, $\alpha_v\beta_5$, $\alpha_5\beta_1$ are over-expressed in tumor vessels [73]. We are beginning to exploit the uniqueness of the vasculature markers by utilizing targeted therapy with the use of nanoparticles [74]. There are many newly discovered pathways available in the complex process of angiogenesis. To get success in this field it will be important to focus on the mechanisms specific to a particular organ.

The other important area has been in the study of vessel maturation. Anti-angiogenic therapy which promotes vessel maturation may also increase the delivery of drugs to the cells [75]. It is an exciting challenge to think that an effective treatment of malignant tumors might be achievable by the use of two paradoxically opposing strategies e.g. initially targeting the specific tumor vasculature, once the vasculature starts maturing, targeting the tumor with chemotherapy or trying a combination of both. Long term prospective trials and implementation of translational research with evaluation of limitations and benefits of anti-angiogenic therapy is needed for success in anti-angiogenic therapy.

ACKNOWLEDGEMENTS

Declared None.

CONFLICT OF INTEREST

The authors confirm that this chapter content has no conflict of interest.

DISCLOSURE

The chapter submitted for Patent eBook Series "Topics in Anti-Cancer Research", Volume 2 is an update of our article Recent "Anti-Angiogenic Therapy in Renal Cell Carcinoma", published in the journal 'Recent Patents on Anti-Cancer Drug Discovery', Volume 5, Number 1, January Issue 2010, Page 77 to 83 with modified title, additional text and recent references.

REFERECNES

[1] American Cancer Society Inc. Cancer facts and figures. 2012. Report No.: http://www.cancer.org/acs/groups/content/@epidemiologysurveilance/documents/document/acspc-031941.pdf.

[2] Barriere J, Hoch B, Ferrero JM. New perspectives in the treatment of metastatic renal cell carcinoma. Crit Rev Oncol Hematol 2011; 84(Suppl 1): e16-23.

[3] Herbert SP, Stainier DY. Molecular control of endothelial cell behaviour during blood vessel morphogenesis. Nat Rev Mol Cell Biol 2011; 12(9): 551-64.

[4] Boisset JC, van Cappellen W, Andrieu-Soler C, Galjart N, Dzierzak E, Robin C. *In vivo* imaging of haematopoietic cells emerging from the mouse aortic endothelium. Nature 2010; 464(7285): 116-20.
[5] Patan S, Munn LL, Jain RK. Intussusceptive microvascular growth in a human colon adenocarcinoma xenograft: A novel mechanism of tumor angiogenesis. Microvasc Res 1996; 51(2): 260-72.
[6] Fox SB. Tumor angiogenesis and prognosis. Histopathology 1997; 30(3): 294-301.
[7] Nikitenko L, Boshoff C. Endothelial cells and cancer. In: Moncada S, Higgs A, editors. The Vascular Endothelium II (Handbook of Experimental Pharmacology). 176th ed. Springer-Verlag Berlin Heidelberg; 2010, p. 307-34.
[8] Rocha SF, Adams RH. Molecular differentiation and specialization of vascular beds. Angiogenesis 2009; 12(2): 139-47.
[9] Ruoslahti E, Rajotte D. An address system in the vasculature of normal tissues and tumors. Annu Rev Immunol 2000; 18: 813-27.
[10] Ruoslahti E. Vascular zip codes in angiogenesis and metastasis. Biochem Soc Trans 2004; 32(Pt3): 397-402.
[11] Grandinetti CA, Goldspiel BR. Sorafenib and sunitinib: Novel targeted therapies for renal cell cancer. Pharmacotherapy 2007; 27(8): 1125-44.
[12] Lodish H, Berk A, Matsudaira Pea. Control of cell fates by graded amounts of regulators. In: Lodish H, Berk A, Matsudaira Pea, editors. Molecular Cell Biology 2004th ed. Freeman WH Company, New York; 2004, p. 620-1.
[13] Grothey A, Ellis LM. Targeting angiogenesis driven by vascular endothelial growth factors using antibody-based therapies. Cancer J 2008; 14(3): 170-7.
[14] Veeravagu A, Hsu AR, Cai W, Hou LC, Tse VC, Chen X. Vascular endothelial growth factor and vascular endothelial growth factor receptor inhibitors as anti-angiogenic agents in cancer therapy. Recent Pat Anticancer Drug Discov 2007; 2(1): 59-71.
[15] Lodish H, Berk A, Matsudaira Pea. Receptor tyrosine kinases and activation of ras. In: Lodish H, Berk A, Matsudaira Pea, editors. Molecular Cell Biology 5th ed. New York: Freeman WH Company: 2004, 587-98.
[16] Gunningham SP, Currie MJ, Han C, Turner K, Scott PA, Robinson BA, *et al.* Vascular endothelial growth factor-B and vascular endothelial growth factor-C expression in renal cell carcinomas: Regulation by the von hippel-lindau gene and hypoxia. Cancer Res 2001; 61(7): 3206-11.
[17] Ahmad SA, Liu W, Jung YD, Fan F, Wilson M, Reinmuth N, *et al.* The effects of angiopoietin-1 and -2 on tumor growth and angiogenesis in human colon cancer. Cancer Res 2001; 61(4): 1255-9.
[18] Carlson TR, Feng Y, Maisonpierre PC, Mrksich M, Morla AO. Direct cell adhesion to the angiopoietins mediated by integrins. J Biol Chem 2001; 276(28): 26516-25.
[19] Pal SK, Williams S, Josephson DY, Carmichael C, Vogelzang NJ, Quinn DI. Novel therapies for metastatic renal cell carcinoma: Efforts to expand beyond the VEGF/mTOR signaling paradigm. Mol Cancer Ther 2012; 11(3): 526-37.
[20] Folgueras AR, Pendas AM, Sanchez LM, Lopez-Otin C. Matrix metalloproteinases in cancer: From new functions to improved inhibition strategies. Int J Dev Biol 2004; 48(5-6): 411-24.
[21] Murphy EA, Majeti BK, Barnes LA, Makale M, Weis SM, Lutu-Fuga K, *et al.* Nanoparticle-mediated drug delivery to tumor vasculature suppresses metastasis. Proc Natl Acad Sci USA 2008; 105(27): 9343-8.

[22] Pantuck AJ, Thomas G, Belldegrun AS, Figlin RA. Mammalian target of rapamycin inhibitors in renal cell carcinoma: Current status and future applications. Semin Oncol 2006; 33(5): 607-13.

[23] Atkins MB, Hidalgo M, Stadler WM, Logan TF, Dutcher JP, Hudes GR, *et al.* Randomized Phase II study of multiple dose levels of CCI-779, a novel mammalian target of rapamycin kinase inhibitor, in patients with advanced refractory renal cell carcinoma. J Clin Oncol 2004; 22(5): 909-18.

[24] Pinto Marin A, Redondo Sanchez A, Espinosa Arranz E, Zamora Aunon P, *et al.* mTOR pathway inhibition in renal cell carcinoma. Urol Oncol 2012; 30(4): 356-61. doi: 10.1016/j.urolonc.2009.11.008 [Epub 2010 Mar].

[25] Kapoor A, Figlin RA. Targeted inhibition of mammalian target of rapamycin for the treatment of advanced renal cell carcinoma. Cancer 2009; 115(16): 3618-30.

[26] Murakami M, Simons M. Fibroblast growth factor regulation of neovascularization. Curr Opin Hematol 2008; 15(3): 215-20.

[27] Cenni E, Perut F, Granchi D, Avnet S, Amato I, Brandi ML, *et al.* Inhibition of angiogenesis via FGF-2 blockage in primitive and bone metastatic renal cell carcinoma. Anticancer Res 2007; 27(1A): 315-9.

[28] Saylor PJ, Escudier B, Michaelson MD. Importance of fibroblast growth factor receptor in neovascularization and tumor escape from antiangiogenic therapy. Clin Genitourin Cancer 2012; 10(2): 77-83.

[29] Choueiri TK, Bukowski RM, Rini BI. The current role of angiogenesis inhibitors in the treatment of renal cell carcinoma. Semin Oncol 2006; 33(5): 596-606.

[30] Rini BI, Halabi S, Rosenberg JE, Stadler WM, Vaena DA, Ou SS, *et al.* Bevacizumab plus interferon alfa compared with interferon alfa monotherapy in patients with metastatic renal cell carcinoma: CALGB 90206. J Clin Oncol 2008; 26(33): 5422-8.

[31] Escudier B, Pluzanska A, Koralewski P, Ravaud A, Bracarda S, Szczylik C, *et al.* Bevacizumab plus interferon alfa-2a for treatment of metastatic renal cell carcinoma: A randomised, double-blind Phase III trial. Lancet 2007; 370(9605): 2103-11.

[32] Escudier B, Szczylik C, Porta C, Gore M. Treatment selection in metastatic renal cell carcinoma: expert consensus. Nat Rev Clin Oncol 2012; 9(6): 327-37.

[33] Escudier B, Eisen T, Stadler WM, Szczylik C, Oudard S, Siebels M, *et al.* Sorafenib in advanced clear-cell renal-cell carcinoma. N Engl J Med 2007; 356(2): 125-34.

[34] Rini BI, Small EJ. Biology and clinical development of vascular endothelial growth factor-targeted therapy in renal cell carcinoma. J Clin Oncol 2005; 23(5): 1028-43.

[35] Motzer RJ, Escudier B, Oudard S, Hutson TE, Porta C, Bracarda S, *et al.* Efficacy of everolimus in advanced renal cell carcinoma: A double-blind, randomised, placebo-controlled Phase III trial. Lancet 2008; 372(9637): 449-56.

[36] Motzer RJ, Hutson TE, Tomczak P, Michaelson MD, Bukowski RM, Oudard S, *et al.* Overall survival and updated results for sunitinib compared with interferon alfa in patients with metastatic renal cell carcinoma. J Clin Oncol 2009; 27(22): 3584-90.

[37] Motzer RJ, Hutson TE, Olsen MR, Hudes GR, Burke JM, Edenfield WJ, *et al.* Randomized Phase II trial of sunitinib on an intermittent versus continuous dosing schedule as first-line therapy for advanced renal cell carcinoma. J Clin Oncol 2012; 30(12): 1371-7.

[38] Rixe O, Bukowski RM, Michaelson MD, Wilding G, Hudes GR, Bolte O, *et al.* Axitinib treatment in patients with cytokine-refractory metastatic renal-cell cancer: A Phase II study. Lancet Oncol 2007; 8(11): 975-84.

[39] Rini BI, Escudier B, Tomczak P, Kaprin A, Szczylik C, Hutson TE, *et al.* Comparative effectiveness of axitinib versus sorafenib in advanced renal cell carcinoma (AXIS): A randomised Phase 3 trial. Lancet 2011; 378(9807): 1931-9.

[40] Pick AM, Nystrom KK. Pazopanib for the treatment of metastatic renal cell carcinoma. Clin Ther 2012; 34(3): 511-20.

[41] Sternberg CN, Davis ID, Mardiak J, Szczylik C, Lee E, Wagstaff J, *et al.* Pazopanib in locally advanced or metastatic renal cell carcinoma: Results of a randomized Phase III trial. J Clin Oncol 2010; 28(6): 1061-8.

[42] Hudes G, Carducci M, Tomczak P, Dutcher J, Figlin R, Kapoor A, *et al.* Temsirolimus, interferon alfa, or both for advanced renal-cell carcinoma. N Engl J Med 2007; 356(22): 2271-81.

[43] Strimpakos AS, Karapanagiotou EM, Saif MW, Syrigos KN. The role of mTOR in the management of solid tumors: An overview. Cancer Treat Rev 2009; 35(2): 148-59.

[44] Motzer RJ, Escudier B, Oudard S, Hutson TE, Porta C, Bracarda S, *et al.* Phase 3 trial of everolimus for metastatic renal cell carcinoma: Final results and analysis of prognostic factors. Cancer 2010; 116(18): 4256-65.

[45] Verheul HM, Hammers H, van Erp K, Wei Y, Sanni T, Salumbides B, *et al.* Vascular endothelial growth factor trap blocks tumor growth, metastasis formation, and vascular leakage in an orthotopic murine renal cell cancer model. Clin Cancer Res 2007; 13(14): 4201-8.

[46] Schwartz JD, Rowinsky EK, Youssoufian H, Pytowski B, Wu Y. Vascular endothelial growth factor receptor-1 in human cancer: Concise review and rationale for development of IMC-18F1 (human antibody targeting vascular endothelial growth factor receptor-1). Cancer 2010; 116(4 Suppl): 1027-32.

[47] Keyes KA, Mann L, Sherman M, Galbreath E, Schirtzinger L, Ballard D, *et al.* LY317615 decreases plasma VEGF levels in human tumor xenograft-bearing mice. Cancer Chemother Pharmacol 2004; 53(2): 133-40.

[48] Mukohara T, Nagai S, Koshiji M, Yoshizawa K, Minami H. Phase I dose escalation and pharmacokinetic study of oral enzastaurin (LY317615) in advanced solid tumors. Cancer Sci 2010; 101(10): 2193-9.

[49] Sawhney R, Kabbinavar F. Angiogenesis and angiogenic inhibitors in renal cell carcinoma. Curr Urol Rep 2008; 9(1): 26-33.

[50] Heng DY, Kollmannsberger C, Chi KN. Targeted therapy for metastatic renal cell carcinoma: Current treatment and future directions. Ther Adv Med Oncol 2010; 2(1): 39-49.

[51] Kuwada SK. Drug evaluation: Volociximab, an angiogenesis-inhibiting chimeric monoclonal antibody. Curr Opin Mol Ther 2007; 9(1): 92-8.

[52] Chan LS, Daruwalla J, Christophi C. Selective targeting of the tumor vasculature. ANZ J Surg 2008; 78(11): 955-67.

[53] Murphy EA, Majeti BK, Barnes LA, Makale M, Weis SM, Lutu-Fuga K, *et al.* Nanoparticle-mediated drug delivery to tumor vasculature suppresses metastasis. Proc Natl Acad Sci USA. 2008; 105(27): 9343-8.

[54] Sipkins DA, Cheresh DA, Kazemi MR, Nevin LM, Bednarski MD, Li KC. Detection of tumor angiogenesis *in vivo* by alphaVbeta3-targeted magnetic resonance imaging. Nat Med 1998; 4(5): 623-6.

[55] Dupont, E., Brazeau, P., Juneau, C. Extracts of shark cartilage having an anti-angiogenic activity and an effect on tumor regression; process of making thereof. US5618925 (**1997**).

[56] Batist G, Patenaude F, Champagne P, Croteau D, Levinton C, Hariton C, *et al.* Neovastat (AE-941) in refractory renal cell carcinoma patients: Report of a Phase II trial with two dose levels. Ann Oncol 2002; 13(8): 1259-63.

[57] Escudier B, Choueiri TK, Oudard S, Szczylik C, Negrier S, Ravaud A, *et al.* Prognostic factors of metastatic renal cell carcinoma after failure of immunotherapy: New paradigm from a large Phase III trial with shark cartilage extract AE 941. J Urol 2007; 178(5): 1901-5.

[58] Muraishi Y, Mitani N, Fuse H, Saiki I. Effect of a matrix metalloproteinase inhibitor (ONO-4817) on lung metastasis of murine renal cell carcinoma. Anticancer Res 2001; 21(6A): 3845-52.

[59] Haraldsson, B., Nilsson, U., Buvall, L., Nystrom, J. Treatment of renal cell carcinoma. US8053430 (**2011**), US20120077846 (**2012**) & US8349823 (**2013**).

[60] Mertins, S.D., Bates, S.E., Covell, D.G., Patton, G.W., Hollingshead, M.G., Vishnuvajjala, R. Treating renal cancer using a 4-[bis[2-[(methylsulfonyl)oxy]ethyl]amino]-benzaldehyde. US7989501 (**2011**).

[61] Terret, J.A. Methods for diagnosis and treatment of epithelial-derived cancers. US7745156 (**2010**).

[62] Massfelder, T., Lang, H., Schordan, E., Helwig, J.J. Use of PTHrP antagonists for treating renal cell carcinoma. US7727526 (**2010**).

[63] Baca, M., Wells, J.A., Presta, L.G., Lowman, H.B., Chen, Y.M.Y. Anti-VEGF antibodies. US7375193 (**2008**).

[64] Holash, J., Jaffe, R., Hu, L., Yancopoulos, G. D. Method of treating cancer with a VEGF antagonist and an anti-proliferative agent. US7354579 (**2008**).

[65] Thompson, J.W., Fetter, R.J., Bellet, R.E., Li, H. Methods for treatment of renal cell carcinoma. US6538029 (**2003**).

[66] Creaven, J.P. Method for the treatment of renal cell carcinoma. US4994440 (**1991**).

[67] Hirsch, F., Angevin, E. Monoclonal antibody directed against cells of human renal cell carcinoma. US7074613 (**2006**).

[68] Luxon, A.B., Copland, A.J., Wood, G.C. Methods for detecting, diagnosing and treating human renal cell carcinoma. US20050130193 (**2005**).

[69] Nakamura, Y., Katagiri, T. Hypoxia-inducible protein 2 (hig2), a novel therapeutic potential target of renal cell carcinoma (RCC). US20070059814 (**2007**).

[70] Heavner, A.G., Giles-Kornor, M.J., Knight, M.D., Scallon, J.B., Shealy, J.D. Treating renal cell carcinoma with an anti-TNF human antibody or fragment. US20070160606 (**2007**).

[71] Folkman J, Browder T, Palmblad J. Angiogenesis research: Guidelines for translation to clinical application. Thromb Haemost 2001; 86(1): 23-33.

[72] Ebos JM, Lee CR, Cruz-Munoz W, Bjarnason GA, Christensen JG, Kerbel RS. Accelerated metastasis after short-term treatment with a potent inhibitor of tumor angiogenesis. Cancer Cell 2009; 15(3): 232-9.

[73] Ruoslahti E. Drug targeting to specific vascular sites. Drug Discov Today 2002; 7(22): 1138-43.

[74] Ruoslahti E, Bhatia SN, Sailor MJ. Targeting of drugs and nanoparticles to tumors. J Cell Biol 2010; 188(6): 759-68.

[75] Jain RK. Molecular regulation of vessel maturation. Nat Med 2003; 9(6): 685-93.

Send Orders of Reprints at reprints@benthamscience.net
Topics in Anti-Cancer Research, Vol. 2, 2013, 299-319

CHAPTER 9

Anti-Angiogenic Therapy for Cancer: Past, Present and Future

Boel De Paepe*

Ghent University Hospital, Neurology and Pathology, UZ 1K12A, De Pintelaan 185, 9000 Ghent, Belgium

Abstract: Tumors are dependent upon neovascularization to feed their massive demand for nutrients and oxygen. To uphold the nutrient influx, cancer cells produce growth factors and activators that stimulate and shape the blood vessel network around the tumor. Therapies aimed at reducing the blood flow to the cancer cells can slow down tumor growth and reduce metastasis. This chapter focuses on tumor neovascularization as a target for anti-cancer therapy. An overview of long standing and novel anti-angiogenic agents is given, which includes antibodies directed against vascular growth factors and angiotensin II, pharmaceutical compounds and natural metabolites, and combination therapy. The relevant patents are discussed. Anti-angiogenic therapy has every potential of becoming indispensible, as a supplement to chemo- and radiation-cancer therapy.

Keywords: Angiogenesis, angiopoietin inhibitors, angiotensin-converting enzyme inhibitors, angiotensin II receptor 1 antagonists, antibody therapy, combination therapy, epigallocatechin-3-gallate, hepatocyte growth factor inhibitors, intergrins, liposomes, matrix metalloproteinases, mitocans, opioids, phytochemicals, polymers, polyphenols, thrombospondins, troponin I, tyrosine kinase inhibitors, vascular endothelial growth factor inhibitors.

INTRODUCTION

The process of angiogenesis is regulated by both activator and inhibitor molecules. In adult tissues blood vessels are quiescent structures, and the inhibitors of angiogenesis predominate. When the need arises for neovascularization, the balance tips over to the activators, which prompts vascular endothelial cells to divide and form new blood vessels. This occurs only in specific physiological processes such as wound healing and during the menstrual cycle. Angiogenesis is a multi-step process tightly regulated through a myriad of

***Address correspondence to Boel De Paepe:** Ghent University Hospital, Neurology and Pathology, UZ 1K12A, De Pintelaan 185, 9000 Ghent, Belgium; Tel: 0032 9 3324391; Fax: 0032 93324971; E-mail: boel.depaepe@ugent.be

Atta-ur Rahman and Khurshid Zaman (Eds)

cellular factors. The cascade of angiogenesis is initiated by the release of pro-angiogenic mediators that bind and activate endothelial cells. Through subsequent enzyme production, the basement membrane is degraded and the extracellular matrix (ECM) is remodeled, permitting endothelial cells to divide and migrate to the surrounding tissues. Endothelial cells are then positioned by means of adhesion molecules or integrins, organized into tubular structures, and formed into functional blood vessels.

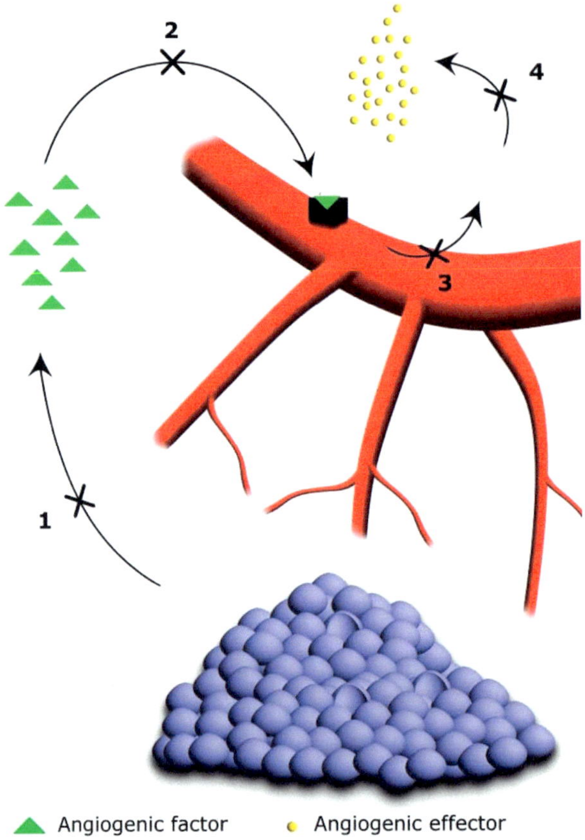

Figure 1: Theoretical anti-angiogenic therapeutic strategies for cancer, and examples of strategies targeting vascular endothelial growth factor (VEGF) signaling. (1) Diminishing the expression of angiogenic factors: VEGF/VEGF receptor small interfering RNA, selective proteases, (2) Diminishing ligand-receptor interaction: VEGF-neutralizing fragments (pegatanib, ranibizumab), anti-VEGF/VEGF receptor antibodies (bevacizumab,), (3) Inhibiting signaling pathways: Tyrosine kinase inhibitors (vatalanib, AE-941, sorafenib, sunitinib) and (4) Inhibiting effector expression: prostaglandin inhibitors (cyclooxygenase inhibitors (celecoxib, rofecoxib, valdecoxib), non-steroidal anti-inflammatory drugs, inhibitors of terminal prostaglandin synthases).

In cancerous tissues, angiogenesis is promoted. To accommodate their growth, solid tumors release signal molecules to the surrounding host tissue that encourage the formation of new blood vessels. The newly formed network of blood vessels penetrates the cancerous growth, supplying the tumor with nutrients and oxygen, and enabling the removal of waste products. Continuous neovascularization is a prerequisite for sustained tumor growth and metastasis. Taking this into account, anti-angiogenic therapy, which can be achieved through different strategies, Fig. (**1**), is an amenable approach for anti-cancer treatment. This chapter focuses on anti-angiogenic cancer therapy, offering a concise listing of the most amenable targets, each illustrated by a selection of compounds and relevant patents.

TARGETING ENDOTHELIAL GROWTH FACTORS

Tumor growth requires the continuous maintenance and expansion of its vascular network, which relies on the influx of endothelial cells. Activating endothelial cells is accomplished when the inhibiting factors that dominate under normal physiological conditions are overruled by stimulating factors. Tumor cells create such a pro-angiogenic micro-environment by producing endothelial growth factors. Vascular endothelial growth factor (VEGF) in particular appears to be of primordial importance for sustained tumor growth. The VEGF pathway includes five distinct ligands, VEGF-A to D and placental growth factor (PlGF), that can bind three VEGF receptors. In response to ligand binding, the VEGF receptor tyrosine kinase activity triggers a network of signaling events, that lead to prostaglandin production, and that effect vascular cell survival, permeability and migration. VEGF-A is a key regulator of tumor vascularization, VEGF-B and PlGF also appear to play major roles.

Tyrosine Kinase Inhibitors

A successful strategy to affect angiogenesis is to target the tyrosine kinase activities of pro-angiogenic receptors. Many of the available multi-targeted pharmaceutical tyrosine kinase inhibitors block signal transduction via VEGF receptors. The first compound tested was semoxinal, but anti-tumor response in renal and skin cancer was poor [1]. AZD2171 is an orally bioavailable VEGF receptor-2 tyrosine kinase inhibitor with potent anti-cancer activity [2]. Results of a Phase I clinical study in patients with advanced solid tumors refractory or unsuited to standard treatment were encouraging, and demonstrated a dose-related control of tumor growth [3]. Sunitinib (sutent®, Pfizer) is a multitargeted tyrosine kinase inhibitor, which is efficient and safe in patients with advanced gastro-intestinal stromal tumors after failure of imatinib [4]. Sunitinib has become standard treatment for metastatic renal-cell carcinoma, and a retrospective study showed increased overall survival in treated patients [5]. Sorafenib (nexavar®, Bayer) is a small molecular inhibitor of several protein kinases including VEGF-receptors that has been FDA approved for the treatment of renal and liver cancers in 2005. Pazopanib (votrient®, GSK) has been approved for advanced renal-cell carcinoma. Vatalinib is another potent oral tyrosine kinase inhibitor, but in a clinical trial this compound did not meet the primary objectives [6]. ABT-869 (linifanib) is a selective inhibitor of VEGF and platelet-derived growth factor. It has been shown active in Phase II trials in patients with advanced non-small cell lung cancer [7] and advanced renal-cell cancer [8].

VEGF Inhibitors

The central role played by VEGF in tumor vascularization makes it an attractive target for more selective anti-cancer therapy. VEGF receptor blocking antibodies could be a solid alternative for the multi-targeted tyrosine kinase inhibitors [9]. The anti-VEGF antibody bevacizumab (avastin™, Genentech) has been shown to delay tumor growth and extend the life of cancer patients [10]. Based on a Phase III clinical trial that showed benefit in first-line treatment of metastatic colorectal cancer when added to standard chemotherapy [11], avastin™ was FDA approved. At this moment, new VEGF antibodies are continuously being developed [12-16].

Soluble decoy receptors that are able to neutralize circulating VEGF are also being developed and evaluated [17]. Aflibercept, also known as VEGF-Trap, is a recombinant decoy receptor that contains extracellular VEGF receptor domains fused to the Fc region of IgG_1 [18]. Aflibercept binds VEGF-A, VEGF-B and PlGF, preventing activation of angiogenic pathways. Preclinical and clinical tests evaluating the therapeutic efficacy of aflibercept for treating cancer, have been reviewed recently [19]. The compound demonstrates an acceptable safety profile and evidence of clinical activity. Different Phase II and Phase III clinical trials are ongoing, of which publication of data is expected in the near future.

An alternative 'molecular' approach would be the elimination of VEGF or the VEGF receptor at the mRNA level, by administering short interfering RNA [20, 21], or at the protein level, through cleavage by selective proteases [22, 23]. Another alternative is the use of ribozymes, which are RNA molecules that lead to recognition and cleavage of other RNA molecules that can target VEGF receptor mRNAs. In a recently reported open-label Phase II trial however, angiozyme (RPI.4610) lacked efficacy for treating metastatic breast cancer [24].

HGF Inhibitors

Hepatocyte growth factor (HGF) signaling via the MET receptor promotes the formation of new blood vessels by stimulating endothelial cell proliferation and migration, through induction of VEGF expression [25]. Many agents have been developed that can neutralize HGF through different strategies:

(i) Direct inhibition of the receptor by anti-MET antibodies: The combination of two human anti-MET antibodies, termed R13 and R28, was shown to abrogate HGF-induced activation of MET, leading to a significant reduction of tumor growth in a colon tumor xenograft model [26].

(ii) Inactivation of its ligand HGF: A fully humanized anti-HGF antibody, AMG102, and an anti-HGF antibody, L2G7, have been developed. In transgenic mice overexpressing human HGF in the airways, L2G7-treatment significantly reduced the mean number of tumors per mouse [27].

(iii) Interfering with HGF binding to MET: NK4 is a fragment of HGF that binds the receptor but does not activate it, thereby functioning as a competitive inhibitor [28]. NK4 suppresses HGF-induced in-gel invasion of pleural mesothelioma cells [29].

(iv) Inhibiting MET kinase activity: The tyrosine kinase inhibitors PHA-665752 and SU11274 have been developed. A published review gives an overview of patents filed for small molecule MET kinase inhibitors [30].

Angiopoietin Inhibitors

Angiopoietins (Ang) are important regulators of angiogenesis, blood vessel maturation and integrity of the vascular endothelium. The two variants termed Angl and Ang2, are ligands of the Tie2 receptor and activate an angiogenic pathway separate from the VEGF axis. MEDI3617, a human anti-Ang2 monoclonal antibody reduces tumor angiogenesis in xenograft tumor models [31]. The Angl/2 neutralizing peptide-Fc fusion protein AMG386 shows anti-tumor activity in Phase I clinical trials in advanced solid cancers [32, 33]. A family of proteins structurally similar to angiopoietins, and co-regulators of angiogenesis, has been designated angiopoietin-like proteins. Inhibitors of angiopoietin-like 4 have been put forward as possible modulators of tumor angiogenesis [34].

ADMINISTERING ANGIOSTATIC COMPOUNDS

Several agents have been shown to selectively induce apoptosis in actively proliferating endothelial cells, thus suppressing tumor angiogenesis without much harm to the arrested endothelial cells of normal blood vessels present in the healthy tissues. The compounds therefore represent amenable anti-cancer agents.

Thrombospondins

Thrombospondins (TSP) are an important family of naturally occurring angiogenesis inhibitors that act by targeting fibroblast growth factor (FGF), preventing fibroblast-mediated deposition of tumor-friendly ECM. TSP-1 affects angiogenesis both directly, through its interaction with the endothelial CD36 receptor inducing apoptosis [35], and indirectly, through interactions with other cell types involved in the angiogenic process, including vascular smooth muscle cells and lymphocytes. TSP-1 interferes with FGF-2 binding to ECM receptors, preventing FGF-2-mediated activation of endothelial cells [36]. Synthetic peptides based upon the active sequence of TSP have been generated that have anti-angiogenic and anti-cancer activity. ABT-510 and the related peptide ABT-526 inhibit tumor growth and vascularization *in vivo* [37]. Phase II studies with ABT-510 so far have, however, been disappointing [38]. Second generation anti-angiogenic TSP mimetic peptides are currently being developed. ABT-898 is active at much lower concentrations [39] and has been shown to reduce ovarian tumors in an animal model [40].

Mitocans

Mitocans are anti-cancer agents that act through the mitochondria of tumor cells. Cancer cells display various alterations in the energy metabolism, which include increase in aerobic glycolysis, elevated levels of reactive oxygen species, and resistance to apoptosis [41]. Mitocans provide strategies for the targeting of mitochondrial metabolism and apoptotic processes. The vitamin E analog alpha-tocopheryl succinate (alpha-TOS) is a mitocan that inhibits the mitochondrial electron redox chain by interfering with the ubiquinone-binding sites of complex II [42]. This results in the suppression of processes that are essential for endothelial cell proliferation and maintenance [43, 44]. Mitochondrial targeting of alpha-TOS analogs can be achieved by a delivery moiety, for instance a lipophilic cation [45]. The mitochondrially targeted analog of alpha-TOS, termed MitoVes, is more potent in preventing tumor neovascularization and suppressing cancer growth. This selectivity is attributed to the greater mitochondrial inner membrane potential of proliferating endothelial cells, and translates in reduced tumor progression in an *in vivo* breast cancer model [46].

PREVENTING ECM BREAKDOWN AND ADHESION

The breakdown of ECM is an essential event for endothelial cell migration and blood vessel formation. Matrix metalloproteinases (MMP) are key enzymes in these processes. MMP are produced as inactive pro-enzymes and are activated when necessary by cleavage of the amino terminal domain. The activated MMP are regulated individually by endogenous inhibitors among which the tissue inhibitors of MMP (TIMP). TIMP2 for instance, has been described as a specific MMP2 inhibitor [47]. Endogenous MMP inhibitors often have multiple anti-angiogenic properties, and TIMP3 has been shown to be a direct antagonist of the VEGF receptor [48]. Neovastat is a shark cartilage extract that contains the biologically active AE-941 molecule with strong anti-angiogenic activity, which appears also to act through multiple targets. AE-941 strongly inhibits the gelatinolytic and elastinolytic activity of MMP2, inhibits VEGF binding to its receptor [49], and induces apoptosis of endothelial cells [50]. Cartilage is a rich source of natural inhibitors of angiogenesis, as it is a site of poor blood supply that does not undergo neovascularization. Unfortunately, many naturally occurring

MMP inhibitors have a poor oral bioavailability. Therefore, synthetic inhibitors are being developed better suited for clinical purposes. Batimastat, marimistat (both by British Biotech), CGS27023A (Novartis), prinomastat (Agouron), tanomastat (Bayer) and BMS-275291 (Bristol Myers Squibb) are competitive inhibitors that bind reversibly to the active site of MMP [51]. Although these synthetic MMP inhibitors worked well in animal models, results of clinical trials in cancer patients have been mostly disappointing [52]. The use of more potent MMP inhibitor derivatives could be further explored. A substituted pheryl-pyridine compound that acts as an MMP inhibitor has been developed [53].

Integrins are cell surface adhesion molecules that promote cell-cell or cell-matrix interactions. They mediate cell attachment to ECM proteins and to the intracellular cytoskeleton. Tumor cells often display upregulated integrin expression, which has been correlated with their ability to metastasize [54]. It is the crosstalk between integrins and activated cytokine or growth-factor receptors that will determine cell survival, migration and invasion. Integrin inhibitors could thus be of therapeutic use for their anti-angiogenic activity, as well as for preventing the spread of cancer cells to other tissues. Functional alpha-5-beta-1-integrin is an essential requisite for the adherence of endothelial cells to the extracellular fibronectin network. When this interaction is blocked, migration of endothelial cells and the subsequent formation of new blood vessels is hampered [55]. The monoclonal anti-alpha-5-beta-1-integrin antibody volociximab (PDL BioPharma and Biogen Idec) has entered Phase II clinical trials in cancer patients [56]. The therapeutic use of chimeric and humanized alpha-5-beta-1 integrin antibodies is currently being explored further [57]. In addition, several anti-alpha-2-beta-1-integrin antibodies have become commercially available that may also be suited as anti-tumor agents [58]. Vicrostatin is a chimeric recombinant disintegrin that competes for the integrin receptors, that way inhibiting endothelial cell migration and tube formation dose-dependently. Vicrostatin inhibits breast cancer cell motility *in vitro* [59].

TARGETING THE RENIN-ANGIOTENSIN SYSTEM

The renin-angiotensin system has a fundamental role in controlled vasoconstriction and blood pressure regulation. Through the action of renin,

Angiotensin I is generated from angiotensinogen, which is later converted to active angiotensin II (AngII) by the angiotensin-converting enzyme (ACE). An alternative AngII-generating pathway exists in which other enzymes, such as chymase, are involved [60]. AngII positively regulates endothelial cell migration [61] and angiogenesis, the latter via upregulation of VEGF [62]. AngII acts through at least two high-affinity G-protein coupled receptors: AngII receptors 1 (ATR1) and 2 (ATR2). Most of the vascular effects of AngII, such as vasoconstriction and growth, are mediated via ATR1. Evidence implicating ATR1 signaling in the neovascularization, proliferation and invasion of tumors is compelling [63]. A mouse model has shown that the enhanced reduction of vascularization in response to a combination of radiation and the AT1 blocker TCV-116 is due to reduced levels of VEGF [64].

Angiotensin II Receptor Antagonists

ATR1 is the dominant receptor involved in various aspects of cancer progression [65], and many studies have become available that provide evidence of the involvement of ATR1 in breast cancer in particular [66]. Our own studies have revealed differential ATR1 expression in the breast epithelium of controls and breast cancer patients [67]. The upregulation of ATR1 in hyperplastic acini, a precursor of malignity, might be an important stepping stone for the development of breast carcinoma. It has been recognized that angiogenesis commences during the premalignant stages of breast cancer [68]. Selective pharmaceutical ATR1 antagonists have been in use to treat hypertension since the 1990s [69]. A long list of compounds have been developed that posses high affinity for ATR1: losartan, valsartan, irbesartan, eprosartan, telmisartan, candesartan and tranilast. The use of these compounds has been shown beneficial to patients with hormone-refractory prostate cancer [70]. The anti-cancer action of ATR1 blocking antibodies has been explored through *in vitro* and *in vivo* studies with breast cancer cells. R6313/G2, a recombinant short-chain variable fragment form of the monoclonal ATR1 antibody was found to be more effective in suppressing cell proliferation *in vitro* and tumor growth *in vivo* than the ATR1 antagonist losartan [71].

ACE Inhibitors

ACE inhibitors prescribed for hypertension or other cardiovascular and renal diseases may reduce the risk of cancer in users, most particularly the risk of developing breast cancer [72], but data of epidemiological studies have not been consistent on this point. Nevertheless, ACE inhibition does display remarkable tumor-suppressive effects in experimental models [73] and ACE polymorphisms have been linked to either increased [74] or decreased [75] breast cancer predisposition. High expression levels of ACE correlate significantly with tumor VEGF expression in pancreatic ductal adenocarcinoma [76]. Many compounds exhibiting ACE inhibitory effects have been developed, and include quinapril, captopril, perindopril and enalapril. The inhibitory effect of captopril on tumor angiogenesis has been shown in an animal model more than a decade ago [77], and a Phase II randomized trial is ongoing in patients with lung cancer.

NATURAL COMPOUNDS & DERIVATIVES

The large spectrum of natural anti-angiogenic metabolites continues to offer basis for the development of novel anti-cancer therapies. When developing natural anti-cancer agents, elaborate and in-depth studies are necessary to elucidate the mechanisms of actions and to isolate the active compound(s).

One of the best known success stories in cancer therapy is that of paclitaxel (taxol®). This plant alkaloid with anti-microtubule characteristics was originally prepared from the bark of the Western or Pacific yew. It can now also be synthetized in large quantities and researchers are currently seeking to modify the drug further, to create and test even more effective and selective derivates [78]. The anti-cancer characteristics of phytochemicals in spices have been reviewed in [79]. Gingerol, a pungent compound of ginger, for instance inhibits VEGF-induced angiogenesis *in vitro* and *in vivo* [80] and inhibits metastasis of breast cancer cells through interference with MMP activity [81]. Jojoba seed-derived simmondsins, which were earlier reported to be non-toxic food intake and body weight reducers [82], have angiostatic properties [83]. Morphine, an opioid derivative originally extracted from poppies, has been shown to stimulate microvascular endothelial cell proliferation and angiogenesis. The use of opioid antagonists as anti-cancer agents has been put forward [84], and could be explored further [85]. From the non-oxidized, non-fermented leaves of Camellia sinensis, green tea is prepared of which consumption has been linked to reduced cancer risk [86]. Green tea polyphenols inhibit angiogenesis and metastasis, and epigallocatechin-3-gallate (EGCG) in particular reduces VEGF and MMP expression in human cancer cell lines [87, 88]. EGCG inhibits angiogenesis *in vitro* [89] and triggers mitochondria-related cell death events [90]. Clinical trials are ongoing assessing the anti-cancer activities of EGCG [91]. In line with these findings, substituted phenols are potential inhibitors of VEGF expression [92].

Animals also, are a potential source of angiostatic compounds. The shark troponin I gene product inhibits endothelial cell proliferation and angiogenesis. The polypeptide from Lys91 to Leu123 inhibits tumor growth in a murine breast carcinoma xenograft model [93]. Arenobufagin, one of the main active ingredients of toad venom, targets the VEGF receptor signaling pathway, and inhibits endothelial cell migration *in vitro* [94].

CURRENT & FUTURE DEVELOPMENTS

It has been noted that tumors may escape or become resistant to individual anti-angiogenic compounds. The acquired resistance includes tumor adaptation to growth in an angiogenesis-independent manner, hypoxia-induced selection of more malignant and invasive tumor cells and compensation by increased expression of angiogenic factors. Also, anti-angiogenic therapy can be associated with important side-effects. Toxicity of anti-angiogenic drugs is variable in severity and incidence both within the same class of molecules and between the different types of tumors. Most frequently reported side effects include thrombotic and hemorrhagic complications, hypertensia, proteinuria, gastrointestinal perforation and impaired wound healing. The safety for treating breast cancer with bevacizumab for instance, has been reviewed recently, pinpointing serious side effects [95]. Yet, Phase III trials so far have shown increased response rates and progression-free survival in subgroups of patients. Side effects could be partly prevented by optimization of schedule of administration and length of treatment. In addition, different strategies may aid to prevent resistance, and could boost the clinical benefits.

Combined Therapy that includes Anti-Angiogenic Agents

Only few examples support the efficacy of anti-angiogenic monotherapy: Sorafenib [96] and sunitinib [97] have been shown efiicacious for treating advanced renal cell carcinoma. However, in most cases, simultaneous targeting of different tumor-promoting pathways will be a more potent therapeutic approach. The combination of anti-MET agent NK4 with another signal transduction inhibitor, epidermal growth factor receptor inhibitor gefitinib, is explored for treating gastric cancer [98]. Combining anti-VEGF antibodies with cytotoxic chemotherapy is also an amenable approach [99-101]. The soluble VEGF receptor FP3 demonstrates synergistic antitumor effects when combined with 5-fluorouracil [17]. HGF inhibitor ABT-510 (200mg/day) in combination with radiation and temozolomide slowed down the progression of glioblastoma [102]. Combining different anti-angiogenic compounds is another option. Aflibercept combined with paclitaxel inhibits ovarian cancer metastasis in a xenograft model [103]. Also, the potential of a combination of an ACE inhibitor with a non-steroidal anti-inflammatory drug [104], could be beneficial to patients.

Optimized Agent Stability and Delivery

Approaches to increase compound stability have a strong impact on their therapeutic potential. The short half-life of many compounds, such as ABT-510, implies the need for repeated injections. Conjugating active agents to a polymer, which increases resistance to degradation and allows controlled release [105], could be an attractive innovation. The development of small interfering RNA (siRNA)-based therapy in particular, is hampered by their poor *in vivo* stability and inefficient cellular uptake. In this respect, VEGF siRNA conjugated through disulfide linkage to polyethylene glycol (PEG), shows greater stability than bare VEGF siRNA [106]. Biomembrane covering of the angiostatic vitamin E analog alpha-TOS has been put forward as a means to prevent decomposition in body fluids [107]. Along the same line, liposome-based formulations of vitamin E analogs [108] and polymerosomes [109] could protect the active compound from premature degradation. Intravenous administration of integrin-binding vicrostatin packaged in liposomes significantly delays tumor growth in an animal model [59].

Polymeric nanoparticles and liposomes contain functional groups at their surface, that can be conjugated to targeting ligands allowing tumor-specific drug delivery. The cyclic Arg-Gly-Asp (RGD) peptide is such a targeting ligand, and RGD-targeted PEGylated liposome-polycation-DNA particles containing VEGF receptor 2 siRNA have been shown promising *in vitro* [110]. The efficacy of chitosan/siRNA VEGF or VEGF receptor nanoplexes has been evaluated in a rat breast cancer model. Marked reduction of tumor volumes was observed in complex-injected rats, while injection of bare siRNA showed a much more modest reduction [111]. Improved targeting of anti-angiogenic agents to tissue tumor sites could be achieved through protein fusion. A recombinant fusion protein consisting of the *N*-terminal region of TSP-2 and an IgG-Fc1 fragment inhibits breast cancer growth and metastasis [112]. In the CVX-045 compound, two TSP-1 peptides are covalently attached to the Fab binding site of a humanized antibody [113]. VEGF decoy receptor fused with the IgG Fc region (FP3) is more potent as an inhibitor of tumor growth than bevacizumab [17].

Anti-angiogenic agents have themselves been implicated in improved delivery of anti-cancer therapeutics. Possibly, they maneuver toward vascular normalization, away from the tortuous vessels typically associated with tumor growth, fortifying the blood vessel walls in the process. These changes could render the tumor vasculature less leaky, and facilitate uniform delivery of therapeutic agents [114].

Questions Remaining

In view of the overwhelming evidence of neovascularization being an essential part of tumor progression and metastasis, continuous exploration of angiostatic therapy for cancer is warranted. However, the clinical efficacy of anti-angiogenic agents has so far been less than anticipated. Bevacizumab for instance, increases progression-free survival of breast cancer patients, yet this does not translate into increased overall survival [115]. In general, the success of bevacizumab in treating colorectal cancer contrasts with more disappointing results in breast cancer patients [116]. In addition, the mechanisms by which tumorigenesis can progress during anti-VEGF treatment, are still poorly understood. Metastases appear to rely on alternative mechanisms to promote angiogenesis that are able to continue with ongoing VEGF blockade [117]. One can also foresee that developing more optimal therapeutic strategies will also require identification of patient subpopulations, hence the need for reliable predictive biomarkers. Plasma concentrations of VEGF-A have been put forward as a predictive value for overall survival in Phase III trials assessing bevacizumab efficacy [118]. Research in these areas remains of primordial importance for developing better therapies in the future.

ACKNOWLEDGEMENTS

The author thanks Sophie D'hose for graphics.

CONFLICT OF INTEREST

The author declares to have no conflict of interest.

DISCLOSURE

The chapter submitted for Patent eBook Series "Topics in Anti-Cancer Research", Volume 2 is an update of the article "Anti-Angiogenic Agents and Cancer: Current Insights and Future Perspectives", published in the journal 'Recent Patents on Anti-Cancer Drug Discovery', Volume 4, Number 2, June, 2009, Page 180 to 185 with modified title, additional text and references.

REFERENCES

[1] Kuenen BC, Tabernero J, Baselga J, Cavalli F, Pfanner E, Conte PF, *et al.* Efficacy and toxicity of the angiogenesis inhibitor SU5416 as a single agent in patients with advanced renal cell carcinoma, melanoma, and soft tissue carcinoma. Clin Cancer Res 2003; 9(5): 1648-55.

[2] Wedge SR, Kendrew J, Hennequin LF, Valentine PJ, Barry ST, Brave SR, *et al.* AZD2171: A highly potent, orally bioavailable, vascular endothelial growth factor receptor-2 tyrosine kinase inhibitor for the treatment of cancer. Cancer Res 2005; 65(10): 4389-400.

[3] Drevs J, Siegert P, Medinger M, Mross K, Strecker R, Zingiebel U, *et al.* Phase I clinical study of AZD2171, an oral vascular endothelial growth factor signaling inhibitor, in patients with advanced solid tumors. J Clin Oncol 2007; 25(21): 3045-54.

[4] Demetri GD, van Oosterom AT, Garrett CR, Blackstein ME, Shah MH, Verweij L, *et al.* Efficacy and safety of sunitinib in patients with advanced gastrointestinal stromal tumor after failure of imatinib: A randomized controlled trial. Lancet 2006; 368(9544): 1329-38.

[5] Keizman D, Huang P, Eisenberger MA, Pili R, Kim JJ, Antonarakis ES, *et al.* Angiotensin system inhibitors and outcome of sunitinib treatment in patients with metastatic renal cell carcinoma: A retrospective examination. Eur J Cancer 2011; 47(13): 1955-61.

[6] Scott EN, Meinhardt G, Jacques C, Laurent D, Thomas AL. Vatalinib: The clinical development of a tyrosine kinase inhibitor of angiogenesis in solid tumors. Exp Opin Invest Drugs 2007; 16(3): 367-79.

[7] Tan EH, Goss GD, Salgia R, Besse B, Gandara DR, Hanna NH, *et al.* Phase 2 trial of linifanib (ABT-869) in patients with advanced non-small cell lung cancer. J Thorac Oncol 2011; 6(8): 1418-25.

[8] Tannir NM, Wong YN, Kollmannsberger CK, Ernstoff MS, Perry DJ, Appleman LJ, *et al.* Phase 2 trial of linifanib (ABT-869) in patients with advanced renal cell cancer after sunitinib failure. Eur J Cancer 2011; 47(18): 2706-14.

[9] Fyfe, G., Holmgren, E., Mass, R.D., Novotny, W. Treatment with anti-VEGF antibodies. US2008267968 (**2008**).

[10] Yang JC, Haworth L, Sherry RM, Hwu P, Schwartzentruber DJ, Topalian SL, *et al.* A randomized trial of bevacizumab, an anti-vascular endothelial growth factor antibody, for metastatic renal cancer. N Engl J Med 2003; 349(5): 427-34.

[11] Hurwitz H, Fehrenbacher L, Novotny W, Cartwright T, Hainsworth J, Heim W, *et al.* Bevacizumab plus irinotecan, fluorouracil, and leucovorin for metastatic colorectal cancer. New Engl J Med 2004; 350 (23): 2335-42.

[12] Fuh, G., Gerber, H.P., Liang, W.C., Fellouse, F.A., Sidhu, S.S., Wiesmann, C. Anti-VEGF antibodies. US8092797 (**2012**) & US20110020346 (**2011**).

[13] Kavlie, A. Schlunegger, K. Anti-VEGF antibody compositions and methods. US8034905 (**2011**).

[14] van Bruggen, N., Ferrara, N. Vascular endothelial cell growth factor antagonists and uses thereof. US7998931 (**2011**) & EP1140173 (**2013**).

[15] Fuh, G., Lee, C.V. Anti-VEGF antibodies. US20110159009 (**2011**) & US7910098 (**2011**).

[16] Sullivan LA, Carbon JG, Roland CL, Toombs JE, Nyquist-Andersen M, Kavlie A, *et al.* R84, a novel therapeutic antibody against mouse and human VEGF with potent anti-tumor activity and limited induction. PlosOne 2010; 5(8): e12031.

[17] Yu DC, Lee JS, Yoo JY, Shin H, Deng HX, Wei Q, *et al.* Soluble vascular endothelial growth factor decoy receptor FP3 exerts potent anti-angiogenic effects. Molec Ther 2012; 20(5): 938-47.

[18] Holash J, Davis S, Papadopoulos N, Croll SD, Ho L, Russell M, *et al.* VEGF-Trap, a VEGF blocker with potent antitumor effects. Proc Natl Acad Sci 2002; 99(17): 11393-8.

[19] Gaya A, Tse V. A preclinical and clinical review of aflibercept for the management of cancer. Cancer treat Rev 2012; 38(5): 484-93.

[20] Tolentino, M.J., Reich, S.L. Composition and methods for siRNA inhibition of angiogenesis. EP2345718 (**2011**).

[21] Dejneka, N. Compositions and methods for inhibition of VEGF. US20110142915 (**2011**) & WO2011069155 (**2011**).

[22] Ruggles, S., Nguyen, J. Mutant MT-SP1 proteases with altered substrate specificity or activity. US20110177581 (**2011**) & US7939304 (**2011**).

[23] Ruggles, S.W., Nguyen, J. Cleavage of VEGF and VEGF receptor by wild type and mutant MT-SP1. EP1735439 (**2011**).

[24] Morrow PK, Murthy RK, Ensor JD, Gordon GS, Margolin KA, Elias AD, *et al.* An open-label, Phase 2 trial of RPI.4610 (angiozyme) in the treatment of metastatic breast cancer. Cancer 2012; 118(17):4098-104.

[25] Matsumoto K, Nakamura T. Hepatocyte growth factor and the Met system as a mediator of tumor-stromal interactions. Int J Cancer 2006; 119(3): 477-83.

[26] van der Horst HE, Chinn L, Wang M, Velilla T, Tran H, Madrona Y, *et al.* Discovery of fully human anti-MET monoclonal antibodies with antitumor activity against colon cancer tumor models *in vivo*. Neoplasia 2009; 11(4): 355-64.

[27] Stabile LP, Rothstein ME, Keohavong P, Jin J, Yin J, Land SR, *et al.* Therapeutic targeting of human hepatocyte growth factor with a single neutralizing monoclonal antibody reduces lung tumorigenesis. Mol Cancer Ther 2008; 7(7): 1913-22.

[28] Date K, Matsumoto K, Shimura H, Tanaka M, Nakamura T. HGF/NKY is a specific antagonist for pleiotrophic actions of hepatocyte growth factor. FEBS Lett 1997; 420(1): 1-6.

[29] Suzuki Y, Sakai K, Ueki J, Xu Q, Nakamura T, Shimada H, *et al.* Inhibition of Met/HGF receptor and angiogenesis by NK4 leads to suppression of tumor growth and migration in malignant pleural mesothelioma. Int J Cancer 2010; 127(8): 1948-57.

[30] Porter J. Small molecule c-Met kinase inhibitors: A review of recent patents. Expert Opin Ther Patents 2010; 20(2): 159-77.

[31] Leow CC, Coffman K, Inigo I, Breen S, Czapiga M, Soukharev S, *et al.* MEDI3617, a human anti-angiopoietin 2 monoclonal antibody, inhibits angiogenesis and tumor growth in human tumor xenograft models. Int J Oncol 2012; 40(5): 1321-330.

[32] Herbst RS, Hong D, Chap L, Kurzrock R, Jackson E, Silverman JM, *et al.* Safety, pharmacokinetics, and antitumor activity of AMG 386, a selective angiopoietin inhibitor, in adult patients with advanced solid tumors. J Clin Oncol 2009; 27(12): 3557-65.

[33] Mita AC, Takimoto CH, Mita M, Tolcher A, Sankhala K, Sarantopoulos J, *et al.* Phase I study of AMG 386, a selective angiopoietin 1/2-neutralizing petibody, in combination with chemotherapy in adults with advanced solid tumors. Clin Cancer Res 2010; 16(11): 3044-56.

[34] Gerber, H., Ferrara, N., Liang, X.H. Inhibitors of angiopoietin-like 4 protein, combinations, and their use. US20110311524 (**2011**).

[35] Jimenez B, Volpert OV, Crawford SE, Febbraio M, Silverstein RL, Bouck N. Signals leading to apoptosis-dependent inhibition of neovascularization by thrombospondin-1. Nature Med 2000; 6(1): 41-8.

[36] Margosio B, Marchetti D, Vergani V, Giavazzi R, Rusnati M, Presta M, *et al.* Thrombospondin1 as a scavenger for matrix-associated fibroblast growth factor 2. Blood 2003; 102(13): 4399-406.

[37] Anderson JC, Grammer JR, Wang W, Nabors LB, Menkin J, Stewart JE, *et al.* ABT-510, a modified type 1 repeat peptide of thrombospondin, inhibits malignant glioma growth *in vivo* by inhibiting angiogenesis. Cancer Biol Ther 2007; 6(3): 454-62.

[38] Henkin J, Volpert OV. Therapies using anti-angiogenic peptide mimetics of thrombospondin-1. Expert Opin Ther Targets 2011; 15(12): 1369-86.

[39] Garside SA, Henkin J, Morris KD, Norvell SM, Thomas FH, Fraser HM. A thrombospondin mimetic peptide, ABT-898, suppresses angiogenesis and promotes follicular atresia in pre- and early-antral follicles *in vivo*. Endocrinology 2010; 151(12): 5905-15.

[40] Campbell N, Greenaway J, Henkin J, Petrik J. ABT-898 induces tumor regression and prolongs survival in a mouse model of epithelial ovarian cancer. Mol Cancer Ther 2011; 10(10): 1876-85.

[41] Chen G, Wang F, Trachootham D, Huang P. Preferential killing of cancer cells with mitochondrial dysfunction by natural compounds. Mitochondrion 2010; 10(6): 614-25.

[42] Dong LF, Low P, Dyason JC, Wang XF, Porchazka L, Witting PK, *et al.* Alpha-tocopheryl succinate induces apoptosis by targeting ubiquinonen-binding sites in mitochondrial respiratory complex II. Oncogene 2008; 27(31): 4324-35.

[43] Ralph SJ, Neuzil J. Mitochondria as targets for cancer therapy. Mol Nutr Food Res 2009; 53(1): 9-28.

[44] Ralph, S.J. Neuzil, J. Pro-oxidant anti-cancer compounds. US0059898 (**2011**).

[45] Ralph, S.J., Neuzil, J. Mitochondrially delivered anti-cancer compounds. US20110105437 (**2011**).

[46] Rohlena J, Dong LF, Kluckova K, Zobalova R, Goodwin J, Tilly D, *et al.* Mitochondrially targeted alpha-Tocopheryl succinate is antiangiogenic: Potential benefit against tumor angiogenesis but caution against wound healing. Antioxid Redox Signal 2011; 15(12): 2923-35.

[47] Itoh Y, Ito A, Iwata K, Tanzawa K, Mori Y, Nagase H. Plasma membrane-bound tissue inhibitor of metalloproteinases (TIMP)2 specifically inhibits matrix metalloproteinase 2 (gelatinase A) activated on the cell surface. J Biol Chem 1998; 273(1): 24360-7.

[48] Qi JH, Ebrahem Q, Moore N, Murphy G, Claesson-Welsh L, Bond M, *et al.* A novel function for tissue inhibitor of metalloproteinases-3 (TIMP3): Inhibition of angiogenesis by blockage of VEGF binding to VEGF receptor-2. Nat Med 2003; 9(4): 407-15.

[49] Cho JJ, Kim YT. Sharks: A potential source of antiangiogenic factors and tumor treatments. Mar Biotechnol 2002; 4(6): 521-5.

[50] Boivin D, Gendron S, Beaulieu E, Gingras D, Beliveau R. The antiangiogenic agent Neovastat (AE-941) induces endothelial cell apoptosis. Mol Cancer Ther 2002; 1(10): 795-802.

[51] Glasspool RM, Twelves CJ. Matrix metalloproteinase inhibitors: Past lessons and future prospects in breast cancer. The Breast 2001; 10(5): 368-378.

[52] Coussens LM, Fingleton B, Matrisian LM. Cancer therapy - Matrix metalloproteinase inhibitors and cancer: Trials and tribulations. Science 2002; 295(5564): 2387-92.

[53] Hoekstra, W.J. Schotzinger, R.J., Rafferty, S.W. Metalloenzyme inhibitor compounds. US20110306644 (**2011**).

[54] Felding-Habermann B, O'Toole T, Smith JW, Fransvea E, Ruggeri ZM, Ginsberg MH, *et al.* Integrin activation controls metastasis in human breast cancer. Proc Natl Acad Sci 2001; 98(4): 1853-8.

[55] Kim S, Harris M, Varner JA. Regulation of integrin avb3-mediated endothelial cell migration and angiogenesis by integrin a5b1 and protein kinase A. J Biol Chem 2000; 275(43): 33920-8.

[56] Almokadem S, Belani CP. Volociximab in cancer. Exp Opin Biol Ther 2012; 12(2): 251-7.

[57] Ramakrishnan, V., Powers, D., Johnson, D.E., Jeffry, U., Bhadkar, V. Chimeric and humanized antibodies to alpha5beta1 integrin that modulate angiogenesis. US20080260732 (**2008**).

[58] Zutter, M. Anti-angiogenic targets for cancer therapy. US20080267978 (**2008**).

[59] Minea R, Helchowski C, Rubino B, Brodmann K, Swenson S, Markland F Jr. Development of a chimeric recombinant disintegrin as a cost effective anticancer agent with promising translational potential. Toxicon 2012; 59(4): 472-86.

[60] Li M, Liu K, Michalicek J, Angus JA, Hunt JE, Dell'Italia LJ, *et al.* Involvement of chymase-mediated angiotensin II generation in blood pressure regulation. J Clin Invest 2004; 114(1): 112-20.

[61] Nadal JA, Scicli GM, Carbini LA, Scicli AG. Angiotensin II stimulates migration of retinal microvascular pericytes involvement of TGF-beta and PDGF-beta. 2002; 282(2): H739-48.

[62] Chua CC, Hamdy RC, Chua BH. Upregulation of vascular endothelial growth factor by angiotensin II in rat heart endothelial cells. Biochim Biophys Acta 1998; 1401(2): 187-94.
[63] Egami K, Murohara T, Shimada T, Sasaki K, Shintani S, Surgaya T, *et al.* Role of host angiotensin II type 1 receptor in tumor angiogenesis and growth. J Clin Invest 2003; 112(1): 67-75.
[64] Ohnuma Y, Toda M, Fujita M, Hosono K, Suzuki T, Ogawa Y, *et al.* Blockade of angiotensin type I receptor enhances effects of radiation on tumor growth and tumor-associated angiogenesis by reducing vascular endothelial growth factor expression. Biomed Pharmacother 2009; 36(2): 136-45.
[65] Smith GR, Missailidis S. Cancer, inflammation and the AT1 and AT2 receptors. J Inflamm 2004; 1: 3.
[66] Puddefoot JR, Udeozo UK, Barker S, Vinson GP. The role of angiotensin II in the regulation of breast cancer cell adhesion and invasion. Endocr Relat Cancer 2006; 13(3): 895-903.
[67] De Paepe B, Verstraeten VLRM, De Potter CR, Vakaet LAML, Bullock GR. Growth stimulatory angiotensin II type-1 receptor is upregulated in breast hyperplasia and *in situ* carcinoma but not in invasive carcinoma. Histochem Cell Biol 2001; 116(3): 247-54.
[68] Bluff JE, Menakuru SR, Cross SS, Higham SE, Balasubramanian SP, Brown NJ, *et al.* Angiogenesis is associated with the onset of hyperplasia in human ductal breast disease. Br J Cancer 2009; 101(4): 666-72.
[69] Burnier M. Angiotensin II type 1 receptor blockers. Circulation 2001; 103(6): 904-12.
[70] Yamagishi T, Uemura H, Nakaigawa N, Noguchi K, Kubota Y. Angiotensin II blocker reduced serum PSA in hormone refractory prostate cancer. J Urol 2005; 173(2): 441.
[71] Redondo-Muller MA, Stevanovic-Walker M, Barker S, Puddefoot JR, Vinson GP. Anti-cancer actions of a recombinant antibody (R6313/G2) against the angiotensin II AT1 receptor. Endocr Rel Cancer 2008; 15(1): 277-88.
[72] Lever AF, Hole DJ, Gillis CR, McCallum IR, McInnes GT, MacKinnon, *et al.* Do inhibitors of angiotensin-I- converting enzyme protect against risk of cancer? Lancet 1998; 352(9123): 179-84.
[73] Lindberg H, Nielsen D, Jensen BV, Eriksen J, Skovsgaard T. Angiotensin converting enzyme inhibitors for cancer treatment? Acta Oncol 2004; 43(2): 142-52.
[74] Gonzales-Zuloeta Ladd AM, Arias Vasquez A, Sayed-Tabatabaei FA, Coebergh JW, Hofman A, Njajou O, *et al.* Angiotensin-converting enzyme gene insertion/deletion polymorphism and breast cancer risk. Cancer Epidemiol Biomarkers Prev 2005; 14(9): 2143-6.
[75] Koh WP, Yvan JM, Van Den Berg D, Lee HP, Yu MC. Polymorphisms in angiotensin II type 1 receptor and angiotensin I-converting enzyme genes and breast cancer risk among Chinese women in Singapore. Carcinogenesis 2005; 26(2): 459-64.
[76] Arafat HA, Gong Q, Chipitsyna G, Rizvi A, Saa CT, Yeo CJ. Antihypertensives as novel antineoplastics: Angiotensin-I-converting enzyme inhibitors and angiotensin II type 1 receptor blockers in pancreatic ductal adenocarcinoma. J Am Coll Surg 2007; 204(5): 996-1006.
[77] Volpert OV, Ward WF, Lingen MW, Chesler L, Solt DB, Johnson MD, *et al.* Captopril inhibits angiogenesis and slows the growth of experimental tumors in rats. J Clin Invest 1996; 98(3): 671-9.
[78] Dieras V, Limentani S, Romieu G, Tubiana-Hulin M, Lorthdary A, Kaufman P, *et al.* Phase II multicenter study of larotaxel (XRP9881) a novel taxoid, in patients with metastatic

breast cancer who previously received taxane-based therapy. Ann Oncol 2008; 19(7): 1255-60.

[79] Aggarwal BB, Kunnumakkara AB, Harikumar KB, Tharakan ST, Sung B, Amand P. Potential of spice-derived phytochemicals for cancer prevention. Planta Medica 2008; 74(13): 1560-9.

[80] Kim EC, Min JK, Kim TY, Lee SJ, yang HO, Han S, *et al.* 6-Gingerol, a pungent ingredient of ginger, inhibits angiogenesis *in vitro* and *in vivo*. Biochem Biophys Res Commun 2005; 335(2): 300-8.

[81] Lee HS, Seo EY, Kang NE, Kim WK. 6-Gingerol inhibits metastasis of MDA-MB-231 human breast cancer cells. J Nutr Biochem 2008; 19(5): 313-9.

[82] Boozer CN, Herron AJ. Simmondsin for weight loss in rats. Int J Obes 2006; 30(7): 1143-8.

[83] D'Oosterlynck, A., Raes, S. Simmondsin for use as angiogenesis inhibitor. US7387999 (**2008**).

[84] Gupta K, Kshirsagar S, Chang L, Schwartz R, Law PY, Yee D, *et al.* Morphine stimulates angiogenesis by activating proangiogenic and survival-promoting signaling and promotes breast tumor growth. Cancer Res 2002; 62(15): 4491-8.

[85] Moss, J., Lingen, M., Singleton, P.A., Garcia, J.G.N. Use of opioid antagonists to attenuate endothelial cell proliferation and migration. US20080274119 (**2008**).

[86] Stich HF. Teas and tea components as inhibitors of carcinogen formation in model systems and man. Prev Med 1992; 21(3): 377-84.

[87] Shankar S, Ganapathy S, Srivastava RK. Green tea polyphenols: Biology and therapeutic implications in cancer. Front Biosci 2007; 12: 4881-99.

[88] Sartippour MR, Shao ZM, Heber D, Beatty P, Zhang LP, Liu CH, *et al.* Green tea inhibits vascular endothelial growth factor (VEGF) induction in human breast cancer cells. J Nutr 2002; 132(8): 2307-11.

[89] Lamy S, Gingras D, Beliveau R. Green tea catechins inhibit vascular endothelial growth factor receptor phosphorylation. Cancer Res 2002; 62(2): 381-5.

[90] Nakazato T, Ito K, Ikeda Y, Kizaki M. Green tea component, catechin, induces apoptosis of human malignant B cells via production of reactive oxygen species. Clin Cancer Res 2005; 11(2): 6040-9.

[91] Shanafelt TD, Call TG, Zent CS, LaPlant B, Bowen DA, Roos M, *et al.* Phase I trial of daily oral polyphenon E in patients with asymptomatic Rai stage 0 to II chronic lymphocytic leukemia. J Clin Oncol 2009; 27(23): 3808-14.

[92] Choi, S., Moon, Y.C., Tamilarasu, N. Substituted phenols as active agents inhibiting VEGF production. US20080261956 (**2008**).

[93] Xie Q, Yao S, Chen X, Xu L, Peng W, Zhang L. A polypeptide from shark troponin I can inhibit angiogenesis and tumor growth. Mol Biol Rep 2012; 39(2): 1493-501.

[94] Li M, Wu S, Liu Z, Zhang W, Xu J, Wang Y. Arenobufagin, bufadienolide compound from toad venom, inhibits VEGF-mediated angiogenesis through suppression of VEGFR-2 signaling pathways. Biochem Pharmacol 2012; 83(9): 1251-60.

[95] Kumber I, Nielsen DL. Trials of bevacizumab in breast cancer - a safety review. Exp Opin Drug Safety 2012; 11(S1): 37-48.

[96] Escudier B, Eisen T, Stadler WM, Szczylik C, Oudard S, Siebels M, *et al.* Sorafenib in advanced clear-cell renal-cell carcinoma. N Engl J Med 2007; 356(2):125-34.

[97] Motzer R, Hutson TE, Tomczak P, Michaelson MD, Buckowski RM, Rixe O, *et al.* Sunitinib vs. interferon alpha in metastatic renal-cell carcinoma. N Engl J Med 2007; 356: 115-24.

[98] Namiki Y, Namiki T, Yoshida H, Date M, Yashiro M, Matsumoto K, *et al.* Preclinical study of a "tailor-made" combination of NK4-expressing gene therapy and gefitinib (ZD1839, Iressa) for disseminated peritoneal scirrhous gastric cancer. Int J Cancer 2006; 118(6): 1545-55.

[99] Dupont, J., Irl, C. Anti-angiogenesis therapy for the treatment of ovarian cancer. WO20110106300 (**2011**) & EP2539367 (**2013**).

[100] Fyfe, G., Holmgren, E., Moss, R.D., Novotny, W. Treatment with anti-VEGF antibodies. US20110123494 (**2011**).

[101] Rajeshwari, S., Hambleton, J. Anti-angiogenesis therapy for the treatment of previously treated breast cancer. WO2011022264 (**2011**) & US0047103 (**2011**).

[102] Nabors LB, Fiveash JB, Markert JM, Kekan MS, Gillespie GY, Huang Z, *et al.* A Phase I trial of ABT-510 concurrent with standard chemoradiation for patients with newly diagnosed glioblastoma. Arch Neurol 2010; 67(3): 313-9.

[103] Hu L, Hofmann J, Holash J, Yancopoulos GD, Sood AK, Jaffe RB. Vascular endothelial growth factor trap combined with pactitaxel strikingly inhibits tumor and ascites, prolonging survival in a human ovarian cancer model. Clin Cancer Res 2005; 11(19): 6966-71.

[104] Young, F., Maki, J., Bascomb, N. Combination of an ACE inhibitor and an NSAID for use in ameliorating cachexia/SIRS. EP2374458 (**2011**).

[105] Farokhzad, O.C., Kolishetti, N., Dhar, S., Lippard, S.J., Langer, R.S., Valencia, P.M. Particles for multiple agent delivery. WO2011084620 (**2011**).

[106] Kim SH, Jeong JH, Lee SH, Kim SW, Park TG. PEG conjugated VEGF siRNA for anti-angiogenic gene therapy. J Control Release 2006; 116(2): 123-9.

[107] Vader P, Crielaard BJ, van Dommelen SM, van der Meel R, Storm G, Schiffelers RM. Targeted delivery of small interfering RNA to angiogenic endothelial cells with liposome-polycarion-DNA particles. J Control Release 2012; 160(2): 211-6.

[108] Salva E, Kabasakal L, Eren F, Ozkan N, Cakalagaoglu F, Akbuga J. Local delivery of chitosan/VEGF siRNA nanoplexes reduces angiogenesis and growth of breast cancer *in vivo*. Nucleic Acid Ther 2012; 22(1): 40-8.

[109] Cao, G., Wei, C., Qihua, N., Xiaoliang, N., Weijian, T. Preparation method of d-alpha-tocopheryl succinate monioester biomembrane covering. CN101785866 (**2010**).

[110] Turanek J, Wang XF, Knotigova P, Koudelka S, Dong LF, Vrublova E, *et al.* Liposomal formulation of alpha-tocopheryl maleamide: *In vitro* and *in vivo* toxicological profile and anticancer effect against spontaneous breast carcinomas in mice. Toxicol Appl Pharmacol 2009; 237(3): 249-57.

[111] You, H.B., Halqing, Y. Polymerosomes and methods of making and using thereof. US20110027347 (**2011**).

[112] Koch M, Hussein F, Woeste A, Grundker C, Frontzek K, Emons G, *et al.* CD36-mediated activation of endothelial cell apoptosis by an *N*-terminal recombinant fragment of thrombospondin-2 inhibits breast cancer growth and metastasis *in vivo*. Breast Cancer Res Treat 2011; 128(2): 337-46.

[113] Li LN, Leedom TA, Do J, Huang HH, Lai JY, Johnson K, *et al.* Antitumor efficacy of a thrombospondin 1 mimetic CovX-Body. Translat Oncol 2011; 4(4): 239-47.

[114] Tong RT, Boucher Y, Kozin SV, Winkler F, Hicklin DJ, Jain RK. Vascular normalization by vascular endothelial growth factor receptor 2 blockade induces a pressure gradient

across the vasculature and improves drug penetration in tumors. Cancer Res 2004; 64(11): 3731-6.

[115] Stevenson CE, Nagahashi M, Ramachandran S, Yamada A, Bear HD, Takabe K. Bevacizumab and breast cancer: What does the future hold? Future Oncol 2012; 8(4): 403-14.

[116] Rosen LS. VEGF-targeted therapy: Therapeutic potential and recent advances. Oncologist 2005; 10(6): 382-91.

[117] Trinh XB, van Dam PA, Vermeulen PB, Van Laere SJ, Van den Eynden GG, Tjalma WAA, *et al.* VEGF-A-independent and angiogenesis-dependent tumor growth in patients with metastatic breast cancer. Clin Transl Oncol 2011; 13(11): 805-8.

[118] Jayson GC, Hicklin DJ, Ellis LM. Antiangiogenic therapy-evolving view based on clinical trial results. Nature Rev Clin Oncol 2012; 9(5): 297-303.

Send Orders of Reprints at reprints@benthamscience.net

CHAPTER 10

Paradigm Shift in the Therapeutic Potential of Endogenous Angiogenesis Inhibitors for Cancer Therapy: Historical Perspective and Future Direction

Mohanraj Dhanabal[1,*] and Natarajan Sethuraman[2]

[1]EMD Serono Research Institute Inc., 45A Middlesex Turnpike, Billerica, MA 01821, USA; [2]GlycoFi, 21 Lafayette Street, Suite 200, Lebanon, NH 03766, USA

Abstract: Angiogenesis, the formation of new blood vessels from preexisting microvasculature is a highly regulated process. Angiogenesis is controlled by both positive and negative factors thus providing several targets for drug discovery. Targeting tumor endothelial cells has gained much attention with the notion that tumors can be starved to death by cutting the lifeline of tumor cells, i.e. vascular endothelial cells. In this regard, the inhibition of angiogenesis represents a new approach to cancer therapy and several agents and approaches are in different stages of clinical development. A paradigm shift is expected in the treatment of malignancies because of the recent introduction of mechanism-based systemic therapies that may be more specific, less toxic, and more effective. These inhibitors were recently shown to constitute a new modality for cancer treatment. In this chapter, we will review the recent angiogenesis inhibitors-related patent literature. This review will cover specifically the discovery and development disclosures of endogenous inhibitors. The scope of this chapter is to give the reader a well structured patent literature overview of agents targeting different steps of the angiogenic process. Finally, we have summarized the key attributes of the emerging endogenous angiogenesis inhibitors that make them a potent antitumor agents.

Keywords: Angiogenesis, angiostatin, anti-angiogenesis inhibitors, cancer, endostatin, receptor tyrosine kinase and kringle, vascular target, VEGF.

INTRODUCTION

Cancer is the second most common cause of death in the United States accounting for approximately 23 % of all death. In 2005, it is estimated that approximately a total of 1,372,910 new cases of cancer will be diagnosed and that approximately 570,280 Americans will die of cancer, corresponding to more than 1500 deaths

***Address correspondence to Mohanraj Dhanabal:** EMD Serono Research Institute Inc., 45A Middlesex Turnpike, Billerica, MA 01821, USA; Tel: 978-294-1483; Fax: 978-294-1407; E-mails: mohanraj.dhanabal@emdserono.com; mdhanabal@hotmail.com

Atta-ur Rahman and Khurshid Zaman (Eds)

per day [1]. The heterogeneity in the genetic make up which influences cancer development and progression coupled with metastasis makes cure difficult for majority of cancer. Despite the remarkable progress made over the past two decades in understanding the molecular, cellular and tissue processes involved in the progression of cancer, though translated into effective therapies for a majority of cancers, further research is needed to obtain cure in a greater percentage of cancers. Though major advances have been made with chemotherapeutics, singular breakthroughs are unlikely given the complexity and adaptive nature of cancer.

Historically, surgery has been the mainstay for the treatment of solid tumor [2]. Following surgery, chemotherapy or radiotherapy approaches remain the second line of cancer treatment for tumors that cannot be cured solely by surgical excision. Recent work suggests that a sub-population of cancer cells with stem-cell-like properties may be critical for triggering metastatic tumor development [3]. The term targeted therapy is often used to describe new generation of cancer drugs designed to interfere with a specific molecular target that are believed to play a critical role in the tumor growth or progression [4]. These novel drugs differ with respect to the mode of action (MOA) and are amenable for combination therapy with traditional chemotherapeutic drugs. Hormonal therapy is an effective option for cancers that are influenced by hormones and exert their therapeutic action by blocking the effect of body's hormone which promote tumor growth through the use of tumor growth inhibiting hormones or analogues [2]. Traditional therapies are generally more effective against the primary tumor than against the metastatic tumor [5-9]. During the metastatic process there is cross talk between stroma and tumor cells thereby altering the local extracellular matrix (ECM) resulting in enhanced migration, invasion, proliferation and survival of tumor cells. This process which is unique for cancer cells is an attractive target for the development of a novel anti-cancer strategy to achieve long-term therapeutic control.

Recently, much attention has been devoted to the notion that tumor can be starved of blood supply through the use of anti-angiogenic agents [10-13]. Substantial preclinical and clinical evidence suggests that angiogenesis plays an important role in the development and progression of tumor malignancies [4, 14-23]. The approval of a monoclonal antibody directed against the vascular endothelial growth factor (VEGF) for the treatment of colon cancer has given a boost to the concept of developing anti-angiogenic therapy as a viable approach for the treatment of a range of pathologies, such as diabetic retinopathy, rheumatoid arthritis, glaucoma and psoriasis [24-28]. It has been estimated that > 200 companies are working in the area of angiogenesis and several of the compounds that modulate angiogenesis are currently being evaluated in clinical trials [29]. Currently, there are 329 different Molecular Targeted Therapy (MTTs) in developmental pipelines. Of these, 44 (13%) are grouped as angiogenesis inhibitors, 45 (14 %) are single-targeted signal transduction inhibitors followed by 65 (20%) multi-targeted inhibitors [30]. A list of approved anti-angiogenic inhibitors is shown in Table **1**. Although there are limited reviews covering the patent applications published between 1999 - 2002, to date there has not been an exhaustive review on this specific topic [30, 31]. The scope of this chapter is focused on patent applications published between 2000-2005 describing inhibitors of angiogenesis. Patent landscape on cancer-related angiogenesis is too broad and thus difficult to cover the entire field in this short review and consequently this review has been restricted to cover patent applications specifically related to endogenous inhibitors of angiogenesis. Furthermore, this chaper will not discuss the applications covering the mechanism-based approaches such as matrix metalloproteinase inhibitors (MMPI's) and inhibitors of growth factor signaling pathways or natural products derived inhibitors, a topic which has been reviewed elsewhere [31-34]. The aim of this chapter is to give the reader a well structured collection of patent applications covering endogenous inhibitors including the emerging inhibitors of angiogenesis being developed for targeted therapy for cancer.

Table 1: List of antiangiogenic drugs approved for clinical use.

Brand	**Drug**	**Target**	**Company**	**Indication**
Bevacizumab	Avastin	VEGF	Genentech	mCRC, NSCLC, Advanced breast cancer
*Cetuximab	Erbitux	EGFR	Imclone	mCRC & Head and Neck cancer
*Panitumumab	Vectibix	EGFR	Amgen	mCRC
Ranibizumab	Lucentis	VEGF	Genentech	Wet Age-related macular regeneration

Table 1: cont….

Pegaptanib	Macugen	VEGF	OSI Pharmaceuticals	Wet Age-related macular regeneration
Endostatin	Endostar	Angiogenesis inhibitor	Shangdong Simcere Medgen	Lung Cancer
*Nexavar	Sorafenib	VEGFR, PDGFR & Raf	Bayer AG/Onyx	Advanced RCC
*Sutent	Sunitinib	VEGFR, PDGFR & c-Kit	Pfizer	Advanced RCC & GIST
Thalidomide	Thalomid	Angiogenesis inhibitor	Celgene Corporation	Multiple myeloma
*Nexavar	Sorafenib	PDGFR, VEGFR & c-Kit	Bayer AG/Onyx	Advanced RCC
*Sutent	Sunitinib	PDGFR & VEGFR	Pfizer	Advanced RCC & GIST
*Sprycel	Dasatinib	Bcr-Abl & Src	Bristol-Myers squibb	Gleeve-resistant CML or Ph+ ALL
*Tykerb	Lapatinib	EGFR & Her2/neu	GlaxoSmithKline	Advanced metastatic HER2+ breast cancer
*Bortezomib	Velcade	Proteosome inhibitor	Millennium Pharmaceuticals	Multiple myeloma
*Erlotinib	Tarceva	EGFR	Genentech/OSI	Lung cancer

* Indirect anti-angiogenic inhibitors

Angiogenesis

Angiogenesis, the formation of new blood vessels from the pre-existing microvasculature, is among the key events for embryonic development, the menstrual cycle and wound healing [17, 18, 35]. Angiogenesis also plays a vital role in the development of many diseases including atherosclerosis, rheumatic disease, psoriasis and cancer [18, 19, 21]. In the past three decades, our understanding of angiogenesis in general, and tumor angiogenesis in particular, has grown exponentially, resulting in the approval of the first anti-angiogenic agent, bevacizumab (Avastin), for the treatment of advanced colorectal cancer [27, 28, 36]. Virchow in 1863 first proposed that growth of tumor beyond few mm^3 is dependent on angiogenesis and this concept was developed further by Folkman [14, 37, 38]. Under normal physiological conditions, there is a perfect balance between numerous pro and anti-angiogenic molecules which orchestrate the different steps of blood vessel formation [39-43]. The list of identified pro and anti-angiogenic factors continues to grow. Table **2** presents a partial listing of some of these factors. For tumor growth to occur, the effect of proangiogenic factors must outweigh that of anti-angiogenic factors. This process has been described as the angiogenic switch, which fosters the development of new vessels and allows tumor progression [44]. Hence, the inhibition of angiogenesis has been demonstrated to be one of the potentially more promising new approaches to anti-cancer therapy.

Table 2: Representative proangiogenic and anti-angiogenic factors are listed below.

Proangiogenic factors	Antiangiogenic factors
Angiogenin	Antithrombin III
Angiopoietin-1	Angiostatin (Plasminogen fragment)
Epidermal growth factor	Arresten (Fragment of α1 chain of Type IV collagen)
Ephrin	Canstatin (Fragment of α2 chain of Type IV collagen)
Fibroblast growth factor	Endostatin (C-terminal fragment of Type XVIII collagen)
Hepatocyte growth factor	Interferon-α
Interleukin-8	Interferon inducible protein- IP 10
Leptin	Interleukin-12
Placental-derived growth factor	Maspin
Platelet-derived growth factor	Pigment-epithelium derived factor
Transforming growth factor	Platelet factor-4
Vascular endothelial growth factor	Prolactin
	PEX (MMP-2 fragment)
	Restin (C-terminal fragment of Type XV collagen)
	Tumstatin (Fragment of α3 chain of Type IV collagen)
	Thrombospondin-1
	Vasostatin (Calreticulin fragment)
	Vasculostatin

Anti-angiogenic treatment strategies focus on endothelial compartment and offer several advantages over conventional chemotherapeutic strategies [13, 45]. Firstly, they target endothelial cells which represent a genetically stable, normal and homogenous cell type that is unlikely to develop drug-resistance. Secondly, endothelial cells are readily accessible to systemically administered selective angiogenesis inhibitors. Thirdly, tumor endothelium expresses high levels of specific molecular targets and antigens that may be targeted by selective inhibitors. Fourthly, the growth of a tumor beyond a certain size requires the acquisition of new blood vessels, thus the inhibitors of angiogenesis would be sufficient to prevent the expansion of tumor mass. Fifthly, in contrast to the conventional use of chemotherapeutics to target tumor cells, destruction of all the target cells is not needed. Finally and most importantly, they are particularly suited for combination therapy with cytotoxic chemotherapeutics or radiotherapy because their target is entirely different from these therapies.

Angiogenesis inhibitors have been classified into different groups depending upon the parameter used for grouping. One research group has classified angiogenesis inhibitors (AIs) into three groups: direct, indirect or mixed inhibitors [45]. Folkman proposed a classification system based on the efficacy of angiogenesis inhibitors in preclinical tumor models - first generation AIs, such as interferons, TNP-470. thalidomide, and matrix metalloproteinases inhibitors (MMPIs), only slow tumor growth; second-generation AIs, such as anti-VEGF and anti-integrin $\alpha_v\beta_3$ antibodies, frequently produce regression; third-generation AIs, such as angiostatin, endostatin and TSP-1, can be curative in experimental tumors [46]. AIs can also be classified by the mechanism of action: inhibitors of angiogenic factors secretion, inhibitors of endothelial intracellular signaling transduction, inhibitors of endothelial cell proliferation, inhibitors of MMPs, agents cytotoxic toward endothelial cells, and inhibitors of mobilization of endothelial precursor cells (EPC) from bone marrow [47-54]. In the previous reviews, the patent applications covering anti-angiogenesis agents have been organized into four different categories- (i) mechanism-based approaches, (ii) endogenous inhibitor or inhibitors of unknown mechanisms, (iii) natural products based approaches and (iv) vascular targeting strategies [31, 32]. A representative key players involved in interaction of vascular endothelial cell-associated integrins and their intracellular partners for endogenous inhibitors are depicted in Fig. (**1**). In the following chapter, we discuss the recent patent applications of various endogenous inhibitors of angiogenesis targeting different steps of angiogenic process.

Paradigm Shift in Cancer Therapy

The traditional paradigm of systemic cancer therapy calls for the use of maximally tolerated doses of drugs to shrink tumors (i.e., obtain objective responses), with the ultimate goal of improving survival time or quality of life or both. According to this paradigm, objective responses are used as surrogate markers for drug efficacy. Although there are situations in which objective responses are correlated with improvement in tumor-related symptoms, as has been demonstrated in metastatic breast cancer, [55] objective responses are not always correlated with survival time or overall quality of life. In addition, response evaluation is problematic in certain situations, such as pancreatic cancer

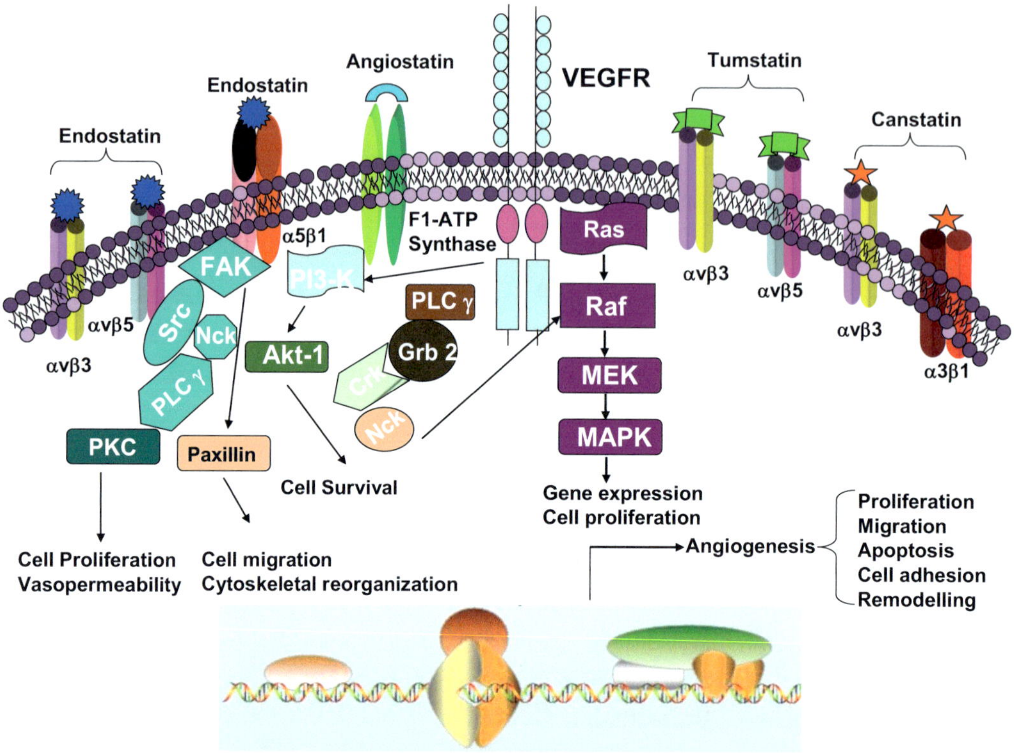

Interaction of vascular endothelial cell-associated integrins with matrix-derived angiogenesis inhibitors. The cryptic ligands for various integrins are generated from basement membrane collagen-derived matrix fragments which acts on the proliferating endothelial cells. Some of the endogenous angiogenesis inhibitors derived from basement membrane- endostatin, arresten, canstatin and tumstatin interact with various forms of integrins expressed on the surface of human endothelial cells. Both endostatin and tumstatin, both basement membrane collagen-derived inhibitors, function via distinct integrins to negative regulate proliferating endothelial cells through unique signaling paths.

Figure 1: Schematic illustration of vascular endothelial cell and associated integrins interaction with endogenous inhibitors.

[56] Another limitation of response evaluation is that certain subsets of patients with advanced cancer may also benefit from disease stabilization caused by systemic treatment. This concept has been verified in patients with metastatic breast cancer treated with hormonal therapies or chemotherapy [57, 58]. Despite the limitations of this "cytotoxic paradigm," according to which response evaluation is based on morphological and radiographic criteria, this method has stood the test of time and applies relatively well to many clinical settings in

oncology. However, the cytotoxic paradigm may not be adequate for assessing responses to molecularly targeted drugs, many of which seem to exert cytostatic rather than cytotoxic effects. Although objective responses have been seen with TKIs used in isolation [59-61], there is a growing recognition among investigators that objective tumor measurement may not be a good surrogate marker for the evaluation of many of the novel drugs. For example, anti-angiogenic agents are not expected to produce rapid objective responses; some randomized trials have suggested that the pattern of disease progression differs between patients given chemotherapy with or without anti-angiogenic agents, the former having a smaller tumor burden at the time of progression [62]. These considerations have arisen mainly from the analysis of Phase I and Phase II trials of targeted agents, and they bear on the decision to move such drugs to Phase III evaluation. If a shift from the cytotoxic to the cytostatic paradigm is contemplated, the endpoints chosen in clinical trials may need to be revisited. As already mentioned, objective responses may not be the best way to evaluate the activity of predominantly cytostatic agents [62]. Survival and quality of life after treatment with these agents may still be evaluated according to the usual methods employed with chemotherapy and other therapeutic interventions

Endogenous Inhibitors

The endogenous inhibitors of angiogenesis include various anti-angiogenic peptides, hormones, metabolites and apoptosis modulators [19, 63]. To date numerous endogenous inhibitors have been identified and their roles in inhibiting angiogenesis have been elucidated. The endogenous inhibitors of angiogenesis have been divided into two major classes (Table **3**) - matrix-derived and non-matrix derived inhibitors [41]. In this section, we will highlight the patent applications covering the most important endogenous inhibitors (Table **4**).

Angiostatin

Angiostatin is a 38- kDa fragment of plasminogen containing either kringle domains 1 to 4 or kringle 1 to 3 or kringle 5 fragment [64]. Angiostatin is a cryptic fragment of plasminogen that possesses anti-angiogenic properties, a property not shared by the parent molecule- plasminogen. Angiostatin was

Table 3: Representative endogenous inhibitor either matrix- derived or non-matrix derived are listed below.

Endogenous inhibitors of angiogenesis

Matrix derived factors	**Non-matrix derived factors**
Collagen IV- α1chain Arresten	**Growth factors and Cytokines**
Collagen IV- α2 chain Canstatin	Interferons
Collagen IV- α3 chain Tumstatin	Interleukins
Collagen fragments	Pigment-epithelium derived factor (PEDF)
Collagen XV fragment-Restin	Platelet factor-4 (PF-4)
Collagen XV fragment-Apomigren	**Others**
Collagen XVIII fragment-Endostatin	Angiostatin
Endorepellin	Antithrombin- III (AT-III)
Fibronectin fragment- ED-B	Chondromodulin
Fibulin	2-Methoxyestradiol
Thrombospondin- TSP-1 & TSP-2	PEX (MMP-2 fragment)
	Kringle-5 (Plasminogen fragment)
	Prolactin fragment
	Prothrombin kringle 2
	Maspin
	sFlt-1
	TIMPs
	Troponin I
	Vasostatin
	Vasculostatin
	Vasohibin

Table 4: Summary of Representative Endogenous Inhibitor-Mechanism of Action and Relevant Patent Applications are listed below.

Drug/Target	**Mechanism of Action**	**Characterization & Biological Functions**	**Patent Application**	**References**
Angiostatin	Proliferation & migration	Isolation & purification	US5639725, WO0158912, WO0158912, US6538103, US6723536, US6444431, WO995920, WO0056299	[14-17,19-21 66-69]
		Biology	WO0056299, US6908898, US6638502, WO9939702, WO9926480	[70, 73, 76, 78, 82-85]
		Therapy	US6420335, WO03086178, WO002368, WO00660945, WO0058498, US20090075369, US7510714, US7365159, US20070009538, US7306803	[58-64]
Endostatin	Proliferation & migration	Isolation & purification	WO0242319, US6852691, US6797488	[95-97, 101, 107, 110, 111]
		Biology	WO04104227, WO0063249, WO9939702, US63446510, WO03066085	[83, 103-106, 112]

Table 4: contd….

		Therapy	WO03102148, US6759047, US7524811, US7495089, US20090191224, US20090175893, US20090137518, US7470667, US20080269135, US20070100468	[96, 100, 88-91, 93, 94]
Type IV collagen	Proliferation & migration	Isolation & purification	WO030599257, US6759047	[116, 117]
		Biology	WO30599257, US6759047, WO9949885, US6358735, US6361994	[116-119]
		Therapy	US6432706, WO0059532, WO4073649, US7488792, US7122517, US20090221494, US20090214488, US20090054344	[119-125]
Thrombospondin	Proliferation & migration	Isolation & purification	WO0057899, WO2078606, WO00771577	[151-152]
		Biology	WO0191781	[142]
		Therapy	WO05007193, US7517522, US20090208448, US20090131314, US20080312146, US7223731, US20070020234	[145-147]
Antithrombin III	Proliferation & migration	Isolation & purification	US6451978, US6607724	[156, 160]
		Therapy	US68778813, US7482139, US20090176246, US20080139459	[157-161]
Kininogen	Proliferation & migration	Isolation & purification	WO00274415, WO0027866, WO0035407	[133, 119]
		Therapy	US6869931, US686552691, US6797488, WO99229878, US20060159620	[171, 172 174, 175]
Platelet factor-4	Proliferation & migration	Isolation & purification	WO9929856, US6919309, US6288024, US6391850	[207-210]
		Therapy	US6670333, US6797691, US20060193833, US20070243539	[212-214]

originally purified from serum and urine of mice bearing subcutaneous Lewis lung carcinoma (LLC), where the growth of metastases was inhibited by tumor-generated angiostatin. The patents covering angiostatin includes identification, method of production and characterization are described in the following section. The isolation and purification of angiostatin from the serum and urine of mice bearing subcutaneous Lewis lung carcinoma is described in patent application filed by Children's Hospital Medical Center [65]. The claims on the issued patent cover angiostatin wherein the amino acid sequence is plasminogen fragment of human, murine, porcine, Rhesus monkey or bovine origin and where the plasminogen fragment has endothelial growth inhibitory activity and tumor inhibitory activity. Following this patent, Children's Hospital medical center has filed several patent applications with claims to fragments derived from plasminogen as endothelial cell growth inhibitors that could be used to inhibit angiogenesis of tumor and for treating angiogenesis-dependent diseases [14-17, 19-21, 46, 51, 66-69]. The deglycosylated angiostatin derivatives are claimed along with methods for their recombinant production [70]. The method for inhibition of angiogenesis using increasing concentration of a deglycosylated fragment of a kringle 1-5 region has been disclosed. The isolation, recombinant preparation and use of angiostatin and related analogues are disclosed in the application from Northwestern University [71]. Kringle 4 fragment of plasminogen derived from murine, human rhesus, porcine and bovine sources and the use of the polypeptide or DNA encoding Kringle 4 to treat cancer, macular degeneration and diabetic retinopathy are specifically cited in the application [72]. A patent from Bristol-Myers has narrow claims to lysine binding fragments of human plasminogen and Fc-fusion proteins for treatment of cancer [73]. The process for expressing recombinant version of the protein using desirable host has been disclosed. A patent from Lexingen Pharmaceutical claims DNA coding for fusion protein consisting of angiostatin-a plasminogen fragment having angiostatin activity, endostatin-a collagen XVIII fragment having endostatin activity, and combinations thereof with Fc, the fusion protein, method of production and use of DNA or fusion protein for treating disease condition mediated by angiogenesis [67]. The Fc portion of the fusion increases the serum half-life and provides a purification tag for one step purification. A patent application from EntreMed claims methods for identifying angiogenesis-inhibiting protein receptors, DNA and protein sequences and their use in inducing angiogenesis [74]. Another patent application from EntreMed claims method of inhibiting angiogenesis using Kringle domain containing proteins and peptides for treating angiogenesis mediated diseases [75]. In particular, methods of administration of low doses of endostatin, angiostatin and TNP-470 especially scheduling one or more therapeutic agents are disclosed. A patent from Pharmacia-Upjohn claims an angiostatin-binding protein [76] and use of this protein for screening and identification of small molecule agonists of angiostatin as well as a pharmaceutical composition consisting of the angiostatin-binding protein or fragment there of and the therapeutic compositions isolated using the angiostatin-binding protein. A patent from Duke University claims the receptor for angiostatin and the use of this receptor for identifying agonist or antagonist [77]. They claim that angiostatin binds directly to the ATP synthase on the surface of endothelial cells, leading to a drop in the intracellular pH triggering apoptotic events in endothelial cells. They claim methods for screening compounds which disrupt this interaction leading to the identification of angiostatin agonist, partial agonists or allosteric modulators. Such compounds can be conjugated to or combined with various cytotoxic agents. The compounds which regulate angiostatin levels have been claimed in the patent application [78]. Among the several compounds, amifostine injection resulted in a four-fold enhancement of angiostatin levels found in control mice. The application claims a method for reducing the number of metastasis in an animal exhibiting a primary tumor. The generation of angiostatin *in vivo* from plasminogen with a plasminogen activator and a sulfhydryl donar or interaction of plasmin with a sulfhydryl donar was initially disclosed [79]. A patent assigned to Gencell SAS claims anti-angiogenic gene therapy vector for delivering nucleic acid molecule which expresses anti-angiogenesis polypeptides-comprises an amino terminal fragment of urokinase that comprises an EGF-like domain [80]. A patent application filed by Genetix Pharmaceuticals, Inc., claims gene therapy using a nucleic acid molecule which expresses an anti-angiogenic polypeptide selected from the group consisting of human angiostatin, murine angiostatin, human endostatin, murine endostatin, and angiogenesis-inhibiting fragments thereof for inhibiting tumor growth in a human patient harboring a solid tumor [81]. A method of regulating the size and/or growth of normal vasculature in normal tissue including adipose tissue, intestinal polyps and muscle tissue using angiogenesis inhibitors such as TNP-470, angiostatin, endostatin and thalidomide was disclosed in the application from Children's hospital [82]. An issued patent assigned to Dana Farber Cancer Institute, Arch Development Corporation and Beth Israel Deaconess Medical Center, Inc. claims a method of sensitizing cells to radiation therapy using angiogenesis inhibitors such as angiostatin and endostatin [83].

A patent from Karolinska Innovation claims proteins and nucleic acid encoding for proteins containing kringle domains 1, 2 or 3 with kringle 5 as inhibitors of angiogenesis. It claims the synergistic activity observed when kringle 5 is used in combination with other domains [84]. A patent from Conjuchem claims a derivative of kringle 5 peptide where the derivative comprises a reactive group which reacts with amino group, hydroxyl group or thiols on blood protein to form a stable bond to increase the circulating half life of kringle 5 [85]. An application from Northwestern University claims method for producing angiostatin by treatment of plasminogen with a plasminogen activator and a sulfhydryl donor [71]. A method of modulating angiogenesis using modified plasminogen activator inhibitor-1 (PAI-1) has been claimed in an application by Dartmouth College. The modified version of plasminogen activator inhibitor-1 (PAI-1) has also been shown to inhibit cell proliferation, migration and also produce proteolytic fragment corresponding to angiostatin kringle 1-3 or kringle 1-4 [68]. A method of inhibiting disorders associated with vascular hyper permeability by administering effective amount of an anti-angiogenic compound consisting of endostatin, thrombospondin, angiostatin, tumstatin, arresten recombinant EPO, and polymer conjugated TNP-470 has been claimed in the patent application assigned to Children's Medical Center [86]. The patent from Pfizer relates to feline angiostatin genes. The invention includes nucleic acids sequence, angiostatin variants or antibodies directly against such product [87]. It relates more to methods for diagnostic evaluation, genetic testing and prognosis of angiogenesis-related diseases. The invention from EntreMed provides method for recombinant production, recovery and purification of angiostatin protein. It provides details for large scale recovery and purification of recombinantly-produced human angiostatin [88]. Finally, the patent from Karolinska Institute provides the sequence of a protein capable of acting as an angiostatin receptor as well as the nucleic acid sequence thereof. The invention also relates to the use of the receptor in screening methods wherein novel substances could be created exhibiting similar biological properties as angiostatin [89].

Endostatin

Endostatin is an endogenous collagen XVIII-derived angiogenesis inhibitor identified and purified from murine hemangioendothelioma cell line (EOMA) and later characterized in mice [90]. Recombinant endostatin efficiently blocks different processes of angiogenesis and has been shown to suppress primary tumor growth and metastasis in experimental animal models without any apparent side effects, toxicity or development of drug resistance [91]. Endostatin mediates its effect on cell adhesion and cell structure components through down regulation of many signaling pathways associated with proangiogenic activity and at the same time up-regulating many anti-angiogenic genes. Endostatin patents include those describing initial identification, characterization and mechanisms of action are described as follows [91-98]. The patent application from Children's hospital listing Prof. Judah Folkman and O'Reilly as inventors claims protein and DNA sequences of endostatin as well as their use in treating angiogenesis related diseases such as cancer [94]. Two patents filed by Merck claims methods for preparing soluble endostatin, one expressing it in *Streptomyces* and second describes methods for preparing recombinant form of endostatin linked to a cleavable linker with an isolation tag [99, 100]. A patent from Novartis claims an adenoviral vector-mediated delivery of endostatin for the treatment of cancer cell metastases [101]. A patent from Burnham Institute claims peptide variants of endostatin containing 4 - 7 amino acids residues for inhibiting angiogenesis [102]. Separate claims for endostatin variants containing the amino acids sequence RGD are also included in the application [52, 94, 98, 103]. A patent from the Universities of Milan and Florence claims fragments of endostatin 10-60 amino acids with anti-angiogenic activity. It also describes a process for the preparation as well as pharmaceutical formulation of the said peptide [104]. Patents filed by MIT and Children's hospital show the effects of angiogenesis inhibitor using an animal model for obesity, intestinal polyps, cardiac hypertrophy and endometriosis. Methods for regulating the growth and size of normal vascular tissues and reducing obesity through the use of angiogenesis inhibitors is covered by patents filed by Children's Medical Center [82, 94]. Another patent filed by Children's Medical Center claims the sequence of endostatin and method of producing endostatin using recombinant DNA technology [95]. An issued patent application assigned to Dana Farber Cancer Institute, Arch Development Corporation and Beth Israel Deaconess Medical Center, Inc. claims a method of sensitizing cells to radiation therapy using angiogenesis inhibitors such as angiostatin and endostatin [83].

Patents from EntreMed disclose that endostatin may act through a structural epitope that is common with PITSLRE protein kinase and claim a method of regulating angiogenesis through a protein that is homologous to PITSLRE kinase including endostatin which is an angiogenic factor and its use in treating angiogenic-related diseases [105-107]. An albumin fusion protein comprising angiogenesis inhibiting protein such as endostatin or fragment thereof wherein the albumin fusion extends the *in vivo* half-life of angiogenesis inhibiting factor is claimed by a patent assigned to Aventis Behring GMBH and Delta Biotechnology

Ltd. The invention further relates to the composition and methods for preventing primary tumor or metastatic growth as well as for treating diabetic retinopathy, progressive macular degeneration or rheumatic arthritis [108, 109]. A patent application assigned to Pfizer claims methods and compositions for diagnosing and treating disorder involving angiogenesis. The invention relates to feline endostatin gene. It describes methods for the identification of compounds that modulated the expression of endostatin genes [87].

Diagnostic methods and kits for the detection and quantitation of endostatin in biological fluids and tissues were described in the patent filed by Children's hospital [95]. The application claims the usefulness of angiogenesis inhibitors in benign tumor diseases, rheumatoid arthritis, psoriasis and ocular diseases. An approved patent assigned to Searle and Co. claims methods for the isolation of endostatin expressed in a prokaryotic expression system from inclusion bodies [110]. Also it describes method for refolding the protein isolated from inclusion after solubulizing in denaturant. The nuclcic acid sequence encoding endostatin and related sequences and their use in gene therapy or recombinant expression for the treatment of angiogenesis-related diseases are claimed in a granted patent assigned to The Children's Medical Center [96]. Following this, a patent from Children's Medical center claims endostatin derived from collagen protein and therapeutic compositions containing endostatin and their use as anti-angiogenic agent [97]. A patent from Pfizer Inc., claims endostatin comprising amino acids 1-175 or fusion protein comprising the isolated polypeptide for the diagnostic evaluation, genetic testing and prognosis of angiogenesis-related disorders [111]. US Patents granted to Beth Israel Deaconess Medical Center claim the expression of biologically active soluble endostatin protein using a yeast expression system as well as a deletion mutant of endostatin (EM-1) for the treatment of cancer [112, 113]. Finally, the patent from Milano University claims polypeptides with sequence prepared by solid phase synthesis corresponding or homologous to endostatin for the treatment of angiogenesis-dependent tumors. A patent granted to Milano University claims a polypeptide prepared by solid phase synthesis which is pentacontapeptide IV having the sequence Cys-Glu-Thr-Trp-Arg-Thr-Glu-Thr-Thr-Gly-Ala-Thr-Gly-Gln-Ala-Ser-Ser-Leu-Ser-Gly-Arg-Leu-Leu-Glu-Gln-Lys-Ala-Ala-Ser-Cys-His-Asn-Ser-Tyr-Ile-Val-Leu-Cys(tBu)-Ile-Glu-Asn-Ser-P and a method of inhibiting angiogenesis using the said peptide [105, 114].

Type IV Collagen-Derived Fragments

The main component of vascular basement membrane is Type IV collagen, forming a mesh-like structure with other macromolecules, such as laminin, heparan sulfate proteoglycans (HSPG), fibronectin, and entactin [115]. Type IV collagen is composed of six distinct gene products (α1- α6). It has been reported that the fragments isolated from these gene products are found to have inhibitory effect on endothelial cells [116]. The NC1 domains of collagen IV- α1, α2, α3 αvδ α6 exert anti-angiogenic activity by regulating endothelial cell adhesion, proliferation and migration [40, 117-133]. Patent applications from BIDMC claim three anti-angiogenic proteins, arresten, canstatin and tumstatin having anti-angiogenic properties [121, 122]. Arresten is an endogenous inhibitor, a protein comprising NC-1 domain of the α-1 chain, canstatin comprises the NC-1 domain of the α-2 chain and tumstatin, the NC-1 domain of α-3 domain of Type IV collagen. The patents claim tumstatin and its peptide fragments with particular sequence formula for inhibition of cap-dependent protein synthesis or endothelial cells expressing $\alpha_v\beta_3$. Patent applications from University of Kansas Medical Center describe methods for inhibiting angiogenesis, tumor growth and metastasis using an isolated Type IV collagen NC-1 domain of α-1, α-2, α-3 or α-6 chain monomer or protein construct [118, 119]. Following this, Biostratum patent describes methods and kits for inhibiting angiogenesis, tumor growth and metastasis [134]. The invention describes the use of domains of Type IV collagen to inhibit the interactions with the ECM or to a specific integrin receptor. The patent from Peter Brook's group describes the use of an antagonist that binds specifically to a proteolyzed or denatured form of collagen. The antagonists include monoclonal antibodies referred to as HU177, HUIV26 and XL313 [135]. The crystal structure of NC-1 domain hexamer of Type IV collagen was disclosed in patent application filed by University of Kansas [136]. It provides a rational drug design methods based on the analysis of Type IV collagen NC-1 hexamer structure as well as specific compositions of matter derived by utilizing the rational drug design method described in the patent. The patent application from New York University describes method for inhibiting angiogenesis using an antagonist specific for proteolyzed or denatured form of Type IV collagen for therapeutic treatment of tumor growth, metastasis or of restenosis as well as specific peptide antagonists against denatured or proteolyzed forms of Type IV collagen [137]. Also, methods to use such antagonist as diagnostic markers of angiogenesis in normal or diseases both *in vitro* and *in vivo* are described. The use of 7S domain of Type IV collagen to disrupt cell aggregation or tissue development was disclosed in patent application filed by University of Kansas [120, 138]. The claims encompass either the 7S domain or the NC-1 domain of Type IV collagen or substantially homologous protein construct which contain the specific structural elements within the 7S and NC-1domain. The granted patents claim methods for inhibiting tumor growth by using Type IV collagen α-2 NC-1 domain, antibody against such a domain and methods of treating angiogenesis mediated diseases with Type IV collagen α- 3 NC-1 domain.

Thrombospondin

Thrombospondin-1 (TSP-1) was the first protein to be recognized as a naturally occurring inhibitor of angiogenesis [139]. It is a large multifunctional ECM glycoprotein that regulates various biological events, such as cell adhesion, angiogenesis, cell proliferation and survival, transforming growth factor-β (TGF-β) activation and protease activation [140]. Studies have suggested that TSP may possess dual activity (proangiogenic and anti-angiogenic) depending on proteases that generate fragments of TSP-1 [95, 141-150]. TSP regulates various biological events like cell adhesion, angiogenesis, cell proliferation and survival, transforming growth factor-β activation and protease activation. TSP has been shown to inhibit tumor growth and metastasis, thus making it a potent inhibitor of *in vivo* neovascularization and tumorigenesis. A patent from Massachusetts General Hospital (MGH) features method for treating disorders characterized by unwanted angiogenesis by increasing TSP-2 activity [151, 152]. The invention also claims methods for identifying compounds which might modulate TSP-2 activity. The patents also claim synthetic peptides or fragments of TSP-2 with anti-angiogenic activity for the treatment of unwanted angiogenesis. A patent from Human Genome Sciences claims nucleic acids coding for proteins related to thrombospondin, human METH1 and METH 2 as well as methods of producing the proteins by recombinant DNA technology, the polypeptide sequences and their use for inhibiting angiogenesis [142]. A patent from BIDMC elucidates the molecular mechanism involved in the inhibition of tumor growth by the Type I repeats of TSP-1 [145]. The method for making recombinant version of these motifs have been claimed and demonstrated to inhibit the growth of experimental B16F10 and Lewis lung carcinomas in a xenograft model. The polypeptides, variants, fragments generated either by recombinant DNA technology or chemical synthesis have been claimed in the filing. A patent from Children's Hospital describes methods for decreasing or inhibiting disorders associated with vascular hyper permeability and a method for screening compounds that affect vascular permeability [86]. The method includes administration of anti-angiogenic compound selected from the group consisting of endostatin, thrombospondin, angiostatin, tumstatin, arresten and polymer conjugated to TNP-470. It claims methods for assessing bioeffectiveness of anti-angiogenic compounds in a patient treated with above compounds. A patent application by Zhang describes the therapeutic utility of TSP-1, TSP-1-agonist, peptides and mimics as well as inducers of TSP-1 when used in conjunction with inhibitors of VEGF [153]. This application also discloses the important mechanism of action of TSP in modulating the role of HGF/SF in tumor development. Furthermore, the patent discloses that the ectopic expression of TSP-1 markedly inhibits tumor formation through the suppression of angiogenesis.

Antithrombin III Fragment (AT-III)

The circulating clotting factors in the blood seems to play an important role in angiogenesis [154]. Antithrombin III (AT-III) is a member of the serpin family and functions as an inhibitor of the clotting cascade. An issued patent from Biovitrum describes protein purification processes for the preparation of substantially pure AT-III, the antithrombin isoforms- AT-III α and AT-III β and histidine-rich glycoprotein (HRGP) [155]. The invention claims a process for the preparation of pure AT-III and its isoforms using a cation exchange chromatography wherein the cation exchange groups are attached to a gel matrix. Children's Hospital claims in its issued patent a method for inhibiting tumor growth using a non-native conformation of AT-III. The non-native conformation of AT-III comprises the *N*-terminal half of the reactive center loop, or a portion thereof, inserted as a sixth strand into the A-beta sheet of AT-III [156]. The administration of non-native conformation of AT-III from the L-form was shown to inhibit tumor growth, an effect reported in a recent publication [157-160]. Modified versions of AT-III which is resistant to elastase is claimed in a patent granted to Temple University. The patent describes methods for producing elastase-resistant AT-III by introducing specific modifications at positions P4 and P5 of AT-III. The patent further claims AT-III that has enhanced heparin binding activity. The compounds may have applicability in treating or reducing pathological symptoms due to sepsis, trauma, acute respiratory distress syndrome, thrombosis and stroke [161].

Kininogen

Kininogen is a 120- kDa glycoprotein containing heavy and light chains comprising of domains 1-3 and domains 5-6 respectively [162-170]. The mechanism by which high molecular weight kininogen (Hka) exerts its anti-angiogenic activity remains controversial, but appears to involve binding to cell surface tropomyosin and induction of apoptosis of proliferating endothelial cells. A role for tropomyosin in mediating the anti-angiogenic signals of other anti-angiogenic proteins such as endostatin and histidine-proline-rich glycoprotein (HPRG) has also been reported. Three applications from Temple University refer to peptide analogues of high and low molecular weight kininogen (LK and HK). The first and second applications, have claims to peptide analogues of the light chain domain 5 comprising segment of *N*-terminal or *C*-terminal truncated fragments. The peptide analogues have the formula X1-His-Lys-X-Lys-X2 wherein X is any amino acid, X1 is from zero to twelve amino acids and X2 is from zero to twelve amino acids. Methods for inhibiting endothelial cell proliferation and angiogenesis are specifically claimed using the peptides analogues derived from the above formula [171, 172]. A series of synthetic peptide analogues of HK domain 3 is claimed in another patent application assigned to Temple University (137). Similar to HK domain 5 peptide analogues, the patent provides specific peptide formulae including biologically active fragments of high molecular weight kininogen domain as well as claims for methods for inhibiting endothelial cell proliferation and angiogenesis using the peptide analogues to HK domain 3. [173]. Six peptides were evaluated for inhibitory activity in subnanomolar concentration. In addition to the generic claims, five specific amino acid sequences ranging in length from 10-185 amino acids are claimed. Similarly, methods of inhibiting angiogenesis using antibodies directed against an antigenic determinant of high molecular weight kininogen domain 5 containing amino acid Gly 440 to Lys 502 are claimed in another patent application assigned to Temple University [174]. Peptides corresponding to the human kininogen D5 (domain 5), fusion peptides containing peptide sequences corresponding to human kininogen D5 and antibodies directed against the kininogen D5 are claimed to in another PCT application [139]. The use of these peptides for diagnosis as well as therapy of diseases associated with endothelial cell migration and proliferation are also claimed in the application as well as nucleic acid sequences encoding the peptides, recombinant cells expressing the peptides and methods for isolating D5 from such cells [175]. In parallel, peptides from kringle domain 5 having the formula X sub.1-His-Lys-X-Lys-X sub.2 wherein X is any amino acid, X sub.1 is from zero to 12 amino acid and X sub.2 is from zero to 12 amino acids more preferably from zero to six amino acids and most preferably from zero to three amino acids as well as method of using the above peptides to inhibit endothelial cell proliferation and angiogenesis are claimed in a granted US patent [176]. Similar to D5, human kininogen domain 3 (HK-D3) polypeptide or biologically active variants and derivatives of HK-D3 as well as methods of inhibiting angiogenesis using such compounds have been claimed in a PCT application [177]. Because of anti-angiogenic function of HK-D3, these molecules could be potentially used to treat cancer by inhibiting or reversing the growth of primary or metastatic tumors. Similar claims of peptide analogs to high molecular weight kininogen domain 3 as potent inhibitors of angiogenesis have been claimed by a group from Temple University [142]. They claim specifically peptide analogs of high molecular weight kininogen domain 3 derived from the peptide formula or *N*-terminal and *C*-terminal biologically active fragments for inhibition of endothelial cell proliferation and angiogenesis [178].

Prolactin Fragment

The intact prolactin (23-kDa) is an enzymatically cleaved in different tissues to generate a 16-kDa and a 8-kDa fragments [179-181]. The 16-kDa fragment inhibits VEGF-induced activation of Ras in capillary endothelial cells. Fusion protein derivatives consisting of a soluble anti-angiogenic polypeptide such as 16-kDa fragment of prolactin covalently attached to a membrane binding domain to target the anti-angiogenic peptide to site of active angiogenesis is claimed in a PCT application assigned to Adprotech [146]. A method of multimerizing anti-angiogenic polypeptides including the fragments containing prolactin by creating a fusion protein with a portion of *N*-terminal region of human cartilage oligomeric matrix protein (COMP) which allows pentamer formations thereby making an effective anti-angiogenic molecule has been disclosed in the patent application by Beth Israel Deaconess Medical Center [144]. The use of nucleic acid molecules, vectors and host cells for the expression and production of these chimeric proteins have been claimed in this patent filed by BIDMC. Similarly, novel fusion proteins comprising a receptor antagonizing domain such as prolactin-antagonist domain coupled to an angiogenesis inhibitor domain such as human endostatin have been claimed in a PCT application by Greenville Hospital System. The patent also has claims to methods of treatment using a number of such fusion proteins [109].

Fibronectin Fragment

The ED-B domain of fibronectin which is inserted by alternative splicing specifically accumulate around neovascular site and could be potentially used as a target for molecular intervention [182]. Antibodies with subnanomolar affinity to the epitope of the ED-B domain of fibronectin or fusion proteins have been claimed by numerous patents [183-186] including conjugates consisting of an antibody against ED-B domain fused to a group of proteins such as IL-2 or IL-12 or TNF-α or IFN-γ. Selective targeting of tumor vasculature using an antibody or antibody fragments with binding affinity for ED-B have been claimed by a patent filed by Schering Plough AG. The patent also claims different diagnostic and therapeutic applications of these antibodies and antibody fragments [187]. In contrast to the anti-angiogenic approach, ECM containing fibronectin or fragment there of have been used to deliver VEGF 165 or VEGF 121 to a site to promote angiogenesis as a method to stimulate angiogenesis with potential utility in wound healing process [188].

Endorepellin

Perlecan is a HSPG (heparan sulfate proteoglycan) of basement membrane that plays an important role in vascular growth [189, 190]. The COOH- terminal end of perlecan, called endorepellin or perlecan domain V, potently inhibits several processes of angiogenesis. Endorepellin binds to endothelial cells as well as to squamous cell carcinoma via a high affinity receptor. The exact mechanism of by which endorepellin exerts its anti-angiogenic effect is not yet known. The anti-angiogenic function of endorepellin has been described in the patent applications from Thomas Jefferson University and which claims its utility for the treatment of tumors or angiogenesis-mediated diseases. The patents claim endorepellin protein or its fragments or derivatives as well as methods for inhibition of the growth of tumor-associated blood vessels comprising administration of endorepellin protein or its fragments or derivatives. Also claimed in the applications are the use of anti-endorepellin antibody for detection, diagnosis and monitoring the process of angiogenesis involved in tumor growth and angiogenesis-mediated disease conditions [191, 192]

Endostatin-Like Fragment from Type XV Collagen

A fragment related to endostatin was identified by homology based search [193]. The 22-kDa fragment of collagen XV was named as restin and reported to inhibit migration of endothelial cells with no effect on proliferation [193-196]. Systemic administration of recombinant protein suppressed the growth of renal cell carcinoma (786-0) in a xenograft model [193]. Patent application filed by BIDMC discloses that one of the fragments of non-collagenous domain of Type XV named Restin is an anti-angiogenic molecule with activity equal to or superior to that endostatin [101]. The use of restin and apomigren to induce apoptosis of endothelial cells and inhibition of angiogenic response in mammalian tissues are disclosed in the patent application [113]. The patent has claims directed towards, methods for making recombinant restin with anti-angiogenic properties using yeast expression systems. The patent claims method for producing biologically active anti-angiogenic protein or biologically active mutant, fragment, derivatives or fusion proteins there of using the yeast including *Pichia pastoris* [112, 113, 197, 198].

Pigment Epithelium-Derived Factor

In 1999, the pigment epithelium-derived factor (PEDF), the most potent inhibitor of angiogenesis in the mammalian eye, was identified to be responsible for the avasculairty of ocular compartment, [199, 200]. PEDF possesses several physiological properties of which its selective anti-angiogenic effect restricted to only new vessel growth without affecting the preexisting vessel is the hallmark for this factor [201, 202]. Methods of inhibiting angiogenesis within a tissue by proving PEDF to endothelial cells associated with the said tissue such as tissue near tumor, eyes, joints, skin, etc., as a soluble protein or by viral-mediated gene transfer has been claimed by patent applications filed by Bouck, *et al.* NorthWestern University. The patent also has claims to methods for using it as a diagnostic factor for determining the severity of tumor which shows a nice correlation to the presence of PEDF within the tumor [203, 204]. Issued patent assigned to Genvec Inc., claims methods for the delivery of PEDF using an adenoviral vector or an adeno-associated viral vector [205, 206].

Platelet Factor- 4 (PF- 4)

PF- 4, a protein released from platelet α-granule during platelet aggregation has been shown to have anti-angiogenic properties both *in vitro* and *in vivo* [159, 207-210]. A patent assigned to Curative Technologies claims octapeptide derived from PF- 4 and seven structurally related peptides which are capable of inducing an angiogenic response *in vivo* [211]. The angiogenic peptide of the invention may be particularly useful in promoting wound healing including incisional healing, bone repair and burn healing. In contrast, patents from Eli Lilly & Co claim methods of inhibiting angiogenesis and tumor growth using two modified forms of human PF- 4 named as MPF- 4 and CPF- 4 which are approximately 10 - 100 fold more potent than native or recombinant PF- 4 in inhibiting endothelial cell growth [212, 213]. The minor modification in the active site of PF- 4 by the addition of ERL domain significantly improves its anti-angiogenic potential. Finally, a patent from JCR Pharmaceuticals Co., claims a process for isolation of native PF- 4 using a more readily available sulfated chitin which significantly improved the purification as well as its yield [214].

Miscellaneous Inhibitors

The patent landscape involving angiogenesis continues to show robust growth. Selected subsets of various endogenous angiogenesis inhibitors in clinical development are illustrated in Table **5**. Applications related to MMPIs continues to grow in number and in complexity [215-220]. The patent application from University of Southern California claims methods and compositions for inhibiting

Table 5: List of selected anti-angiogenic inhibitors including endogenous inhibitors in Clinical trials (Source NCI-PDQ Clinical Trial Database).

Drug/ Target	Sponsor/ Company	Mechanism	Clinical Devel. Status
I Endogenous inhibitors of angiogenesis			
Alphastatin	Novartis	Proliferation	Preclinical
Angiostatin	EntreMed	Proliferation & Migration	Phase II
Arresten	Ilex Oncology	Proliferation & Migration	Preclinical
Antithrombin- III	Children's Hospital	Proliferation & Migration	Preclinical
Canstatin	Ilex Oncology	Proliferation & Migration	Preclinical
Endostatin	EntreMed	Proliferation & Migration	Phase II
Fibulin-5	NIH	Proliferation	Preclinical
Interferon-beta	Biogen	Proliferation	Phase III
2-methoxyestradiol	EntreMed	Proliferation	Phase II
PEDF	GeneVec Inc.,	Proliferation	Phase I
Platelet factor-4	Eli Lilly	Proliferation	Phase I
Thrombospondin-1	Abbot Laboratories	Proliferation & Migration	Phase II
TIMP-2	NIH	Proliferation	Phase I
Tumstatin	Ilex Oncology	Proliferation & adhesion	Preclinical
HRGP		Proliferation	Preclinical
II Inhibitors of extracellular matrix breakdown (MMPI)			
Marimastat/ Batismastat	British Biotech	Broadspectrum MMPI	Phase III- breast, lung
Prinomastat	Agouron/Warner	MMP-2 & MMP-9	Phase III NSCLC
Neovastat (AE- 941)	Aeterna Lab	Naturally occuring MMPI	Phase III- colon,& kidney
BAY 12-9566	Bayer	MMP-2 & MMP-9 inhibitor	Phase III- lung, ovary
COL-3/CMT-3	CollaGenex	Tetracycline derived MMPI	Phase I
BMS-275291	Bristol-Myers Squibb	Broadspectrum MMPI	Phase II- Kaposi's
CGS-27023A	Novartis	Broadspectrum MMPI	Phase II Discontinued
Captopril	Bristol-Myers Squibb	MMPI	Phase II-solid tumor
III Inhibitors of endothelial cell proliferation and migration			
TNP-470	TAP Pharmaceuticals	Inhibits EC growth	Phase II-solid tumor
Thalidomide	Celgene	Inhibits GF mediated growth	Phase II/III-Head & neck
2-Methoxyestradiol	EntreMed	Inhibits EC growth	Phase I solid tumor
Combretastatin	Oxigene	Induction of EC apoptosis	Phase I/II
Squalamine	Genera	Inhibits NHE 3 exchanger	Phase III-NSCLC
Farnesyl Transferase	NCI & Merck	Blocks EC proliferation	Phase I solid tumor
IV Inhibitors of endothelial cell receptor tyrosine kinase			
SU 5416	SUGEN/Pfizer	Blocks VEGFR2 receptor	Phase I/II Kaposi's
SU 6668	SUGEN/Pfizer	Blocks VEGFR, FGFR& PDGF	Phase I
SU11248	SUGEN/Pfizer	Blocks VEGFR1& VEGFR2	Phase I ongoing
PTK 787/ZK22584	Schering/Novartis	Blocks VEGF receptor	Phase I
ZD 6474	Astra Zeneca	Blocks VEGFR2 & EGFR	Phase I- II
CP547, 632	Pfizer	Blocks VEGFR2& EGFR	Phase I
PD173074		Blocks FGFR1	Phase I

angiogenesis using a peptide that contains a specific amino acid sequence of MMP-2 [217]. It describes methods for detecting angiogenesis in tumor tissue, metastasis and tumor invasion and provides screening approaches to detect those processes. A patent from Exelixis Inc., describes the role of ADAM-10 (A disintegrin and metalloproteinase domain 10) (Mammalian disintegrin-metalloprotease) protein in biological processes and claims compositions and methods for modulating the activity of ADAM-10 and their utility for the treatment of cancer, arthritis and disease related to angiogenesis [218]. The patent from US Department of Health claims composition such as calreticulin fragments and variants, methods for producing the composition and method of use for the compositions for inhibiting endothelial cell growth [221]. Such approaches are useful for the treatment of cancer and diseases associated with unwanted angiogenesis [221]. The fragment of calreticulin *N*-domain and fusion protein there of have been claimed to have anti-endothelial activity. The efficacy of calreticulin fragment on inhibiting tumor growth including the growth of Burkitt lymphoma, breast adenocarcinoma, colon, lung and melanoma have been described.

Interleukins (IL) are a family of leukocyte-derived protein with broad-ranging effects on multiple physiological processes including angiogenesis [222]. IL-12 and IL-18 are interferon (IFN-γ) inducing cytokines. IL-12 has been shown to inhibit angiogenesis through downstream chemokines such as IFN- inducible protein -10 (IP-10) and monokine induced by IFN-γ [160, 223]. A patent from Wistar Institute claims composition and methods for co-administration of synergistic amounts of IL-12 and IL-18 for the prevention or retardation of tumor cell growth [224]. A patent from Centocor describes a method of using IL-6 antagonist to treat pathological processes associated with cancer specifically neovascularization. It relates to the use of IL-6 antagonist such as antibodies directed toward IL-6 protein or fragments there of in an amount sufficient to inhibit angiogenesis [225]. Interferons, pleiotropic cytokines known to regulate numerous biological processes were the first endogenous anti-angiogenic regulators identified [226]. A PCT application claims virus particles that replicate exclusively in tumor cells and express high levels of interferon exclusively in tumor cells [194]. The patent claims that the presence of high levels of interferon around the tumor site evokes immune reaction resulting in inhibition of both growth and metastasis of tumor [227].

Emerging Targeted Therapies

The emerging concept of targeted therapy for cancer related to angiogenesis can be grouped into three categories - vascular targeted therapy, stem-cell targeted therapy and compounds derived from natural products. A number of emerging inhibitors belonging to different catogories in various stages of clinical development are shown in Table **6** [228-236] followed by potential molecules in the late stage of clinical development Table **7**. Although the idea of targeted therapy towards tumor vasculature as an anticancer therapy has been around for some time, Burrows and Thorpe were the first to provide experimental evidence of efficacy by targeting the toxin ricin to the tumor vasculature in an experimental mouse model [237]. Anti-vascular tumor therapy represents a promising new strategy for cancer treatment. It differs from the aforementioned anti-angiogenic therapies since the target for vascular disrupting agents (VDA's) is pre-existing vasculature, whereas traditional anti-angiogenic therapy is based on inhibition of neovascularization [238-242]. The issued US patents related with VDAs have increased from 9 in 2001 to 20 in 2005 and there are > 10 issued patents covering VDAs from January to September of 2006. Although some single agent activities have been observed with VDAs, such as OXi-4503, VDAs have shown the best efficacy when in combination with other anticancer agents. The success of Oxigene's vascular damaging agent CA4P has generated interest in the area of neovascular targeting strategies [243]. There is growing evidence that some, if not all, tumors derive from a small number of stem-cell-like cells that either retain or acquire capacity for self-renewal. Based on the unique cell-surface expression, monoclonal antibodies may be designed to target them specifically [3]. The blockage of signaling pathways required for stem-cell function could be potentially exploited using pharmacological blockers. But the performance of such inhibitors in clinical trials is still being debated. Nevertheless, there is still significant activity in the natural product front, where analogues of existing compounds are disclosed or new utilities of existing agents are identified. Numerous cytotoxic agents derived from natural products are being identified and evaluated for their ability to inhibit endothelial cell proliferation, tumor growth and metastasis as a method of controlling angiogenesis.

Table 6: Selected list of candidates in the VDA field in preclinical and clinical development.

Compound name	Sponsor	Reference
CA4P	Arizona State University/OxiGENE	[228]
OXi-493	Arizona State University/OxiGENE	[229]
DMXAA	University of Auckland	[230]
MN-029	Angiogene Pharmaceuticals	[231]
ZD6126	AstraZeneca	[232]
AVE8062	Sanofi-Aventis/Ajinomoto	[233]
NPI-2358	Nereus Pharmaceuticals	[234]
EPC2407	EpiCept	[235]
4,5 Diaryl-		
isoxazole	Synta Pharmaceuticals	[236]

Table 7: List of late phases (Phase II & Phase III) anti-angiogenic agents.

Brand	Drug	Target	Company	Indication	Phase
Not known	Aflibercept (VEGF-TRAP)	VEGF	Sanofi Aventis/Regenron	NSCLC and ovarian cancer	III
Recentin	Cediranib (AZD2171)	VEGFR1,2 & 3	AstraZeneca	CRC, NSCLC, GBM	III
Not known	Pazopanib	PDGFR, Kit & VEGFRs	GlaxoSmithKline	RCC, ovarian & breast cancer	III
Angiostatin	K1-4	Angiogenesis inhibitor	EntreMed	NSCLC	II
Apilidin	Plitidepsin	VEGFR1	PharmaMar	SCLC, AML, ALL & MM	II
Endostatin	NSC704805	Angiogenesis inhibitor	EntreMed	Melanoma & NET	II
Everolimus	mTOR inhibitor		Novartis	Neuroendocrine tumor, breast & lung	II
AMG 386	Ang-2 Peptibody	Angiopoietin	Amgen	RCC, metastatic breast cancer	II
Vitaxin	MEDI-522	Integrin	AstraZeneca	Melanoma, CRC & prostate	II
Not known	ATN-161	Integrin RTK	Attenuon	Gliomas	II
Not known	Cilengitide	Integrin RTK	Merck Serono	NSCLC, glioma & pancreatic	II

Table 7: cont....

Not known	Combrestastati n	Cadherin 5	OXiGENE	CRC, NSCLC & head and neck	II
Not known	ORA-101	Angiognesis inhibitor	Yeda	NSCLC	II
Not known	SU14813	VEGFR	Pfizer	Breast cancer	II
Not known	Volociximab	Integrin cMab	PDL Biopharma	NSCLC, RCC & melanoma	II
Not known	ABT 510	Thrombospondin	Annptt :anpratproes	NSCLC, RCC & sarcoma	II

Side-Effects and Resistance to Anti-Angiogenic Therapies

Although, anti-angiogenic agents were felt initially to lack significant toxicity, it is becoming increasingly clear that these agents are not without toxicity. Bevacizumab therapy - particularly at high doses may lead to severe hypertension, proteinuria and renal thrombotic microangiopathy (TMA) features that resemble human preeclampsia in 10-20% of the subjects [244]. These complications are class effects as similar pathologies have been observed in rodents rendered VEGF deficient [245, 246]. Other small molecule inhibitors of VEGF signaling such as sunitinib and sorafenib have also been associated with similar side effects [247]. Although rare, bevacizumab can also lead to life threatening cerebral edema with reversible posterior leucoencephalopathy that can be detected with MRI scans of the central nervous [248, 249]. Bowel perforations and thyroid dysfunction has also been noted in subjects exposed VEGF inhibitors chronically [250, 251]

The mechanisms of resistance to anti-VEGF therapies are beginning to be understood. One important pathway that is up-regulated in the tumors resistant to anti-VEGF therapies is notch-delta like ligand 4 (DLL4) [23, 252, 253]. Interestingly, DLL4 inhibition leads paradoxically to more abnormal vessels, but tumor growth is decreased. Other angiogenic pathways that may contribute to tumor progression include the up-regulation of Angiopoietin-2 (Ang-2), vasoinhibin and bFGF [254]. Phenotypic resistance to functional-blockade of VEGFR antibodies was mediated through reactivation of tumor pro-angiogenesis growth factors, in particular VEGF-A, several FGF-family members, Ephrin-A1 and Angiopoietin-1[255]. Hence, a tumor cell could be envisioned to become resistant to a particular insult by up-regulation of other growth factors. The role of tumor suppressor genes or oncogenes may influence how tumors respond to certain anti-angiogenic agents by making changes in tumor cells to be less dependent on angiogenesis [256, 257]. It has also been reported that infiltration of tumor tissue by myeloid cells ($CD11b^{+}Gr1^{+}$) may contribute to VEGF refractoriness [258]. It has been speculated that the myelosuppression associated with standard chemotherapy may contribute to the success of bevacizumab therapy when used in combination with chemotherapy.

A functional role of tumor associated stromal cells in the progression of cervical carcinoma was demonstrated by pharmacological blockade of PDGF receptor signaling (imatinib) [259]. The combined synergestic effect of targeting both VEGFR (SU5416) and PDGFR (Gleevec) has shown promising results compared to individual treatment in pancreatic islet cancer, the RIP1Tag2 mouse model [260]. Anti-angiogenic molecules in addition to their predominant effect on tumor-associated endothelial cells can also play a role in immunomodulation, as were demonstrated in combination treatment schedules. Studies have shown that a metronomic cytoxan anti-angiogenic regimen used in patients with advanced chemotherapy resistant cancers also decreased the number of circulating T-reg cells and restored T cell proliferation and NK cell effector function [261, 262]. These studies provide evidence for combining conventional chemotherapeutic modalities with immunotherapeutic agents.

CURRENT & FUTURE DEVELOPMENTS

The availability of global gene expression analyses technology coupled with sequencing of human genome has led to the exponential growth in the identification of novel drug targets in the last 5 years. The relative lack of serious side effects compared to traditional chemotherapy makes angiogenesis inhibitors an extremely attractive option. The discovery of numerous endogenous inhibitors of angiogenesis represents an important step which might constitute a critical line of defense against the conversion of dormant tumor into a malignant phenotype. Currently, at least 27 different proteins and small molecules are known to exist in the body which influences the growth and functions as inhibitors of angiogenesis. The field of anti-angiogenesis therapy related to exploiting the endogenous inhibitors continues to dominate the field. The sheer numbers of applications that claim these inhibitors continue to rise. Early results from clinical trials with angiostatin, endostatin and TSP suggest that further studies are required to understand the mechanism of action and dosing regiments. The optimal dosing of anti-angiogenic therapy is another key issue for further research. Preclinical and recent clinical data suggest that concept of using the maximum tolerated dose may not be applicable for this line of therapy. The early clinical data suggest that these agents are primarily cytostatic, hence greater emphasis on patient survival relative to the objective response may be more appropriate. The patents covering the angiogenesis inhibitors will continue to remain robust as the research is so exciting and unprecedented in cancer drug discovery. Though there are increasing number of applications directed towards a single agent, the time will tell whether these agents live up to their potential as a single agent or works better in combination with established cytotoxics. Finally, future research with anti-angiogenic therapy either alone or in combination will focus on determining the tumor type and stage of cancer that is most vulnerable for therapy using this approach.

ACKNOWLEDGEMENTS

We gratefully acknowledge support from the EMD Serono Inc. management team including colleagues from Lead Discovery Technologies for their support.

CONFLICT OF INTEREST:

We declare no conflict of interest.

DISCLOSURE

The chapter submitted for Patent eBook Series "Topics in Anti-Cancer Research, Volume 2 is an update of our article "Endogenous Angiogenesis Inhibitors as Therapeutic Agents: Historical Perspective and Future Direction", published in the journal "Recent Patents on Anti-Cancer Drug Discovery", Volume 1, Number 2, June Issue 2006, Page 223 to 236 with modified title, additional text and references.

REFERENCE

[1] Jemal AMT, Ward E, Samuels A, Tiwari RC, Ghafoor A, Feur EJ, *et al*. Cancer statistics. CA Cancer J Clin 2005; 55: 10-30.

[2] Fleming S, Lucas F, Schofield M. A therapeutic area review of oncology products and players. Expert Opin Emerging Drugs 2001; 6(2): 317-29.
[3] Sawyers C. Targeted cancer therapy. Nature 2004;432: 294-7.
[4] Sawyers CL. Opportunities and challenges in the development of kinase inhibitor therapy for cancer. Genes Dev 2003; 17: 2998-3010.
[5] Kerbel RS. Inhibition of tumor angiogenesis as a strategy to circumvent acquired resistance to anti-cancer therapeutic agents. Bioessays 1991; 13(1): 31-6.
[6] Kerbel RS. A cancer therapy resistant to resistance. Nature 1997; 390(6658): 335-6.
[7] Kerbel RS, Kamen BA. The anti-angiogenic basis of metronomic chemotherapy. Nat Rev Cancer 2004; 4(6): 423-36.
[8] D'Amore PA. Anti-angiogenesis as a strategy for antimetastasis. Semin Thromb Hemost 1988; 14(1): 73-8.
[9] Cristofanilli M, Hortobagyi GN. New horizons in treating metastatic disease. Clin Breast Cancer 2001; 1(4): 276-87.
[10] Jain RK. Anti-angiogenic therapy for cancer: Current and emerging concepts. Oncology (Huntingt) 2005; 19(4): 7-16.
[11] Lenz H-J. Anti-angiogenic agents in cancer therapy. Oncology (Huntingt) 2005; 19(4): 17-25.
[12] Kremmidiotis G, Lavranos TC. Discovery and validation of drug targets for tumor angiogenesis. Expert Opin Ther Targets 2005; 9(2): 211-5.
[13] Ziche M, Donnini S, Morbidelli L. Development of new drugs in angiogenesis. Curr Drug Targets 2004; 5(5): 485-93.
[14] Folkman J. Tumor angiogenesis: Therapeutic implications. N Engl J Med 1971; 285(21): 1182-6.
[15] Folkman J. Tumor angiogensis: Role in regulation of tumor growth. Symp Soc Dev Biol 1974; 30: 43-52.
[16] Folkman J. Tumor angiogenesis. Adv Cancer Res 1974; 19: 331-58.
[17] Folkman J. Angiogenesis-retrospect and outlook. Exs 1992; 61: 4-13.
[18] Folkman J, Shing Y. Angiogenesis. J Biol Chem 1992; 267(16): 10931-4.
[19] Folkman J. Angiogenesis in cancer, vascular, rheumatoid and other disease. Nat Med 1995; 1(1): 27-31.
[20] Folkman J. Angiogenesis and angiogenesis inhibition: An overview. Exs 1997; 79: 1-8.
[21] Folkman J. Angiogenesis inhibitors: A new class of drugs. Cancer Biol Ther 2003; 2(4 Suppl 1): S127-33.
[22] Harris AL. Anti-angiogenesis for cancer therapy. Lancet 1997; 349 (Suppl 2): SII13-5.
[23] Jansen M, de Witt Hamer PC, Witmer AN, Troost D, van Noorden CJ. Current perspectives on anti-angiogenesis strategies in the treatment of malignant gliomas. Brain Res Brain Res Rev 2004; 45(3): 143-63.
[24] O'Connell MJ. Current status of adjuvant therapy for colorectal cancer. Oncology (Huntingt) 2004; 18(6): 751-5.
[25] Slevin M, Payne S. New treatments for colon cancer. BMJ 2004; 329(7458): 124-6.
[26] Wilson JF. Angiogenesis therapy moves beyond cancer. Ann Intern Med 2004; 141(2): 165-8.
[27] Ferrara N, Hillan KJ, Gerber HP, Novotny W. Discovery and development of bevacizumab, an anti-VEGF antibody for treating cancer. Nat Rev Drug Discov 2004; 3(5): 391-400.
[28] Ferrara N, Alitalo K. Clinical applications of angiogenic growth factors and their inhibitors. Nat Med 1999; 5(12): 1359-64.

[29] Birch S. Angiogenesis inhibitors: Recent disappointments and long term prospects; 2000. Report No.: BDHC0269.

[30] Datamonitor. Pipeline insight: Molecular targeted cancer therapies, can anything else revolutionize the market? ; 2007.

[31] Connell RD. Cancer chemotherapeutics-angiogenesis agents. Expert Opin Ther Patents 2000; 10(6): 767-86.

[32] Connell RD, Beebe JS. Patent focus on cancer chemotherapeutics. II Angiogenesis agents. Expert Opin Ther Patents 2001; 11(1): 77-114.

[33] Connell RD, Beebe JS. Patent focus on cancer chemotherapeutics. III Angiogenesis agents. Expert Opin Ther Patents 2001; 11(7): 1171-203.

[34] Connell RD. Patent focus on cancer chemotherapeutics V. Angiogenesis agents. Expert Opin Ther Patents 2002; 12(12): 1763-81.

[35] Mantovani A, Sozzani S, Vecchi A, Introna M, Allavena P. Cytokine activation of endothelial cells: New molecules for an old paradigm. Thromb Haemost 1997; 78(1): 406-14.

[36] Ferrara N, Hillan KJ, Novotny W. Bevacizumab (Avastin), a humanized anti-VEGF monoclonal antibody for cancer therapy. Biochem Biophys Res Commun 2005; 333(2): 328-35.

[37] David H. Rudolf Virchow and modern aspects of tumor pathology. Pathol Res Pract 1988; 183(3): 356-64.

[38] Gimbrone MA Jr., Aster RH, Cotran RS, Corkery J, Jandl JH, Folkman J. Preservation of vascular integrity in organs perfused *in vitro* with a platelet-rich medium. Nature 1969; 221(188): 33-6.

[39] Hamano Y, Kalluri R. Tumstatin, the NC1 domain of alpha3 chain of type IV collagen, is an endogenous inhibitor of pathological angiogenesis and suppresses tumor growth. Biochem Biophys Res Commun 2005; 333(2): 292-8.

[40] Folkman J, Kalluri R. Cancer without disease. Nature 2004; 427(6977): 787.

[41] Nyberg P, Xie L, Kalluri R. Endogenous inhibitors of angiogenesis. Cancer Res 2005; 65(10): 3967-79.

[42] Giovannoni, L. Process for selecting anti-angiogenesis antibody fragments, anti-angiogenesis antibody fragments thus obtained and their use. US7723269 (**2010**).

[43] Matsuoka, H., Nishimura, K., Seike, H., Aono, H., Murai, M. Angiogenesis inhibitor. US7741346 (**2010**).

[44] Tanaka S, Sugimachi K, Yamashita Y, Shirabe K, Shimada M, Wands JR. Angiogenic switch as a molecular target of malignant tumors. J Gastroenterol 2003; 38 (Suppl 15): 93-7.

[45] Gasparini G, Longo R, Fanelli M, Teicher BA. Combination of anti-angiogenic therapy with other anticancer therapies: Results, challenges, and open questions. J Clin Oncol 2005; 23(6): 1295-311.

[46] Folkman J. Looking for a good endothelial address. Cancer Cell 2002; 1(2): 113-5.

[47] Kerbel RS. Clinical trials of anti-angiogenic drugs: Opportunities, problems and assessment of initial results. J Clin Oncol 2001; 19: 45s-51s.

[48] Brooks, P.C., Zu, J., E P. Antagonists and methods for inhibiting angiogenesis. US8025883 (**2011**).

[49] Byzova, T., Maha, B., Ganapati, H., Feng, W. Compounds and methods of modulating angiogenesis. US8080252 (**2011**).

[50] Isner, J.M., Linda, A., Takayuki, L., Douglas, W. Composition and methods for regulating angiogenesis. US8075880 (**2011**).

[51] Brown, M.L., Laurel, M.D. Dual small molecule inhibitors of cancer and angiogenesis. US8178545 (**2012**).

[52] Imhof, B.A., Aurran-Lions, M. Angiogenesis inhibiting molecules, their selection, production and their use in the treatment of cancer. US8093010 (**2012**).

[53] Li, D.Y., Park, K.W. Methods for inhibiting angiogenesis. US8097253 (**2012**).

[54] Neufeld, G., Akiri, G., Vadasz, Z., Gengrinovitch, S. Methods and compositions for modulating angiogenesis. US8168180 (**2012**).

[55] Eisenhauer EA. From the molecule to the clinic-inhibiting HER2 to treat breast cancer. N Engl J Med 2001; 344(11): 841-2.

[56] Rothenberg ML, Abbruzzese JL, Moore M, Portenoy RK, Robertson JM, Wanebo HJ. A rationale for expanding the endpoints for clinical trials in advanced pancreatic carcinoma. Cancer 1996; 78(3 Suppl): 627-32.

[57] Blum JL, Jones SE, Buzdar AU, LoRusso PM, Kuter I, Vogel C, *et al.* Multicenter Phase II study of capecitabine in paclitaxel-refractory metastatic breast cancer. J Clin Oncol 1999; 17(2): 485-93.

[58] Howell A, Mackintosh J, Jones M, Redford J, Wagstaff J, Sellwood RA. The definition of the "no change" category in patients treated with endocrine therapy and chemotherapy for advanced carcinoma of the breast. Eur J Cancer Clin Oncol 1988; 24(10): 1567-72.

[59] Demetri GD, von Mehren M, Blanke CD, Van den Abbeele AD, Eisenberg B, Roberts PJ, *et al.* Efficacy and safety of imatinib mesylate in advanced gastrointestinal stromal tumors. N Engl J Med 2002; 347(7): 472-80.

[60] Hidalgo M, Siu LL, Nemunaitis J, Rizzo J, Hammond LA, Takimoto C, *et al.* Phase I and pharmacologic study of OSI-774, an epidermal growth factor receptor tyrosine kinase inhibitor, in patients with advanced solid malignancies. J Clin Oncol 2001; 19(13): 3267-79.

[61] van Oosterom AT, Judson I, Verweij J, Stroobants S, Donato di Paola E, Dimitrijevic S, *et al.* Safety and efficacy of imatinib (STI571) in metastatic gastrointestinal stromal tumours: A Phase I study. Lancet 2001; 358(9291): 1421-3.

[62] Stadler WM, Ratain MJ. Development of target-based antineoplastic agents. Invest New Drugs 2000; 18(1): 7-16.

[63] Folkman J. Angiogenesis and apoptosis. Semin Cancer Biol 2003; 13: 159-67.

[64] O'Reilly MS, Holmgren L, Shing Y, Chen C, Rosenthal RA, Cao Y, *et al.* Angiostatin: A circulating endothelial cell inhibitor that suppresses angiogenesis and tumor growth. Cold Spring Harb Symp Quant Biol 1994; 59: 471-82.

[65] O'Reilly, M.S., Folkman, M.J. Angiostatin protein. US5639725 (**1997**).

[66] Folkman, M.J., O'Reilly, M.S. Aggregate angiostatin and method of use. US5861372 (**1999**).

[67] Lo, K.-M., Li, Y., Gillies, S.D. Expression and export of angiostain and endostatin as immunofusion. WO0011033 (**2000**).

[68] Mulligan-Kehoe, M.J., Powell, R.J. Methods for modulating angiogenesis via VEGF. WO03084483 (**2003**).

[69] O'Reilly, M.S., Folkman, M.J. Method of detecting angiogenic protein. US5776704 (**1998**).

[70] Pirie-Shepherd, S., Folkman, M.J., Liang, H., MacDonald, N., Sim, K.L. Deglycosylated kringle 1-5 region fragments of plasminogen and methods of use. WO0047729 (**2000**).

[71] Soff, G., Gately, S.T., Twardowski, P. Methods and compositions for generating angiostatin. WO0158921 (**2001**).

[72] Shing, Y.W., O'Reilly, M.S., Folkman, M.J. Plasminogen kringle 4 region fragments and methods of use. WO0044391 (**2000**).

[73] Ji, R.-W.-D., Trail, P.A. Lysine binding fragments of angiostatin. WO0003726 (**2000**) & US6538103 (**2003**).

[74] MacDonald, N.J., Sim, K.L. Compositions amd methods of using proteins and peptides that bind angiogenesis inhibiting proteins. WO0032631 (**2000**).

[75] Liang, H., Sim, K.L. Compositions and methods for inhibiting endothelial cell proliferation. WO0144294 (**2001**).

[76] Holmgren, L., Troyanovsky, B., Mazzini, G. Angiostatin-binding protein. WO9966038 (**1999**).

[77] Moser, T.L., Pizzo, S.V., Stack, M.S. Angiostatin receptor. US6444431 (**2002**) & WO00326631 (**2000**).

[78] Grdina, D.J., Milas, L., Shishima, G. A method for protection against tumor metastasis formation. WO0056299 (**2000**).

[79] Soff, G., Gately, S.T., Twardowski, P. Methods and compositions for generating angiostatin. US6576609 (**2003**).

[80] Li, H., Lu, H., Griscelli, F., Opolon, P., Soria, C., Ragot, T., Legrand, Y., Soria, J., Mabilat, C., Perricaudet, M., Yeh, P. Adenovirus mediated intratumoral delivery of angiogenesis antagonist for the treatment of tumors. US6638502 (**2003**).

[81] Leboulch, P., Rawliuk, R.J., Bachelot, T. Anti-angiogenic gene therapy vectors and their use in treating angiogenesis-related diseases. WO9926480 (**1999**).

[82] Rupnick, M., Langer, R.S., Folkman, M.J. Method for regulating size and growth of vascularized normal tissue. WO9939702 (**1999**).

[83] Weichselbaum, R.R., Sukhatme, V.P., Kufe, D.W. Combination of radiotherapy and anti-angiogenic factors. US6420335 (**2002**).

[84] Cao, Y. Kringle domains of plasminogen, capable of modulating angiogenesis *in vivo*. WO0061179 (**2000**).

[85] Bridon, D.P., Rasamoelisolo, M., Thibaudeau, K., Huang, X., Beliveau, R. Long lasting anti-angiogenic peptides. WO0070665 (**2000**).

[86] Soker, S., Satchi-Fainaro, R. Methods for inhibiting vascular hyperpermeability. WO03086178 (**2003**).

[87] Cai, J.H., Tong, X. Methods and compositions for diagnosing and treating disorders involving angiogenesis. WO2004104227 (**2004**).

[88] Madsen, J., Liang, H., Sim, K.L., Zhou, X., Chang-Murad, A., Boerner, R.J., Bermejo, L.L., Mistry, F.R., Schrimsher, J.L., Shepard, S.R., Johnston, J. Method of producing and purifying angiostatin. US6723536 (**2004**).

[89] Holmgren, L., Troyanovsky, B. Angiogenesis related molecules. US6908898 (**2005**).

[90] O'Reilly MS, Boehm T, Shing Y, Fukai N, Vasios G, Lane WS, *et al.* Endostatin: An endogenous inhibitor of angiogenesis and tumor growth. Cell 1997; 88(2): 277-85.

[91] Boehm T, Folkman J, Browder T, O'Reilly MS. Anti-angiogenic therapy of experimental cancer does not induce acquired drug resistance. Nature 1997; 390(6658): 404-7.

[92] Boehm T, O'Reilly MS, Keough K, Shiloach J, Shapiro R, Folkman J. Zinc-binding of endostatin is essential for its anti-angiogenic activity. Biochem Biophys Res Commun 1998; 252(1): 190-4.

[93] Lee TH, Rhim T, Kim SS. Prothrombin kringle-2 domain has a growth inhibitory activity against basic fibroblast growth factor-stimulated capillary endothelial cells. J Biol Chem 1998; 273(44): 28805-12.

[94] O'Reilly, M.S., Folkman, M.J. Therapeutic anti-angiogenic endostatin compositions. WO0026368 (**2000**), US6346510 (**2002**) & US7867978. (**2010**).

[95] O'Reilly, M.S., Folkman, M.J. Methods for expressing endostatin protein. US6544758 (**2003**).

[96] O'Reilly, M.S., Folkman, M.J. Nucleic acids encoding for endostatin protein. US6746865 (**2004**).

[97] O'Reilly, M.S., Folkman, M.J. Endostatin protein and fragments thereof. US6764995 (**2004**).

[98] O'Reilly, M.S., Folkman, M.J. Nucleic acid molecules encoding endostatin protein and peptide fragments thereof. US7655458 (**2010**).

[99] Desanti, C.L., Strohl, W.R. Soluble recombinant endostatin and method of making same from Streptomyces sp. WO0060945 (**2000**).

[100] Boice, J.A., Leiting, B., O'Connell, J.F., Pompliano, D.L. Soluble recombinant endostatin. WO0058498 (**2000**).

[101] Hallenbeck, P.L., Chen, C.T., Becker, K. Adenoviral vectors including DNA sequences encoding angiogenic inhibitors. WO0112830 (**2001**).

[102] Vuori, K., Gay, D.A. Anti-angiogenic endostatin peptides, endostatin variants and methods of use. WO0067771 (**2000**).

[103] Bottaro, D.P., Giubellino, A., Atabey, S.N., Soriano, J.V., Breckenridge, D.E., Burke, Jr. T.R. Inhibition of cell motility, angiogenesis and metastasis. US7871981 (**2011**).

[104] Chillemi, F., Francescato, P., Ziche, M., Minoja, F. Polypeptides derived from endostatin exhibiting anti-angiogenic activity. WO0063249 (**2000**).

[105] Agoston, G., Shah, J.H., Hunsucker, K.A., Pribluda, V., Lavallee, T., Green, S.J., Herbstrritt, C.J., Zhan, X.H., Treston, A. Anti-angiogenic agents. WO0242319 (**2002**).

[106] Sim, K.L., MacDonald, N., Kulkarni, S. Angiostatin and endostatin binding proteins and methods of use. WO01093897 (**2001**).

[107] Sim, K.L., Liang, H. Angiogenesis-inhibiting peptides and proteins and methods of use. WO0230982 (**2002**).

[108] Mertins, P., Celik, I., Kisker, O., Sleep, D., Hay, J., Hauser, H.-P. Albumin-fusion anti-angiogenesis peptides. WO03066085 (**2003**).

[109] Chen, W.Y., Schill, C.F. Human prolactin antagonist-Angiogenesis inhibitor fusion proteins. WO03102148 (**2003**).

[110] Violand, B.N., Harding, E.I. Method of producing mouse and human endostatin. US6653098 (**2003**).

[111] Tong, X., Sheppard, M.G. Methods and compositions for diagnosing and treating disorders involving angiogenesis. US6803211 (**2004**).

[112] Sukhatme, V.P. Anti-angiogenic peptides and methods of use thereof. US6852691 (**2005**).

[113] Sukhatme, V.P. Methods of producing anti-angiogenic proteins. US6797488 (**2004**).

[114] Chillemi, F., Francescato, P., Ziche, M. Polypeptides derived from endostatin exhibiting anti-angiogenic activity. US6921749 (**2005**).

[115] Timpl R. Macromolecular organization of basement membrane. Curr Opin Cell Biol 1996; 8: 618-24.

[116] Madri JA. Extracellular matrix modulation of vascular cell behavior. Transpl Immunol 1997; 5: 179-83.

[117] Burgess JK, Boustany S, Moir LM, Weckmann M, Lau JY, Grafton K, *et al.* Reduction of tumstatin in asthmatic airways contributes to angiogenesis, inflammation, and hyperresponsiveness. Am J Respir Crit Care Med 2010; 181(2): 106-15.

[118] Hudson, B.G., Sarras, J., Michael, P. The use of isolated domains of type IV collagen to modify cell and tissue interaction. WO9949885 (**1999**).

[119] Hudson, B.G., Sarras, J., Michael, P. Method for inhibiting angiogenesis and tumors with the isolated NC1.alpha.6. chain monomer of type IV collagen. US6432706 (**2002**), US6358735 (**2002**) & US6361994 (**2002**).

[120] Hudson, B.G., Sarras, Jr. M.P. Use of isolated domains of type IV collagen to modify cell and tissue interactions. US6689746 (**2004**).

[121] Kalluri, R. Anti-angiogenic proteins and fragments and methods of use thereof. WO03059257 (**2003**).

[122] Kalluri, R. Anti-angiogenic proteins and methods of use thereof. US6759047 (**2004**).

[123] Cooke VG, Kalluri R. Chapter 1. Molecular mechanism of type IV collagen-derived endogenous inhibitors of angiogenesis. Methods Enzymol 2008; 444: 1-19.

[124] Cosgrove D, Rodgers K, Meehan D, Miller C, Bovard K, Gilroy A, *et al.* Integrin alpha1beta1 and transforming growth factor-beta1 play distinct roles in alport glomerular pathogenesis and serve as dual targets for metabolic therapy. Am J Pathol 2000; 157(5): 1649-59.

[125] Iglesias-de la Cruz MC, Ziyadeh FN, Isono M, Kouahou M, Han DC, Kalluri R, *et al.* Effects of high glucose and TGF-beta1 on the expression of collagen IV and vascular endothelial growth factor in mouse podocytes. Kidney Int 2002; 62(3): 901-13.

[126] LeBleu V, Sugimoto H, Mundel TM, Gerami-Naini B, Finan E, Miller CA, *et al.* Stem cell therapies benefit Alport syndrome. J Am Soc Nephrol 2009; 20(11): 2359-70.

[127] MacDonald BA, Sund M, Grant MA, Pfaff KL, Holthaus K, Zon LI, *et al.* Zebrafish to humans: Evolution of the alpha3-chain of type IV collagen and emergence of the autoimmune epitopes associated with Goodpasture syndrome. Blood 2006; 107(5): 1908-15.

[128] Sudhakar A, Nyberg P, Keshamouni VG, Mannam AP, Li J, Sugimoto H, *et al.* Human alpha1 type IV collagen NC1 domain exhibits distinct anti-angiogenic activity mediated by alpha1beta1 integrin. J Clin Invest 2005; 115(10): 2801-10.

[129] Sugimoto H, Mundel TM, Sund M, Xie L, Cosgrove D, Kalluri R. Bone-marrow-derived stem cells repair basement membrane collagen defects and reverse genetic kidney disease. Proc Natl Acad Sci USA 2006; 103(19): 7321-6.

[130] Sund M, Maeshima Y, Kalluri R. Bifunctional promoter of type IV collagen COL4A5 and COL4A6 genes regulates the expression of alpha5 and alpha6 chains in a distinct cell-specific fashion. Biochem J 2005; 387(Pt 3): 755-61.

[131] Tanjore H, Kalluri R. The role of type IV collagen and basement membranes in cancer progression and metastasis. Am J Pathol 2006; 168(3): 715-7.

[132] Zeisberg M, Bonner G, Maeshima Y, Colorado P, Muller GA, Strutz F, *et al.* Renal fibrosis: Collagen composition and assembly regulates epithelial-mesenchymal transdifferentiation. Am J Pathol 2001; 159(4): 1313-21.

[133] Zeisberg M, Khurana M, Rao VH, Cosgrove D, Rougier JP, Werner MC, *et al.* Stage-specific action of matrix metalloproteinases influences progressive hereditary kidney disease. PLoS Med 2006; 3(4): e100.

[134] Brooks, P., Hudson, B.G. The use of domains of type IV collagen to inhibit angiogenesis and tumor growth. WO0059532 (**2000**).

[135] Brooks, P., PetitClerc, E., Xu, J. Method and composition for angiogenesis inhibition. WO0040597 (**2000**).

[136] Sundaramoorthy, M., Hudson, B.G. Crystallized structure of Type IV collagen NC1 domain hexamer. WO2004067762 (**2004**) & WO03012122 (**2003**).

[137] Brooks, P., Roth, J.M. CLK-peptide and SLK-peptide. WO2004073649 (**2004**).

[138] Sarras, J., Michael, P., Hudson, B.G. Use of isolated domains of type IV collagen to modify cell and tissue interaction. US6384012 (**2002**) & US6680293 (**2004**).

[139] Good DJ, Polverini PJ, Rastinejad F, Le Beau MM, Lemons RS, Frazier WA, *et al.* A tumor suppressor-dependent inhibitor of angiogenesis is immunologically and functionally indistinguishable from a fragment of thrombospondin. Proc Natl Acad Sci USA 1990; 87(17): 6624-8.

[140] Chen H, Herndon ME, Lawler J. The cell biology of thrombospondin-1. Matrix Biol 2000; 19(7): 597-614.

[141] Agah A, Kyriakides TR, Lawler J, Bornstein P. The lack of thrombospondin-1 (TSP1) dictates the course of wound healing in double-TSP1/TSP2-null mice. Am J Pathol 2002; 161(3): 831-9.

[142] Iruela-Arispe, M.L., Hastings, G.A., Ruben, S.M., Jonak, Z.L. METH1 and METH2 polynucleotides and polypeptides. WO0071577 (**2000**).

[143] Iruela-Arispe ML, Luque A, Lee N. Thrombospondin modules and angiogenesis. Int J Biochem Cell Biol 2004; 36(6): 1070-8.

[144] Lawler, J.W. COMP/TSP-1, COMP/TSP-2 and other chimeric proteins. WO0044908 (**2000**).

[145] Lawler, J.W. Thrombospondin-1 type I repeat polypeptides. WO0191781 (**2001**).

[146] Dudek AZ, Pawlak WZ, Kirstein MN. Molecular targets in the inhibition of angiogenesis. Expert Opin Ther Targets 2003; 7(4): 527-41.

[147] Punekar S, Zak S, Kalter VG, Dobransky L, Punekar I, Lawler JW, *et al.* Thrombospondin 1 and its mimetic peptide ABT-510 decrease angiogenesis and inflammation in a murine model of inflammatory bowel disease. Pathobiology 2008; 75(1): 9-21.

[148] Yang Q, Tian Y, Liu S, Zeine R, Chlenski A, Salwen HR, *et al.* Thrombospondin-1 peptide ABT-510 combined with valproic acid is an effective anti-angiogenesis strategy in neuroblastoma. Cancer Res 2007; 67(4): 1716-24.

[149] Zhang X, Galardi E, Duquette M, Delic M, Lawler J, Parangi S. Anti-angiogenic treatment with the three thrombospondin-1 type 1 repeats recombinant protein in an orthotopic human pancreatic cancer model. Clin Cancer Res 2005; 11(6): 2337-44.

[150] Zhong H, Bowen JP. Anti-angiogenesis drug design: Multiple pathways targeting tumor vasculature. Curr Med Chem 2006; 13(8): 849-62.

[151] Detmar, M., Streit, M. Thrombospondin-2 and uses thereof. WO0057899 (**2000**).

[152] Streit, M., Detmar, M. Thrombospondin-2 and the uses there of. WO02078606 (**2002**).

[153] Zhang, Y.-W. Inhibition of tumor angiogenesis by combination of thrombospondin-1 and inhibitors of vascular endothelial growth factor. WO2005007193 (**2005**).

[154] O'Reilly MS, Pirie-Shepherd S, Lane WS, Folkman J. Anti-angiogenic activity of the cleaved conformation of the serpin antithrombin. Science 1999; 285(5435): 1926-8.

[155] Winge, S. Purification of antithrombin-III. alpha and beta. US6451978 (**2002**).

[156] O'Reilly, M.S., Folkman, M.J. Compositions and methods for inhibiting angiogenesis. US6607724 (**2003**).

[157] Pal N, Kertai MD, Lakshminarasimhachar A, Avidan MS. Pharmacology and clinical applications of human recombinant antithrombin. Expert Opin Biol Ther 2010; 10(7): 1155-68.

[158] Freedman MD. Pharmacodynamics, clinical indications, and adverse effects of heparin. J Clin Pharmacol 1992; 32(7): 584-96.

[159] Voest EE. Inhibitors of angiogenesis in a clinical perspective. Anticancer Drugs 1996; 7(7): 723-7.

[160] Voest EE, Kenyon BM, O'Reilly MS, Truitt G, D'Amato RJ, Folkman J. Inhibition of angiogenesis *in vivo* by interleukin 12. J Natl Cancer Inst 1995; 87(8): 581-6.

[161] Bock, S.C., Picard, V., Zendehrough, P. Human antithrombin IIIs and methods related there to. US6878813 (**2005**).

[162] Coffman LG, Parsonage D, D'Agostino R, Jr., Torti FM, Torti SV. Regulatory effects of ferritin on angiogenesis. Proc Natl Acad Sci USA 2009; 106(2): 570-5.

[163] Colman RW. Inhibition of angiogenesis by a monoclonal antibody to kininogen as well as by kininostatin which block proangiogenic high molecular weight kininogen. Int Immunopharmacol 2002; 2(13-14): 1887-94.

[164] Colman RW, Jameson BA, Lin Y, Johnson D, Mousa SA. Domain 5 of high molecular weight kininogen (kininostatin) down-regulates endothelial cell proliferation and migration and inhibits angiogenesis. Blood 2000; 95(2): 543-50.

[165] Colman RW, Pixley RA, Sainz IM, Song JS, Isordia-Salas I, Muhamed SN, *et al.* Inhibition of angiogenesis by antibody blocking the action of proangiogenic high-molecular-weight kininogen. J Thromb Haemost 2003; 1(1): 164-70.

[166] Donate F, McCrae K, Shaw DE, Mazar AP. Extracellular tropomyosin: A novel common pathway target for anti-angiogenic therapy. Curr Cancer Drug Targets 2004; 4(7): 543-53.

[167] Liu Y, Cao DJ, Sainz IM, Guo YL, Colman RW. The inhibitory effect of HKa in endothelial cell tube formation is mediated by disrupting the uPA-uPAR complex and inhibiting its signaling and internalization. Am J Physiol Cell Physiol 2008; 295(1): C257-67.

[168] Liu Y, Sainz IM, Wu Y, Pixley R, Espinola RG, Hassan S, *et al.* The inhibition of tube formation in a collagen-fibrinogen, three-dimensional gel by cleaved kininogen (HKa) and HK domain 5 (D5) is dependent on Src family kinases. Exp Cell Res 2008; 314(4): 774-88.

[169] Wu Y, Rizzo V, Liu Y, Sainz IM, Schmuckler NG, Colman RW. Kininostatin associates with membrane rafts and inhibits alpha(v)beta3 integrin activation in human umbilical vein endothelial cells. Arterioscler Thromb Vasc Biol 2007; 27(9): 1968-75.

[170] Zhang JC, Donate F, Qi X, Ziats NP, Juarez JC, Mazar AP, *et al.* The anti-angiogenic activity of cleaved high molecular weight kininogen is mediated through binding to endothelial cell tropomyosin. Proc Natl Acad Sci USA 2002; 99(19): 12224-9.

[171] Colman, W.R., Mousa, A.S., Monaco, D.A. Inhibition of angiogenesis by peptide analogs of high molecular weight kininogen domain 5. WO0027415 (**2000**).

[172] McCrae, R.K., Monaco, D.A. Inhibition of angiogenesis by high molecular weight kininogen and peptide analogs thereof. WO0027866 (**2000**).

[173] McCrae, R.K., Monaco, D.A. Inhibition of angiogenesis by hight molecular weight kininogen domain e peptide analogs. WO0035407 (**2000**).

[174] Colman, W.R., Mousa, A.S., Monaco, D.A. Inhibition of angiogenesis by antibodies against high molecular weight kininogen domain 5. WO0134195 (**2001**).

[175] Mazar, A.P., Juarez, J.C., Livnat, S. Human kininogen D5 domain polypeptides. WO0214369 (**2002**).

[176] McCrae, K.R. Inhibition of angiogenesis by high molecular weight kininogen and peptide analogs thereof. US6767889 (**2004**).

[177] Donate, F., Mazar, A., Livnat, S. Human kininogen D3 domain polypeptide as an anti-angiogenic and anti-tumor agent. WO2004024877 (**2004**).

[178] McCrae, K.R. Inhibition of angiogenesis by high molecular weight kininogen domain 3 peptide analogs. US6869931 (**2005**).

[179] Corbacho AM, Martinez De La Escalera G, Clapp C. Roles of prolactin and related members of the prolactin/growth hormone/placental lactogen family in angiogenesis. J Endocrinol 2002; 173(2): 219-38.

[180] Ferrara N, Clapp C, Weiner R. The 16K fragment of prolactin specifically inhibits basal or fibroblast growth factor stimulated growth of capillary endothelial cells. Endocrinology 1991; 129(2): 896-900.

[181] Pan H, Nguyen NQ, Yoshida H, Bentzien F, Shaw LC, Rentier-Delrue F, *et al.* Molecular targeting of anti-angiogenic factor 16K hPRL inhibits oxygen-induced retinopathy in mice. Invest Ophthalmol Vis Sci 2004; 45(7): 2413-9.

[182] Carnemolla B, Neri D, Castellani P, Leprini A, Neri G, Pini A, *et al.* Phage antibodies with pan-species recognition of the oncofoetal angiogenesis marker fibronectin ED-B domain. Int J Cancer 1996; 68(3): 397-405.

[183] Pasqualini, R., Rusolahti, E., Ramos, R.T. Methods of ameliorating cancer and of inhibiting angiogenesis by using fibronectin. WO9812226 (**1998**).

[184] Neri, D., Gervasi, G. Specific binding molecules for scintigraphy, conjugates containing them and therapeutic method for treatment of angiogenesis. WO9958570 (**1999**).

[185] Wijelath, E.S., Murray-Wijelath, J., Hammond, W.P. Endothelial cell stimulation by a complex of fibronectin and vascular endothelial growth Factor. WO0055206 (**2000**).

[186] Zardi, L., Neri. D., Carnemolla, B., Nilsson, F., Tarli, L., Borsi, L., Halin, C. Compositions and methods for treatment of angiogenesis in pathological lesions. WO0162298 (**2001**).

[187] Borsi, L., Carnemolla, B., Balza, E., Castellani, P., Zardi, L., Friebe, M., Hilger, C.-S. Selective targeting of tumor vasculature using antibody molecules. WO03076469 (**2003**).

[188] Nugent, M.A, Georges, A.L., Eisenstein, R.I. Method for stimulating angiogenesis and wound healing. WO2004091370 (**2004**).

[189] Mongiat M, Sweeney SM, San Antonio JD, Fu J, Iozzo RV. Endorepellin, a novel inhibitor of angiogenesis derived from the C terminus of perlecan. J Biol Chem 2003; 278(6): 4238-49.

[190] Yurchenco PD, O'Rear JJ. Basal lamina assembly. Curr Opin Cell Biol 1994; 6(5): 674-81.

[191] Iozzo, R.V., Monaco, D.A. Endorepellin compositions and methods for inhibiting angiogenesis. WO03048333 (**2003**).

[192] Iozzo, R.V. Endorepellin: Methods and compositions for inhibiting angiogenesis. US6821947 (**2004**).

[193] Ramchandran R, Dhanabal M, Volk R, Waterman MJ, Segal M, Lu H, *et al.* Anti-angiogenic activity of restin, NC10 domain of human collagen XV: Comparison to endostatin. Biochem Biophys Res Commun 1999; 255(3): 735-9.

[194] Xu R, Xin L, Zhang JM, Li ZP, Gan RB. Restin expressed *in vivo* suppresses the growth of tumors in nude mice. Sheng Wu Hua Xue Yu Sheng Wu Wu Li Xue Bao (Shanghai) 2002; 34(5): 571-5.

[195] Sasaki T, Larsson H, Tisi D, Claesson-Welsh L, Hohenester E, Timpl R. Endostatins derived from collagens XV and XVIII differ in structural and binding properties, tissue distribution and anti-angiogenic activity. J Mol Biol 2000; 301(5): 1179-90.
[196] Marneros AG, Olsen BR. The role of collagen-derived proteolytic fragments in angiogenesis. Matrix Biol 2001; 20(5-6): 337-45.
[197] Sukhatme, V.P. Methods of producing anti-angiogenic proteins: Endostatin, angiostatin or restin using a Pichia yeast expression system. WO9929878 (**1999**).
[198] Sukhatme, V.P. Restin and methods of use thereof. WO9929856 (**1999**).
[199] Dawson DW, Volpert OV, Gillis P, Crawford SE, Xu H, Benedict W, *et al.* Pigment epithelium-derived factor: A potent inhibitor of angiogenesis. Science 1999; 285(5425): 245-8.
[200] Bouck N. PEDF: Anti-angiogenic guardian of ocular function. Trends Mol Med 2002; 8(7): 330-4.
[201] Duh EJ, Yang HS, Haller JA, De Juan E, Humayun MS, Gehlbach P, *et al.* Vitreous levels of pigment epithelium-derived factor and vascular endothelial growth factor: Implications for ocular angiogenesis. Am J Ophthalmol 2004; 137(4): 668-74.
[202] Yamagishi S, Inagaki Y, Amano S, Okamoto T, Takeuchi M, Makita Z. Pigment epithelium-derived factor protects cultured retinal pericytes from advanced glycation end product-induced injury through its antioxidative properties. Biochem Biophys Res Commun 2002; 296(4): 877-82.
[203] Bouck, N.P., Dawson, D.W., Gillis, P.R. Methods and compositions for inhibiting angiogenesis. US6288024 (**2001**), US6391850 (**2002**) & US6670333 (**2003**).
[204] Bouck, N.P., Dawson, D.W., Gillis, P.R., Volpert, O., Crawford, S.E., Stellmach, V.M. Methods and compositions for inhibiting angiogenesis. US6797691 (**2004**) & US6919309 (**2005**).
[205] Kovesdi, I., Brough, D.E., McVey, D.L., Wei, L. Viral vector encoding pigment epithelium-derived factor. US6821775 (**2004**).
[206] Kovesdi, I. Method of modulating neovascularization. US6753321 (**2004**).
[207] Bikfalvi A. Platelet factor 4: An inhibitor of angiogenesis. Semin Thromb Hemost 2004; 30(3): 379-85.
[208] Borgstrom P, Discipio R, Maione TE. Recombinant platelet factor 4, an angiogenic marker for human breast carcinoma. Anticancer Res 1998; 18(6A): 4035-41.
[209] Perollet C, Han ZC, Savona C, Caen JP, Bikfalvi A. Platelet factor 4 modulates fibroblast growth factor 2 (FGF-2) activity and inhibits FGF-2 dimerization. Blood 1998; 91(9): 3289-99.
[210] Peterson JE, Zurakowski D, Italiano JE, Jr., Michel LV, Connors S, Oenick M, *et al.* VEGF, PF4 and PDGF are elevated in platelets of colorectal cancer patients. Angiogenesis 2012; 15(2): 265-73.
[211] Whitman, R.B., Wohl, R., Duff, R.G. Angiogenic peptide. US5470831 (**1995**).
[212] Gupta, S.K., Singh, J.P. Method for inhibiting angiogenesis with modified platelet factor-4 and cleaved platelet factor-4. US5512550 (**1996**).
[213] Gupta, S.K., Singh, J.P. Modified platelet factor-4. US5935928 (**1999**).
[214] Komurasaki, Y., Shindoh, C., Hirose, T., Koh, K., Nishimuro, S. Process for obtaining platelet factor-4. US5847084 (**1998**).
[215] DeNanteuil, G., Remond, G., Paladino, J., Pierre, A., Tucker, G., Bonnet, J., Sabatini, M. Metalloproteinase inhibitors. US6066633 (**2000**).

[216] Brodt, P., Durko, M. Antisense nucleic acid molecules targeted to type I collagenase (MMP-1) for inhibition of melanoma invasion. WO01070950 (**2001**).

[217] Brooks, P.C., Rodriguez, D. Novel method and compositin for inhibition of angiogenesis and tumor growth using compounds based on a sequence within MMP-2. WO02098351 (**2002**).

[218] Bannen, L.C., Co, E.W., Jammalamadaka, V., Nuss, J.M., Kim, M.H., Le, D.T., Lew, A., Mac, M.B., Mamo, S., Wen, Z., Xu, W. Human ADAM-10 inhibitors. WO03106381 (**2003**).

[219] Panchal, C., Daigneault, L., Hawkins, R., Ruiz, M., Garde, S. Regulation of matrix metalloproteinases by PSP94 family members. WO2005033141 (**2005**).

[220] Fong, T., Lazarov, M.E., Welihinda, A. RDP58 compositins and methods for inhibiting vascularization of cell populations. WO2005009457 (**2005**).

[221] Tosata, G., Pike, S.E., Yao, L. Use of Calreticulin and Calreticulin fragments to inhibit endothelial cell growth and angiogenesis, and suppress tumor growth. WO0020577 (**2000**) & US6867180 (**2005**).

[222] Strieter RM, Polverini PJ, Kunkel SL, Arenberg DA, Burdick MD, Kasper J, *et al.* The functional role of the ELR motif in CXC chemokine-mediated angiogenesis. J Biol Chem 1995; 270(45): 27348-57.

[223] Sgadari C, Angiolillo AL, Cherney BW, Pike SE, Farber JM, Koniaris LG, *et al.* Interferon-inducible protein-10 identified as a mediator of tumor necrosis *in vivo*. Proc Natl Acad Sci USA 1996; 93(24): 13791-6.

[224] Trinchieri, G., Lee, W.M.F., Coughlin, C.M., Bak, M.E. Method and compositions for inhibiting angiogenesis and treating cancer. WO9922760 (**1999**).

[225] Trikha, M., Zhou, Z., Dow, K.J. Anti-angiogenic uses of IL-6 antagonists. WO2004045507 (**2004**).

[226] Lingen MW, Polverini PJ, Bouck NP. Retinoic acid and interferon alpha act synergistically as anti-angiogenic and antitumor agents against human head and neck squamous cell carcinoma. Cancer Res 1998; 58(23): 5551-8.

[227] Qian, Q., Che, X., Shan, S., Wu, M. Virus high effectively expressing the tumor interferon and specifically reproduction in tumor cells and the use thereof. WO02095041 (**2002**).

[228] Petit, G.R. Combrestatin A-4 prodrug. US5561122 (**1996**).

[229] Petit, G.R., Lippert, J.W. Combretastatin A-1 phosphate and combretastatin B-1 phosphate prodrugs. WO0181355 (**2001**).

[230] Denny WA, Baguley BC, Atwell GJ, Rewcastle, G.W. Compounds having antitumor and antibacterial propertis. US5281620 (**1994**).

[231] Davis PD, Dougherty GJ, Blakey DC, Galbraith SM, Tozer GM, Holder AL, *et al.* ZD6126: A novel vascular-targeting agent that causes selective destruction of tumor vasculature. Cancer Res 2002; 62(24): 7247-53.

[232] Dougherty, G. Use of colchinol derivatives as vascular damaging agents. US6423753 (**2002**).

[233] Hatanaka, T., Ohsumi, K., Tsuji, T., Nihei, Y, Nakagawa, R., Ohishi, K. Stilbene compounds and pharmacecutical compositions containing them. US5674906 (**1997**).

[234] Hayashi K, Madri JA, Yurchenco PD. Endothelial cells interact with the core protein of basement membrane perlecan through beta 1 and beta 3 integrins: An adhesion modulated by glycosaminoglycan. J Cell Biol 1992; 119(4): 945-59.

[235] Drewe, J.A., Cai, S.X., Wang, Y. Substituted 4H-chromene and analogs as activators of caspases and inducers of apoptosis and the use thereof. US6906203 (**2005**).
[236] Sun, L., Borella, C., Li, H., Jian, J., Chen, S., Koya, K., Inoue, T., Du, Z., Foley K., Wu, Y., Zhang, M., Ying, W. Compounds for the treatment of proliferative disorder. WO06089177 (**2006**).
[237] Burrows FJ, Thorpe PE. Vascular targeting-a new approach to the therapy of solid tumors. Pharmacol Ther 1994; 64(1): 155-74.
[238] Denekamp J. Endothelial cell proliferation as a novel approach to targeting tumour therapy. Br J Cancer 1982; 45(1): 136-9.
[239] Denekamp J. Review article: Angiogenesis, neovascular proliferation and vascular pathophysiology as targets for cancer therapy. Br J Radiol 1993; 66(783): 181-96.
[240] Thorpe PE. Vascular Targeting agents as cancer therapeutics. Clin Cancer Res 2004; 10: 415-27.
[241] Thorpe PE, Burrows FJ. Antibody-directed targeting of the vasculature of solid tumors. Breast Cancer Res Treat 1995; 36(2): 237-51.
[242] Thorpe PE, Chaplin DJ, Blakey DC. The first international conference on vascular targeting: Meeting overview. Cancer Res 2003; 63(5): 1144-7.
[243] Dark GG, Hill SA, Prise VE, Tozer GM, Pettit GR, Chaplin DJ. Combretastatin A-4, an agent that displays potent and selective toxicity toward tumor vasculature. Cancer Res 1997; 57(10): 1829-34.
[244] Eremina V, Jefferson JA, Kowalewska J, Hochster H, Haas M, Weisstuch J, *et al.* VEGF inhibition and renal thrombotic microangiopathy. N Engl J Med 2008; 358(11): 1129-36.
[245] Gerber HP, Wu X, Yu L, Wiesmann C, Liang XH, Lee CV, *et al.* Mice expressing a humanized form of VEGF-A may provide insights into the safety and efficacy of anti-VEGF antibodies. Proc Natl Acad Sci USA 2007; 104(9): 3478-83.
[246] Maynard SE, Min JY, Merchan J, Lim KH, Li J, Mondal S, *et al.* Excess placental soluble fms-like tyrosine kinase 1 (sFlt1) may contribute to endothelial dysfunction, hypertension, and proteinuria in preeclampsia. J Clin Invest 2003; 111(5): 649-58.
[247] Patel TV, Morgan JA, Demetri GD, George S, Maki RG, Quigley M, *et al.* A preeclampsia-like syndrome characterized by reversible hypertension and proteinuria induced by the multitargeted kinase inhibitors sunitinib and sorafenib. J Natl Cancer Inst 2008; 100(4): 282-4.
[248] Glusker P, Recht L, Lane B. Reversible posterior leukoencephalopathy syndrome and bevacizumab. N Engl J Med 2006; 354(9): 980-2.
[249] Ozcan C, Wong SJ, Hari P. Reversible posterior leukoencephalopathy syndrome and bevacizumab. N Engl J Med 2006; 354(9): 980-2.
[250] Desai J, Yassa L, Marqusee E, George S, Frates MC, Chen MH, *et al.* Hypothyroidism after sunitinib treatment for patients with gastrointestinal stromal tumors. Ann Intern Med 2006; 145(9): 660-4.
[251] Heinzerling JH, Huerta S. Bowel perforation from bevacizumab for the treatment of metastatic colon cancer: Incidence, etiology, and management. Curr Surg 2006; 63(5): 334-7.
[252] Noguera-Troise I, Daly C, Papadopoulos NJ, Coetzee S, Boland P, Gale NW, *et al.* Blockade of Dll4 inhibits tumour growth by promoting non-productive angiogenesis. Nature 2006; 444(7122): 1032-7.
[253] Ridgway J, Zhang G, Wu Y, Stawicki S, Liang WC, Chanthery Y, *et al.* Inhibition of Dll4 signalling inhibits tumour growth by deregulating angiogenesis. Nature 2006; 444(7122): 1083-7.

[254] Kerbel RS. Tumor angiogenesis. N Engl J Med 2008; 358(19): 2039-49.
[255] Casanovas O, Hicklin DJ, Bergers G, Hanahan D. Drug resistance by evasion of anti-angiogenic targeting of VEGF signaling in late-stage pancreatic islet tumors. Cancer Cell 2005; 8(4): 299-309.
[256] Rak J, Mitsuhashi Y, Bayko L, Filmus J, Shirasawa S, Sasazuki T, *et al.* Mutant RAS oncogenes upregulate VEGF/VPF expression: Implications for induction and inhibition of tumor angiogenesis. Cancer Res 1995; 55(20): 4575-80.
[257] Yu JL, Rak JW, Coomber BL, Hicklin DJ, Kerbel RS. Effect of p53 status on tumor response to anti-angiogenic therapy. Science 2002; 295(5559): 1526-8.
[258] Shojaei F, Wu X, Malik AK, Zhong C, Baldwin ME, Schanz S, *et al.* Tumor refractoriness to anti-VEGF treatment is mediated by CD11b+Gr1+ myeloid cells. Nat Biotechnol 2007; 25(8): 911-20.
[259] Pietras K, Pahler J, Bergers G, Hanahan D. Functions of paracrine PDGF signaling in the proangiogenic tumor stroma revealed by pharmacological targeting. PLoS Med 2008; 5(1): e19.
[260] Bergers G, Song S, Meyer-Morse N, Bergsland E, Hanahan D. Benefits of targeting both pericytes and endothelial cells in the tumor vasculature with kinase inhibitors. J Clin Invest 2003; 111(9): 1287-95.
[261] Ghiringhelli F, Menard C, Puig PE, Ladoire S, Roux S, Martin F, *et al.* Metronomic cyclophosphamide regimen selectively depletes CD4+CD25+ regulatory T cells and restores T and NK effector functions in end stage cancer patients. Cancer Immunol Immunother 2007; 56(5): 641-8.
[262] Hermans IF, Chong TW, Palmowski MJ, Harris AL, Cerundolo V. Synergistic effect of metronomic dosing of cyclophosphamide combined with specific antitumor immunotherapy in a murine melanoma model. Cancer Res 2003; 63(23): 8408-13.

Send Orders of Reprints at reprints@benthamscience.net
Topics in Anti-Cancer Research, Vol. 2, 2013, 363-406

CHAPTER 11

Ribonucleotide Reductase as a Target to Control Cancer Proliferation

Nuno M.F.S.A. Cerqueira*, Narayana S.H.N. Moorthy, Pedro A. Fernandes and Maria J. Ramos

REQUIMTE / Faculdade de Ciências do Porto, Rua Campo Alegre, 687, 4169-007 Porto, Portugal

Abstract: Ribonucleotide Reductase (RNR) plays a critical role in DNA synthesis, and is a well-recognized target for cancer chemotherapeutic and antiviral agents. RNR inhibition precludes DNA transcription and repair, from which results cell apoptosis. Many regulation checkpoints concerning RNR activity have been unravelled through the last two decades, with potential use to inhibit enzyme activity. This was accomplished by researchers from different but complementary areas from which several and different inhibitors have resulted. The volume of these studies has generated over 5000 articles since the discovery of RNR in 1960. Some of these compounds have already been approved by FDA and EMEA for the treatment of specific types of cancer, as it is the case of gemcitabine, fluoromethylene and hydroxyurea. This chapter summarizes patents and papers during the period 1958 - 2012 dealing with the present understanding of ribonucleotidereductase biochemistry, mechanism of action and the most relevant data concerning RNR inhibition. Special attention is given to the inhibitors that have been patented and are currently in clinical use.

Keywords: Allosteric, antisense, cancer, clinical trials, dimerization, DNA, FDA, gemcitabine, GTI-2040, HIV, hydroxyurea, inhibitors, iron chelators, mechanisms, nucleotides, radical-scavengers, ribonucleotide reductase, substrate analogues, tezacitabine, theoretical results.

1. INTRODUCTION

Cancer cells devote most of their energy to ensure that precursors are available. Among different precursors, the deoxyribonucleotides (dNTPs) are essential for the synthesis of DNA and therefore cancer cells must have high levels of dNTPs in order to sustain high rates of cell division. Because imbalanced or high levels

***Address correspondence to Nuno M. F. S. A. Cerqueira:** REQUIMTE / Faculdade de Ciências do Porto, Rua Campo Alegre, 687, 4169-007 Porto, Portugal; Tel: 351-22 340 14 00; Fax: 351- 22 200 86 28; E-mail: nscerque@fc.up.pt

Atta-ur Rahman and Khurshid Zaman (Eds)

of dNTPs are highly mutagenic, stochastic genetic transitions within the cancer cell population are increased, favoring overall cancer cell survival. Moreover, high levels of dNTPs benefit cancer cells by reducing the accuracy of DNA polymerases, generating a self-perpetuating circle of mutations.A central enzyme that controls the production of dNTPs in mammalian cells is the Ribonucleotide Reductase (RNR) [1].

RNR is a ubiquitous radical-containing enzyme, which belongs to a small family of enzymes that are involved in the conversion of both purine and pyrimidines ribonucleotides diphosphates into their corresponding deoxyribonucleotides. Ribonucleotide reductase is the name by which the enzyme is normally referred to but its systematic name is 2'-deoxyribonucleoside-diphos-phate: thioredoxin-disulfide 2'-oxidoreductase (Scheme 1).The reaction catalysed by RNR involves the replacement of the C 2'-hydroxyl group on the ribose moiety by a hydrogen atom. After phosphorylation, the resulting molecules are the precursors needed for both synthesis and repair of the deoxyribonucleic acid (DNA). In each turnover, the reductive potential ultimately comes from NADH, and intermediately by reductants such as thioredoxin (Scheme **1**).

Several studies indicate that there is a close relationship between tumor growth rate and the hightspecific activity of ribonucleotide Reductase. Having this in mind, RNR inhibition and the resulting events have become a primarily target for therapeutic intervention for a number of human diseases, in which cell proliferation is abnormal and responsible for pathological diseases, such as anti-tumor, anti-viral and even anti-bacterial therapies [2, 3].

In recent years, several RNR inhibitors, including Triapine, Gemcitabine, and GTI-2040, have entered clinical trial or application. However, the mechanism of action of most of these inhibitors remains unkmown to date.

Currently, the volume of data available regarding RNR, including its inhibitors is extensive. The number of articles published till 2011 has already overcome 5000, and it can be observed in Fig. (**1**) that a great boost was given by Nordlund *et al.* [4] in 1990 when the three-dimensional structure of the enzyme was depicted.

In this chapter, a detailed overview of the enzyme is presented. The document has been divided into three main sections that try to summarize the background of RNR biochemistry as well as its mechanism of action and enzyme inhibition. The first section gives a general overview of all RNRs including their division into three classes, and special attention is given to the biochemistry and mechanism of action of class I. In the second section, RNR inhibition is reviewed in detail and the inhibitors have been divided into two main groups according to their mechanism of action, i.e. the inhibitors that preclude the formation of an active RNR and the inhibitors that once RNR is active preclude its activity. In each group, the inhibitors are grouped into several classes and when appropriate the corresponding patents and currently undergoing clinical trials are discussed. The final section gives the current opinion of the authors concerning the current and future developments of RNR taking into account the discussed data.

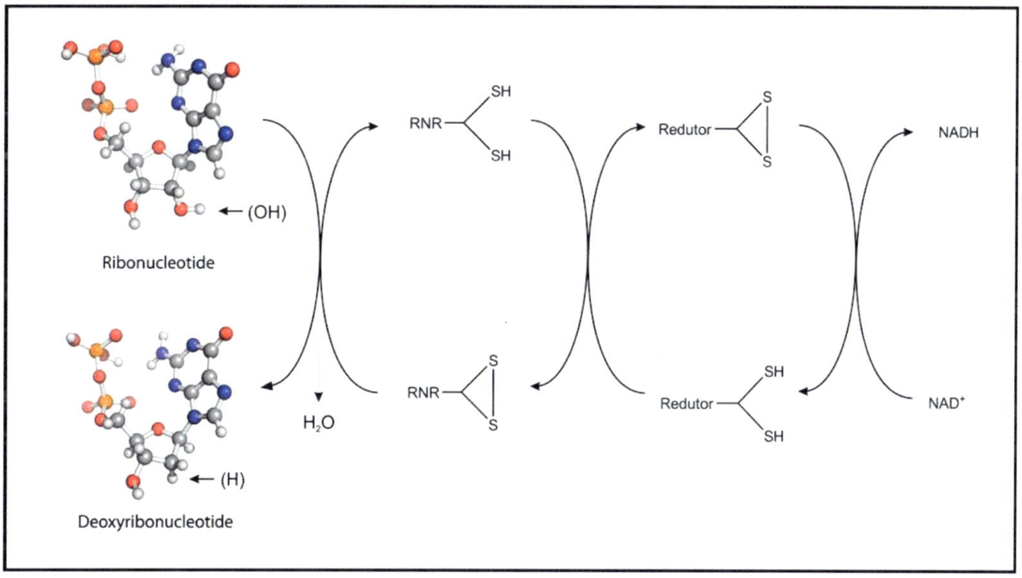

Scheme 1: Ribonucleotide reduction catalyzed by RNR.

1.1. Classes of RNR

A number of RNRs of different species have already been disclosed, pointing to a common radical-based reaction mechanism [5]. Intriguingly, despite their central and common metabolic functions, these enzymes have different amino acid sequences, metallic cofactors, substrate specificity and reducing equivalents to accomplish the same chemistry. Their classification into three classes was based on the quaternary structure and activation mechanisms (Table **1**).

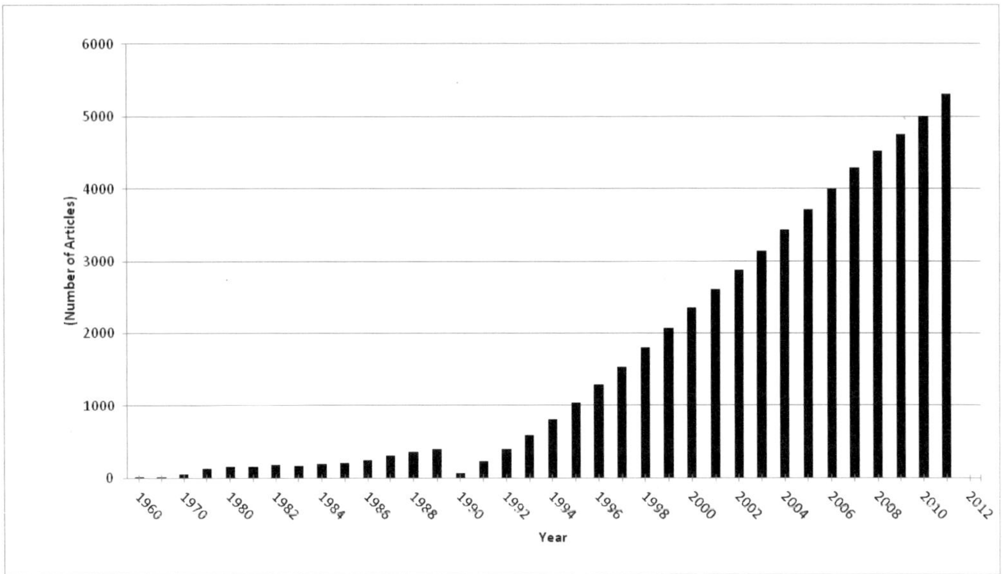

Figure 1: Number of articles that have been published since 1960 related to RNR (source: ISI Web of Science).

All RNR enzymes contain two components: a radical generator and a reductase [6]. These components can be located in different subunits or in the same one. The radical generator, the place where the radical is produced and stored, is not the same within all the RNR enzymes and is deeply buried inside the protein, in order to be protected from the environment. The reductase component is somewhat similar between all RNR classes and is where the reduction takes place. It is believed that upon substrate binding, the radical is transferred through a net of hydrogen atoms to the active site, where it is used to oxidize the substrate to a radical form that is followed by the reduction of the substrate at C2′ position.

Class I RNRs are found in both prokaryotes and eukaryo-tes with few exceptions Fig. (**2**). They are characterized by a tyrosyl radical that is stabilized by an oxo-bridged binuclear Fe(III) complex and requires oxygen for its generation. The enzyme is a holoenzyme $\alpha 2$ $\beta 2$, being the R1 protein com-posed by two identical monomers (761 residues per monomer) each one lodging one active site (for reduction of purines and pyrimidines), constituted by five conserved residues,

Cys439, Cys225, Cys462, Glu441 and Asn437, and three independent allosteric sites named s-site (specificity site), a-site (adenine specific site) and h-site (hexamerization site) that control the activity of the enzyme. The other dimer β_2, named R2 has 375 residues in each monomer, each one containing a stable neutral tyrosyl free radical at position 122, coupled to a binuclear iron (Fe_2O_2) cluster required for generation and stabilization of the radical. The X-ray structures of each subunit have already been determined [7].

Table 1: Overview of the characteristics from each class of ribonucleotide reductase.

	Class I	**Class II**	**Class III**
Genes	*nrdAB/EF*	*NrdJ*	*nrdDG*
Metal Cofactor	Fe^{3+}-O^{2-}-Fe^{3+}	AdenosylCobalmin	[Fe-S] S-adenosin-methionine
Subunit Structure	$\alpha_2\beta_2$	αorα_2	$\alpha_{2\,+}\beta_2$
Radicals involved	Tyr … Cys	AdB12 … Cys	AdoMet … Cys
Substrate	NDP	NDP/NTP	NTP
Reductant	Theioredoxin, Glutaredoxin	Thioredoxin	Formate
Occurrence	Eukaryotes Eubacteria Bacteriophages Viruses	Archaebacteria Eubacteria	Archaebacteria Eubacteria Bacteriophages

*Adapted from Jordan and Reichard, 1998 [3].

Class II RNRs are restricted to prokaryotes (both aerobic and anaerobic) and use adenosylcobalamine to generate a free radical. In this class of enzymes, the radical generator and a reductase are located in the same subunit, and α or α_2 proteins can be found. The radical is produced by adenosyl-cobalamin.

Class III RNRs, only function in anaerobic conditions and require a glycyl radical that is generated by a process that involves a [4Fe-4S] cluster and an S-adenosyl methionine. The α_2 dimer is the active form and contains the active glycyl radical and the binding sites for the aerobic reductases. The β_2 subunit is a small iron sulfur containing protein, which is essential for glycyl radical production.

It is interesting to note that despite the large differences between RNR classes, the common catalytic and similar allosteric mechanisms, as well as retention of critical residues in the protein sequence, suggest similar structures. Although these facts indicate a common origin of RNR during evolution, this subject is still under discussion and recently it was found that some organisms contain genes that encode different reductases [8].

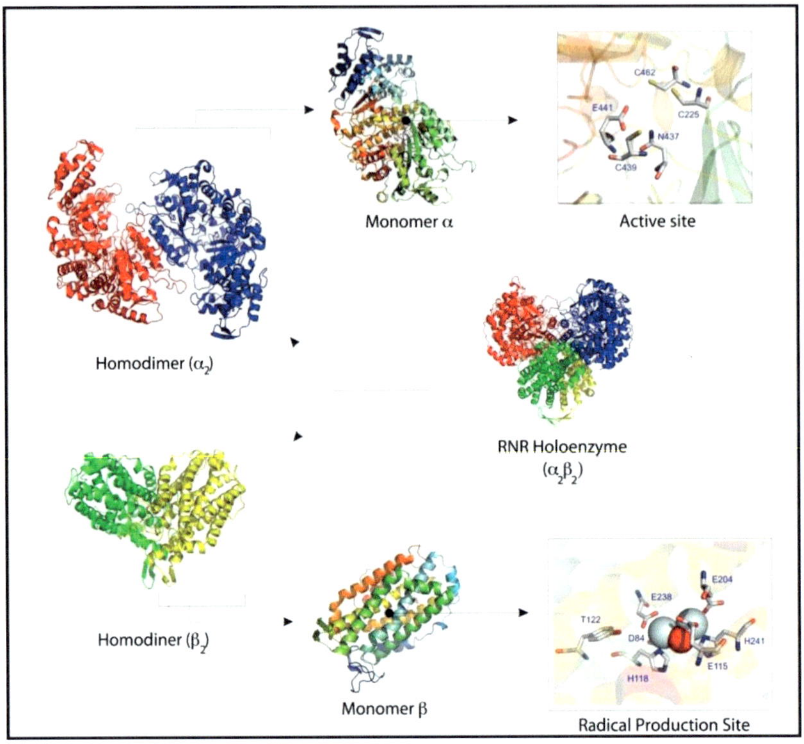

Figure 2: X-Ray structure of protein R1 and R2 of RNR class Ia.

As the aerobic bacteria *E. coli* RNR is the archetype for all Class Iaribonucleotidediphosphatereductase and as it serves as a prototype for the mammalian protein, we will dedicate the rest of this review to this class of enzymes. Therefore, whenever RNR is mentioned in the review it is linked to the enzymes of class Ia otherwise it will be specifically mentioned in the text.

1.2. RNR Regulation

The levels and activity of RNR are highly regulated by the cell cycle and DNA checkpoints which maintain optimal dNTP pools required for genetic fidelity. The enzyme can be regulated by two factors: by transcription of the genes or by allosteric control of RNR by triphosphate effectors.

The genes of each subunit are located on separate chromosomes and the corresponding mRNAs are similarly expressed during the S-Phase of the cell cycle. During the normal cell cycle the levels of the R1 protein do not appear to change substantially and can be detected throughout the whole cycle. In contrast, protein R2 can only be truly detected between the S Phase, where it slowly accumulates, up to late mitosis, where it is rapidly degraded. This mechanism ensures an adequate supply of dNTPs for replication and/or repair during the S and G2 Phase of the cell cycle. What appends next, during the remaining Phases of the cell cycle is still obscure. In fact, the absence of protein R2 during the G1 Phase would lead to the inactivation of protein R1, which precludes the formation of the necessary dNTPs for DNA repair. Some light into these aspects was added by Guittet *et al.* [9], who found that when DNA damage occurs, a transcriptional induction of a new protein called p53R2 (regulated by p53) is observed [10]. This study demonstrated that protein R1 can form a functional complex either with protein R2 or protein p53R2. It is believed that such induction is activated by the cell cycle checkpoints ATM/ATR and CHK2 that promotes the increase of the RNR activity in order to prevent DNA damage. Accordingly, R2 protein appears to be responsible for the maintenance of dNTPs levels for replication, whereas p53R2 is responsible for production of dNTPs is response to DNA damage [11]. It is also suggested that p53R2 together with protein R1 may also have a relevant role in supplyingdNTPs for basal levels of DNA repair and mitochondrial DNA synthesis in Go/G1 cells [10].

These results suggest that blocking of p53R2 in cases of highly malignant cancer with resistance to anti-cancer agents and radiation therapy would be a highly effective treatment with few side-effects. Moreover, because p53R2 may act as a homodimer (as R2 does), it might be possible to confer a dominant negative effect and suppress the activity of the enzyme by introducing mutated p53R2 genes or p53R2 protein into cancer cells, so both mutated p53R2 genes and p53R2 protein should be useful as therapeutic agents for highly malignant cancers with resistance to anti-cancer agents and radiation therapy. In addition, investigation of mutations to this gene should be useful in cancer diagnosis and prevention [12].

It has been reported also that the binding requirements of R1 for more than one radical generator complex may explain the nature of the uncoupled expression of proteins R1 and R2 (R1 gene is located at chromosome 11, R2 at chromosome 2 and p53R2 at chromosome 8 [13]).

Although protein R1 has a longer life (>24h) when compared to protein R2 (3h), it has been speculated also what would happen with protein R1 if DNA synthesis was not required [14]. Some light was shed, in 1999, by Ghabes *et al.* that found a protein in yeast (named Sml1) that was able to bind to protein R1 and inhibit it. These studies have shown also that Sml1p could bind to the mouse ribonucleotide reductase R1 protein too. However, the inhibition was shown to be less pronounced than in yeast, occurring probably via a different mechanism [15].

RNR is also regulated by allosteric control. This regulatory process is able to inhibit or activate the enzyme whenever it is needed, ensuring a balance of deoxyribonucleotide monomores for DNA replication. In 1979, Reichard and Thelander [16] proposed an allosteric cycle from which the activity of the enzyme was dependent. This theory supported the existence of an activity (a-site) and specificity (s-site) sites and correlated the reduction of specific NDPs according to the occupancy of these sites. It was shown that ATP and dATPcan bind to both allosteric sites, while dTTP and dGTP bind only to the s-site. Furthermore, ATP stimulates the reduction of CDP and UDP, dTTP stimulates the reduction of GDP, dGTP stimulates the reduction of ADP and dATP serves as a general inhibitor.

A better allosteric control model has been established by Kashlan, Cooperman and Scott since 2001 [17-19], where the existence of a third allosteric site is presented, the hexamerization site (h-site). Its exact location has however not been disclosed yet. Besides the correlated reduction of NDPs, this new model takes into account the influence of the allosteric ligand effects on the quaternary structure of RNR. These studies resorted to murine RNR. Within this theory the binding of ATP, dATP, dGTP, or dTTP to the s-site drives the formation of $R1_2$ dimer (whose monomers are inactive) that complexes with $R2_2$ dimer generating an active form, $R1_2R2_2$. The binding of ATP or dATP to the a-site drives the formation of a tetramer named $R1_4$, that isome-rizes into an inactive form named Rl_{4b}. If the concentration of ATP is sufficiently high, it will bind to the h-site which favors the conversion of Rl_{4b} into an $R1_6$hexamer. This hexamer will complex with an

$R2_6$ protein generating an $R1_6R2_6$ complex, which is believed to be the major active form of RNR in the cytosol of normal cells *in vivo*.

1.3. Catalytic Mechanism

The mechanism of generation of the radical as well as the reduction pathway has already been extensively studied [20-31]. However, although a great effort is being made toward the understanding of the reactivity of the di-iron cluster and the tyrosyl radical generation and pathway, the overall process still remains elusive, and further studies need to be performed.

The tyrosyl radical of the R2 component is remarkably stable and can exist in the purified enzyme for an extended period of up to one week [32]. This stability comes from the central position of the radical inside the R2 subunit that behaves like a shell and assures its protection from the surrounding environment.

Upon substrate binding the catalytic mechanism is initiated by Cys439 once protein R1 receives the radical from Tyr122. The radical located in the R2 subunit is transferred from Tyr122 to Cys439 through a ~35Å long hydrogen bonds network. This pathway and behaviour are however still obscure.

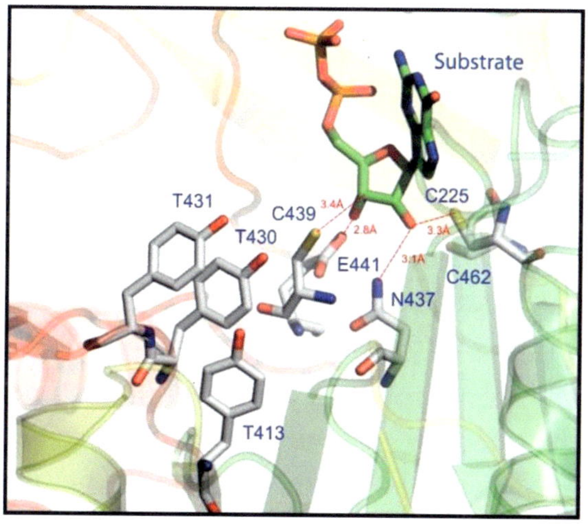

Figure 3: Representation of the active siteof RNR with the bounded substrate(PDB entry 4R1R). In this image are highlighted all the residues that participate directly on the reaction (C439, E441, N437, C462 and C225). Additionally, are also represented several tyrosine residues (T413, T430, T431) that are very close to cysteine C439 that holds the radical and is responsible for the initiation of the catalytic mechanism.

Contrarily, the reduction mechanism is better understood. Although apparently simple, this reaction has been shown to occur in a surprisingly complicated sequence of steps (Scheme**2**). A set of kinetic [33], spectroscopic [34-36], X-ray

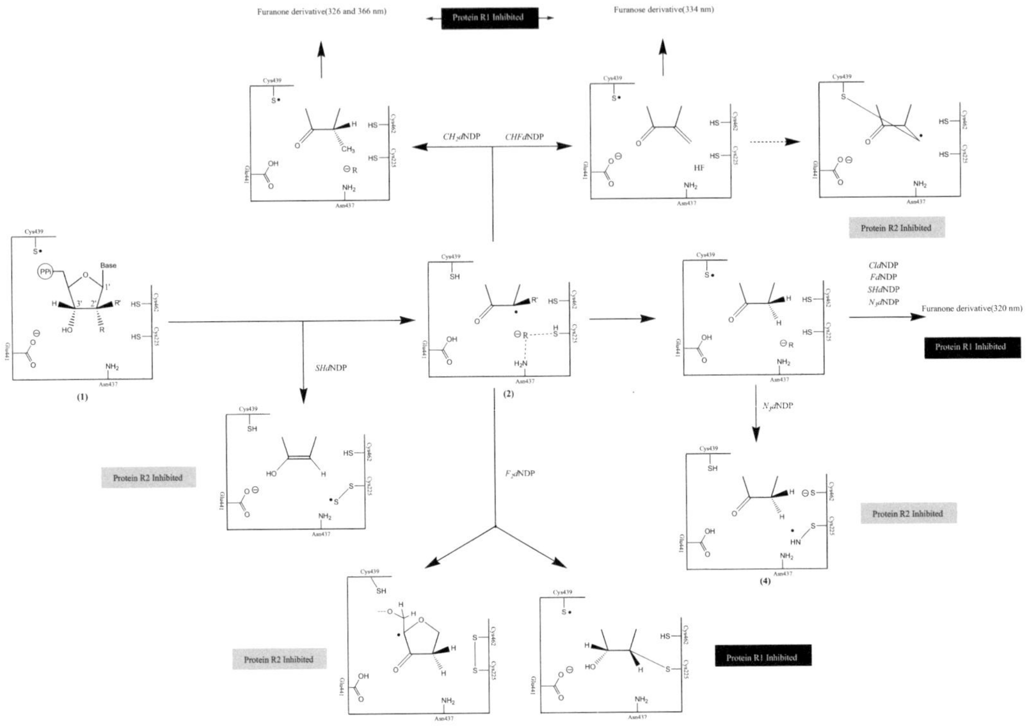

Scheme 2: Catalytic mechanism and inhibitory mechanisms of some RNR substrate analogues inhibitors (adapted from [42]).

crystallographic [4, 37], isotopic labeling [38], site-directed mutagenesis experiments [39, 40], and theoretical calculations [20-22, 24, 26, 41] have shed some light on the chemical events of the catalysis; the key amino acid residues involved were identified and a five-step hypothesis for the reaction mechanism was proposed. The active site is composed by a set of five aminoacids namely, Cys225, Asn437, Cys439, Glu441 and Cys462 and the radical is allocated at Cy439 Fig. (**3**). In the first step, the 3′-H atom is abstracted by the radical sulfur of Cys439; this is followed by the transfer of a proton from the 3′-OH group to Glu441, with concomitant protonation of the 2′-OH group by Cys225 and elimination of a water molecule; the third step corresponds to the abstraction of an H atom from the thiol group of

Cys462 by carbon C2′ - directly or with mediation of the closer Cys225; the resulting disulfide radical anion is subsequently reduced to a standard disulfide bond and a proton is transferred from Glu441 to the 3′-*O* atom, which replaces the charge in the glutamate residue and the spin density in the C3′ carbon; the final step consists of the donation of the H atom by Cys439 back to that carbon; thus, the 2′-deoxyribonucleotide is formed and the essential tyrosyl radical is regenerated. In the end of this process the disulfide bridge is oxidized by Thioredoxin and the enzyme is ready for a new reduction cycle.

A better understanding of the chemical mechanisms involved in normal catalysis is fundamental in order to understand crucial checkpoints that may allow the inhibition of the enzyme. This is important for the rational design of more specific and effective inhibitor compounds.

Several inhibition mechanisms concerning several inhibitors (that are going to be described below) are now better understood. To unravel these puzzling pathways, the available experimental data together with computational methods [20-22, 24-26], particularly quantum chemical calculations and QM/MM calculations have shown to be powerful and valuable tools. The involvement of computational methods allowed structural information of transient events, such as transition states and snapshots of molecules in the act of reaction, that are not possible to detect by normal physical methods. This is particularly important in the case of RNR, in which unstable intermediates such as radical species, are involved.

A review concerning the synthesis of recent work, using computational methods and experimental data, on the action and inhibition mechanisms of class I ribonucleotidereductase (RNR) was performed by Perez *et al.* [42]. Scheme **2** shows a diagram where the catalytic mechanism of the natural substrate is compared with the different pathways that are followed by the substrate analogues that induce enzyme inactivity. This scheme is based on experimental and theoretical works.

2. RNR INHIBITION

RNR inhibition knowledge is increasing substantially. In the last decade, a considerable increase in the intellectual propriety concerning this enzyme has been observed. Its importance in cancer and HIV therapies has motivated many research groups into the study and development of specific and powerful inhibitors that can inhibit this enzyme.

The variety of inhibitors currently known is extensive [43] and in this chapter, they will be divided in two main groups. The first group includes all the inhibitors that hinder the formation of an active RNR and the second group contains all the inhibitors that only inhibit the enzyme when it is already formed and active. Special attention will be addressed to the first group of inhibitors since they are the latest ones and possibly the next generation of RNR inhibitors.

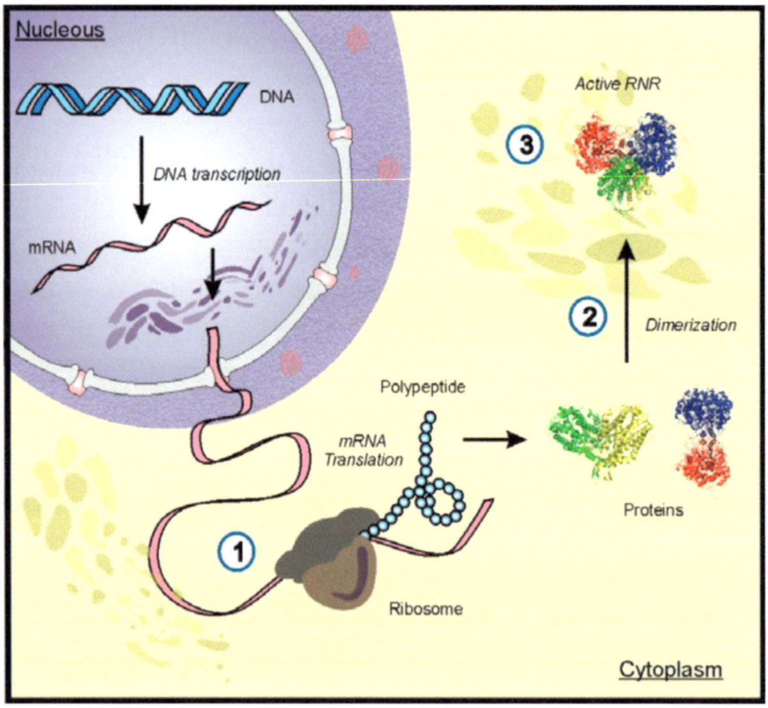

Figure 4: Image describing different regions on the cell where several inhibitors try to inhibit the formation or the activity of RNR.(1- translation inhibitors, 2- dimerization inhibitors and 3- Inhibitors that Preclude Enzyme Activity).

2.1. Inhibitors that Preclude the Formation of an Active RNR

These inhibitors do not allow the formation of an active RNR. They can be divided in two groups: The first group contains the inhibitors that hinder the translation and therefore the formation of the proteins R1 and R2; the second group contains all the inhibitors that do not preclude the formation of proteins R1 and/or R2 but hinder their dimerization, inactivating the enzyme in this way.

2.1.1. Translation Inhibitors

Translation inhibitors are the new generation of RNR inhibitors. The targets of these inhibitors are certain parts of the mRNA or DNA strand that upon binding prevent the expression of specific genes. The building blocks of these inhibitors are generally ribonucleotides or deoxyribonucleotides, depending on the target molecule (mRNA or DNA respectively). These inhibitors are designed to halt a biological event, such as transcription, translation or splicing.

The common name by which these inhibitors are named is antisense inhibitors and they can be widely found in several cells. In fact, some cells can produce naturally antisense RNA molecules that interact with complementary mRNA molecules and inhibit the expression of certain proteins.

Many forms of these inhibitors have been developed and can be broadly categorized into three main categories, compromising different types of oligonucleotides: The first type of oligonucleotide is the classic antisense compound which compromises short gene-specific sequences of nucleic acids, that has as target specific strands of mRNA that prevent the production of that RNA's protein. Some of these antisense compounds have the ability to activate RNase H that allows the antisense to target and bind with another strand of RNA. This process can be repeated over and over, allowing one oligonucleotide to bind with, and destroy, many strands of faulty RNA.

The second type of oligonucleotide is similar to the previous compounds. However, instead of using RNase H to destroy the RNA strand which has combined with the antisense, these oligonucleotides block other processes, such as regulatory binding proteins, ribosso-mes and/or spliceosomes, that hinder mRNA translation. Just as in the classical antisense compounds, this allows a single oligonucleotide to target and bind to numerous strands of RNA.

The third type of oligonucleotide is a triple-helix DNA. Many researchers do not consider this a true antisense compound. The first two types of oligonucleotides target specific strands of RNA to prevent the production of faulty proteins. Triple-helix DNA, however, targets the double-helix DNA strand itself. These triple-helix oligonucleotides are designed to bind with a specific section of the DNA, preventing its transcription into RNA. Triple-helix oligonucleotides truly serve the same purpose as classical antisense. These oligonucleotides simply attack the problem in a different manner, by preventing faulty proteins even earlier in their production process.

The potential of the antisense technology was discovered by Zamecnik and Stephenson in 1978 [44], when they found that a tridecamer d(A-A-T-G-G-T-A-A-A-A-T-G-G), which was complementary to 13 nucleotides of the 3'- and 5'-reiterated terminal sequences of *Rous sarcoma* virus 35S RNA, was able to induce the inhibition of virus production. Since then, antisense technology is an attractive alternative for target validation and therapeutic purposes. Its importance gathers more relevance with the completion of sequencing of the human genome and it is estimated that at least 5000 diseases related with genes are potential candidates for antisense therapy. Currently, the antisense therapies are under evaluation as therapeutic agents for a variety of diseases, including cancer [41, 45] and AIDS [46], and the FDA has already approved a phosphorothioate antisense oligonucleotide, fomivirsen (Vitravene^{TM}), for human therapeutic use [47].

One of the major challenges for antisense approaches is the stabilization of oligonucleotides, since unmodified oligonucleotides are rapidly depredated by biological fluids and in cells by both exonucleases and endonucleases. In early stages, the antisense backbones were made from natural genetic materials and linkages [48]. These compounds were easily degraded or broken down by enzymes in the blood and within cells, and had difficulty crossing cellular membranes to enter the cells that contained their genetic target. Subsequently, modified backbones were designed, which resist degradation by enzymes, and provide enhanced entry to tissues and cells. In fact several companies are working in this field, e.g. Isis Pharmaceuticals that has an impressive patent portfolio built upon its ability to synthesise modified oligonucleotides in large amounts [49]. In general, three types of modifications can be distinguished: altered phosphate backbones, analogues with un-natural bases and analogues with sugars (especially at the 2′ position of the ribose). These groups of modifications are normally known as first, second and third generation of oligonucleotides, respectively. A comprehensive review dealing with the antisense-oligonucleotides modifications and their respective patents was made by Jens Kurreck [50].

Proteins R1 and R2 from RNR are encoded in different chromosomes. In humans, the R1 gene has been mapped to chromosome 11, band p15, [51, 52] and the R2 gene in chromosome 2 [9]. Interestingly, it was found that the R2 gene is composed by two promoters which produce two major mRNAs with 5′-untranslated regions (50-UTRs) of different lengths [53, 54]. However, it is unknown whether both mRNA species can be translated andhow their translations are regulated.

Several studies have been addressed to RNR genes in order to preclude their transcription. For example, in 2000, Chen and co-workers [55] reported that antisense oligonucleotides could be successfully used to inhibit human cancer cell growth by the translation inhibition of both RNR subunits. The study involved the incubation of human oropharyngeal KB cells with human antisense oligonucleotides of both subunits, R1 and R2, by isopropylthiogalactose. Although, it was observed that the antisense of subunit R1 does not reveal a significant inhibition of the cell growth, the antisense of subunit R2 was capable of decreasing the formation of subunit R2, thus reducing the enzyme activity and inhibiting cell growth. In the same year, Aurelian *et al.* [56] reported that in the case of the *herpes simplex virus*, type 2, the growth and latency reactivation by cocultivation could also be inhibited by RNR inactivation with antisense oligonucleotides, but in this case complementary to subunit R1 from RNR.

The successes of these progresses gathered the attention of several companies that started to develop several antisense drugs with RNR as a target [57-60]. Lorus Therapeutics Inc. (Toronto) is developing a line of antisense drugs, with GTI-2040 [61] and GTI-2051 [62] as leading candidates. These oligonucleotides are 20-mer phosphorothioate oligonucleotides that have anti-tumor capabilities and their aim targets are both subunits, R1 and R2, respectively.

These drugs have demonstrated target gene down-regulation and anticancer activity in preclinical models of cancer and are currently being evaluated in a total of eight clinical trials against a range of cancer indications, including kidney cancer, breast cancer, hormone refractory prostate cancer, non-small cell lung cancer, acute myeloid leukemia, colorectal cancer and a variety of solid tumors. The lead antisense drug, GTI-2040, is currently being evaluated in a Phase II clinical trial program sponsored and coordinated by the U.S. National Cancer Institute.

GTI-2040 is a 20-mer phosphorothioate oligonucleotide complementary to the mRNA of the R2 subunit of RNR. *in vitro* GTI-2040 decreases mRNA and protein levels of R2 in a sequence- and target-specific manner. When GTI-2040 is used *in vivo*, as monotherapy, it promotes a highly significant reduction in tumor growth in all nine human cancers tested to date in animal models [63]. In the preclinical toxicology program, no major clinical toxicity has been observed to date. The significant antitumor activity against many different human tumors observed in preclinical studies has promoted this drug to Phase I clinical trial in the U.S., which has already been successfully completed [64].

GTI-2040 is currently the subject of a clinical trials agreement with the United States National Cancer Institute (NCI) under which GTI-2040 is being tested in combination chemotherapy in six different clinical trials. A Phase II study of GTI 2040 in combination with chemotherapy for the treatment of renal cell carcinoma was recently completed. In this study of late stage patients, 52% of the patient population displayed disease stabilizations with few unexpected side effects and tumor regressions were observed in some patients.

The patent application for this antisense drug has been filed in numerous additional international jurisdictions, e.g. Canada, Europe, United States, Singapore, Australia and New Zealand [58,59].

GTI-2501 is a 20-mer oligonucleotide that is comple-mentary to a coding region in the mRNA of R1, the large subunit of RNR. When compared with GTI-2040, GTI-2501 has produced similar results in animal models for a broad range of human cancers and has produced complete tumor regression in all animals in two human cancer models (breast cancer and renal cell carcinoma) [65]. *In vitro* studies have demonstrated that GTI-2501 decreases mRNA and protein levels of

R1 in a sequence-specific and dose-dependent manner. *In vivo* studies have shown that GTI-2501 significantly inhibit the growth of standard mouse models with a variety of different human cancers (lung, liver, ovary, brain, melanoma, breast and pancreatic tumor). This inhibitor has shown specific inhibition of metastasis of human melanoma cells to the lungs in CD-1 athymic nude mice and prolongs the survival of mice bearing human lymphoma.

To date, GTI-2501 has concluded a Phase I clinical trial, and is currently in a Phase II clinical trial, in combination with docetaxel for the treatment of prostate cancer. Initial testing of GTI-2501 demonstrated strong antitumor activity in preclinical studies of prostate cancer and a variety of other human tumor types. With respect to patents, GTI-2501 is under evaluation in the United States and Europe.

In 2010, Davis and coworkers have also found that a small interfering RNAs (siRNAs; approximately 21-base-pair double-stranded RNA) can elicit RNAi in mammalian cells without producing an interferon response [66]. They conducted the first in-human Phase I clinical trial involving the systemic administration of siRNA to patients with solid cancers using a targeted, nanoparticle delivery system. In these studies, they found that tumor biopsies from melanoma patients obtained after treatment show the presence of intracellularly localized nanoparticles in amounts that correlate with dose levels of the nanoparticles administered. Additionally, they have observed a reduction in both the specific messenger RNA (of protein R2 of RNR) and the protein R2 of RNR levels when compared to pre-dosing tissue. This data is very promising as it demonstrates that siRNA administered systemically to a human can produce a specific gene inhibition (reduction in mRNA and protein) by an RNAi mechanism of action.

All these results of the antisense technology allow to conclude that the inhibition of RNR can be performed in a pre-translation Phase, which has several advantages over the other types of inhibition: i) it becomes very specific for the corresponding mRNA of that protein and therefore of each organism, and ii) taking this specificity into account it may decrease the toxicity or even the number of secondary effects that normally follows the other kind of inhibitors [67].

2.1.2. Dimerization Inhibitors

The dimerization inhibitors prevent the complexation of two or more proteins that are crucial for the enzyme activity. In RNR, these inhibitors bind very tightly to protein R1 precluding the complexation with protein R2 [68]. As a result, the enzyme becomes inactive. These inhibitors are peptides, non-peptides or peptidomimetics with similar sequences to the flexible C-terminus of subunit R2, which is responsible for interaction with the R1 subunit [69, 70] (Table **2**).

Table 2: Some examples of dimerization inhibitors and their homology (in bold) to the r2 *C*-terminus sequence of several organisms.

Organism and Class	**R2 C-Terminus Sequence**	**Inhibitor**
Herpes-simplex virus	YAGAVVNDL	STSYAGAVVNDL YVVNDL BILD 1357
Mammalian - 1a	NSFTLDADF	N-Ac-NSFTLDADF N-Ac-FTLDADF N-Ac-AGAFTFNEDF N-Ac-FTFNEDF
Saccharomyces cerevisiae	AGAFTFNEDF	N-Ac-AGAFTFNEDF N-Ac-FTLDADF Sml1
Mycobacterium tuberculosis - 1b	VTEDDDWDF	N-Ac-DDDWDF EDDDWDF N-Ac-VTEDDDWDF
Escherichia coli - la	YLVGQIDSEVDTDDLSNFQL	LVGQIDSEVDTDDLSNFQL N-Ac-DDLSNFQL

* Sequences were obtained from the protein sequence database (EMBL, Switzerland).

Dimerization inhibitors that are able to disrupt RNR quaternary structure still remain an attractive goal in RNR inhibitory research [69, 71]. The main advantage in these kind of inhibitors is the little homology of the R2 *C*-terminus within different organisms. This allows specific inhibition of a parasite RNR without interfering with the host RNR [72]. Some examples of this feature were demonstrated by Chabes *et al.* [15] in which the Sml-1 protein was shown to be an efficient physiological inhibitor of RNR in yeast, whereas in mammalians, it is poorly effective.

RNR dimerization inhibitors were pointed out for the first time by Dutia *et al.* in 1986 [73]. They found that the interaction between the large and small subunits

(subunits R1 and R2, respectively) of Herpes simplex virus (HSV) is highly conserved [54]. Furthermore it was shown that, *in vitro*, it was possible to bind a synthetic peptide that interferes with the complexation of both subunits and from which resulted the enzyme inactivity [74]. The nonpeptideYAGAVVNDL, corresponds to the carboxyl-terminal region of HSV-R2. The interest with these inhibitors increased shortly after because this inhibitor is specific to RNRs of all herpes viruses studied to date (because their R2 carboxyl terminus are homologous) but substantially different from those of other species [75, 76].

However, evaluation and use of this nonpeptide as a potential antiviral agent *in vivo* has not been possible, presumably because the peptide is too large to enter eukaryotic cells. Nevertheless, these findings attracted the attention of several investigators that started to perform detailed structure analysis [77, 78] including NMR studies [79] and mutagenic experiences [80-82], that allowed the extrapolation of new conclusions. For example, these studies allowed concluding that the complementarity of the peptide is not absolutely required and several group substitutions in the five C-terminal residues, along with combination of large hydrophobic groups at the *N*-terminus, optimize the inhibitory effect.

The first patent concerning these type of inhibitors was made by R. Friedinger *et al.* in 1987 [83]. Merck continued these studies and have subsequently showed that the shortest peptide that is able to inhibit the activity of *Herpes simplex* virus RNR *in vitro*, (VVAAL), could be modified to build longer peptides with the same rate of inhibition.

In vivo studies with some of the inhibitors developed by Moss *et al.* [84], were even more stimulating since the inhibition was able to effectively reduce the severity of the virus in most of the cases, without interfering with the infected host. From this group of inhibitors, BILD 1357(Fig. (**5**)) has shown to be the most potent antiherpetic agent (in fact, the most potent dimerization inhibitor known till today) and the pentapeptide H-Val-Val-Asn-Asp-Leu-OH showed promising properties since it was able to increase the inhibition potency up to 4000 times. Currently, BILD 1357 is being used together with other compounds in the development of a new treatment for Human Immunodeficiency Virus (HIV) infection [85].

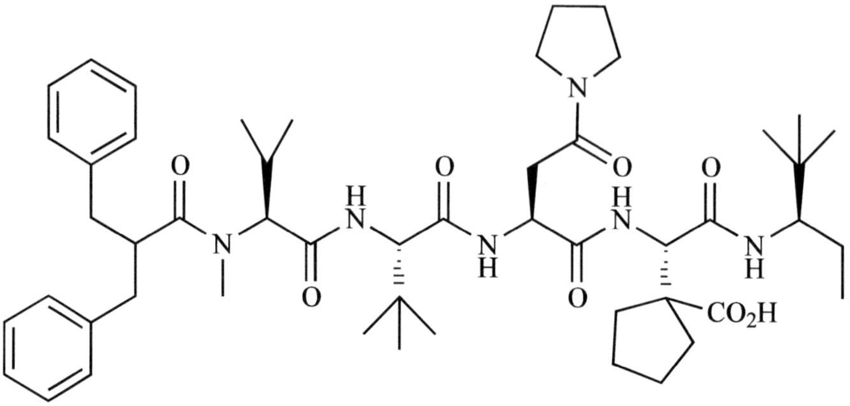

Figure 5: Example of a dimerization Inhibitor (BILD 1357).

Although most of studies were performed with the Herpes simplex virus, some work has also been done with other organisms, such as mammalian [75], *E. coli*, *M. tuberculosis* and *S. cerevisiae*. Some of these inhibitors are represented in Table **2** and are compared with the R2 C-terminus of the corresponding organisms. The first patent concerning peptides that were able to inhibit mammal RNRa was reported by Guindon *et al.* in 1991 [86]. In this report, it was shown that the *C*-terminal of R2 is very similar within mammals, but very different from the viruses. This was a great achievement since the difference between the RNR sequences can lead to the inactivation of the parasite virus without interfering with the host cells.

Taking into account the results obtained with the Herpes simplex virus, several systematic structure-function studies [87], including residues modification and deletions [88, 89], were also performed with these organisms in order to understand the inhibition mechanism and to achieve better inhibitory activity. These studies led to the conclusion that for inhibition it is only necessary a small peptide and that the acetylation [76] of these inhibitors improves, in most of the cases, ligand affinity and therefore the inhibition efficacy. Together with NMR trNOE techniques studies [90, 91], it was also observed that there are two crucial phenylalanine residues upon which the inhibitory activity is dependent ($Phe^1$and Phe^7). Pender *et al.* [88] showed that these Phe residues interact with two distinct positions in subunit R1 with which they have dominant interactions, the F7 subsite which is narrow and deep and very specific for Phe groups (Phe1), and the

F1 subsite, a shallow and broad subsite that can satisfy a wide range of groups and interacts strongly with Phe7.

Another kind of studies was performed by Gao [92, 93] with small molecules. He found that Fmoc-tripeptides (Fmoc: a-fluorenylmethyoxycarbonyl) were also capable of inhibiting the dimerization of the mammalian RNR subunits. The inhibition was shown to occur in both subunits and with higher affinity than with the R2 *C*-terminus polipeptide derivatives. It was also shown that these molecules bind to another site in addition to the ones targeted by the R2 *C*-terminus peptide derivatives. Although, its precise location is still unclear, the fact that these inhibitors strongly inhibit only the $R1_2R2_2$ form and not the $R1_6R2_6$ form, suggests that it may be located on a part of the R1 surface that becomes unavailable for binding after hexamerization [94, 95].

In 1991, Guindon [86] *et al.* showed that several peptides were indicated for preventing or ameliorating abnormal cell proliferation.

Cooperman from the University of Pennsylvania has patented a composition of linear peptides, cyclic peptides, peptide analogs, and peptidomimetics that successfully inhibit ribonucleotide reductase enzymes from mammalians [96]. This composition has shown to be a valuable tool in the treatment of cancer, viral and bacterial infections.

These studies were also extended to some procaryotes (*M. tuberculosis, Plasmodium falciparum* and *E. coli)* and fungi *(S. cerevisiae)*[87, 90, 97]. Although, it was observed that RNR inhibition could also be accomplished by mimicking the R2 C-terminal sequence, the conclusions acquired from some eukaryotes and Herpes simplex virus could not be directly applied to some of these organisms. For example, although in *M. tuberculosis* and *S. cerevisiae* the acetylated R2 C-terminus heptapeptide maximizes the inhibitory efficacy, as in eukaryotes, in *E. coli* it has the opposite effect [68]. Moreover in *E. coli,* the peptides must be longer since the two sites of the R2 *C*-terminus peptide that interact with R1 are not contiguous, contrarily to what happens with mammalians [98]. A patent concerning these inhibitors was published in 1988 by Dobrogosz *et al.* where the inhibition of bacteria, yeast and protozoa was reported with success

[99]. Another patent concerning several oligopeptides that are indicated to prevent bacterial infections was published by Rakhit in 1992 [100]. In 1995, Cooperman have also shown that compounds comprising peptides derived from the C-terminus sequence of the R2 subunit from *Plasmodium falciparum* could hinder its activity. This has shown to be particularly useful in the prevention and treatment of malaria caused by *Plasmodium Falciparum* [101].

Recent work has pointed out that in the murine RNR some small hydrophobic peptides are much more effective as inhibitors of $R1_2R_2$ than of $R1_6R_6$. This raises important questions and these inhibitors must be checked to see if the binding site competes with the oligomerization of RNR or not, as it was observed with the Fmoc-tripeptide inhibitors. Nevertheless, this point is important because, for instance, in tumor cells where the ATP concentration is very low (and where the $R1_2R2_2$ form is more expressed), the action of specific $R1_2R2_2$ inhibitors may be an advantage [102].

As it was mentioned before p53R2 plays a crucial role in supplying dNTPs for DNA repair, mtDNA synthesis, and protection against oxidative stress. p53R2, is a 351-amino acid peptide (39 kDa) homolog (~80%) of protein R2 that is capable of dimerizing with protein R1 when protein R2 of RNR is not available.

The expression of p53R2 is induced by DNA-damaging agents in a p53-dependent manner and p53R2 translocates to the nucleus upon DNA damage. Several studies have shown that there is a positive correlation between the level of this protein and tumor invasiveness [103]. Indeed, several studies have revealed that an increase in p53R2 expression by gene transfection significantly reduced the cellular invasion potential to 54% and 30% in KB and PC-3 cells, respectively, whereas inhibition of p53R2 by short interfering RNA resulted in a 3-fold increase in cell migration [104]. This means that overexpression of P53R2 may open possibilities for more effective therapy of certain types of tumors.

2.2. Inhibitors that Preclude Enzyme Activity

These inhibitors interact with the enzyme and inhibit its function either by destroying the radical that is lodged in subunit R2 or inactivating subunit R1.

Since most of the inhibitors have R1 or R2 as a specific target, these inhibitors are divided in two groups: specific R1 binding inhibitors that bind directly at subunit R1 and can inhibit one or both subunits, and specific R2 binding inhibitors, that bind directly and inhibit subunit R2.

2.2.1. Specific Binding R1 Inhibitors

These inhibitors interact specifically with subunit R1, but can also inhibit protein R2 in some cases. The first inhibitors were produced taking into account RNR allosteric regulation (Table **3**). Therefore, several changes to nucleoside triphosphates were induced to this type of molecules in order to interfere with enzyme activity. This was a challenging process since the substrates of the allosteric control had to compete with the products of the catalytic process. Nevertheless, it was shown by Harrington *et al.* [105] that RNR tolerates a wide range of modifications on the ATP molecule, including changes in the nucleobase, sugar and phosphate linkages, either in the allosteric or catalytic sites. It was found that some of the modified molecules could activate the enzyme as efficiently as ATP e.g., 3-deazaATP or 5'-adenylimidodiphosphate and some analogues were capable of inhibiting RNR. In this group, we can find several analogues of deoxyadenosine, such as 2-chloro-2'-deoxy-adenosine (clarabine- brand name LEUSTATIN®), developed by Ortho Biotech, 9-beta-D-arabinofuranosyl-2-fluoro-adenine (fludarabine - brand name Fludara®) developted by Schering AG, and 2-chloro-2'-arabino-fluoro-2'-deoxyade-nosine (clofarabine), developed by Genzyme Corp. in the US and by Bioenvision in Europe.

Cladribine has been known since the 1960's as an intermediate for the synthesis of 2-deoxynucleotides and its potential for the treatment of leukaemia was disclosed in 1984. It is now used to treat a type of blood cancer known as hairy cell leukaemia [106]. Cladribine was synthesised by Christensen *et al.* [107] and was launched by Ortho Biotech in collaboration with The Scripps Research Institute [108, 109]. This Institute and the Johnson & Johnson group hold several patents claiming preparation methods, and additional indications, such as multiple sclerosis and rheumatoid arthritis [110]. Fludarabine is distributed by Berlex Laboratories, and over the past decade, has become an effective agent for the treatment of lymphatic disorders (chronic lymphocytic leukaemia, prolymphocytic leukaemia and indolent non-Hodgkins lymphoma) [111-113]. Clofarabine is developed by Bioenvision Inc., and has been shown to be powerful in the treatment of acute and chronic leukemias, as well as other hematological malignancies, and solid tumors.

From these analogues, Clofarabine combines many of the favourable properties of the two most commonly used nucleoside analogs, fludarabine and cladribine, but has several-fold greater potency of damaging the DNA of leukaemia cells when compared to fludarabine. Clofarabine appears to achieve this greater potency by a process of breaking DNA chains besides inhibiting ribonucleotide reductase. Clofarabine distinguishes itself from other drugs by its broader activity, in particular the way in which it damages the cells mitochondria and initiates the process of programmed cell death (apoptosis) [114, 115].

Table 3: Allosteric RNR inhibitors.

Names		**Structure**		
Chemical	**Commercial**			
		Base		
Cladribine	Leustatin	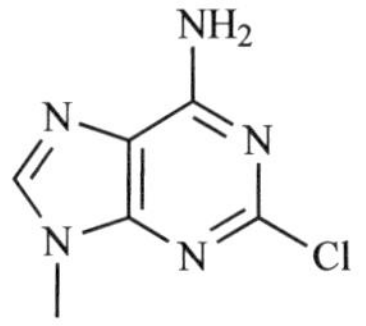	R^1=H R^2=H	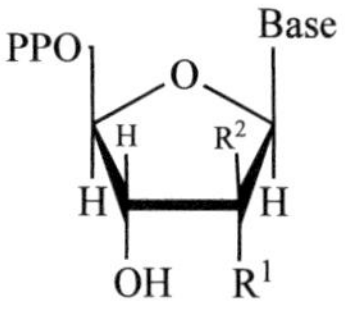
Fludarabine	Fludara	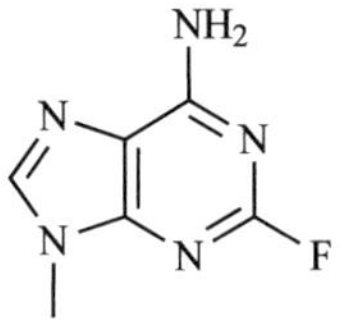	R^1=H R^2=OH	
Clofarabine	Clolar	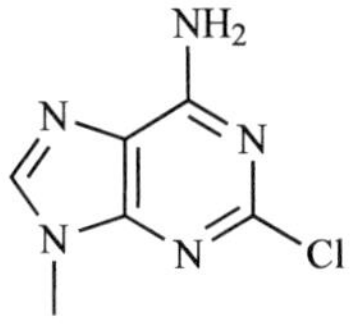	R^1=H R^2=F	

A major problem associated to the effectiveness of these kind of inhibitors is their half-life since, when in excess, they are degraded by adenosine deaminase.

The studies involving these inhibitors have also shown that besides RNR, several enzymes [116, 117] that are involved in DNA replication and repair, can also tolerate a wide range of modifications on the nucleoside triphosphates. Some of the analogues can even hinder their activity and in many cases they can be found incorporated in DNA during the S Phase.

Recently, it was exposed by Hoffer *et al.* that allosteric regulation of RNR in *T. brucei* differs from the mammalian one, which gives hope for the use of allosteric inhibitors in the selective inactivation of parasite RNRs.

Although good results have been obtained with the previous described inhibitors, the most popular ones are the substrate analogues. These inhibitors are administrated as inactive pro-drugs (nucleoside analogues) that only become active (nucleotide analogues) after two phosphorilation steps promoted by the cell kinases. The resulting compounds are recognized by RNR as normal substrates and react in the active site leading to abnormal products that inactivate the enzyme (Table **4**).

Most substrate analogues differ, from the natural one, in the group that is attached to carbon C-2′, since this is the position that is reduced during RNR catalysis. Nevertheless, and similarly to the alosteric binding sites, it was found that the RNR catalytic active site tolerates a wide range of modifications, either on the ribose ring or in the position C-3′ of the nucleotide triphosphate.

The first nucleoside analogue that showed promising anticancer activity was ara-C (arabinosylcytosine, also known as Cytarabine). This compound was developed by Pharmacia & Upjohn and has an arabinose instead of a ribose as central scaffold (the hydroxyl group attached to carbon C-2′ is on the other face of the ring). This compound proved to be a potent drug for the treatment of acute non-lymphocytic leukemia in adults and pediatric patients and was approved by the FDA in 1969. This compound competes with dCTP, for incorporating into DNA, resulting in a block of DNA synthesis and subsequent inhibition of DNA polymerase α and β. In spite of the similarities to cytosine-ribonucleotide, ara-C is not a RNR inhibitor. However, it is generally entitle as the precursor of all RNR inhibitors, since the rapid degradation of this compound by deamination and the ineffectiveness against solid tumors, has promoted the development of other nucleoside analogues, that later one were found to be potent RNR inhibitors. Some examples of such compounds are 2′-chloro-2′-deoxynucleoside-5′-diphosphates (*Cl*dNDP) and 2′-azido-2′-deoxynucleoside-5′-diphosphates (N_3dNDP), which activity was first studied by Thelander and Larsson in 1976, and 2′-deoxy-2′-fluoro-nucleoside-5′-diphosphates (*F*dNDP) studied in 1980 by Stubbe and Kozarich. These inhibitors have a similar mechanistic behavior, and yield a common final product, a ketodeoxyribonucleotide, that leaves the active site, and in solution leads to the formation of a furanone derivative that adds covalently to subunit R1 of RNR (probably to a lysine residue), forming a chromophore with a characteristic UV absorption band. The appearance of this band is normally a consequence of the enzyme inhibition. Within these inhibitors, R2 subunit is also inhibited since after the formation of the ketodeoxyribo-nucleotide the radical becomes lodged at a nitrogen bonded to Cys225 of the active site, precluding tyrosyl radical regeneration.

A similar inhibitor is CH_2dNDP that shows high resistance to cytidinedeaminase, and for which the process of inhibition is believed to be similar, involving the formation of a 2′-methyl furanone derivative. Although, these inhibitors have shown good results in *in vitro* and some *in vivo* studies, it was found that the inhibition is precluded by the presence of reductants such as thioredoxin, dithiothreitol (DDT) or glutathione that are able to intercept the furanone derivative.

(*E*)-2′-Fluoromethylene-2′-deoxycitidine-5′-diphosphate or recently named Tezacitabine (*CHF*dNDP) is another RNR inhibitor [118]. It was developed by Chiron BioPharmaceuticals but it was acquired in January of 2002 by Matrix Pharmaceutical Inc. This inhibitor is able to inactivate both RNR subunits and has shown potent chemotherapeutic efficacy against leukemia and solid tumors [119]. EPR and theoretical studies suggested that the loss of the tyrosyl radical is accompanied by the addition of a substrate analogue to an active site residue (probably a cysteine) which leads to the formation of a chromophore with $\lambda_{max}$of

334nm. Unlike the previous inhibitors, the presence of reductants, such as dithiothreitol does not protect the enzyme against inactivation by *CHF*dNDP, since the substrate analogue binds to the enzyme while it is inside the active site.

Beyond RNR inhibition, some of the substrate analogues are also capable of inhibiting RNA synthesis and/or human DNA elongation, either by their incorporation into the DNA or inhibiting DNA replication. For instance, 2′-deoxy-2′,2′-difluoro-cytidine-5′-diphosphate (F_2dNDP) and 2′-deoxy-2′-methylene-nucleoside-5′-diphosphate (CH_2dNDP) inhibit RNR and are also able to interact with other enzymes that metabolize ribonucleotides and deoxyribonucleotides such as nucleoside and nucleotide kinases, CTP synthethase and DNA polymerases.

F_2dNDP (gemcitabine) is an antimetabolite approved in 1996 by the Food and Drug Administration (FDA) for first-line treatment of locally advanced (nonresectable stage II or stage III) or metastatic (stage IV) adenocarcinoma of the pancreas.

Table 4: RNR substrate analogue inhibitors.

Names			Structure	
Abr.	**Chemical**	**Commercial**		
Ara-C	Cytarabine	Cytosar-U	R^1= OH ; R^2= H ; R^3= OH ; R^4= H	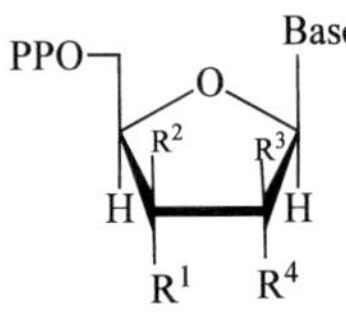
CldNDP		-	R^1= OH ; R^2= H ; R^3= H ; R^4= Cl	
F dNDP		-	R^1= OH ; R^2= H ; R^3= H ; R^4= F	
N_3 dNDP		-	R^1= OH ; R^2= H ; R^3= H ; R^4= N_3	
SHdNDP			R^1= OH ; R^2= H ; R^3= H ; R^4= SH	
F_2 dNDP	Gemcitabine	Gemzar	R^1= OH ; R^2= H ; R^3= F ; R^4= F	
CH_2 dNDP		-	R^1= OH ; R^2= H ; R^3, R^4= CH_2	
CN dNDP		-	R^1= OH ; R^2= H ; R^3= CN ; R^4= H	
CHF dNDP	Fluoromethylene	Tezacitabine	R^1= OH ; R^2= H ; R^3, R^4 = CHF	
C_2H dNDP		-	R^1= OH ; R^2= C_2H ; R^3=H; R^4= OH	

In Europe, it has been approved also for the treatment of patients with cancer of the bladder. Gemcitabine is perhaps one of the most potent compounds that is used nowadays to treat several theses of cancers and is being evaluated for other types of cancer. When compared with other nucleoside analogues, the efficient mode of action of gemcitabine is believed to be dependent on a puzzling metabolic mechanism involving several self-potentiating targets, namely RNR that is inhibited by the diphosphate analogue and DNA polymerase by the triphosphate analogue [43, 120]

Another RNR inhibitor is 2'-cyano-2'-deoxy-arabinosylcytosine (*CN*dNDP). The inhibition effect under RNR is still not known but it is known to delay the progress of further DNA replication similarly to what happens with gemcitabine (F_2dNDP) and other deoxycytidine analogues. However, whereas in gemcitabine the incorporated analogue competes with the natural deoxytidine 5'-triphosphate for incorporation into the replicating DNA, leading to DNA synthesis inactivation at the S Phase, *CN*dNDP also induces DNA strand breaks by a β-elimination-mediated mechanism, that leads to cell cycle arrest at the G2 Phase.

Another kind of RNR inhibitors are the substrate analogues substituted at carbon C-3'. Although less popular there are several compounds of this type. It was suggested that these inhibitors were able to trap the thiyl radical located at Cys439 that is proposed to initiate the reaction, thus quenching the tyrosyl radical and therefore inhibiting RNR. From Matsuda *et al.* [121] studies, it was suggested that ethynyl nucleoside analogues could act as inactivators of RNR, since they share potent anti-tumor activity, both *in vitro* and *in vivo*. However, more studies need to be accomplished with the enzyme *in vivo* and *in vitro*.

As pointed out before, nitric oxide is also an inhibitor of RNR. Taking this idea into account, another class of substrate analogues that are capable of generating $NO^{\bullet}$ was developed by Fallois *et al.* These inhibitors have S-nitro groups attached to carbon C-2′ that spontaneously decompose into nitric oxide, and are capable of inhibiting RNR in both subunits. Although the inhibition with NO is reversible, the remaining radical sulphur of the substrate can interact with the reducing cysteines of the active site and thus modify the course of the reaction, inhibiting irreversibly RNR in subunit R1.

The same group also reported the synthesis of 2'-deoxy-2′-mercaptouridine 5′-diphosphate, a substrate analogue substituted in carbon C-2′ with a SH group, that has been shown to be an efficient inactivator of RNR. The proposed mechanism is still under research [122] but it is known that in the presence of oxygen there is an irreversible inactivation of protein R2 concomitant with the formation of a perthiyl radical (RSS*), whereas in the absence of oxygen no inhibition is observed. This new radical is believed to be located in a cysteine residue of subunit R1, probably in Cys225. Interestingly, the perthiyl radical does not lead to R1 inactivation, suggesting that the presence of reductants such as thioredoxin can regenerate oxidized active site cysteines, as it happens with the natural substrate.

2.2.2. Specific R2 Binding Inhibitors

The target of these inhibitors is protein R2, and from the inhibition results: i) the destruction of the radical that is settled in the tyrosine residue (radical scavengers) or ii) the inactivation of the radical preventing its generation by chelating the iron of the binuclear cluster (iron chelators) (Table **5**).

As the radical is buried *c.a.* 10Å from the surface of the protein, these kind of inhibitors are generally small and planar molecules in order to facilitate their approach to the free radical.

The first inhibitor of this kind that was able to preclude RNR activity was hydroxyurea. Its chemical name is hydroxycarbamide and is trademarked by the commercial name of Hydrea and Droxia®, by Bristol-Myers Squibb Company (BMS).

Hydroxyurea (HU) first started to be investigated, as an antineoplastic agent in humans, in the 1960's. Its synthesis involved many complex crystallization steps [123], but today it is a simple synthesis reaction involving hydroxylamine, HCl and KCN.

This compound is cell cycle Phase-specific (S-Phase) and acts primarily as an inhibitor of RNR. It has already been indicated by the FDA for the treatment of a variety of cancers, e.g., chronic myeloide leukemia, polycythemia vera and hypereosinophilic syndrome. Although its anti-tumor activity is still controversial [124-127], it is a fact that is able to promote temporary remissions in metastatic malignant melanomas and other solid tumors like carcinomas of the head, neck, genitourinary systems, cervix, and lung. Moreover, it has been recently proposed for the treatment of sickle cell anemia and possibly AIDS [128-130]. In small studies combining hydroxyurea with Zerit (d4T) and Videx (ddI), there was noticeable anti-HIV activity [131].

Table 5: RNR radical scavengers and iron chelators inhibitors.

Names		**Structure**
Chemical	**Commercial**	
Hydroxyurea	Hydrea Droxia	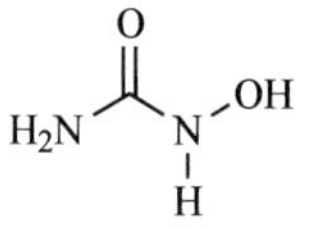
Hydroxamic acid derivatives	-	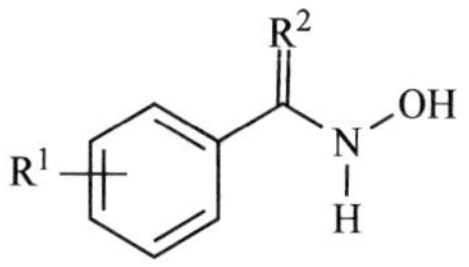
Hydroquinone	-	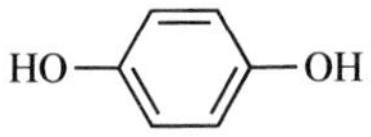
Hydrazine derivatives	-	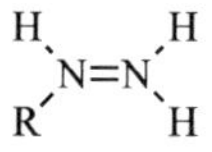 R=H; R=Ph
Hydroxilamine	-	NH_2OH
SNAP	-	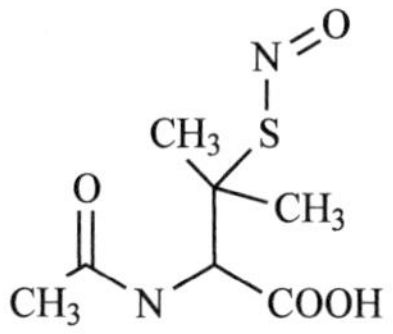
Triapine	Triapine	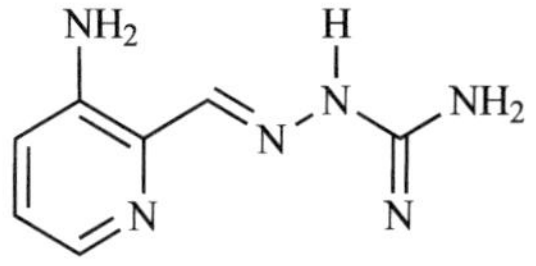

Table 5: contd…

(PIH) and derivatives	Not patentable	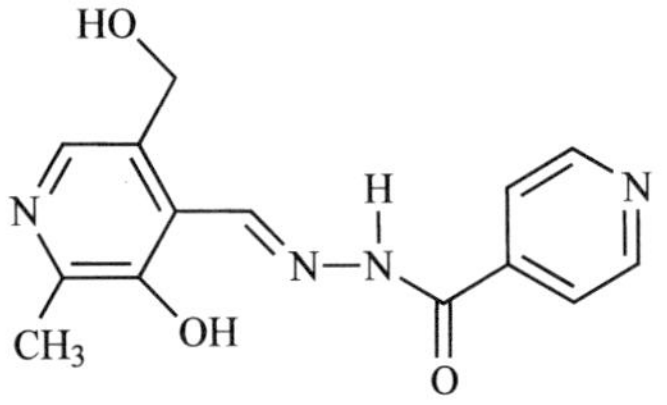
DFO	Desferal	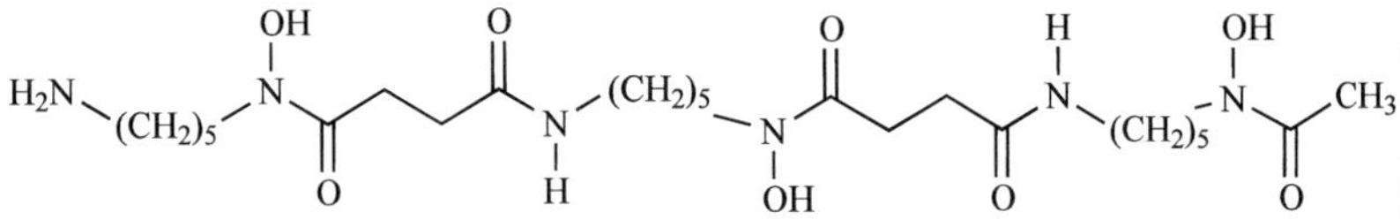

The exact mechanism of HU is still obscure, but it is known to react with the di-iron centers [132]. In fact, it is able to destroy the essential tyrosyl free radical of RNR, turning the enzyme inactive, and therefore consequently stop DNA synthesis.

The most serious side effects of hydroxyurea involve the decrease of blood cells (anemia) [133], platelets (thrombocytopenia) [134], and white blood cell counts (leukopenia, neutropenia [135]), which can decrease patient resistance to infections.

Radical scavengers similar to hydroxyurea [136] such as acetohydroxamate [137], substituted hydroxamic acids [138] or even hydroxylamine, hydroquinones and hydrazine derivatives [139] have shown similar inhibition behavior and some of them have shown to be more potent and/or less toxic than hydroxyurea [140, 141]. Nevertheless, hydroxyurea is still the one that has been more used in cancer therapy.

Since good results were achieved with these inhibitors, similar types of approaches were tried in order to inhibit the enzyme. The iron chelators were the next generation of inhibitors that have shown good properties. These inhibitors are able to bind very tightly to metal ions and form chemically inert complexes, inhibiting the formation of the crucial radical [142]. In addition, many studies have demonstrated that numerous cancer cells types are more susceptible to the effect of the chelators than normal cells.

Several iron chelators such as pyridoxal isonicotinoylhydrazone (PIH), deferoxamine, and thiosemicarbazone derivatives inhibit enzymatic activity, either by chelation of the cofactors, which precludes the incorporation of the cofactor in the enzyme or directly at the enzyme-bound metallic centre. The success of these iron chelators, particularly DFO (Deferrioxaminemesylate), Triapine (3-aminopyridine-2-carboxaldehydethiosemicarbazone) and 2-hydroxy-1-naphthylaldehydeisonicotinoyl hydrazone [143], *in vitro*, *in vivo* and in some clinical trials, together with their selective antitumor activity, confirm their potential as anti-cancer drugs.

Triapine has been developed by Vion Pharmaceuticals, Inc., and has demonstrated a broad spectrum of activity in animal tumor models [144, 145], showing efficacy in both *in vivo* and *in vitro* tests and an ability to inhibit tumor cell growth in the murine L1210 leukemia, murine 109 lung carcinoma and human A2780 ovarian carcinoma models. Tests indicate they are between 65 and 1000 times more potent than FDA's approved Hydroxyurea. Moreover, testing has shown activity against cell lines resistant to Hydrea and Gemzar (see below), which are approved agents for the treatment of cancer.

DFO (desferrioxamine methane sulphonate), developed by Novartis Pharma (brand name Desferal), is a chelating agent used world-wide in the treatment of iron overload conditions, such as hemochromatosis and thalassemia. Desferalis capable of taking up free iron, either in plasma or in cells thereby forming the complex ferrioxamine however, it does not remove iron from transferrin or from hemoglobin or from other heme containing substances. Desferalcan also immobilize and chelate aluminum [146, 147]. However, DFO has some serious disadvantages, including high cost, limited membrane permeability, and long subcutaneous administrations.

Pyridoxal isonicotinoylhydrazone derivatives (PIH) are tridentate chelators and relatively non-toxic drugs, economical to synthesize, orally effective and with high selectivity and affinity for iron. They could be used not only in the treatment of iron overload, but seem to be also effective in the therapy of free radical-mediated injury, malaria and as anti-proliferative agents in some types of cancer. Richarson [148, 149] and Ponka [150] demonstrated that some chelators of the pyridoxal isonicotinoylhydrazone class have antiproliferative activity that is far greater than desferrioxamine(DFO).

The progress in the development of orally effective iron chelators such as PIH has been painfully slow since theseagents are not proprietary (patentable) and therefore their attractiveness for drug industry is severely limited.

Recently, it was also found that the enzyme is rather susceptible to $NO^{\bullet}$ [151]. Studies *in vitro* with several thionitrites, e.g. SNAP (S-nitrosoacetylpenicillamine) manufactured by Alexis Biochemicals, have shown that these $NO^{\bullet}$ donors can inhibit RNR [152], quenching the tyrosyl radical, presumably by forming nitrosotyrosine adducts. However, these adducts have shown to be reversible, which affects the inhibitor efficiency. The reversible behavior should be related with the fact that $NO^{\bullet}$ is also produced physiologically, which suggests that this interaction has an important biological role in the cell regulation.

CURRENT & FUTURE DEVELOPMENTS

Up until now the demise of cancer has relied on surgical resection and the inhibition of tumor cell proliferation, using ionizing radiation or chemotherapeutic drugs designed to perturb DNA synthesis or the mitotic event. The search for new and improved chemotherapeutic agentsagainst cancer cells while leaving normal cells intact is still a hard and constant battle. Different tumors present very different characteristics and one drug can be useful against a certain tumorbut may not be efficient against another. Additionally, cancer cells are also very similar to the normal cells of the host body, and if we target a certain feature common to both cells, we will be not only killing the tumor, but also the host.

The development of RNR inhibitors has become a new hope in this area since several studies indicate that there is a close relationship between tumor growth rate and the hight specific activity of ribonucleotide Reductase. Additionally, several RNR inhibitors have ready shown improvements in the treatment of leukemia, lymphoma, testicular cancer and many other solid tumor types and some of them have already been approved by the FDA and EMEA for clinical use.

Over the last two decades, it has been observed a great increase in the development of potent RNR inhibitors using different strategies. At the same time, important structure-activity relationship studies allowed to point out crucial information that is being used in order to get more efficient substitutions in the general structures of the RNR inhibitors. According to the analysed data, the new generation of inhibitors directed at antisense technology seems to be the most promising one. These inhibitors show many advantages over the others, e.g, rational efficiency in drug design, since they allow shorter timelines to identify lead drug candidates in the discovery Phase of the development as well as reducing the potential for failure in the early stages of development. Furthermore, the rules for creating these drugs are known, the chemistry is constant, and the only modification is the order of the drug's nucleotides, in order to turn the drug target specific. Moreover, the distribution and metabolism of antisense drugs are very similar from drug to drug, resulting in a common and often predictable safety profile across antisense drugs. Dimerization inhibitors have also been showing promising results, since they can inhibit parasite RNRs without interfering with the host RNR. This specific inhibition is already in use and has been showing to be a valuable tool in the treatment of anti-viral and anti-bacterial diseases.

Substrate analogues inhibitors, e.g. gemcitabine that has already been approved by the FDA in the treatment of several kinds of tumor, (as it happened with hydroxyurea) cannot be disclosed from this list. These inhibitors have been in use for longer and successfully employed in several treatments of cancer. However, the toxicity and the inexistence of specificity is a problem with these type of inhibitors. Another limitation of these compounds is that they are admistered as prodrug, which means that need to be activated inside the cell (two phosphorilations) in order to become active. Indeed, the exact mechanism of activation and the inherent side effects of these molecules are still barely known although some of them are already approved by FDA and EMEA for the treatment of several types of tumors.

Although, a great success is being observed with RNR inhibitors, there are two problems that researchers have been facing with: i) the first is the toxicity of the inhibitors, that requires a careful balance between the toxicity of normal tissues vs. cancer cells in order to acquire the desired effect; ii) the second is the resistance to RNR inhibitors that has been observed in several treatments during therapy [153].

The challenge of RNR inhibition now resides in the development of safer and more efficacious inhibitory compounds, which will be surely available soon, taking into account the high potency of the enzyme and the available data.

ACKNOWLEDGEMENTS

NMFSAC, NSHNM, PAF and MJR would like to thank the financial support provided by the Fundaçãopara a Ciência e Tecnologia (BPD/44469/2008 and grant no. Pest-C/EQB/LA0006/2011).

CONFLICT OF INTEREST

The authors confirm that this article content has no conflict of interest.

DISCLOSURE

The chapter submitted for Patent eBook Series entitled "Topics in Anti-Cancer Research", Volume 2 is an update of our article "Ribonucleotide Reductase: A Critical Enzyme for Cancer Chemotherapy and Antiviral Agents", published in the journal 'Recent Patents on Anti-Cancer Drug Discovery', Volume 2, Number 1, January 2007, Page 11 to 29 with modified title, additional text and references.

REFERENCES

[1] Reichard P, Baldesten A, Rutberg L. Formation of deoxycytidine phosphates from cytidine phosphates in extracts from *Escherichia coli*. J Biol Chem 1961; 236: 1150-7.

[2] Jordan A, Reichard P. Ribonucleotide reductases. Annu Rev Biochem 1998; 67: 71-98.

[3] Li J, Zheng LM, King I, Doyle TW, Chen SH. Syntheses and antitumor activities of potent inhibitors of ribonucleotide reductase: 3-Amino-4-methylpyridine-2-carboxaldehyde-thiosemicarbazone (3-AMP), 3-amino-pyridine-2-carboxaldehyde-thiosemicarbazone (3-AP) and its water-soluble prodrugs. Curr Med Chem 2001; 8(2): 121-33.

[4] Nordlund P, Sjoberg BM, Eklund H. 3-Dimensional structure of the free-radical protein of ribonucleotide reductase. Nature 1990; 345: 593-8.

[5] Sjoberg BM. Ribonucleotide reductases - A group of enzymes with different metallosites and a similar reaction mechanism. Struct Bond 1997; 88: 139-73.

[6] Kolberg M, Strand KR, Graff P, Andersson KK. Structure, function, and mechanism of ribonucleotide reductases. Biochim Biophys Acta 2004; 1699: 1-34.

[7] Reichard P. From RNA to DNA, why so many ribonucleotide reductases. Science 1993; 260: 1773-7.

[8] Guittet O, Hakansson P, Voevodskaya N, Fridd S, Gräslund A, Arakawa H, *et al.* Mammalian p53R2 protein forms an active ribonucleotide reductase *in vitro* with the R1 protein, which is expressed both in resting cells in response to DNA damage and in proliferating cells. J Biol Chem 2001; 276: 40647-51.

[9] Pontarin G, Ferraro P, Håkansson P, Thelander L, Reichard P, Bianchi V. p53R2-dependent ribonucleotide reduction provides deoxyribonucleotides in quiescent human fibroblasts in the absence of induced DNA damage. J Biol Chem 2007; 282(23): 16820-8

[10] Shao J, Zhou B, Zhu L, Qiu W, Yuan YC, Xi B, *et al. In vitro* characterization of enzymatic properties and inhibition of the p53R2 subunit of human ribonucleotide reductase. Cancer Res 2004; 64: 1-6.

[11] Hakansson P, Hofer A, Thelander L. Regulation of mammalian ribonucleotide reduction and dNTP pools after DNA damage and in resting cells. J Biol Chem 2006; 281:7834-71.

[12] Nakamura, Y., Arakawa, H., Tanaka, H. Protein having a ribonucleotide reductase activity and a DNA thereof. US6682917 (**2004**).

[13] Elledge SJ, Davis RW. Two genes differentially regulated in the cell cycle and by DNA-damaging agents encode alternative regulatory subunits of ribonucleotide reductase. Genes Dev 1990; 4: 740-51.

[14] Zhao XL, Muller EGD, Rothstein R. A suppressor of two essential checkpoint genes identifies a novel protein that negatively affects dNTP pools. Molecular Cell 1998; 2: 329-40.

[15] Chabes A, Domkin V, Thelander L. Yeast Sml1, a protein inhibitor of ribonucleotide reductase. J Biol Chem 1999; 274: 36679-83.

[16] Thelander L, Reichard P. Reduction of ribonucleotides. Ann Rev Biochem 1979; 48: 133-58.

[17] Kashlan OB, Scott CP, Lear JD, Cooperman BS. A comprehensive model for the allosteric regulation of mammalian ribonucleotide reductase. Functional consequences of ATP- and dATP-induced oligomerization of the large subunit. Biochemistry 2002; 41: 462-74.

[18] Kashlan OB, Cooperman BS. Comprehensive model for allosteric regulation of mammalian ribonucleotide reductase: Refinements and consequences. Biochemistry 2003; 42:1696-706.

[19] Scott CP, Kashlan OB, Lear JD, Cooperman BS. A quantitative model for allosteric control of purine reduction by murine ribonucleotide reductase. Biochemistry 2001; 40: 1651-61.

[20] Cerqueira NMFSA, Fernandes PA, Ramos MJ, Eriksson LA. Dehydration of ribonucleotides catalysed by ribonucleotide reductase: The role of the enzyme. Biophys J 2006; 90: 2109-19.

[21] Cerqueira NMFSA, Fernandes PA, Ramos MJ, Eriksson LA. Ribonucleotide activation by enzyme ribonucleotide reductase: Understanding the role of the enzyme. J Comput Chem 2004; 25: 2031-7.

[22] Cerqueira NMFSA, Fernandes PA, Ramos MJ, Eriksson LA. New insights into a critical biological control step of the mechanism of ribonucleotide reductase. J Mol Struct - Theochem 2004; 53: 53.

[23] Cerqueira NMFSA, Fernandes PA, Ramos MJ. Enzyme ribonucleotide reductase: Unraveling an enigmatic paradigm of enzyme inhibition by furanone derivatives. J Phy Chem B Condens Matter Mater Sruf Interfaces Biophys 2006; 110: 21272-81.

[24] Siegbahn PEM. Theoretical study of the substrate mechanism of ribonucleotide reductase. J Am Chem Soc 1998; 120: 8417-29.

[25] Siegbahn PE. Mechanisms of metalloenzymes studied by quantum chemical methods. Q Rev Biophys 2003; 36: 91-145.

[26] Pelmenschikov V, Cho KB, Siegbahn PE. Class I ribonucleotide reductase revisited: The effect of removing a proton on Glu441. J Comput Chem 2004; 25: 311-21.

[27] Stubbe J, Smith G, Blakley RL. Interaction of 3'-[3H]2'-Chloro-2'-deoxyuridine 5'-triphosphate with ribonucleotide reductase from *Lactobacillus leichmannii*. J Biol Chem 1983; 258: 1619-24.

[28] Stubbe J, Ator M, Krenitsky T. Mechanism of ribonucleoside diphosphate reductase from *Escherichia coli*. Evidence for 3'-C--H bond cleavage. J Biol Chem 1983; 258: 1625-31.

[29] Sjoberg BM, Graslund A, Eckstein F. A substrate radical intermediate in the reaction between ribonucleotide reductase from *Escherichia coli* and 2'-azido-2'-deoxynucleoside diphosphates. J Biol Chem 1983; 258: 8060-7.

[30] Sjoberg BM. The ribonucleotide reductase jigsaw puzzle - a large piece falls into place. Structure 1994; 2: 793-6.

[31] Himo F, Siegbahn PEM. Very stable ribonucleotide substrate radical relevant for class I ribonucleotide reductase. J Phys Chem B 2000; 104: 7502-9.

[32] Bollinger JM Jr, Edmondson DE, Huynh BH, Filley J, Norton JR, Stubbe J. Mechanism of assembly of the tyrosyl radical-dinuclear iron cluster cofactor of ribonucleotide reductase. Science 1991; 253: 292-8.

[33] Stubbe J. Radicals with a controlled lifestyle. Chem Commun (Camb) 2003: 2511-3.

[34] Zipse H. The influence of hydrogen bonding interactions on the C-H bond activation step in class I ribonucleotide reductases. Org Biomol Chem 2003; 1(4): 692-9.

[35] Mohr M, Zipse H. C-H Bond activation in ribonucleotide reductases - Do short, strong hydrogen bonds play a role? Chem Eur J 1999; 5: 3046-54.

[36] Bennati M, Robblee JH, Mugnaini V, Stubbe J, Freed JH, Borbat P. EPR distance measurements support a model for long-range radical initiation in *E. coli* ribonucleotide reductase. J Am Chem Soc 2005; 127: 15014-5.

[37] Strand KR, Karlsen S, Kolberg M, Rohr AK, Gorbitz CH, Andersson KK. Crystal structural studies of changes in the native dinuclear iron center of ribonucleotide reductase protein R2 from mouse. J Biol Chem 2004; 279: 46794-801.

[38] van der Donk WA, Yu GX, Perez L, Sanchez RJ, Stubbe J, Samano V, *et al*. Detection of a new substrate-derived radical during inactivation of ribonucleotide reductase from *Escherichia coli* by gemcitabine 5'-diphosphate. Biochemistry 1998; 37: 6419-26.

[39] Persson AL, Eriksson M, Katterle B, Potsch S, Sahlin M, Sjoberg BM. A new mechanism-based radical intermediate in a mutant R1 protein affecting the catalytically essential Glu(441) in *Escherichia coli* ribonucleotide reductase. J Biol Chem 1997; 272: 31533-41.

[40] Lawrence CC, Bennati M, Obias HV, Bar G, Griffin RG, Stubbe J. High-field EPR detection of a disulfide radical anion in the reduction of cytidine 5'-diphosphate by the E441Q R1 mutant of *Escherichia coli* ribonucleotide reductase. Proc Natl Acad Sci USA 1999; 96: 8979-84.

[41] Crooke ST. Antisense strategies. Curr Mol Med 2004; 4: 465-87.

[42] Perez MAS, Cerqueira NM, Fernandes PA, Ramos MJ. Ribonucleotide reductase: A mechanistic portrait of substrate analogues inhibitors. Curr Med Chem 2010; 17: 2854-72.

[43] Cerqueira NMFSA, Pereira S, Fernandes PA, Ramos MJ. Overview of ribonucleotide reductase inhibitors: An appealing target in anti-tumor therapy. Curr Med Chem 2005; 12: 1283-94.

[44] Zamecnik PC, Stephenson ML. Inhibition of *Rous sarcoma* virus-replication and cell transformation by a specific oligodeoxynucleotide. Proc Nat Acad Sci USA 1978; 75: 280-4.

[45] Holmlund JT, Monia BP, Kwoh TJ, Dorr FA. Toward antisense oligonucleotide therapy for cancer: ISIS compounds in clinical development. Curr Opin Mol Ther 1999; 1: 372-85.

[46] Field AK. Oligonucleotides as inhibitors of human immunodeficiency virus. Curr Opin Mol Ther 1999; 1: 323-31.

[47] Highleyman L. Fomivirsen. Beta 1998; 29: 31.

[48] Grunweller A, Wyszko E, Bieber B, Jahnel R, Erdmann VA, Kurreck J. Comparison of different antisense strategies in mammalian cells using locked nucleic acids, 2'-*O*-methyl RNA, phosphorothioates and small interfering RNA. Nucleic Acids Res 2003; 31: 3185-93.

[49] Agrawal S, Kandimalla ER. Antisense and/or immunostimulatory oligonucleotide therapeutics. Curr Cancer Drug Targets 2001; 1: 197-209.

[50] Kurreck J. Antisense technologies. Improvement through novel chemical modifications. Eur J Biochem 2003; 270: 1628-44.

[51] Yang-Feng TL, Barton DE, Thelander L, Lewis WH, Srinivasan PR, Francke U. Ribonucleotide reductase M2 subunit sequences mapped to four different chromosomal sites in humans and mice: Functional locus identified by its amplification in hydroxyurea-resistant cell lines. Genomics 1987; 1: 77-86.

[52] Brissenden JE, Caras I, Thelander L, Francke U. The structural gene for the M1 subunit of ribonucleotide reductase maps to chromosome 11, band p15, in human and to chromosome 7 in mouse. Exp Cell Res 1988; 174: 302-8.

[53] Park JB, Levine M. Characterization of the promoter of the human ribonucleotide reductase R2 gene. Biochem Biophys Res Commun 2000; 267: 651-7.

[54] Dong Z, Liu Y, Zhang JT. Regulation of ribonucleotide reductase M2 expression by the upstream AUGs. Nucleic Acids Res 2005; 33: 2715-25.

[55] Chen S, Zhou B, He F, Yen Y. Inhibition of human cancer cell growth by inducible expression of human ribonucleotide reductase antisense cDNA. Antisense Nucleic Acid Drug Dev 2000; 10: 111-6.

[56] Aurelian L, Smith CC. *Herpes simplex* virus type 2 growth and latency reactivation by cocultivation are inhibited with antisense oligonucleotides complementary to the translation initiation site of the large subunit of ribonucleotide reductase (RR1). Antisense Nucleic Acid Drug Develop 2000; 10: 77-85.

[57] Wright, J.A., Young, A.H. Antitumor antisense sequences directed against R1 and R2 components of ribonucleotide reductase. WO9805769 (**1999**).

[58] Wright, J.A., Young, A.H. Antisense oligonucleotides directed to ribonucleotide reductase R2 and uses thereof in the treatment of cancer. EP1597365 (**2005**).

[59] Wright, J.A., Young, A.H., Dugourd, D. Antisense oligonucleotide sequences as inhibitors of microorganisms. WO9902673 (**1999**).

[60] Orr RM. GTI-2040. Lorus therapeutics. Curr Opin Invest Drugs 2001; 2: 1462-6.

[61] Tu GC, Tu X. GTI-2501. Lorus therapeutics. Curr Opin Investig Drugs 2001; 2:1467-70.

[62] Lee Y, Vassilakos A, Feng NP, Lam V, Xie H, Wang M, *et al.* GTI-2040, an antisense agent targeting the small subunit component (R2) of human ribonucleotide reductase, shows potent antitumor activity against a variety of tumors. Cancer Res 2003; 63: 2802-11.

[63] Desai AA, Schilsky RL, Young A, Janisch L, Stadler WM, Vogelzang NJ, *et al.* A Phase I study of antisense oligonucleotide GTI-2040 given by continuous intravenous infusion in patients with advanced solid tumors. Ann Oncol 2005; 16: 958-65.

[64] Lee, Y, Vassilakos, A, Feng, N, Jin H, Wang M, Xiong K, *et al.* GTI-2501, an antisense agent targeting R1, the large subunit of human ribonucleotide reductase, shows potent anti-tumor activity against a variety of tumors. Int J Oncol 2006; 28: 469-78.

[65] Davis, ME, Zuckerman JE, Choi CHJ, Seligson D, Tolcher A, Alabi CA, *et al.* Evidence of RNAi in humans from systemically administered siRNA via targeted nanoparticle. Nature 2010; 464: 1067-70.

[66] Davies AM, Gandara DR, Lara PNJr, Mack PC, Lau DH, Gumerlock PH. Antisense oligonucleotides in the treatment of non-small-cell lung cancer. Clin Lung Cancer 2003; 4 (Suppl 2): S68-73.

[67] Climent I, Sjoberg BM, Huang CY. Carboxyl-terminal peptides as probes for *Escherichia coli* ribonucleotide reductase subunit interaction - kinetic-analysis of inhibition studies. Biochemistry1991; 30: 5164-71.

[68] Climent I, Sjoberg BM, Huang CY. Carboxyl terminal peptides as probes for *Escherichia coli* ribonucleotide reductase subunit interaction. FASEB J 1991; 5: A1151.

[69] Cohen EA, Gaudreau P, Brazeau P, Langelier Y. Specific-inhibition of herpesvirus ribonucleotide reductase by a nonapeptide derived from the carboxy terminus of subunit-2. Nature 1986; 321: 441-3.

[70] Lycksell PO, Ingemarson R, Davis R, Graslund A, Thelander L. H-1-NMR studies of mouse ribonucleotide reductase - the R2 protein carboxyl-terminal tail, essential for subunit interaction, is highly flexible but becomes rigid in the presence of protein R1. Biochemistry 1994; 33: 2838-42.

[71] Cooperman BS, Gao Y, Tan C, Kashlan OB, Kaur J. Peptide inhibitors of mammalian ribonucleotide reductase. Adv Enzyme Regul 2005; 45: 112-25.

[72] Deziel, R., Guindon, Y. Antiherpes compositions and method of use. US5552384 (**1994**).

[73] Dutia BM, Frame MC, Subaksharpe JH, Clark WN, Marsden HS. Specific-inhibition of herpesvirus ribonucleotide reductase by synthetic peptides. Nature 1986; 321: 439-41.

[74] Garsky, V.M., Stein, R.A. Inhibitor of ribonucleotide reductase. US4837304 (**1989**).

[75] Yang FD, Spanevello RA, Celiker I, Hirschmann R, Rubin H, Cooperman BS. The carboxyl terminus heptapeptide of the R2 subunit of mammalian ribonucleotide reductase inhibits enzyme-activity and can be used to purify the R1 subunit. Febs Letters 1990; 272: 61-4.

[76] Cosentino, G, Lavallee, P, Rakhit, S, Plante R, Gaudette Y, Lawetz C, *et al.* Specific-inhibition of ribonucleotide reductases by peptides corresponding to the *C*-terminal of their 2nd subunit. Biochem Cell Biol 1991; 69: 79-83.

[77] Gaudreau P, Michaud J, Cohen EA, Langelier Y, Brazeau P. Structure-activity studies on synthetic peptides inhibiting herpes-simplex virus ribonucleotide reductase. J Biol Chem 1987; 262: 12413-6.

[78] Gaudreau P, Brazeau P, Richer M, Cormier J, Langlois D, Langelier Y. Structure-function studies of peptides inhibiting the ribonucleotide reductase-activity of herpes simplex virus type-I. J Med Chem 1992; 35: 346-50.

[79] Laplante SR, Aubry N, Liuzzi M, Thelander L, Ingemarson R, Moss N. The critical C-terminus of the small-subunit of herpes-simplex virus ribonucleotide reductase is mobile and conformationally similar to c-terminal peptides. Int J Peptide Protein Res 1994; 44: 549-55.

[80] Chang LL, Hannah J, Ashton WT, Rasmusson GH, Ikeler TJ, Patel GF, *et al.* Substituted pentapeptides and hexapeptides as potent inhibitors of herpes-simplex virus type-2 ribonucleotide reductase. Bioorg Med Chem Lett 1992; 2: 1207-12.

[81] LlinasBrunet M, Moss N, Scouten E, Liuzzi M, Deziel R. Peptidomimetic inhibitors of herpes virus ribonucleotide reductase. Correlation between herpes simplex and varicella zoster virus. Bioorg Med Chem Lett 1996; 6: 2881-6.

[82] Moss N, Deziel R, Adams J, Aubry N, Bailey M, Baillet M, *et al.* Inhibition of herpes-simplex virus type-1 ribonucleotide reductase by substituted tetrapeptide derivatives. J Med Chem 1993; 36: 3005-9.

[83] Freidinger, R., Hannah, J., Garsky, V.M., Stein, R.B., Tolman, R.L. Inhibitor of ribonucleotide reductase. US4814432 (**1987**).

[84] Moss N, Beaulieu P, Duceppe JS, Ferland JM, Garneau M, Gauthier J, *et al.* Peptidomimetic inhibitors of herpes simplex virus ribonucleotide reductase with improved *in vivo* antiviral activity. J Med Chem 1996; 39: 4173-80.

[85] Avramis, V.I., Cohen, L. Pharmaceutical compositions comprising PEG-asparaginase for the treatment of HIV infections. EP1053012 (**2000**)

[86] Guindon, Y., Lavallee, P., Rakhit, S., Cosentino, G.P. Ribonucleotide reductase inhibitors. US5071835 (**1991**).

[87] Fisher A, Yang FD, Rubin H, Cooperman BS. R2 C-terminal peptide inhibition of mammalian and yeast ribonucleotide reductase. J Med Chem 1993; 36: 3859-62.

[88] Pender BA, Wu X, Axelsen PH, Cooperman BS. Toward a rational design of peptide inhibitors of ribonucleotide reductase: Structure-function and modeling studies. J Med Chem 2001; 44: 36-46.

[89] Liehr S, Barbosa J, Smith AB, Cooperman BS. Synthesis and biological activity of cyclic peptide inhibitors of ribonucleotide reductase. Org Lett 1999; 1: 1201-4.

[90] Fisher A, Laub PB, Cooperman BS. NMR structure of an inhibitory R2 *C*-terminal peptide bound to mouse ribonucleotide reductase R1 subunit. Nat Struct Biol 1995; 2: 951-5.

[91] Pellegrini M, Liehr S, Fisher AL, Laub PB, Cooperman BS, Mierke DF. Structure-based optimization of peptide inhibitors of mammalian ribonucleotide reductase. Biochemistry 2000; 39: 12210-5.

[92] Gao Y, Liehr S, Cooperman BS. Affinity-driven selection of tripeptide inhibitors of ribonucleotide reductase. Bioorg Med Chem Lett 2002; 12: 513-5.

[93] Gao Y, Tan CH, Cooperman BS. Selection of peptide inhibitors of ribonucleotide reductase. Abstr Pap Am Chem S 2002; 224: U41.

[94] Cooperman BS. Oligopeptide inhibition of class I ribonucleotide reductases. Biopolymers 2003; 71: 117-31.

[95] Cooperman BS, Kashlan OB, Scott, CP. A comprehensive model for the allosteric regulation of mammalian ribonucleotide reductase. FASEB J 2002; 16: A154.

[96] Cooperman, B.S., Hirschmann, R.F., Smith III, A.B., Lau, P., Sasho, S., Sprengeler, P.A., Barwis, B.A., Fisher, A., Nair, S. Peptides peptide analogs peptidomimetics and other small molecules useful for inhibiting the activity of ribonucleotide reductase. US6030942 (**2000**).

[97] Yang FD, Curran SC, Li LS, Avarbock D, Graf JD, Chua MM, *et al.* Characterization of two genes encoding the *Mycobacterium tuberculosis* ribonucleotide reductase small subunit. J Bacteriol 1997; 179: 6408-15.

[98] Climent I, Sjoberg BM, Huang CY. Site-directed mutagenesis and deletion of the carboxyl terminus of *Escherichia coli* ribonucleotide reductase protein R2 - effects on catalytic activity and subunit interaction. Biochemistry1992; 31:4801-7.

[99] Dobrogosz, W.J., Lindgren, S.E. Method for inhibiting microorganism growth. US5849289 (**1995**).

[100] Rakhit, S., Plante, R., Cosentino, G.P. Inhibitors of bacterial ribonucleotide reductase. US5198425 (**1993**).

[101] Cooperman, B.S., Rubin, H., Salem, J., Fisher, A.L. *Plasmodium falciparum* ribonucleotide reductase, encoding DNA, and inhibitors. WO9510526 (**1995**).

[102] Martin DS, Spriggs D, Koutcher JA. A concomitant ATP-depleting strategy markedly enhances anticancer agent activity. Apoptosis 2001; 6: 125-31.

[103] Wang X, Zhenchuk A, Wiman KG, Albertioni F. Regulation of p53R2 and its role as potential target for cancer therapy. Cancer Lett 2001; 276(1): 1-7.

[104] Liu X, Zhou B, Xue L, Shih J, Tye K, Lin W, *et al.* Metastasis-suppressing potential of ribonucleotide reductase small subunit p53R2 in human cancer cells. Clin Cancer Res 2006; 12: 6337.

[105] Harrington JA, Spector T. Human ribonucleotide reductase - activation and inhibition by analogs of ATP. Biochem Pharmacol 1991; 42: 759-63.

[106] Chen, R.H.K. Intermediates useful in a synthesis of 2-chloro-2'-deoxyadenosine. US5208327 (**1992**).

[107] Christensen LF, Broom AD, Robins MJ, Bloch A. Synthesis and biological activity of selected 2,6-disubstituted-(2-deoxy- and -D-erythro-pentofuranosyl)purines. J Med Chem 1972; 15: 735-9.

[108] Piro LD, Ellison DJ, Saven A. The scripps clinic experience with 2-chlorodeoxyadenosine in the treatment of hairy cell leukemia. Leuk Lymphoma 1994; 14 (Suppl 1): 121-5.

[109] Saven A, Piro LD. 2-Chlorodeoxyadenosine: A newer purine analog active in the treatment of indolent lymphoid malignancies. Ann Intern Med 1994; 120: 784-91.

[110] Carson, A.D., Carrera, J.C. 2-Halo-2'-deoxyadenosines in the treatment of rheumatoid arthritis. US5310732 (**1994**).

[111] Montgomery, J.A. Anticancer and antiviral activity of 9-β-D-arabinofuranosyl-2-fluoroadenine. US4188378 (**1980**).

[112] Montgomery, J.A., Shortnacy, A.T. Prodrug derivatives of 9β-D-arabinofuranosyl-2-fluoroadenine. US4357324 (**1982**).

[113] Schinazi, R.F., Liotta, D.C., Chu, C.K., McAtee, J.J., Shi, J., Choi, Y., Lee, K., Hong, J.H. 2′-Fluoronucleosides. US6911424 (**2005**) & US8168583 (**2012**).

[114] Watanabe, K.A., Chu, C.K., Fox, J.J. 2-Fluoro-arabinofuranosyl purine nucleosides. US4751221 (**1988**).

[115] Watanabe, K.A., Fox, J.J. 2'-Fluoro-arabinofuranosyl purine nucleosides. US4918179 (**1990**).

[116] Bontemps F, Delacauw A, Cardoen S, Van den Neste E, Van den Berghe G. Metabolism and cytotoxic effects of 2-chloroadenine, the major catabolite of 2-chloro-2'-deoxyadenosine. Biochem Pharmacol 2000; 59: 1237-43.

[117] Mansson E, Flordal E, Liliemark J, Spasokoukotskajad T, Elforde H, Lagercrantzb S, *et al.* Down-regulation of deoxycytidine kinase in human leukemic cell lines resistant to cladribine and clofarabine and increased ribonucleotide reductase activity contributes to fludarabine resistance. Biochem Pharmacol 2003; 65: 237-47.
[118] Jones, R.E., Li, M.T., Trammel, A., Harrison-Bowman, C.M., Shirley, K.R. Stable compositions comprising tezacitabine. WO03069998 (**2003**).
[119] Rodriguez GI, Jones RE, Orenberg EK, Stoltz ML, Brooks DJ. Phase I clinical trials of tezacitabine [(E)-2'-deoxy-2'-(fluoromethylene)cytidine] in patients with refractory solid tumors. Clin Cancer Res 2002; 8: 2828-34.
[120] Grindey, G.B., Hertel, L.W. Method of treating tumors in mammals with 2',2'-difluoronucleosides. US5464826 (**1995**).
[121] Hattori H, Tanaka M, Fukushima M, Sasaki T, Matsuda A. Nucleosides and nucleotides 158. 1-(3-C-ethynyl-beta-D-ribo-pentofuranosyl)cytosine, 1-(3-C-ethynyl-beta-D-ribo-pento-furanosyl)uracil, and their nucleobase analogues as new potential multifunctional antitumor nucleosides with a broad spectrum of activity. J Med Chem 1996; 39: 5005-11.
[122] Pereira S, Fernandes PA, Ramos MJ. Theoretical study on the inhibition of ribonucleotide reductase by 2'-mercapto-2'-deoxyribonucleoside-5'-diphosphates. J Am Chem Soc 2005; 127: 5174-9.
[123] Dresler WFC, Stein R. Uber den Hydroxylharnstoff. Justus Liebigs Ann Chemie 1869; 150: 242-52.
[124] Blumenreich MS, Kellihan MJ, Joseph UG, Lalley KA, Sherrill EJ, Sullivan DM, *et al.* Long-term intravenous hydroxyurea infusions in patients with advanced cancer. A Phase I trial. Cancer 1993; 71: 2828-32.
[125] Olin BR. Drug Facts and Comparisons. St. Louis: Facts and Comparisons: Pharm.D., ed; 1991.
[126] Tosi P, Visani G, Ottaviani E, Tura S, Darnowski JW. Hydroxyurea enhances 3'-azido-3'-deoxythymidine (AZT) cytotoxicity in human chronic myeloid leukemia models. Eur J Haematol 1994; 52: 291-5.
[127] Anand S, Verma H, Kumar L, Singh N. Induction of apoptosis in chronic myelogenous leukemia lymphocytes by hydroxyurea and adriamycin. Cancer Lett1 995; 88: 101-5.
[128] Lori F, Kelly LM, Foli A, Lisziewicz J. Safety of hydroxyurea in the treatment of HIV infection. Expert Opin Drug Saf 2004; 3: 279-88.
[129] Lori F, Lisziewicz J. Hydroxyurea: Mechanisms of HIV-1 inhibition. Antivir Ther 1998; 3 (Suppl 4): 25-33.
[130] Malley, S.D., Vila, J.R. Method of treating HIV in humans by administration of DDI and hydroxycarbamide. US5521161 (**1996**).
[131] Hydroxyurea - new observations. Proj Inf Perspect 1998: 15-7.
[132] Nyholm S, Thelander L, Graslund A. Reduction and loss of the iron center in the reaction of the small subunit of mouse ribonucleotide reductase with hydroxyurea. Biochemistry 1993; 32: 11569-74.
[133] Jabr FI, Shamseddine A, Taher A. Hydroxyurea-induced hemolytic anemia in a patient with essential thrombocythemia. Am J Hematol 2004; 77: 374-6.
[134] Shammas F, Meyer P, Heikkila R, Apeland T, Gøransson L, Berland J, *et al.* Thrombotic microangiopathy in a patient with chronic myelogenous leukemia on hydroxyurea. Acta Haematol 1997; 97: 184-6.

[135] Finazzi G, Barbui T. Efficacy and safety of hydroxyurea in patients with essential thrombocythemia. Pathol Biol (Paris) 2001; 49: 167-9.
[136] Elford H. Inhibition of ribonucleotide reductase by analogs of hydroxyurea and their effect on L1210 leukemia. Proc Am Assoc Can Res 1977; 18: 177-7.
[137] Mayhew CN, Mampuru LJ, Chendil D, Ahmed MM, Phillips JD, Greenberg RN, *et al.* Suppression of retrovirus-induced immunodeficiency disease (murine AIDS) by trimidox and didox - Novel ribonucleotide reductase inhibitors with less bone marrow toxicity than hydroxyurea. Antiviral Res 2002; 56: 167-81.
[138] Atadja, P.W., Shao, W., Bhalla, K.N. Combination of LBH589 with other therapeutic agents for treating cancer. US20100069458 (**2010**).
[139] Han JY, Graslund A, Thelander L, Sykes AG. Kinetic studies on the reduction of the R2 subunit of mouse ribonucleotide reductase with hydroxyurea, hydrazine, phenylhydrazine and hydroxylamine. J Biol Inorg Chem 1997; 2: 287-94.
[140] Li Q, Kasten-Jolly J, Yen Y, Freed BM. Reversal of hydroquinone-mediated suppression of T cell proliferation by transfection of the M2 subunit of ribonucleotide reductase. Toxicol Appl Pharmacol 1998; 150: 154-7.
[141] Elford H, Sumpter R, Inayat M, Gallicchio V. The potential of novel ribonucleotide reductase inhibitors, Didox and Trimidox, compared to hydroxyurea to enhance abacavir antiviral activity *in vivo*. Antiviral Res 2002; 53: A46.
[142] Nyholm S, Mann GJ, Johansson AG, Bergeron RJ, Graslund A, Thelander L. Role of ribonucleotide reductase in inhibition of mammalian cell growth by potent iron chelators. J Biol Chem 1993; 268: 26200-5.
[143] van Reyk D, Sarel S, Hun N. Inhibition of *in vitro* lymphoproliferation by three novel iron chelators of the pyridoxal and salicyl aldehyde hydrazone classes. Biochem Pharmacol 2000; 60: 581-7.
[144] Finch RA, Liu MC, Cory AH, Cory JG, Sartorelli, AC. Triapine (3-aminopyridine-2-carboxaldehyde thiosemicar-bazone; 3-AP): An inhibitor of ribonucleotide reductase with antineoplastic activity. Adv Enzyme Regul 1999; 39: 3-12.
[145] Finch RA, Liu MC, Grill SP, Rose WC, Loomis R, Vasquez KM, *et al.* Triapine (3-aminopyridine-2-carboxaldehydethiosemicarbazone): A potent inhibitor of ribonucleotide reductase activity with broad spectrum antitumor activity. Biochem Pharmacol 2000; 59: 983-91.
[146] Allain P, Chaleil D, Mauras Y, Beaudeau G, Varin MC, Poignet JL, *et al.* Pharmacokinetics of desferrioxamine and of its iron and aluminium chelates in patients on haemodialysis. Clin Chim Acta 1987; 170: 331-8.
[147] Allain P, Mauras Y, Chaleil D, Simon P, Ang KS, Cam G, *et al.* Pharmacokinetics and renal elimination of desferrioxamine and ferrioxamine in healthy subjects and patients with haemochromatosis. Br J Clin Pharmacol 1987; 24: 207-12.
[148] Richardson D, Ponka P, Baker E. The effect of the iron(III) chelator, desferrioxamine, on iron and transferrin uptake by the human malignant melanoma cell. Cancer Res 1994; 54: 685-89.
[149] Richardson DR, Ponka P. The iron metabolism of the human neuroblastoma cell: Lack of relationship between the efficacy of iron chelation and the inhibition of DNA synthesis. J Lab Clin Med 1994; 124: 660-71.
[150] Ponka P, Richardson DR, Edward JT, Chubb FL. Iron chelators of the pyridoxal isonicotinoyl hydrazone class. Relationship of the lipophilicity of the apochelator to its

ability to mobilise iron from reticulocytes *in vitro*. Can J Physiol Pharmacol 1994; 72: 659-66.

[151] Lepoivre M, Fieschi F, Coves J, Thelander L, Fontecave M. Inactivation of ribonucleotide reductase by nitric oxide. Biochem Biophys Res Commun 1991; 179: 442-8.

[152] Lemaire G, Alvarez-Pachon FJ, Beuneu C, Lepoivre M, Petit JF. Differential cytostatic effects of NO donors and NO producing cells. Free Radic Biol Med 1999; 26: 1274-83.

[153] Mansson E, Spasokoukotskaja T, Sallstrom J, Eriksson S, Albertioni F. Molecular and biochemical mechanisms of fludarabine and cladribine resistance in a human promyelocytic cell line. Cancer Res 1999; 59: 5956-63.

Send Orders of Reprints at reprints@benthamscience.net
Topics in Anti-Cancer Research, Vol. 2, 2013, 407-436

CHAPTER 12

Enhancing the Anticancer Activity of Erlotinib in Glioblastoma

Georg Karpel-Massler*, Christian R. Wirtz and Marc-Eric Halatsch

Department of Neurosurgery, University of Ulm School of Medicine, Albert-Einstein-Allee 23, D-89081 Ulm, Germany

Abstract: Glioblastoma multiforme (GBM) is the most common malignant intrinsic brain tumor in adults. Especially in this disease, qualitative and quantitative aspects render the dysregulated epidermal growth factor receptor (HER1/EGFR) an outstanding therapeutic target. A variety of therapeutic compounds was developed to target HER1/EGFR among which the clinically most advanced agents are small molecule tyrosine kinase (TK) inhibitors. Unfortunately, clinical studies examining their therapeutic efficacy have so far failed to document a major therapeutic break-through in the setting of GBM. Thus, the targeted approach against HER1/EGFR likely requires a synergistic drug combination strategy to ultimately become successful in this disease. This patents chapter focuses on innovative therapeutic strategies combining HER1/EGFR-targeted TK inhibitors with novel agents which for the most part have not been evaluated for the treatment of GBM yet but which constitute interesting candidates for further evaluation in this setting.

Keywords: Angiogenesis, combination therapy, erlotinib, glioblastoma, HER1/EGFR, high-grade glioma, histone deacetylase inhibitors, IGF1R, Kit, multi-targeting, neurooncology, oncogene, pralatrexate, radiotherapy, romidepsin, targeted therapy, temozolomide, tumorigenesis, tyrosine kinase inhibitor, vascular disrupting agents.

INTRODUCTION

Even with the best available standard of care, many human malignant diseases, including high-grade gliomas, are still associated with a poor clinical outcome [1]. Therefore, much hope and effort were invested in the search for new therapeutic strategies based on the discovery of molecular targets that are involved in malignant transformation and maintenance of the malignant cellular phenotype.

***Address correspondence to Georg Karpel-Massler:** Department of Neurosurgery, University of Ulm School of Medicine, Albert-Einstein-Allee 23, D-89081 Ulm, Germany; Tel: +49-(0)731-500-55003; Fax: +49-(0)731-500-55002; E-mail: georg.karpel@uniklinik-ulm.de

The epidermal growth factor receptor (HER1/EGFR) was shown to be over expressed in about 50% of glioblastoma which is the most common and the most malignant subtype of high-grade glioma [2-4]. Subsequently, a lot of interest evolved for the creation of HER1/EGFR-targeted agents.

HER1/EGFR tyrosine kinase (TK) inhibitors such as erlotinib (Tarceva®, Genentech Inc., San Francisco, CA, USA) or gefitinib (Iressa®, AstraZeneca Pharmaceuticals, Wilmington, DE, USA) are the most clinically advanced HER1/EGFR-targeted agents for the treatment of high-grade glioma. The molecular mechanism of these molecules is based on a reversible binding to the intracellular catalytic TK domain of HER1/EGFR and subsequent inhibition of autophosphorylation of the receptor as well as further downstream signaling involving phosphatidylinositol 3-kinase/murine thymoma viral oncogene homolog (PI3-K/AKT) and mitogen-activated protein kinase (MAPK) pathways [5-7]. Both gefitinib and crlotinib specifically inhibit HER1/EGFR, while erlotinib also inhibits EGFRvIII, the most frequent mutant form of HER1/EGFR which is characterized by constitutive, i.e. ligand-independent activation [8]. In the setting of high-grade glioma, gefitinib was shown to exert minor inhibitory effects on glioblastoma cells when compared to erlotinib. This finding might be partly explained by the fact that gefitinib is most effective against tumors expressing HER1/EGFR with mutations in exons 19 and 21 of the TK domain which are frequently present in non-small cell lung cancer (NSCLC) but are lacking in glioblastoma [9, 10].

In experimental studies, erlotinib was shown to significantly diminish EGFRvIII expression in transfected glioblastoma cells upon long-term exposure and to inhibit the expression of genes encoding pro-invasive proteins [11]. In addition, the extent of erlotinib-mediated inhibition of anchorage-independent growth of glioblastoma-derived cell lines was shown to correlate inversely with the cellular capability to induce *HER1/EGFR* mRNA, emphasizing the important role of HER1/EGFR in the pathogenesis of glioblastoma [12]. However, the results of clinical studies examining the effect of erlotinib monotherapy in patients with recurrent glioblastoma were disappointing [13, 14]. In a randomized, controlled Phase II trial, only 11.4% of the patients with recurrent glioblastoma treated with erlotinib were free of progression after 6 months compared to 24.1% of the patients treated with temozolomide and carmustine [14]. Moreover, no significant difference in overall survival was found between the two treatment groups (7.7 months for the erlotinib group vs. 7.3 months for the temozolomide/carmustine group). Thus, existing data suggest the need to upgrade from a single-targeted therapeutic approach with HER1/EGFR TK inhibitors towards a combination of these inhibitors with other targeted agents and/or conventional adjuvant therapies.

The therapeutic efficacy of erlotinib in combination with standard radiochemotherapy in patients with glioblastoma has been examined by several studies [15-17]. Overall, the results appear controversial. One major culprit that is shared by these studies is their non-randomized nature and missing appropriate control groups. Hopefully, randomized controlled trials including appropriate control groups will allow making a clear statement. In Table **1**, a summary is given on selected studies with erlotinib in combination with standard chemotherapy or other agents.

Table 1: Selected clinical trials of erlotinib in high-grade glioma.

Treatment	**Phase**	**Description**	***n* (evaluable)**	**Activity Summary**
Erlotinib *vs.* TMZ or BCNU	II, RCT	Erlotinib 150mg/d escalating up to 200mg/d (no EIAEDs) or 300mg/d escalating up to 500mg/d (with EIAEDs); control: TMZ 150-200mg/d for 5 days every 4 weeks or BCNU 80mg/m^2/d for 3 days every 8 weeks in recurrent GBM [14]	Erlotinib: 54 TMZ/BCNU: 56	Erlotinib: Median PFS: 1.8 months Median OS: 7.7 months TMZ/BCNU: Median PFS: 2.4 months Median OS: 7.3 months No significant activity of erlotinib was observed
Erlotinib +RT +TMZ	II	Erlotinib 100mg/d during RT, 150mg/d after RT (no EIAEDs) or 200mg/d during RT and 300mg/d after RT (with EIAEDs); RT 60 Gy in 30 fractions with concomitant TMZ 75mg/m^2/d, followed by 5 days of 200mg/m^2/d TMZ repeated every 4 weeks and starting 2 weeks after RT in patients with newly diagnosed GBM or GS compared to a historical control [16]	GBM/GS: 65 Control: 128	Median PFS: 8.2 months Median OS: 19.3 months Improvement in PFS and OS

Table 1: contd....

Erlotinib +RT +TMZ	II	Erlotinib 50mg/d increased by 50mg/d every 2 weeks to a maximum dose of 150mg/d, RT 60 Gy in 30 fractions with concomitant TMZ 75mg/m^2/d (42 days) prior to 12 four-week cycles comprising each 5 days of 150-200mg/m^2/d TMZ in patients with newly diagnosed GBM [17]	GBM: 27	22 (81%) Patients came off study 18 (67%) for PD 4 (15%) for AE Median PFS: 2.8 months Median OS: 8.6 months This trial was terminated preterm (three deaths related to treatment)
Erlotinib +Bevacizumab	II	Erlotinib 200 mg/d (no EIAEDs) or 500mg/d (with EIAEDs), bevacizumab 10mg/kg i.v. every 2 weeks in patients with recurrent high-grade glioma [22]	GBM: 25 AG: 32	GBM: Median PFS: 18 weeks Median OS: 42 weeks 1 CR (4%); 11 PR (46%); 10 SD (42%) AG: Median PFS: 23.4 weeks Median OS: 71 weeks 1 CR (3%); 9 PR (28%); 14 SD (44%)
Erlotinib +Sirolimus	II	Erlotinib 150mg/d (no EIAEDs) or 450mg/d (with EIAEDs), sirolimus 5mg/d (no EIAEDs) or 10mg/d (with EIAEDs) in patients with recurrent GBM [21]	32	Median PFS: 6.9 weeks Median OS: 33.8 weeks 0 CR; 0 PR; SD 15 (47%) Negligible anti-tumor activity

Abbreviations: AE: Adverse events; AG: Anaplastic glioma; BCNU: Carmustine; EIAED: Enzyme-inducing anti-epileptic drug; GBM: Glioblastoma multiforme; GS: Gliosarcoma; i.v.: Intravenously; PD: Progressive disease; PFS: Progression-free survival; PR: Partial response; RCT: Randomized controlled trial; RT: Radiotherapy; SD: Stable disease; TMZ: Temozolomide

A different approach that has been employed by experimental and also a few clinical studies involves the inhibition of downstream key regulators such as mammalian target of rapamycin (mTOR) and phosphatidylinositol 3-kinase (PI3-K) in addition to treatment with HER1/EGFR TK inhibitors. Experimental studies showed favorable results. Significantly increased anti-proliferative effects were reported for phosphatase and tensin homolog deleted on chromosome 10 (PTEN)-deficient U87 and SF295 glioblastoma cells subjected to combined treatment with erlotinib and rapamycin, an mTOR inhibitor, when compared to cells receiving erlotinib alone [18]. Proliferation was reduced by 38% in PTEN-deficient SF295 cells treated with both, erlotinib and rapamycin, whereas treatment with erlotinib alone reduced proliferation only by 14%. Treatment with rapamycin alone showed results that were comparable to erlotinib monotherapy. Similar findings were reported by another experimental study [19]. Moreover, antiproliferative efficacy was shown to be even more pronounced in PTEN-mutant glioma cells by additional inhibition of PI3-K using a dual mTOR/PI3-K inhibitor (PI-103) when combined with erlotinib in comparison to erlotinib combined with either mTOR or PI3-K inhibition. With regard to the clinical setting, first steps were taken to evaluate a multi-targeting approach that includes erlotinib. Doherty *et al.* showed 6-months progression-free survival of 25% in a pilot study with 22 recurrent glioblastoma patients who were treated with erlotinib or gefitinib in combination with sirolimus (rapamycine, Rapamune®, Wyeth Pharmaceuticals Inc., Ayerst, PA, USA) [20]. However, in a Phase II clinical trial examining the therapeutic efficacy of combined treatment with erlotinib and sirolimus in 32 patients with recurrent glioblastoma, anti-tumor activity was reported to be negligible with no complete or partial responses [21]. Median progression-free survival and median overall survival were shown to be 6.9 weeks and 33.8 weeks, respectively.

Recently, a Phase II clinical trial evaluated the clinical effects of a combined treatment with erlotinib and bevacizumab, a humanized anti-vascular endothelial growth factor (VEGF) monoclonal antibody (mAb), on patients with recurrent high-grade glioma [22]. For glioblastoma patients, median overall survival and 6-months progression-free survivals were reported (42 weeks and 28%, respectively). Moreover, radiographic response was observed for 48% of the glioblastoma patients. Unfortunately, appropriate control groups were not included in this study. However, comparison to historical data of patients treated with bevacizumab only showed a similar progression-free survival and radiographic response.

Target-specific therapeutics are usually characterized by reduced toxicity when compared to conventional chemotherapeuties. Erlotinib, for example, was shown to fit a reasonable safety profile in Phase I trials and was generally well tolerated [23, 24]. From this point of view, the use of HER1/EGFR-targeted TK inhibitors in combination with other therapeutics seems favorable. In this chapter, we review four different novel drug combination strategies aiming at enhancement of the antitumor effect exerted by erlotinib. None of the combination approaches to be discussed have been evaluated in glioma-specific models; selection of these particular patents is hypothesis-driven, assuming solid tumor analogy and sufficient drug availability at the target site.

ERLOTINIB AND ROMIDEPSIN

Histone deacetylase (HDAC) is an enzyme that influences the regulation of gene expression by modifying the chromatin structure. Eighteen HDACs with varying function and tissue distribution have been identified in humans. According to their homology to yeast proteins, four classes of HDACs are distinguished [25]. In the brain, class I, IIa and IV HDACs are found [26]. By deacetylating the ε-amino groups of lysine residues of core histone proteins, HDACs induce increased packaging of chromatin and subsequent repression of transcriptional activity, a process that is fundamental during embryogenesis and cellular differentiation [25, 27]. Downregulation of genes involved in apoptosis and cell cycle control due to modulation of the chromatin state through enzymatic histone modification is considered a key factor in tumorigenesis [28]. Various human cancers such as hematologic malignancies, breast cancer, colorectal cancer or pancreatic carcinoma were found to overexpress HDAC [25, 29]. In addition, inhibition of HDAC was shown to trigger apoptosis by diverse mechanisms, including up-regulation of death receptor proteins such as Fas, tumor necrosis factor-α or tumor necrosis factor-related apoptosis-inducing ligand receptors [30, 31] and increased expression of the proapoptotic genes *Bmf* and *Bim* in different cancer cell lines [32, 33]. HDAC inhibition was also shown to disrupt the function of the chaperone heat shock protein 90 followed by increased degradation of oncogenic proteins such as BCR-ABL, HER1/EGFR or AKT [34-36]. Moreover, down-regulation of HDAC was shown to be related to increased expression of $p21^{WAF1/CIP1}$ which induces cell cycle arrest and cellular differentiation [37, 38].

Based on these findings, inhibition of HDAC may constitute a promising approach in cancer therapy.

Romidepsin, also termed depsipeptide, FK228 or FR901228, is a bicyclic peptide that was first isolated from a broth culture of *Chromobacterium violaceum* Fig. (**1**) [39]. It was shown to have immunosuppressive, anti-microbial and antineoplastic activities [39, 40]. The molecular mechanisms underlying the therapeutic effects of romidepsin have not yet been completely elucidated. However, there is evidence that one mode of action involves the selective inhibition of deacetylases such as HDAC or tubulin deacetylase Fig. (**2**) [28]. Romidepsin is one of the best studied HDAC inhibitors in clinical trials. Most clinical experience with HDAC inhibitors is available for the treatment of

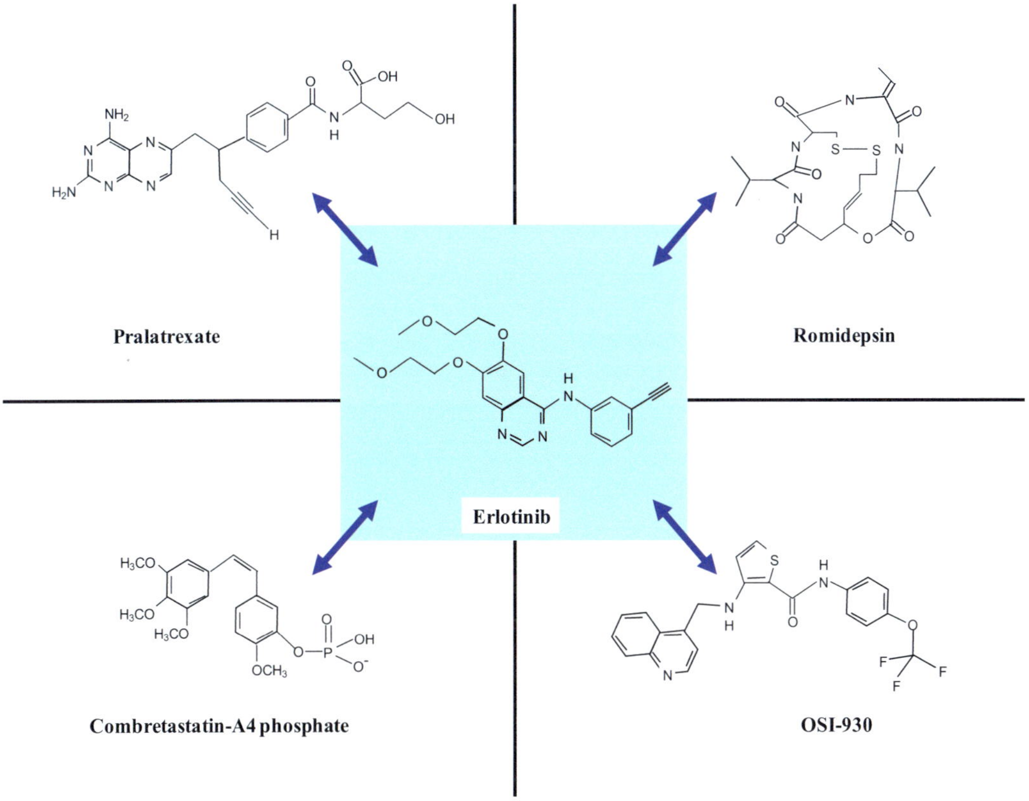

Figure 1: Molecular structures of erlotinib, romidepsin, OSI-930, pralatrexate and combretastatin-A4 phosphate.

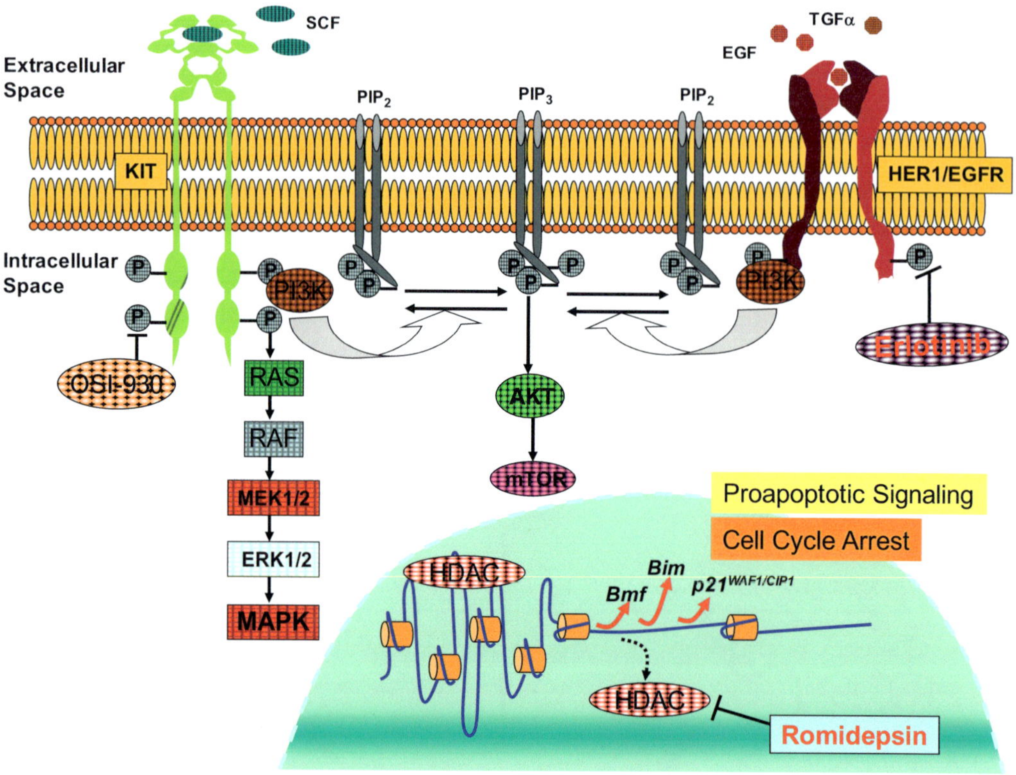

Figure 2: Schematic illustration of some of the agents discussed in this chapter with regard to their site of action. Abbreviations: AKT, Murine thymoma viral oncogene homolog; EGF, Epidermal growth factor; HDAC, Histone deacetylase; HER1/EGFR, Epidermal growth factor receptor; MAPK, Mitogen-activated protein kinase; MEK, Mitogen-activated protein kinase kinase; mTOR, Mammalian target of rapamycin; PI3-K, Phosphatidylinositol 3-kinase; PIP_2, Phosphatidylinositol 3,4 biphosphate; PIP_3, Phosphatidylinositol 3,4,5 Triphosphate; RAF, Murine leukemia viral oncogene homolog; RAS, Rat sarcoma viral oncogene homolog; SCF, Stem cell factor; TGF-α, Transforming growth factor-α.

hematologic malignancies and cutaneous T-cell lymphoma (CTCL) [25, 41]. In an early Phase I trial, Byrd *et al*. examined the effects of romidepsin applied intravenously at a dose of 13 mg/m^2 on day 1, 8, and 15 of a 4-week cycle on 10 patients with chronic lymphocytic leukemia (CLL) and 10 patients with acute myeloid leukemia (AML) [42]. No formal complete or partial responses were observed for any of the patients with AML or CLL. However, in all seven CLL patients who had elevated leukocyte counts at the beginning of the therapy, improvement in peripheral leukocyte counts was observed while in the AML group one patient developed a tumor lysis syndrome. Moreover, in a Phase II study, Odenike *et al.* observed antileukemic activity of romidepsin in 5 of 7 patients with AML as shown by a decrease in bone marrow blasts [43]. However, all 5 patients developed disease progression within 30 days after achieving their best response to romidepsin therapy. Noteworthy, the patients who responded to romidepsin belonged to a subgroup of AML patients with chromosomal abnormalities known to recruit HDACs. Recently, two Phase II clinical trials examining the effects of romidepsin in patients with refractory CTCL were published [44, 45]. Piekarz *et al.* showed an overall response rate of 34% for a group of 71 patients with treatment-refractory or advanced CTCL treated with a starting dose of $14mg/m^2$ romidepsin administered as a 4-h intravenous infusion on days 1, 8, and 15 of a 28-day cycle [44]. Partial response was observed for 26%, complete response for 7% and stable disease for 38% of the patients. Similar results were obtained in the study conducted by Whittacker *et al.* [45]. From 96 patients that were included in this study, 26% had a partial response, 6% a complete response and 47% stable disease.

Romidepsin was generally well tolerated, and serious adverse events reported from clinical trials were shown to be rare [41-45]. Drug-related adverse events included fatigue, nausea, vomiting, pyrexia and electrocardiographic changes, but also signs of myelosuppression such as thrombocytopenia, neutropenia or anemia. Overall, the safety profile of romidepsin has been favorable in Phase I and II trials, especially when compared to traditional chemotherapy.

In the setting of high-grade glioma, there is no clinical data for the use of romidepsin and only sparse clinical data on other HDAC inhibitors. However, in experimental studies, HDAC inhibitors have been shown to exert a radiosensitizing effect on glioblastoma cells. Camphausen *et al.* showed that the fraction of surviving SF539 and U251 glioblastoma cells treated with radiation and valproic acid (VA), an anticonvulsive drug with a known inhibitory effect on HDACs, was significantly lower when compared to cells that were not exposed to VA [46]. In addition, in a heterotopic U251 xenograft model, mice treated with three initial intraperitoneal injections of VA at a dose of 150mg/kg followed by irradiation with 4 Gy and three more intraperitoneal injections of VA showed a significantly greater delay of tumor growth when compared to animals receiving a monotherapy with either VA or irradiation. Similar findings were reported by other groups for various HDAC inhibitors [47, 48]. In a different study, Svechnikova *et al.* showed that treatment with the HDAC inhibitor trichostatin A or 4-phenyl-butyrate induced cellular differentiation and the development of distinct phenotypic characteristics in the human glioblastoma cell lines GBM29, U343MG and U343MGa [27]. In addition, both HDAC inhibitors were shown to exert antiproliferative and proapoptotic effects on the three cell lines.

A single experimental study examined the effects of romidepsin in the setting of glioblastoma. Sawa *et al.* showed that treatment with romidepsin at a concentration of 1 ng/ml resulted in significantly reduced proliferation rates in T98G, U251MG and U87MG glioblastoma cells [49]. In addition, the concentration of the proapoptotic protein Bad was found to be significantly increased whereas the concentration of the antiapoptotic protein Bcl-xL was shown to be significantly decreased. Moreover, cellular invasiveness was significantly reduced in U251MG cells treated with romidepsin when compared to controls. Finally, in a murine heterotopic xenograft model, tumor growth of subcutaneously inoculated U87MG human glioblastoma cells which had been transformed with exogenous EGFRvIII was shown to be significantly inhibited by the treatment with romidepsin.

Both erlotinib and romidepsin are promising anticancer agents fitting a reasonable safety profile. A recently published patent claims that the combination of TK inhibitors such as erlotinib and HDAC inhibitors such as romidepsin may be particularly useful in the treatment of proliferative diseases [50]. In their patent application, the authors show *in vitro* that in 13 out of 16 non-small cell lung cancer cell lines sensitivity towards erlotinib increased 13-fold (median) when romidepsin was coadministered. This effect was especially pronounced on cells expressing wild-type HER1/EGFR and wild-type KRAS. The authors showed that one way allowing romidepsin to enhance the antineoplastic effect of erlotinib may be by facilitating apoptosis. HCC15 NSCLC cells treated with 5μM erlotinib did not undergo apoptosis, and cells treated with 2ng/ml romidepsin showed only a 2.7-fold increase in apoptosis. However, combined treatment with erlotinib and romidepsin yielded a 5.9-fold increase in apoptosis. Moreover, in a murine xenograft model using subcutaneously inoculated NCI-H1299 metastatic NSCLC cells, tumor growth was significantly inhibited by the combined treatment with erlotinib and romidepsin when compared to animals receiving erlotinib and romidepsin treatment alone.

Thus, a therapeutic approach combining the antineoplastic effects of erlotinib and HDAC inhibitors such as romidepsin appears promising based on those preclinical data. Further studies are needed to elucidate if such a combined treatment may provide any clinical benefit in the setting of high-grade glioma.

COMBINED TREATMENT WITH ERLOTINIB AND OSI-930

Kit (CD117) is a receptor tyrosine kinase related to the platelet-derived growth factor receptor (PDGFR) and the macrophage colony stimulating factor receptor (c-fms) [51, 52]. Its encoding gene sequence is located on chromosome 4q12. Kit has a molecular size of 145kDa and consists of an extracellular portion containing a ligand-binding and dimerization domain, a transmembraneous portion and an intracellular portion containing a juxtamembrane inhibitory domain and two tyrosine kinase domains Fig. (**2**). Stem cell factor, also known as steel factor, Kit ligand or mast cell factor, is the physiologic ligand for Kit [53]. Once it binds to the ligand-binding site, receptor dimerization occurs, followed by autophosphorylation and subsequent activation of downstream signaling via PI3K/AKT, MAPK and JAK/STAT pathways [54, 55]. Among the cells that have been shown to express Kit are haemopoietic progenitor cells, mast cells, melanocytes, germ cells and the interstitial cells of Cajal [56-59]. Dysregulation of Kit has been implicated in the pathogenesis of a variety of human cancers including gastrointestinal stromal tumors (GIST), melanoma, NSCLC, mast cell leukemia, AML, breast cancer and germ cell tumors [51, 60, 61].

Kit was also shown to be expressed by glial tumors. Cetin *et al.* reported that 75% of 52 glial tumor specimens of various histologic grades were positive for Kit expression [62]. In addition, Kit was shown to be expressed at significantly higher levels in high-grade gliomas compared to low-grade gliomas. Another study reported that in 47% of primary glioblastoma amplification of Kit was present [63]. Moreover, amplification of Kit was shown to be more frequent in recurrent than in initial disease [64]. In 8 of 16 (50%) recurrent anaplastic astrocytomas, compared to 5 out of 13 (28%) newly diagnosed anaplastic astrocytomas, amplified Kit was found. In accordance with the results of the previously mentioned study, amplification of Kit was shown to be more frequent in high-grade gliomas. These findings support a possible role of Kit in the process of tumorigenesis and malignant transformation of gliomas.

A variety of mutations of Kit have been described, including small in-frame deletions or insertions in the inhibitory juxtamembrane region which cause ligand-independent activation of the receptor [51]. Other alterations such as the D816V mutation confer increased catalytic activity of Kit and an increased affinity to adenosine triphosphate due to changes within the activation loop. For gliomas, such mutations of Kit have not yet been reported. However, in other human malignant diseases such as mast cell leukemia or GIST, these mutations have been shown to be quite common. Thus, the development of Kit-targeted therapeutic agents for the treatment of cancers that bear mutational changes causing dysregulation of Kit appears promising. Mutations of the Kit gene were shown to be present in at least 80% of the tumors studied [60]. Treatment with imatinib mesylate (Gleevec®, Novartis, East Hanover, NJ, USA), a Kit-targeted small molecule TK inhibitor, was shown to significantly increase median overall survival of patients with GIST from 19 months to more than 50 months [65-67]. Moreover, up to 84% of the patients treated with imatinib were shown to attain at least stable disease [66-68].

In the setting of glioblastoma, imatinib was shown *in vitro* to have an antiproliferative effect on certain cell lines [69]. In addition, it was reported that imatinib inhibits proliferation and significantly increases radiosensitivity of the human U87 glioblastoma cell line *in vitro* and *in vivo* [70]. Several clinical Phase I and Phase II studies were conducted to examine the role of imatinib in the treatment of glioblastoma [71, 72]. However, for the most part, only moderate antitumor activity was shown to be conferred by imatinib. A Phase I/II study evaluating the effect of single-agent therapy with imatinib at a dose of 800mg/d in 34 patients with glioblastoma showed that only 6 patients reached stable disease while 2 patients showed partial response and no patient achieved complete response [72]. Progression-free survival at 6 months was only 3%. In another Phase II study, Razis *et al.* evaluated the effect of imatinib on the molecular level. Twenty patients with glioblastoma were diagnosed by tumor biopsy and treated with 400mg imatinib administered twice a day for a period of 7 days prior to re-biopsy or tumor resection. Molecular analysis revealed that treatment with imatinib did not affect tumor proliferation as there was no significant change in Ki67 expression [71]. Median survival was only 6.2 months which may be partly due to the selection of patients with an *a priori* worse prognosis.

One reason explaining the limited antineoplastic activity of single-agent therapy with imatinib in glioblastoma may be that inhibition of Kit and co-targeted TKs such as the PDGFR is not sufficient to suppress tumor growth. Dysregulation of other growth factor receptors such as HER1/EGFR may interfere with the inhibitory effect of Kit-targeted therapeutics and preserve the malignant cellular phenotype. A recently published patent proposes a combined simultaneous or sequential treatment of neoplastic diseases with a HER1/EGFR TK inhibitor (e.g., erlotinib) and an inhibitor of Kit (*e.g.*, OSI-930) in order to yield an additive or synergistic anti-tumor effect [73]. *N*-(4-trifluoromethoxyphenyl) 3-[(quinolin-4-ylmethyl)amino]thiophene-2-carboxamide, also termed OSI-930, is a small molecule TK inhibitor of Kit [74]. In that patent, the authors claim that in female nu/nu CD-1 mice that were subcutaneously inoculated with human H2122 or H441 NSCLC cells, tumor growth was significantly more inhibited by a combined treatment with erlotinib and OSI-930 at a dose of 100mg/kg each when compared to treatment with erlotinib or OSI-930 alone at the same single dosage. For the H2122 NSCLC cell xenografts, combination therapy was reported to reduce tumor volume to 50% of the initial tumor volume, whereas single-agent treatment with erlotinib or OSI-930 resulted only in a reduction of the tumor growth rate (tumor volume of 250% and 120%, respectively, of the initial tumor volume). Similar findings were reported with respect to the H441 NSCLC cell xenografts. Moreover, the authors claim a significant benefit provided by a combinatorial regimen with erlotinib and OSI-930 in an experimental setting of disease progression. In that context, NSCLC NCI-H292 tumor cells with reduced sensitivity to erlotinib were selected and subcutaneously xenografted in mice. After 32 days of treatment with erlotinib alone, mice that had initially responded to erlotinib but then developed tumor re-growth in the sense of progressive disease were either set off further treatment, had maintained treatment with erlotinib alone, replacement therapy with OSI-930 or addition of OSI-930 to the continous treatment with erlotinib. Mice receiving combined therapy with erlotinib and OSI-930 after progression showed a delay in doubling of the tumor volume greater than 56 days. This delay was significantly higher when compared to animals receiving single-agent therapy with either erlotinib or OSI-930 (time to tumor volume doubling 19.6 days and 30 days, respectively).

The promising findings described in this patent require further confirmation. To date, neither preclinical nor clinical data exist concerning a combined therapeutic approach with erlotinib and an inhibitor of Kit in glioblastoma. However, a Phase II study examining the effects of a combined treatment with imatinib and hydroxyurea, a ribonucleotide reductase inhibitor, in the setting of recurrent glioblastoma showed encouraging results [75]. Out of 33 patients enrolled in this study, 27% were free of progression at 6 months with a median progression-free survival of 14.4 weeks. In addition, 9% of patients showed radiographic response, 42% achieved stable disease within a median follow-up of 58 weeks, and median overall survival was 48.9 weeks. Thus, despite rather disappointing results in clinical studies when applied as single agents, Kit inhibitors may prove themselves as valuable partners in combination with other agents such as erlotinib for the treatment of glioblastoma.

ERLOTINIB AND PRALATREXATE

Pralatrexate (Folotyn®, Allos Therapeutics, Inc., Westminster, CO, USA), otherwise known as 10-propargyl-10-deazaaminopterin or PDX, is an inhibitor of dihydrofolate reductase and was shown to have greater affinity to the reduced folate carrier (RFC)-1 and folylpolyglutamate synthetase than other antifolates such as methotrexate [76]. Therefore, cellular uptake and polyglutamylation of pralatrexate are increased, resulting in a higher intracellular concentration and longer intracellular half-life span, which enhances cytotoxicity due to antifolate effects [77].

In experimental studies, pralatrexate was shown to exert superior anti-tumor activity *in vitro* in lung and breast cancer cell lines when compared to methotrexate [77]. Similarly, in xenograft models of lymphoma or NSCLC, pralatrexate was shown to have stronger antineoplastic activity than methotrexate [78, 79]. Pralatrexate has also been examined in several early Phase clinical studies for the treatment of various human cancers including NSCLC, mesothelioma or peripheral T-cell lymphoma (PTCL). In unresectable malignant pleural mesothelioma, Krug *et al.* showed in a Phase II study that treatment with pralatrexate administered intravenously at a biweekly dose of 135mg/m^2 did not exhibit significant antitumoral activity [80]. In contrast, in 109 patients with relapsed or refractory PTCL, a recent Phase II trial of pralatrexate (PROPEL) showed an overall response rate of 29% [81]. In another Phase II study, 39 patients with progressive NSCLC were treated with pralatrexate at a dose of 150mg/m^2 every 2 weeks. Thirty-one patients achieved stable disease, the median time to progression was 3 months, and the median survival was 13.5 months [82]. Clinically, pralatrexate was generally well tolerated and exhibited a favorable safety profile with stomatitis as primary toxicity which could be mitigated by supplementation with vitamin B_{12} and folic acid.

Thus, pralatrexate fulfills important criteria for a successful combination partner in a multi-drug approach. *In vitro,* pralatrexate and bortezomib (Velcade®, Millenium Pharmaceuticals, Inc., Cambridge, MA, USA), a proteasome inhibitor, were shown to exert a synergistic cytotoxic and pro-apoptotic effect on various T-lymphoma cell lines [81]. Moreover, in a xenograft model, HH CTCL cells were implanted subcutaneously into mice prior to treatment with pralatrexate alone, bortezomib alone, or both drugs. Six of the 10 mice that were treated with both agents achieved complete response whereas no complete responses were observed in the mice receiving single-agent treatments. Promising results were also reported from a Phase I study examining the effects of pralatrexate when applied in combination with docetaxel (Taxotere, Sanofi-Aventis, Bridgewater, NJ, USA). Forty patients with metastatic NSCLC were treated with pralatrexate and docetaxel at doses of 120mg/m^2 and 35mg/m^2, respectively, every two weeks. Fifteen percent of the patients achieved partial response, 50% achieved stable disease, and median progression-free survival was 4 months. Notably, 28% of patients had a progression-free survival of greater than 1 year, and median overall survival was 18 months [83].

In addition, a patent describes the combined treatment with erlotinib and pralatrexate for patients with NSCLC [84]. In this patent, the author claims that tumor growth in a murine A549 NSCLC xenograft model was inhibited in a synergistic manner by combined treatment with erlotinib (50mg/kg orally) and pralatrexate (2mg/kg intraperitoneally). The combinatorial regimen with erlotinib and pralatrexate was reported to be significantly more effective at controlling tumor growth than single-agent therapy with either erlotinib or paralatrexate (tumor volumes: 152 $\pm$ 85mm^3, 358 $\pm$ 282mm^3 and 210 $\pm$ 109mm^3, respectively). In conclusion, while the combined therapy with erlotinib and pralatrexate appears promising, preclinical as well as clinical data evaluating the use of pralatrexate in glioblastoma are lacking. Further studies are needed to investigate a possible antineoplastic activity of pralatrexate alone and in combination with erlotinib to allow for a sound judgement on the efficacy of this approach in the setting of glioblastoma.

ERLOTINIB AND INSULIN-LIKE GROWTH FACTOR 1 RECEPTOR (IGF1R) ANTAGONISTS

The IGF1R is a membrane-bound TK receptor which is closely related to the insulin receptor (reviewed in [85]). Biochemically, it consists of an α-subunit containing the ligand-binding domain and a β-subunit containing the transmembraneous portion plus the intracellular TK domain. The IGF1R is formed by the assembly of two of each subunit types, resulting in a heterotetramer. Once its natural ligands, IGF1 or IGF2, bind, autophosphorylation occurs followed by subsequent downward signaling.

There is compelling evidence that IGFR1-mediated signaling is of great importance for the promotion of cellular proliferation and differentiation, the inhibition of apoptosis and most strikingly, the development of human malignancies [86-88]. Several groups have shown that cells with disrupted IGF1R genes were not able to undergo malignant transformation despite treatment with different transforming agents [89, 90]. Moreover, the risk to develop a common cancer was shown to be increased for those individuals displaying "high normal" levels of IGF1 when compared to individuals with "low normal" levels [91].

The use of IGF1R-targeted therapeutic agents in cancer is supported by different studies. Long *et al.* showed that murine carcinoma cells treated with IGF1R small interfering (si) RNA lost their metastatic phenotype [92]. In addition, Rohlik *et al.* showed that the growth of breast cancer cells was significantly impaired when subjected to a treatment with an IGF1R-targeted antibody. Moreover, in various preclinical studies, murine IGF1R-targeted antibodies were shown to inhibit tumor growth *in vivo* [93].

Two patents claim that the combined use of erlotinib and a human IGF1R-targeted antibody enhances the therapeutic efficacy of erlotinib compared to single-agent treatment. In their patent, Juchem *et al.* showed that tumor size in severe combined immunodeficiency mice engrafted with the human NSCLC cell line H332M and subjected to a combination treatment with erlotinib and a humanized mAb against IGF1R (HUMAB Clone 18) was strongly reduced in comparison to control and mice treated with either agent alone [94]. In addition, histologic analysis revealed that invasive growth was absent and the apoptotic index was markedly reduced. Similar to the findings of Juchem *et al.*, Yan *et al.* described that the treatment with MK-0646, a humanized anti-IGF1R IgG1 mAb, and erlotinib resulted in an increased anti-tumor activity in NSCLC mouse xenografts [95]. Moreover, a Phase I trial showed that the combined treatment with MK-0646 (5 or 10mg/kg once per week) and erlotinib (150mg/d) was well tolerated by patients suffering from stage IIIb/IV NSCLC. A randomized Phase II trial comparing the combination treatment *vs.* a treatment with erlotinib alone was stated to be ongoing.

In a recent study, Rosen *et al.* examined the effect of a combined treatment with ganitumab, a fully human anti-IGF1R mAb and different targeted or cytotoxic agents including erlotinib on advanced solid tumors [96]. Combination therapy with erlotinib (150mg/kg/day) and ganitumab (6 or 12mg/kg once every two weeks) was shown to be generally well tolerated, and the additional application of ganitumab did not seem to affect the estimated pharmacokinetic parameters of erlotinib. Out of 12 patients receiving both erlotinib and ganitumab, only one patient receiving the higher dosage of ganitumab developed a dose-limiting toxicity (grade 4 thrombocytopenia) and had to go off the trial. With respect to tumor responses, one patient reached partial response (censored at last assessment) and two patients achieved stable disease. Currently, there is no data on a combined use of erlotinib and an inhibitor of IGFR1 in the setting of glioblastoma. However, using gene expression analysis, Löw *et al.* identified IGF1 to be overexpressed in glioblastoma cell lines with erlotinib-resistant phenotype [97]. These data suggest that treatment with an inhibitor of IGF1-mediated signaling might increase the susceptibility of erlotinib-resistant glioblastoma cells towards a treatment with erlotinib and possibly improves the therapeutic response towards erlotinib in this disease.

COMBINED TREATMENT WITH ERLOTINIB AND DISODIUM COMBRETASTATIN A-4 3-O-PHOSPHATE (CA4P)

Tumor angiogenesis is a process that was found to be of critical importance for the growth and metastasis of solid tumors and encompasses the capability of cancers to develop their own blood supply by different mechanisms [98]. Sprouting angiogenesis represents one such mechanism which is a slow process requiring the proliferation of endothelial cells for the formation of new blood vessels from pre-existing ones. Tumors may also recruit bone marrow-derived endothelial progenitor cells into growing vessels. Another mechanism that enhances tumor vascularisation involves the longitudinal splitting of existing blood vessels called intussusception. The vascular endothelial growth factor represents one of the most important proangiogenic mediators in tumors. Other molecules known to promote tumor angiogenesis are interleukin-8 and fibroblast growth factor.

Different anti-angiogenic compounds have been evaluated for their use in cancer therapy including treatment of high-grade glioma. Thalidomide (Thalomid®, Celgene Corporation, Warren, NJ, USA) was one of the first anti-angiogenic agents to be applied in the setting of recurrent malignant glioma. However, only moderate antitumor activity was reported when applied as a single-agent [99] as well as when given in combination with carmustine [100]. Moreover, supplementary administration of thalidomide with temozolomide and radiotherapy in patients with newly diagnosed glioblastoma did not provide any additional clinical benefit [101]. Consequently, thalidomide and its derivatives are currently not clinically used. However, other anti-angiogenic agents such as bevacizumab

(Avastin®, Genentech Inc., San Francisco, CA, USA), a humanized monoclonal antibody targeted to VEGF, have provided promising clinical results. In a Phase II study, 20 of 35 patients (57%) with recurrent glioblastoma who were treated with bevacizumab in combination with irinotecan showed at least partial response. The 6-months progression-free survival and 6-months overall survival rates were 46% and 77%, respectively [102]. For patients with recurrent WHO grade III gliomas, similar findings were reported [103]. In a randomized Phase II trial, a larger population of patients with recurrent glioblastoma receiving either bevacizumab alone (n = 85) or in combination with irinotecan (n = 82) were compared. In this study, response rates of 28.2 and 37.8%, 6-months progression-free survival rates of 42.6 and 50.3% as well as median overall survival of 9.2 and 8.7 months, respectively, were achieved [104].

Tumor vascularisation may be therapeutically compromised not only by inhibition of the formation of new tumor-supplying blood vessels with anti-angiogenic means but also by disruption of already existing tumor blood vessels. Small molecule microtubule-depolymerising vascular disrupting agents (VDA) such as the combretastatins belong to this class of compounds that cause selective destruction of the vascular tumor network and subsequent tumor necrosis. The combretastatins were extracted from the South African bush willow, *Combretum caffrum*, and are structurally related to colchicine. Currently, CA4P (Zybrestat™, Oxigene Inc., Lund, Sweden) represents the best studied member of this group of anticancer compounds Fig. (**1**). CA4P is a prodrug which is dephosphorylated in plasma prior to gaining complete function and reversibly binding to tubulin.

In preclinical studies, CA4P was shown to significantly reduce blood supply to spontaneous and ortho- and heterotopically transplanted rodent tumors as well as to human xenografted tumors within 10-20 min after application [105]. This effect was reported to last for up to 24 hrs in some tumors [106]. Despite dramatic effects involving up to 80-90% of tumor necrosis that were observed within hours of a single-dose application of CA4P, cells in the outer tumor rim survived, serving as a possible source of tumor regrowth [106, 107]. In a study in rats, BT_4An rat glioma tissue was transplanted subcutaneously, and blood flow was measured by laser Doppler flowmetry [108]. A decrease in tumor blood flow of 47-55% was observed during the first 110 min after administration of CA4P.

Interestingly, treatment with CA4P at a dose of 50mg/kg did not result in significantly reduced tumor growth when compared to controls. However, when applied 3 hrs prior to hyperthermic treatment (44°C, 60 min), tumor growth was significantly delayed in comparison to animals receiving CA4P immediately prior to hyperthermia and animals receiving only hyperthermia. Thus, CA4P enhances thermal damage in this setting if applied with the right timing. Notably, in another study, the same research group observed in four out of six BT_4An tumors of rats treated with CA4P a minor central necrosis, implying at least a slight anti-vascular effect of CA4P when given alone in this setting [109]. To date, clinical studies evaluating the effects of CA4P in high-grade glioma do not exist. In three Phase I clinical trials, CA4P was shown to reduce blood flow and perfusion in advanced solid tumors [110-112]. Despite the fact that the main purpose of these studies was to determine CA4P's safety profile, some clinical benefit was noted. One patient with anaplastic thyroid cancer achieved complete response, remaining free of disease for more than 5 years, and one patient with fibrosarcoma reached partial response. Moreover, in 31 patients (32%) stable disease was observed. Overall, treatment with CA4P was well tolerated. Common side effects included hypertension and pain. Serious adverse side effects were observed in 16 (16.7%) patients, including two patients who developed cardiac ischemia.

In order to eliminate the cancerous cells in the outer rim which survive the treatment with VDAs, a combined therapy with radiation or conventional chemotherapy was attempted. In a clinical study, eight patients with advanced NSCLC received radiotherapy (27 Gy in six fractions, twice a week) accompanied by intravenous application of CA4P at a dose of $50mg/m^2$ starting after the second fraction of radiotherapy [113]. In six patients, a reduction in tumor blood volume of 22.9% and of 29.4% was observed 4 and 72 hrs after application of CA4P, respectively. Notably, the reduction in blood volume was sustained up to 72 hrs and was greater at the rim of the tumor compared with its center (51.4% *vs.* 22.8%). Thus, radiotherapy seems to enhance the antivascular effect of CA4P in NSCLC patients. In a Phase Ib study, patients with various advanced cancers refractory to standard therapy were treated with CA4P followed by a single-agent treatment with carboplatin or paclitaxel 18-22 hrs later or a combined treatment with paclitaxel and carboplatin in sequential order [114]. Seven of 18 patients with primary peritoneal carcinoma, ovarian cancer or cancer of the fallopian tube had a formal response. Another three out of 30 patients with non-ovarian cancer achieved partial remission, demonstrating antitumor activity of this combinatorial regimen in patients with difficult-to-treat cancers.

Moreover, a recent patent claims that a combined treatment with a VDA such as CA4P or combretastatin A-1 diphosphate (CA1P) and a small molecule receptor TK inhibitor such as erlotinib or sorafenib (Nexavar®, Bayer Schering Pharma AG, Leverkusen, Germany) yields antineoplastic activity in cancer patients [115]. In addition, the authors assert that this combinatorial regimen represents a method to prevent tumor regrowth and to inhibit tumor-associated angiogenesis. In one example described in this patent, growth of LOX IMVI human melanoma xenografts in athymic nude mice was inhibited to a greater extent by a combined treatment with CA1P and sorafenib when compared to controls or single-agent treatment with either one of the two compounds. Similar results were reported for C1AP and sorafenib in a murine HEP-G2 human hepatocellular carcinoma xenograft model. The authors also claimed synergistic enhancement of anti-tumor activity against H460 lung cancer xenografts in SCID mice by combining erlotinib at a dose of 50 mg/kg with either CA4P or CA1P at doses of 75mg/kg each. However, these data were not shown.

In summary, VDAs are promising compounds for combination with other anticancer drugs. The shut-down of tumor blood flow not only causes secondary tumor cell death due to ischemia but may also cause local accumulation of other therapeutics in the tumor tissue when used at the right time. Thereby, viable cells in the outer rim of the tumor which had survived the therapy with VDAs may finally be killed, under optimal conditions preventing tumor regrowth. Currently, data on the efficacy of a combinatorial therapy with VDAs and erlotinib for the treatment of high-grade glioma are lacking. Thus, studies are needed to evaluate if a combinatorial regimen of a VDA and erlotinib may provide enhanced overall anti-tumor activity in high-grade glioma.

CURRENT & FUTURE DEVELOPMENTS

Gross total tumor resection, if expected to be achievable without creating new neurological deficits, followed by radiotherapy plus concomitant and adjuvant treatment with temozolomide, represents the current standard of care for patients with glioblastoma. However, this protocol has fallen short of changing the generally dismal prognosis. Despite great research efforts aimed at developing new therapeutic approaches to further improve the limited clinical efficacy of standard therapy for patients with high-grade gliomas, a significant break-through has not yet been achieved. In this context, promising results from preclinical studies with small-molecule TK inhibitors targeted at HER1/EGFR, *e.g.* erlotinib, were not confirmed in clinical settings [14, 15].

New strategies, including the combination of erlotinib with targeted agents able to inhibit key regulators that are located further downstream within the signaling cascade or with agents inhibiting other signaling pathways, are currently being investigated to achieve enhanced therapeutic efficacy against glioblastoma. A Phase II trial investigating the effects of a combined treatment with erlotinib and sorafenib (BAY 54-9085, Bayer HealthCare Pharmaceuticals, Montville, NJ, USA), an inhibitor of murine leukemia viral oncogene homolog (RAF)/mitogen-activated protein kinase kinase (MEK)/extracellular signal-regulated kinase (ERK) and VEGFR-2/PDGFR-β signaling pathways in patients with progressive or recurrent glioblastoma has been completed. The results are pending. Moreover, results are awaited of a Phase I/II clinical trial that was recently completed, studying the effects of concomitant treatment with erlotinib, sorafenib and temsirolimus (CCI-779, Wyeth Pharmaceuticals, Madison, NJ, USA), an inhibitor of mTOR in patients with recurrent glioblastoma or gliosarcoma.

Another approach involves the use of a combinatorial regimen of erlotinib and novel agents, aiming at enhanced overall antineoplastic activity and non-overlapping toxicity. Some of the agents described herein have not yet been evaluated for the treatment of gliomas, but constitute worthy candidates.

ACKNOWLEDGEMENTS

Declared None.

CONFLICT OF INTEREST

The authors confirm that this chapter content has no conflict of interest.

DISCLOSURE

The chapter submitted for Patent eBook Series entitled "Topics in Anti-Cancer Research", Volume 2 is an update of our article "Drug Combinations Enhancing the Antineoplastic Effects of Erlotinib in High-Grade Glioma", published in the journal 'Recent Patents on Anti-Cancer Drug Discovery', Volume 6, Number 3, September, 2011, Page 384 to 394 with modified title, additional text and references.

REFERENCES

[1] Stupp R, Mason W, van den Bent M, Weller M, Fisher B, Taphoom M, *et al.* Radiotherapy plus concomitant and adjuvant temozolomide for glioblastoma. N Engl J Med 2005; 352: 987-96.

[2] Libermann T, Nusbaum H, Razon N, Kris R, Lax I, Soreq H, *et al.* Amplification, enhanced expression and possible rearrangement of EGF receptor gene in primary human brain tumors of glial origin. Nature 1985; 313: 144-7.

[3] Ekstrand A, James C, Cavanee W, Seliger B, Pettersson R, Collins V. Genes for epidermal growth factor receptor, transforming growth factor alpha and epidermal growth factor and their expression in human gliomas *in vivo*. Cancer Res 1991; 51: 2164-72.

[4] Karpel-Massler G, Schmidt U, Unterberg A, Halatsch M. Therapeutic inhibition of the epidermal growth factor receptor in high-grade gliomas - where do we stand? Mol Cancer Res 2009; 7: 1000-12.

[5] Scagliotti G, Selvaggi G, Novello S, Hirsch F. The biology of epidermal growth factor receptor in lung cancer. Clin Cancer Res 2004; 10: 4227s-32s.

[6] Busse D, Doughty R, Ramsey T, Russell W, Price J, Flanagan W, *et al.* Reversible G_1 arrest induced by inhibition of the epidermal growth factor receptor tyrosine kinase requires up-regulation of $p27^{KIP1}$ independent of MAPK activity. J Biol Chem 2000; 275: 6987-5.

[7] Arteaga C. The epidermal growth factor receptor: from mutant oncogene in nonhuman cancers to therapeutic target in human neoplasia. J Clin Oncol 2001; 19: 32S-40S.

[8] Chu C, Everiss K, Wikstrand C, Batra S, Kung H, Bigner D. Receptor dimerization is not a factor in the signaling activity of a transforming variant epidermal growth factor receptor (EGFRvIII). Biochem J 1997; 324: 855-61.

[9] Lynch T, Bell D, Sordella R, Gurubhagavatula S, Okimoto R, Brannigan B, *et al.* Activating mutations in the epidermal growth factor receptor underlying responsiveness of non-small-cell lung cancer to gefitinib. N Engl J Med 2004; 350: 2129-39.

[10] Paez J, Jänne P, Lee J, Tracy S, Greulich H, Gabriel S, *et al.* EGFR mutations in lung cancer: Correlation with clinical response to gefitinib therapy. Science 2004; 304: 1497-500.

[11] Lal A, Glazer C, Martinson H, Friedman H, Archer G, Sampson J, *et al.* Mutant epidermal growth factor receptor up-regulates molecular effectors of tumor invasion. Cancer Res 2002; 62: 3335-9.

[12] Halatsch M-E, Gehrke E, Vougioukas V, Bötefür I, Efferth T, Gebhardt E, *et al.* Inverse correlation of epidermal growth factor receptor messenger RNA induction and suppression

of anchorage-independent growth by OSI-774, an epidermal growth factor receptor tyrosine kinase inhibitor, in glioblastoma multiforme cell lines. J Neurosurg 2004; 100: 523-33.

[13] Raizer J, Abrey L, Lassman A, Chang S, Lamborn K, Kuhn J, *et al.* A Phase II trial of erlotinib in patients with recurrent malignant gliomas and nonprogressive glioblastoma multiforme postradiation therapy. Neurooncol 2010; 12: 95-103.

[14] van den Bent M, Brandes A, Rampling R, Kouwenhoven M, Kros J, Carpentier A, *et al.* Randomized Phase II trial of erlotinib vs. temozolomide or carmustine in recurrent glioblastoma: EORTC brain tumor group study 26034. J Clin Oncol 2009; 27: 1268-74.

[15] Brown P, Krishnan S, Sarkaria J, Wu W, Jaeckle K, Uhm J, *et al.* Phase I/II trial of erlotinib and temozolomide with radiation therapy in the treatment of newly diagnosed glioblastoma multiforme: North central cancer treatment group study N0177. J Clin Oncol 2008; 26: 5603-9.

[16] Prados M, Chang S, Butowski N, DeBoer R, Parvataneni R, Carliner H, *et al.* Phase II study of erlotinib plus temozolomide during and after radiation therapy in patients with newly diagnosed glioblastoma multiforme or gliosarcoma. J Clin Oncol 2009; 27: 579-84.

[17] Peereboom D, Shepard D, Ahluwalia M, Brewer C, Agarwal N, Stevens G, *et al.* Phase II trial of erlotinib with temozolomide and radiation in patients with newly diagnosed glioblastoma multiforme. J Neurooncol 2010; 98: 93-9.

[18] Wang M, Lu K, Zhu S, Dia E, Vivanco I, Shackleford G, *et al.* Mammalian target of rapamycin inhibition promotes response to epidermal growth factor receptor kinase inhibitors in PTEN-deficient and PTEN-intact glioblastoma cells. Cancer Res 2006; 66: 7864-9.

[19] Fan Q-W, Cheng C, Nicolaides T, Hackett C, Knight Z, Shokat K, *et al.* A dual phosphoinositide-3-kinase anti/mTOR inhibitor cooperates with blockade of epidermal growth factor receptor in PTEN-mutant glioma. Cancer Res 2007; 67: 7960-5.

[20] Doherty L, Gigas D, Kesari S, Drappatz J, Kim R, Zimmermann J, *et al.* Pilot study of the combination of EGFR and mTOR inhibitors in recurrent malignant gliomas. Neurology 2006; 67: 156-8.

[21] Reardon D, Desjardins A, Vredenburgh J, Gururangan S, Friedman A, Herndon II J, *et al.* Phase II trial of erlotinib plus sirolimus in adults with recurrent glioblastoma. J Neurooncol 2010; 96: 219-30.

[22] Sathornsumetee S, Desjardins A, Vredenburgh J, McLendon R, Marcello J, Herndon II J, *et al.* Phase II trial of bevacizumab and erlotinib in patients with recurrent malignant glioma. Neurooncol 2010; 12: 1300-10.

[23] Krishnan S, Brown P, Ballmann K, Fiveash J, Uhm J, Giannini C, *et al.* Phase I trial of erlotinib with radiation therapy in patients with glioblastoma multiforme: Results of north central cancer treatment group protocol N0177. Int J Radiat Oncol Biol Phys 2006; 65: 1192-9.

[24] Prados M, Lamborn K, Chang S, Burton E, Butowski N, Malec M, *et al.* Phase I study of erlotinib HCl alone and combined with temozolomide in patients with stable or recurrent malignant glioma. Neurooncol 2006; 8: 67-78.

[25] Lane AA, Chabner BA. Histone deacetylase inhibitors in cancer therapy. J Clin Oncol 2009; 27: 5459-68.

[26] Marsoni S, Damia G, Camboni G. A work in progress: The clinical development of histone deacetylase inhibitors. Epigenetics 2008; 3: 164-71.

[27] Svechnikova I, Almqvist PM, Ekstrom TJ. HDAC inhibitors effectively induce cell type-specific differentiation in human glioblastoma cell lines of different origin. Int J Oncol 2008; 32: 821-7.

[28] Yoo CB, Jones PA. Epigenetic therapy of cancer: Past, present and future. Nat Rev Drug Discov 2006; 5: 37-50.

[29] Nakagawa M, Oda Y, Eguchi T, Aishima S, Yao T, Hosoi F, *et al.* Expression profile of class I histone deacetylases in human cancer tissues. Oncol Rep 2007; 18: 769-74.

[30] Insinga A, Monestiroli S, Ronzoni S, Gelmetti V, Marchesi F, Viale A, *et al.* Inhibitors of histone deacetylases induce tumor-selective apoptosis through activation of the death receptor pathway. Nat Med 2005; 11: 71-6.

[31] Nebbioso A, Clarke N, Voltz E, Germain E, Ambrosino C, Bontempo P, *et al.* Tumor-selective action of HDAC inhibitors involves TRAIL induction in acute myeloid leukemia cells. Nat Med 2005; 11: 77-84.

[32] Zhang Y, Adachi M, Kawamura R, Imai K. BMF is a possible mediator in histone deacetylase inhibitors FK228 and CBHA-induced apoptosis. Cell Death Differ 2006; 13: 129-40.

[33] Zhao Y, Tan J, Zhuang L, Jiang X, Liu ET, Yu Q. Inhibitors of histone deacetylases target the Rb-E2F1 pathway for apoptosis induction through activation of proapoptotic protein Bim. Proc Natl Acad Sci USA 2005; 102: 16090-5.

[34] Bolden JE, Peart MJ, Johnstone RW. Anticancer activities of histone deacetylase inhibitors. Nat Rev Drug Discov 2006; 5: 769-84.

[35] Kovacs JJ, Murphy PJ, Gaillard S, Zhao X, Wu JT, Nicchitta CV, *et al.* HDAC6 regulates Hsp90 acetylation and chaperone-dependent activation of glucocorticoid receptor. Mol Cell 2005; 18: 601-7.

[36] Whitesell L, Lindquist SL. Hsp90 and the chaperoning of cancer. Nat Rev Cancer 2005; 5: 761-72.

[37] Richon VM, Sandhoff TW, Rifkind RA, Marks PA. Histone deacetylase inhibitor selectively induces p21WAF1 expression and gene-associated histone acetylation. Proc Natl Acad Sci USA 2000; 97: 10014-9.

[38] Sandor V, Senderowicz A, Mertins S, Sackett D, Sausville E, Blagosklonny MV, *et al.* P21-dependent G1 arrest with downregulation of cyclin D1 and upregulation of cyclin E by the histone deacetylase inhibitor FR901228. Br J Cancer 2000; 83: 817-25.

[39] Ueda H, Nakajima H, Hori Y, Fujita T, Nishimura M, Goto T, *et al.* FR901228, a novel antitumor bicyclic depsipeptide produced by *Chromobacterium violaceum* No. 968. I. Taxonomy, fermentation, isolation, physico-chemical and biological properties, and antitumor activity. J Antibiot (Tokyo) 1994; 47: 301-10.

[40] Ritchie D, Piekarz RL, Blombery P, Karai LJ, Pittaluga S, Jaffe ES, *et al.* Reactivation of DNA viruses in association with histone deacetylase inhibitor therapy: A case series report. Haematologica 2009; 94: 1618-22.

[41] Prince HM, Bishton MJ, Harrison SJ. Clinical studies of histone deacetylase inhibitors. Clin Cancer Res 2009; 15: 3958-69.

[42] Byrd J, Marcucci G, Parthun M, Xiao J, Klisovic R, Moran M, *et al.* A Phase 1 and pharmacodynamic study of depsipeptide (FK228) in chronic lymphocytic leukemia and acute myeloid leukemia. Blood 2005; 105: 959-67.

[43] Odenike O, Alkan S, Sher D, Godwin J, Huo D, Brandt S, *et al.* Histone deacetylase inhibitor romidepsin has differential activity in core binding factor acute myeloid leukemia. Clin Cancer Res 2008; 14: 7095-101.

[44] Piekarz R, Frye R, Turner M, Wright J, Allen S, Kirschbaum M, *et al.* Phase II Multi-institutional trial of the histone deacetylase inhibitor romidepsin as monotherapy for patients with cutaneous T-cell lymphoma. J Clin Oncol 2009; 27: 5410-7.
[45] Whittaker S, Demierre M-F, Kim E, Rook A, Lerner A, Duvic M, *et al.* Final results from a multicenter, international, pivotal study of romidepsin in refractory cutaneous T-cell lymphoma. J Clin Oncol 2010; 28(29: 4485-91.
[46] Camphausen K, Cerna D, Scott T, Sproull M, Burgan W, Cerra M, *et al.* Enhancement of *in vitro* and *in vivo* tumor cell radiosensitivity by valproic acid. Int J Cancer 2005; 114: 380-6.
[47] Entin-Meer M, Yang X, Van den Berg S, Lamborn K, Nudelman A, Rephaeli A, *et al. In vivo* efficacy of a novel histone deacetylase inhibitor in combination with radiation for the treatment of gliomas. Neurooncol 2007; 9: 82-8.
[48] Lucio-Eterovic AK, Cortez MA, Valera ET, Motta FJ, Queiroz RG, Machado HR, *et al.* Differential expression of 12 histone deacetylase (HDAC) genes in astrocytomas and normal brain tissue: Class II and IV are hypoexpressed in glioblastomas. BMC Cancer 2008; 8: 243.
[49] Sawa H, Murakami H, Kumagai M, Nakasato M, Yamauchi S, Matsuyama N, *et al.* Histone deacetylase inhibitor, FK228, induces apoptosis and suppresses cell proliferation of human glioblastoma cells *in vitro* and *in vivo*. Acta Neuropathol 2004; 107: 523-31.
[50] Frenkel, E.P. Combination therapy for cancer. WO2008127659 (**2008**).
[51] Heinrich MC, Blanke CD, Druker BJ, Corless CL. Inhibition of KIT tyrosine kinase activity: A novel molecular approach to the treatment of KIT-positive malignancies. J Clin Oncol 2002; 20: 1692-703.
[52] Yarden Y, Kuang W-J, Yang-Feng T, Coussens L, Munemitsu S, Dull T, *et al.* Human proto-oncogene c-kit: A new cell surface receptor tyrosine kinase for an unidentified ligand. EMBO J 1987; 11: 3341-51.
[53] Nocka K, Buck J, Levi E, Besmer P. Candidate ligand for the c-kit transmembrane kinase receptor: KL, a fibroblast derived growth factor stimulates mast cells and erythroid progenitors. EMBO J 1990; 9: 3287-94.
[54] Duensing A, Medeiros F, McConarty B, Joseph NE, Panigrahy D, Singer S, *et al.* Mechanisms of oncogenic KIT signal transduction in primary gastrointestinal stromal tumors (GISTs). Oncogene 2004; 23: 3999-4006.
[55] Mol CD, Lim KB, Sridhar V, Zou H, Chien EY, Sang BC, *et al.* Structure of a c-kit product complex reveals the basis for kinase transactivation. J Biol Chem 2003; 278: 31461-4.
[56] Ishikawa K, Komuro T, Hirota S, Kitamura Y. Ultrastructural identification of the c-kit-expressing interstitial cells in the rat stomach: A comparison of control and Ws/Ws mutant rats. Cell Tissue Res 1997; 289: 137-43.
[57] Natali PG, Nicotra MR, Sures I, Santoro E, Bigotti A, Ullrich A. Expression of c-kit receptor in normal and transformed human nonlymphoid tissues. Cancer Res 1992; 52: 6139-43.
[58] Nocka K, Majumder S, Chabot B, Ray P, Cervone M, Bernstein A, *et al.* Expression of c-kit gene products in known cellular targets of W mutations in normal and W mutant mice - evidence for an impaired c-kit kinase in mutant mice. Genes Dev 1989; 3: 816-26.
[59] Turner AM, Zsebo KM, Martin F, Jacobsen FW, Bennett LG, Broudy VC. Nonhematopoietic tumor cell lines express stem cell factor and display c-kit receptors. Blood 1992; 80: 374-81.

[60] Duensing S, Duensing A. Targeted therapies of gastrointestinal stromal tumors (GIST) - the next frontiers. Biochem Pharmacol 2010; 80: 575-83.

[61] Woodman SE, Davies MA. Targeting KIT in melanoma: A paradigm of molecular medicine and targeted therapeutics. Biochem Pharmacol 80: 568-74.

[62] Cetin N, Dienel G, Gokden M. CD117 expression in glial tumors. J Neurooncol 2005; 75: 195-202.

[63] Joensuu H, Puputti M, Sihto H, Tynninen O, Nupponen NN. Amplification of genes encoding KIT, PDGFRalpha and VEGFR2 receptor tyrosine kinases is frequent in glioblastoma multiforme. J Pathol 2005; 207: 224-31.

[64] Puputti M, Tynninen O, Sihto H, Blom T, Maenpaa H, Isola J, *et al.* Amplification of KIT, PDGFRA, VEGFR2, and EGFR in gliomas. Mol Cancer Res 2006; 4: 927-34.

[65] Blanke CD, Demetri GD, von Mehren M, Heinrich MC, Eisenberg B, Fletcher JA, *et al.* Long-term results from a randomized Phase II trial of standard- vs. higher-dose imatinib mesylate for patients with unresectable or metastatic gastrointestinal stromal tumors expressing KIT. J Clin Oncol 2008; 26: 620-5.

[66] Blanke CD, Rankin C, Demetri GD, Ryan CW, von Mehren M, Benjamin RS, *et al.* Phase III randomized, intergroup trial assessing imatinib mesylate at two dose levels in patients with unresectable or metastatic gastrointestinal stromal tumors expressing the kit receptor tyrosine kinase: S0033. J Clin Oncol 2008; 26: 626-32.

[67] Gold JS, van der Zwan SM, Gonen M, Maki RG, Singer S, Brennan MF, *et al.* Outcome of metastatic GIST in the era before tyrosine kinase inhibitors. Ann Surg Oncol 2007; 14: 134-42.

[68] Verweij J, Casali PG, Zalcberg J, LeCesne A, Reichardt P, Blay JY, *et al.* Progression-free survival in gastrointestinal stromal tumors with high-dose imatinib: Randomised trial. Lancet 2004; 364: 1127-34.

[69] Hagerstrand D, Hesselager G, Achterberg S. Characterization of an imatinib-sensitive subset of high-grade human glioma cultures. Oncogene 2006; 25: 4913-22.

[70] Oertel S, Krempien R, Lindel K, Zabel A, Milker-Zabel S, Bischof M, *et al.* Human glioblastoma and carcinoma xenograft tumors treated by combined radiation and imatinib (Gleevec®). Strahlenther Onkol 2006; 7: 400-7.

[71] Razis E, Selviaridis P, Labropoulos S, Norris JL, Zhu MJ, Song DD, *et al.* Phase II study of neoadjuvant imatinib in glioblastoma: Evaluation of clinical and molecular effects of the treatment. Clin Cancer Res 2009; 15: 6258-66.

[72] Wen P, Yung W, Lamborn K, Dahia P, Wang Y, Peng B, *et al.* Phase I/II study of imatinib mesylate for recurrent malignant gliomas: North American braintumor consortium study 99- 08. Clin Cancer Res 2006; 12: 4899-907.

[73] Garton, A.J., Franklin, M.R. Combined treatment with an EGFR kinase inhibitor and an inhibitor of c-kit. WO2009073139 (**2009**).

[74] Garton AJ, Crew AP, Franklin M, Cooke AR, Wynne GM, Castaldo L, *et al.* OSI-930: A novel selective inhibitor of Kit and kinase insert domain receptor tyrosine kinases with antitumor activity in mouse xenograft models. Cancer Res 2006; 66: 1015-24.

[75] Reardon D, Egorin M, Quinn J, Rich Sr J, Gururangan I, Vredenburgh J, *et al.* Phase II study of imatinib mesylate plus hydroxyurea in adults with recurrent glioblastoma multiforme. J Clin Oncol 2005; 23: 9359-68.

[76] O'Connor OA. Pralatrexate: An emerging new agent with activity in T-cell lymphomas. Curr Opin Oncol 2006; 18: 591-7.

[77] Izbicka E, Diaz A, Streeper R, Wick M, Campos D, Steffen R, *et al.* Distinct mechanistic activity profile of pralatrexate in comparison to other antifolates in *in vitro* and *in vivo* models of human cancers. Cancer Chemother Pharmacol 2009; 64: 993-9.

[78] Wang E, O'Connor O, She Y, Zelenetz A, Sirotnak F, Moore M. Activity of a novel anti-folate (PDX, 10-propargyl 10-deazaaminopterin) against human lymphoma is superior to methotrexate and correlates with tumor RFC-1 gene expression. Leuk Lymphoma 2003; 44: 1027-35.

[79] Sirotnak FM, DeGraw JI, Colwell WT, Piper JR. A new analogue of 10-deazaaminopterin with markedly enhanced curative effects against human tumor xenografts in mice. Cancer Chemother Pharmacol 1998; 42: 313-8.

[80] Krug LM, Heelan RT, Kris MG, Venkatraman E, Sirotnak FM. Phase II trial of pralatrexate (10-propargyl-10-deazaaminopterin, PDX) in patients with unresectable malignant pleural mesothelioma. J Thorac Oncol 2007; 2: 317-20.

[81] Marchi E, Paoluzzi L, Scotto L, Seshan VE, Zain JM, Zinzani PL, *et al.* Pralatrexate is synergistic with the proteasome inhibitor bortezomib in *in vitro* and *in vivo* models of T-cell lymphoid malignancies. Clin Cancer Res 2010; 16: 3648-58.

[82] Krug LM, Azzoli CG, Kris MG, Miller VA, Khokhar NZ, Tong W, *et al.* 10-Propargyl-10-deazaaminopterin: An antifolate with activity in patients with previously treated non-small cell lung cancer. Clin Cancer Res 2003; 9: 2072-8.

[83] Azzoli CG, Krug LM, Gomez J, Miller VA, Kris MG, Ginsberg MS, *et al.* A Phase 1 study of pralatrexate in combination with paclitaxel or docetaxel in patients with advanced solid tumors. Clin Cancer Res 2007; 13: 2692-8.

[84] Steffen, R.P. Combination of 10-propargyl-10-deazaaminopterin and erlotinib for the treatment of non-small cell lung cancer. US20090048262 (**2009**).

[85] Tao Y, Pinzi V, Bourhis J, Deutsch E. Mechanisms of disease: Signalling of the insulin-like growth factor 1 receptor pathway - therapeutic perspectives in cancer. Nat Clin Pract Oncol 2007; 4: 591-602.

[86] Ouban A, Muraca P, Yeatman T, Coppola D. Expression and distribution of insulin-like growth factor-1 receptor in human carcinomas. Hum Pathol 2003; 34: 803-8.

[87] Khandwala H, McCutcheon I, Flyvbjerg A, Friend K. The effects of insulin-like growth factors on tumorigenesis and neoplastic growth. Endocr Rev 2000; 21: 215-44.

[88] Baserga R, Peruzzi F, Reiss K. The IGF-1 receptor in cancer biology. Int J Cancer 2003; 107: 873-7.

[89] Sell C, Rubini M, Rubin R, Liu J, Efstratiadis A, Baserga R. Simian virus 40 large tumor antigen is unable to transform mouse embryonic fibroblasts lacking type 1 insulin-like growth factor receptor. Proc Natl Acad Sci USA 1993; 90: 11217-21.

[90] Coppola D, Ferber A, Miura M, Sell C, D'Ambrosio C, Rubin R, *et al.* A functional insulin-like growth factor I receptor is required for the mitogenic and transforming activities of the epidermal growth factor receptor. Mol Cell Biol 1994; 14: 4588-95.

[91] Rosen C, Pollak M. Circulating IGF-I: New perspectives for a new century. Trends Endocrinol Metab 1999; 10: 136-41.

[92] Long L, Rubin R, Baserga R, Brodt P. Loss of the metastatic phenotype in murine carcinoma cells expressing an antisense RNA to the insulin-like growth factor receptor. Cancer Res 1995; 55: 1006-9.

[93] Rohlik Q, Adams D, Kull FJ, Jacobs S. An antibody to the receptor for insulin-like growth factor I inhibits the growth of MCF-7 cells in tissue culture. Biochem Biophys Res Commun 1987; 149: 276-81.

[94] Juchem, R., Künkele, K.-P., Wartha, K. Combination therapy of erlotinib with an anti-IGF-1R antibody, which does not inhibit binding of insulin to the insulin receptor. EP2236139 (**2010**).

[95] Yan, L., Chastain, M., Hsu, K. Combination therapy using an anti-EGFR agent(s) and IGF-1R specific antibodies. WO2010096289 (**2010**).

[96] Rosen L, Puzanov I, Friberg G, Chan E, Hwang Y, Deng H, *et al.* Safety and pharmacokinetics of ganitumab (AMG 479) combined with sorafenib, panitumumab, erlotinib, or gemcitabine in patients with advanced solid tumors. Clin Cancer Res 2012; 18(12): 3414-27.

[97] Löw S, Vougioukas V, Hielscher T, Schmidt U, Unterberg A, Halatsch M-E. Pathogenic pathways leading to glioblastoma multiforme: Association between gene expressions and resistance to erlotinib. Anticancer Res 2008; 28: 3729-32.

[98] Heath VL, Bicknell R. Anticancer strategies involving the vasculature. Nat Rev Clin Oncol 2009; 6: 395-404.

[99] Fine HA, Figg WD, Jaeckle K, Wen PY, Kyritsis AP, Loeffler JS, *et al.* Phase II trial of the antiangiogenic agent thalidomide in patients with recurrent high-grade gliomas. J Clin Oncol 2000; 18: 708-15.

[100] Fine HA, Wen PY, Maher EA, Viscosi E, Batchelor T, Lakhani N, *et al.* Phase II trial of thalidomide and carmustine for patients with recurrent high-grade gliomas. J Clin Oncol 2003; 21: 2299-2304.

[101] Chang SM, Lamborn KR, Malec M, Larson D, Wara W, Sneed P, *et al.* Phase II study of temozolomide and thalidomide with radiation therapy for newly diagnosed glioblastoma multiforme. Int J Radiat Oncol Biol Phys 2004; 60: 353-357.

[102] Vredenburgh JJ, Desjardins A, Herndon JE, 2nd, Marcello J, Reardon DA, Quinn JA, *et al.* Bevacizumab plus irinotecan in recurrent glioblastoma multiforme. J Clin Oncol 2007; 25: 4722-4729.

[103] Desjardins A, Reardon DA, Herndon JE, Marcello J, Quinn JA, Rich JN, *et al.* Bevacizumab plus irinotecan in recurrent WHO grade 3 malignant gliomas. Clin Cancer Res 2008; 14: 7068-73.

[104] Friedman H, Prados M, Wen P, Mikkelsen T, Schiff D, Abrey L, *et al.* Bevacizumab alone and in combination with irinotecan in recurrent glioblastoma. J Clin Oncol 2009; 27: 4733-40.

[105] Kanthou C, Tozer GM. Tumor targeting by microtubule-depolymerizing vascular disrupting agents. Expert Opin Ther Targets 2007; 11: 1443-57.

[106] Tozer GM, Prise VE, Wilson J, Cemazar M, Shan S, Dewhirst MW, *et al.* Mechanisms associated with tumor vascular shut-down induced by combretastatin A-4 phosphate: Intravital microscopy and measurement of vascular permeability. Cancer Res 2001; 61: 6413-22.

[107] Dark GG, Hill SA, Prise VE, Tozer GM, Pettit GR, Chaplin DJ. Combretastatin A-4, an agent that displays potent and selective toxicity toward tumor vasculature. Cancer Res 1997; 57: 1829-34.

[108] Eikesdal HP, Schem BC, Mella O, Dahl O. The new tubulin-inhibitor combretastatin A-4 enhances thermal damage in the BT4An rat glioma. Int J Radiat Oncol Biol Phys 2000; 46: 645-52.

[109] Eikesdal HP, Bjerkvig R, Raleigh JA, Mella O, Dahl O. Tumor vasculature is targeted by the combination of combretastatin A-4 and hyperthermia. Radiother Oncol 2001; 61: 313-20.

[110] Dowlati A, Robertson K, Cooney M, Petros WP, Stratford M, Jesberger J, *et al.* A Phase I pharmacokinetic and translational study of the novel vascular targeting agent combretastatin a-4 phosphate on a single-dose intravenous schedule in patients with advanced cancer. Cancer Res 2002; 62: 3408-16.

[111] Rustin GJ, Galbraith SM, Anderson H, Stratford M, Folkes LK, Sena L, *et al.* Phase I clinical trial of weekly combretastatin A4 phosphate: Clinical and pharmacokinetic results. J Clin Oncol 2003; 21: 2815-22.

[112] Stevenson JP, Rosen M, Sun W, Gallagher M, Haller DG, Vaughn D, *et al.* Phase I trial of the antivascular agent combretastatin A4 phosphate on a 5-day schedule to patients with cancer: Magnetic resonance imaging evidence for altered tumor blood flow. J Clin Oncol 2003; 21: 4428-38.

[113] Ng Q-S, Goh V, Carnell D, Meer K, Padhani A, Saunders M, *et al.* Tumor antivascular effects of radiotherapy combined with combretastatin A4 phosphate in human non-small-cell lung cancer. Int J Radiat Oncol Biol Phys 2007; 67: 1375-80.

[114] Rustin GJ, Shreeves G, Nathan PD, Gaya A, Ganesan TS, Wang D, *et al.* A Phase Ib trial of CA4P (combretastatin A-4 phosphate), carboplatin, and paclitaxel in patients with advanced cancer. Br J Cancer 102: 1355-60.

[115] Chaplin, D., Silm, B. Methods and compositions for enhancing the efficacy of RTK inhibitors. WO2009103076 (**2009**).

Send Orders of Reprints at reprints@benthamscience.net
Topics in Anti-Cancer Research, Vol. 2, 2013, 437-494

CHAPTER 13

Nanodrugs: Magic Bullets in Cancer Chemotherapy

Kishwar Saleem[1], Waseem A. Wani[1], Ashanul Haque[1], Archana Milhotra[2] and Imran Ali[1,*]

[1]Department of Chemistry, Jamia Millia Islamia (Central University), New Delhi-110025, India; [2]Department of Chemistry, Deshbandhu College, University of Delhi, India

Abstract: Cancer is a disease which brings about a huge sense of terror. It has therefore, been a threat to human beings globally. Many organic and metallo chemotherapeutics are currently available in the market for the treatment of different sorts of cancers, but, still there is no drug which can curb this disease at late stages completely and worse, most drugs exhibit severe side effects. The choice for cancer treatment seems to be nanodrugs, which are effective at much lower concentrations and with much less side effects. Nanodrugs are the magic bullets, designed to be selective for tumor tissue and to act only on cancer cells. Nanodrugs are macromolecules or nanoparticles that function as targeted carrier systems to deliver active anticancer drug exclusively at the site of cancer. The well known anticancer chemotherapeutics cisplatin, carboplatin, 5-fluorouracil, bleomycin, paclitaxel, doxorubicin, vinblastin and topotecan etc., but also novel drugs including nucleic acids and proteins can be incorporated into these delivery systems. Drugs become active only at the site of cancer cells. A consideration of the unique properties of nanodrugs seems to bring about a revolution in cancer treatment which is the urgent need of time. The present chapter describes the huge diversity of nanodrugs and highlights the few principles of their mechanisms. Moreover, the superiority of nano anticancer modalities in comparison to the conventional chemotherapeutic anticancer drugs will be discussed. Recent patents in the field have been discussed under different sections of the chapter. Recent rocketing developments in the field will be introduced and emphasis has been laid on future perspectives.

Keywords: Cancer epidemiology, chemotherapeutics, chemotherapy, conventional anticancer drugs, dendrimers nanodrugs, drug delivery, future perspectives, inorganic material containing nanodrugs, liposomal nanodrugs, magic bullets, mechanism of action of nanodrugs, micellar nanodrugs, nanodrug diversity, nanodrugs, nanotechnology, organic material based nanodrugs, polymeric nanodrugs, recent developments, scope of nanodrugs, targeted medical tools.

***Address correspondence to Imran Ali:** Department of Chemistry, Jamia Millia Islamia (Central University), New Delhi-110025, India; Tel: 011-2698717 (Ext: 3253); Fax: 9971847086; E-mail: drimran_ali@yahoo.com, drimran.chiral@gmail.com

Atta-ur Rahman and Khurshid Zaman (Eds)

1. INTRODUCTION

Cancer is a terrible havoc for the entire world as almost 7.6 million people die due to this disease annually [1]. Approximations predict that around 1,660,290 new cancer cases will be diagnosed by the end of 2013. The data from the American Cancer Society suggests that about 580,250 Americans may die due to cancer in 2013. Only next to cardiovascular diseases, cancer is the cause of maximum deaths in the US, and accounts for almost 1 of every 4 deaths [2]. Approximately, 70% of the deaths in the developing countries occur due to cancer as a result of its poor prevention, diagnosis and treatment. Developing countries are witnessing an explosively increased incidence of cancers [3]. A hope in the chemotherapy of cancer was brought about by the discovery of the chemotherapeutics such as cisplatin and the development of its second and third generation analogues [4]. Other chemotherapeutics such as bleomycin, 5-fluorouracil, doxorubicin, dactinomycin, 6-mercaptopurine, paclitaxel, topotecan, vinblastine, etoposide etc. in single or combination therapy have been used for the treatment of various cancers [5]. These treatments are effective but are associated with certain limitations; renal impairment, neurotoxicity and ototoxicity, fast drug release, short blood circulation time and non-target specificity. These drawbacks and the dose limitation due to the side effects decrease their therapeutic efficiency considerably. Because these chemotherapeutics must be applied systemically, they have serious side effects by harming normal cells [6]. An obvious improvement would be to concentrate drugs in malignant tissue, while avoiding healthy tissue.

Nanotechnology brought about this innovative achievement. The new innovation included the loading of anticancer drugs onto nanocarrier molecules either by chemical bonds that are cleaved within cancer tissue or by encapsulation within nanosized suprastructures. These nanoparticle based drugs ensure their controlled release and enhanced permeability into their sites of action by recognition of tumor specific vessel morphology and tumor marker molecules on the surface of tumor cells. These drugs exhibit no or little side effects on normal cells and have the potential to cross the barriers of cancer cells easily. The efficacy of various nano anticancer drugs is much higher than their non-nano counterparts [7]. Nano drug delivery systems are safe and effective transporters which can be tailored to treat in principle any type of cancer by combining known drugs with molecules that specifically target malignant tissue/cells of interest [8]. This versatile interdisciplinary field has been termed "nanomedicine". By using the new attributes, nanomedicine seeks to circumvent unsatisfying properties of conventional anticancer drugs by harnessing novel physical and chemical properties of nano drug delivery systems, such as targeting and encapsulation to control pharmacokinetics and pharmacodynamics that cannot be achieved with conventional drugs [9]. Particle size, molecular weight, ionic strength, monomer concentration, pH and surface charge are the most important features of these drugs. The most commonly used polymers for the preparation of nanoparticle based anticancer drugs include linear biopolymers (e.g. polymalic acid) [10] or synthetic polymers (e.g. HPMA) [11], multivalent polymers [12], block copolymers [13], graft copolymers (copolymers with polymer side chains) [14], star polymers [15], dendrimers [16], dendronized polymers [17], and besides polymers, inorganic materials such as gold and mesoporous silica [18, 19]. Till now, some naoparticles are primarily in clinical trials and few others have emerged as new nano anticancer drugs in clinics, e.g., Myocet, DaunoXome, Prothecan and Aroplatin.

2. CANCER EPIDEMIOLOGY

Cancer is the second most common disease in India, owing to its poor prevention, diagnosis and treatment [20]. Among the various etiological factors, modernization of our society is a significant factor [21]. It is approximated that the number of deaths due to cancer may rise up to 9.0 million and 11.0 million in 2015 and 2030, respectively [1]. Under age 85 years in United States; cancer is the leading cause of death. It has for the first time surpassed heart diseases as the number one killer [8]. Cancer patient distribution is dependent on several factors imposing a wide variation of mortality rates across the world. Thus, the incidence rate of cancer showed a variation of 2.0 per 1,00,000 patients per year among females in Africa to a 61.2 per 1,00,000 patients per year among the men in North America [22]. Cancer incidence rates are found to be three times higher in developed nations as compared to the under developed geographic regions of the world. For example, the incidence of colorectal cancer was found to be four times higher in developing countries as compared to that in under developing countries.

Primary cancer appears in different types depending on the body tissue. More than 100 different cancer types have been recognized. WHO reports in 2006, indicated that skin cancer had the highest frequency of more than 10,00,000 patients in USA alone whereas lung cancer was the second major class accounting for about 1.3 million people worldwide per year [23]. Colorectal cancer stands as the fourth most common cancer diagnosed in the modern societies of developed countries [24]. Stomach cancer, which stands at fifth place has claimed 6,03,003 and 3,30,290 deaths during 1993 to 2001 [25]. Prostate cancer is the sixth most common cancer found globally. Statistical data from the American Cancer Society, 2012 indicate that around 226,160 new lung cancer cases will be identified in 2012, accounting for 14% of cancer diagnoses. The number of cancer cases estimated to be identified in 2012 are invasive cervical (12,170), breast (226,870), colon (103,170), rectal (40,290), kidney (64,770) and leukemia (47,150) [2]. Number of metastatic tumors in brain is growing and approximately 7 and 14 persons per 100,000 US populations have mctastatic brain tumors [26]. Lung metastatic cancers including non-small-cell lung cancer (NSCLC) account for nearly 80-85% of all lung cancer cases. The incidence of NSCLC drastically differs across different European countries. These incidence rates in men and women vary from 22 to 63 per 100,000 and from 5 to 33 per 100,000 per year, respectively [27].

3. CANCER CHEMOTHERAPY

Basically, chemotherapy refers to the use of conventional, synthetic (small molecula) drugs for the treatment of any disease. However, in general, chemotherapy refers to the use of drugs for the treatment of cancer. In addition, chemotherapy is often described by two other medical terms, viz, antineoplastic (meaning anticancer) therapy and cytotoxic (cell-killing) therapy. The first drug used for the chemotherapy of cancer did not start out as a medicine. Mustard gas (Fig. (**1**)); used as a chemical warfare agent during World War I, was studied further during World War II [28]. An accidental exposure of a group of people to mustard gas during World War II, caused those people to have very low white blood cell counts and, therefore, it was suggested that something had damaged the rapidly growing white blood cells and that agent might have a similar effect on rapidly dividing cancer cells [29]. Therefore, several patients with advanced lymphomas during 1940s were given intravenous doses of the drug. Although the improvements due to intravenous formulations of mustard gas were temporary, this experience was enough for providing the necessary impetus to search for other substances that might have similar effects against cancer. All this led to the development of the first ever chemotherapeutic drug; mustine (Fig. **2**) used for the treatment of prostate cancer. Consequently, a large number of chemical compounds, both organic and metal based were developed with the claim of good anticancer properties. Many anticancer drugs like cisplatin, carboplatin, oxaliplatin, nedaplatin, bleomycin, 5-fluorouracil, doxorubicin, dactinomycin, 6-mercaptopurine, paclitaxel, topotecan, etoposide (Fig. (**3**)) etc. are currently being used for the treatment of various sorts of cancers. In addition, various natural products were screened for their anticancer properties among which many are being used worldwide for the treatment of different cancers. Anticancer compounds obtained from natural products have been considered as more acceptable than the synthetic drugs for the treatment of cancer [30]. The isolation of the vinca alkaloids, vinblastine and vincristine (Fig. **4**) from the Madagascar periwinkle (*Catharanthus roseus*) stimulated the search for the development of natural products as anticancer agents. Vincristine and vinblastine were the first plant based agents those advanced into clinical use for the treatment of cancer. These agents are basically used in combination with other anticancer drugs for the treatment of various cancers, viz. leukemias, lymphomas, advanced testicular cancer, breast and lung cancers and Kaposi's sarcoma [31]. Besides, these two natural products, a large number of other natural products are being explored throughout the world for the treatment of cancer. Furthermore, combination drug therapies are being encouraged for the effective control of cancer. However, still we are not able to control cancer effectively and there are many side effects that the patients suffer from the available anticancer drugs.

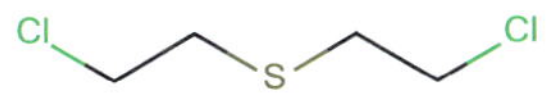

Figure 1: Chemical structure of mustard gas.

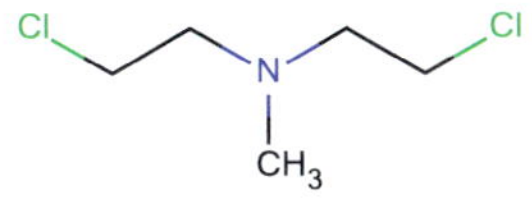

Figure 2: Chemical structure of mustine.

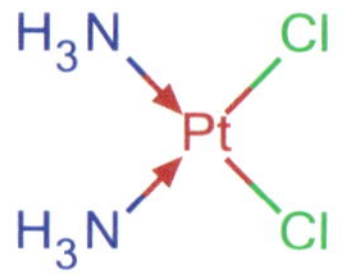

Cis-platin

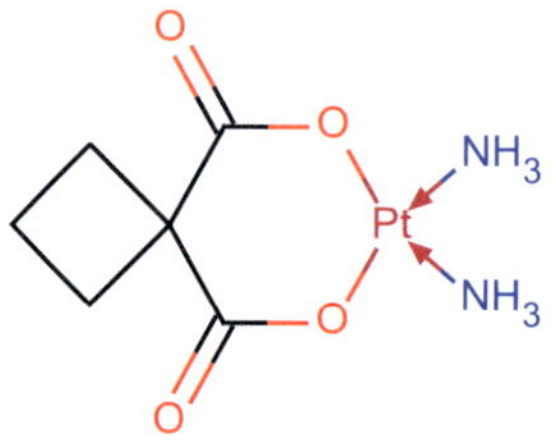

Carboplatin

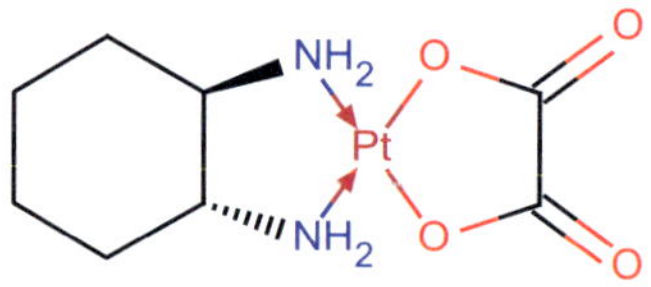

Oxaliplatin

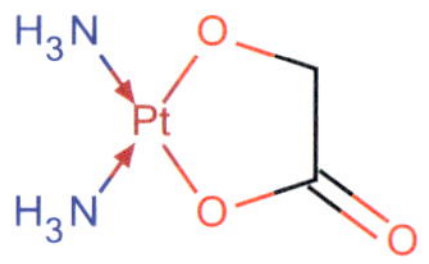

Nedaplatin

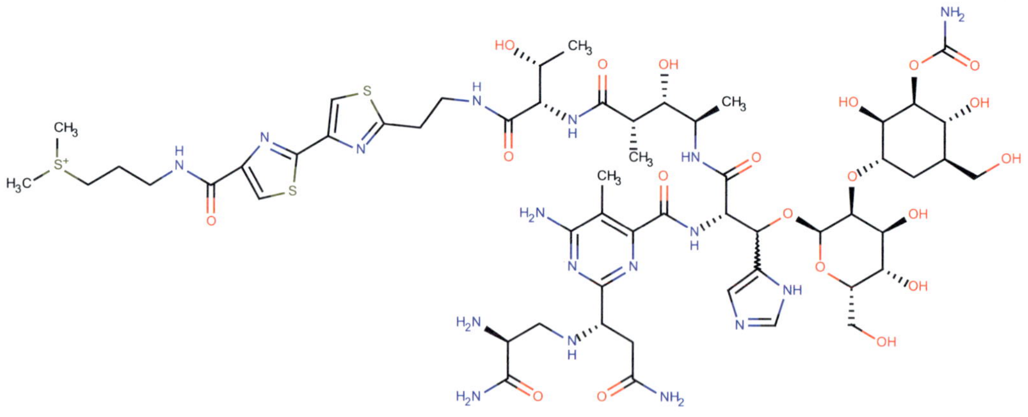

Bleomycin

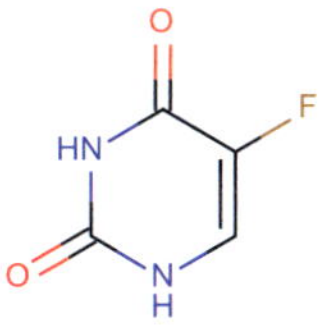

5-Fluorouracil

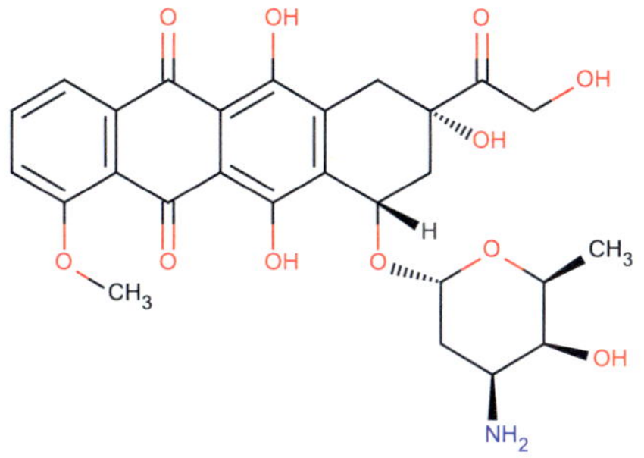

Doxorubicin

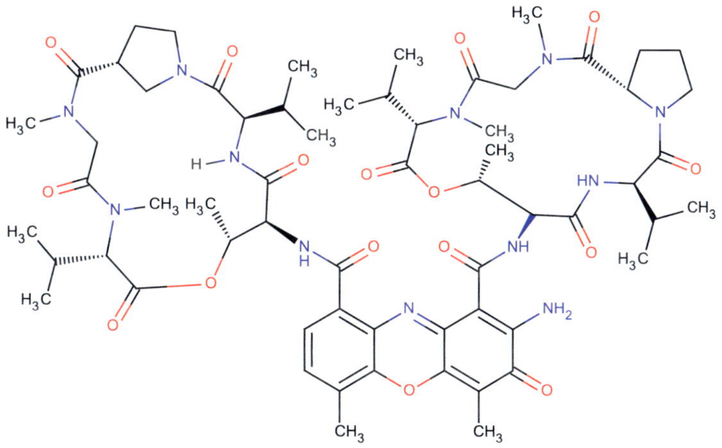

Dactinomycin A

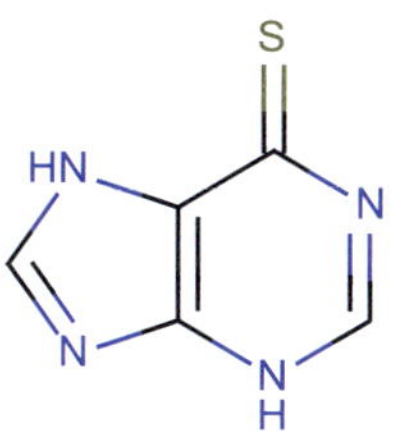

6-Mercaptopurine

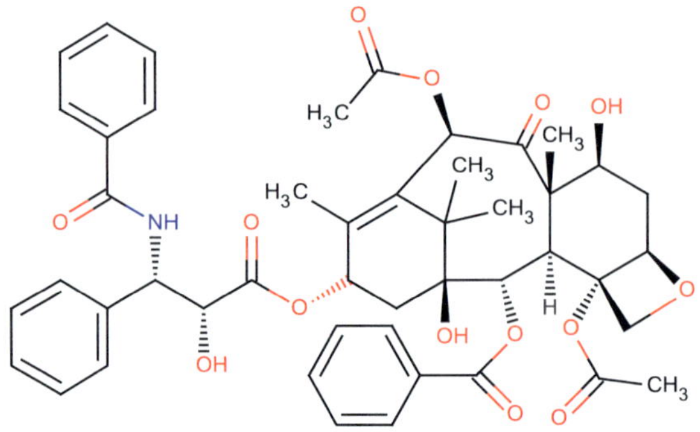

Paclitaxel

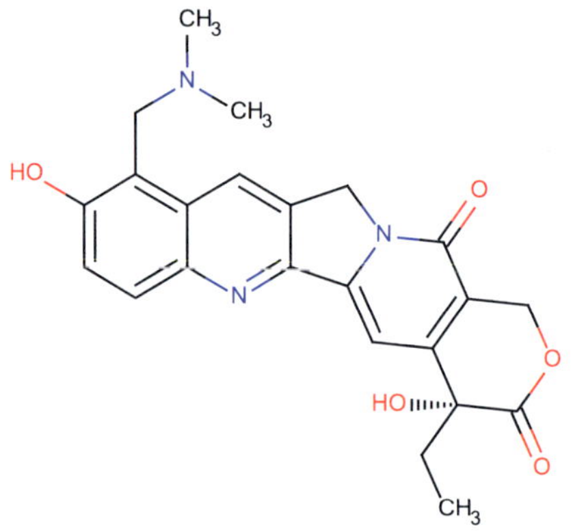

Topotecan

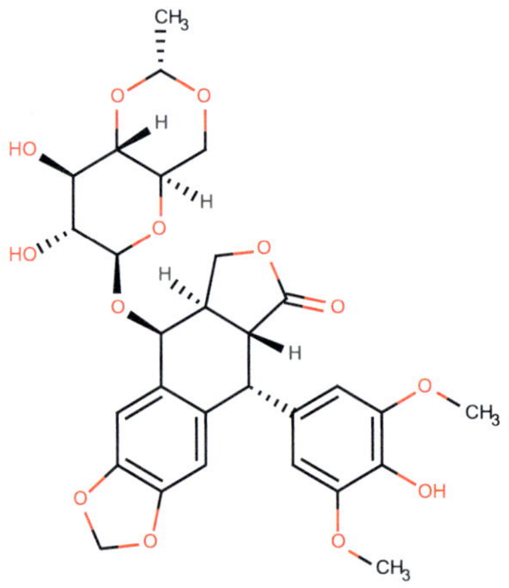

Etoposide

Figure 3: Chemical structures of anticancer drugs presently used for the treatment of different cancers.

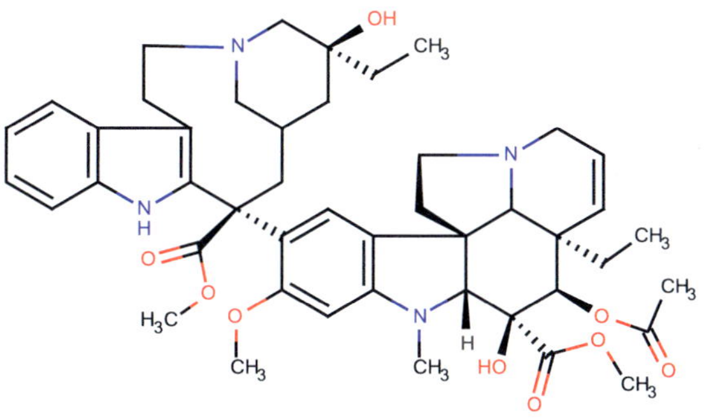

Vinblastine

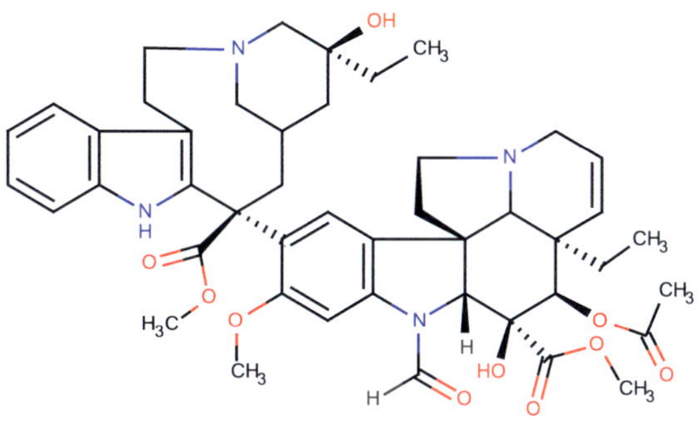

Vincristine

Figure 4: Natural product based anticancer drugs, vinblastine and vincristine obtained from *Catharanthus roseus*.

4. NANODRUGS: TARGETED MEDICAL TOOLS

The visionary idea that, "tiny nanorobots and related machines could be developed and introduced into the human body for carrying out cellular repairs at molecular level" stands as the basis for the birth of the concept of nanomedicine [32]. Reducing the size of medical entities might provide more versatile, accurate, reliable, cost-effective, controllable and quite faster approaches for the improvement of quality of life of mankind. In addition, nanomedicine was expected to solve many crucial medical issues by the use of nanoscale-structured materials and other simple nanodevices over the next 5 to 10 years. Basically, nanomedicine [33] involves diagnosis [34], treatment and prevention of disease and traumatic injury, pain relief and the improvement of human health with the use of the molecular tools and molecular knowledge of the human body.

Nanoscience and nanotechnology deal with the studies of properties and applications of matter at nano-scale. The dimensions of a nanometer measure about one millionth of a millimetre. A single human hair grand measures around 80,000 nm in thickness. Nanomedicine basically operates at the dimensions of about 100 nm or less. At these dimensions, most of the biological molecules and structures inside living cells are known to operate. The size dimensions of various biological entities are given in Fig. (**5**). It is clear from this figure that a typical protein has the dimensions of around 3 to 10 nm, while red blood cells measure about 6000-8000 nm. The sizes of nanoparticulate systems more often range from 10-20 nm (micelles) to several hundreds of nanometers (liposomes). As a matter of fact, drug delivery systems can, therefore, efficiently interact with biomolecules located on surfaces of cells and inside the cells. Therefore, it is quite obvious that the nanodrug is a delivery system that brings drug molecules into the target cells along with their safe transport. Moreover, the specificity of the delivery systems can be quite improved by decorating their surfaces with antibodies for targeting specific tissues [35]. Nanomaterials were initially studied for their physical, mechanical, electrical, magnetic, chemical and biological applications. However, attention has been shifted towards their pharmaceutical applications in the last 15-20 years. Nanostructures protect encapsulated drugs from degradation in the blood system, usually after intravenous injection, (not gastrointenstinal tract except few cases) and allow their delivery to specific sites in the body. Importantly, the technology ensures the delivery of poorly water soluble drugs and can also provide the means of bypassing the reticuloendothelial system (RES) [36-37].

Extensive analyses and observations by Chekman [38] in 2010 indicated that a good nanodrug should have the following properties:

i. Much more expressed effect in comparison with conventional drugs.

ii. Least or no adverse reactions.

iii. No drug-drug interaction in case of multidrug medication.

iv. Bring positive pharmacoeconomic parameters.

v. Usable for different ways of drug administration.

vi. Inexpensive and ecofriendly.

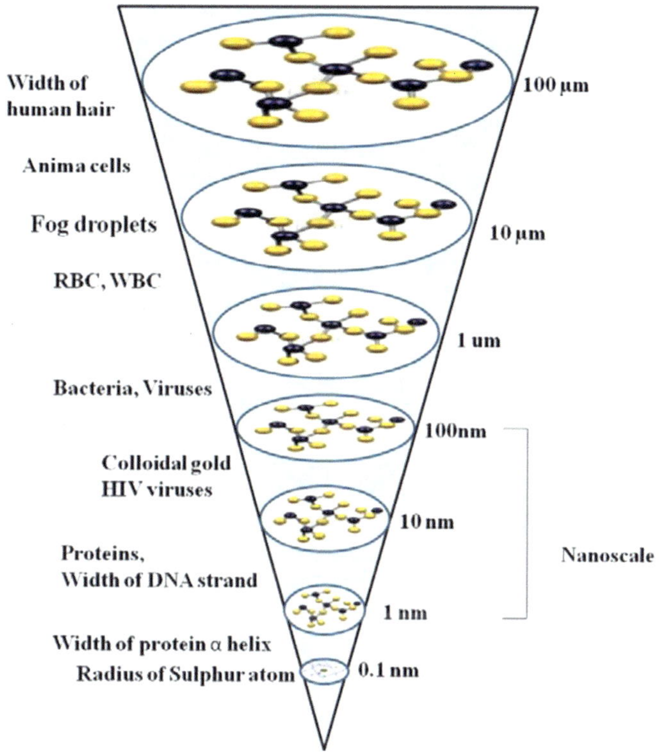

Figure 5: Dimensions of various biochemical entities in nanoscale.

5. SCOPE OF NANODRUGS

Nanotechnology is expected to address several issues of normal chemotherapy. A new generation of effective cancer therapies may be developed by using nanotechnology which may overcome the biological, biophysical and biomedical barriers that the body imposes against a standard intervention. Nanoparticle based drugs are promising in cancer therapy as they selectively gain access to tumors due to their small size and modifiability [39].

The following examples illustrate nanodrug development: Tseng *et al.* [40] developed a polymer-anticancer drug conjugate using gelatin nanoparticles (GPs) as carriers of cisplatin (CDDP), with improved therapeutic effect and significantly reduced side effects. Anticancer activities of CDDP loaded in GPs (GP-Pt) with biotinylated-endothelial growth factor (bEGF) modification (GP-Pt-bEGF) showed that GP-Pt-bEGF was more potent than free CDDP or GP-Pt because of its immediate effect on the cell cycle. In addition, GP-Pt-bEGF had stronger anti-tumor activity and was less toxic than free CDDP *in vivo*. Ding *et al.* [41] reported the *in vivo* antitumor efficiency and tumor cell penetration of cisplatin (CDDP)-loaded gelatin-poly(acrylic acid) (GEL-PAA). CDDP was sustainably released from the nanoparticles with a small initial burst release. Besides, CDDP-loaded nanoparticles had similar cytotoxicity to free CDDP after 48 h co-incubation with human colorectal cancer cell line LoVo. Moreover, the nanoparticle formulation was superior in anticancer effect to free CDDP on murine hepatic H22 tumor-bearing mice model through intraperitoneal administration and displayed a dose-dependent antitumor efficacy. Inoue *et al.* [42] recently reported a novel, targeted, nanobiopolymeric conjugate based on biodegradable, non-toxic, and non-immunogenic PMLA [poly(β-L-malic acid)]. The lead drug significantly inhibited the growth of HER2/neu-positive breast cancer cells *in vitro* and *in vivo* by enhanced apoptosis and inhibition of HER2/neu receptor signaling with suppression of Akt phosphorylation. The reported nanodrug selectively accumulated in tumor cells via an active delivery mechanism. Systemic treatment of human breast tumor-bearing nude mice resulted in more than 90% inhibition of tumor growth and tumor regression, as compared with partial (50%) tumor growth inhibition in mice treated with trastuzumab (Herceptin) or antisense oligonucleotides (AON), either free or attached to PMLA. Wang *et al.* [43] described the co-delivery of doxorubicin and paclitaxel with amphiphilic methoxy PEG-PLGA (poly(ethylene glycol)-poly(lactide-co-glycolide) copolymer nanoparticles. The reported NPs co-delivered hydrophilic doxorubicin (DOX) and hydrophobic paclitaxel (TAX). It was observed that both the delivered drugs were efficiently taken up by the cells and released simultaneously. Besides, the growth of tumor cells was suppressed more efficiently by the co-delivery nanocarrier than the delivery of either DOX or TAX at the same concentrations, which indicated a synergistic effect. Highest anti-tumor activity against the three different types of tumor cells was reported for the NPs with drugs loaded with a DOX/TAX concentration ratio of 2:1. Lawrence and coworkers [44] devised protocols of the compositions and methods for the delivery of agents, including therapeutic compounds, pharmaceutical agents, drugs, detection agents, nucleic acid sequences and biological factors for the treatment of chronic and acute diseases, infectious diseases, cancer, solid tumors and angiogenic states as well as other physiological disorders. The compositions of the developed nanotherapeutic system comprised of a colloidal metal sol (gold), PEG as a stealth agent and prodrug, and one or more agents (TNF). The colloidal gold was employed as a sol containing gold particles with a wide range of sizes. However, the most preferred particle size was 1 to 40 nm. The reported nanotherapeutic was highly effective as it did not allow the hydrolysis and conversion of the prodrug to its active form until the target (tumor) is reached. The presence of TNF as the targeting ligand further contributed to its effectiveness as it contributes in limiting the biodistribution of the nanoparticles primarily to the site of disease and enables them to simultaneously kill the host stromal cells that support and promote the tumor growth. Therefore, nanotherapy as a result of targeted delivery and the generation of active drug over time also improves the safety of the drug by facilitating the use of lower doses of drug.

Presently, various anticancer drugs as nano identities are under clinical trials whereas few others are in market for the treatment of various types of cancers. Table **1** [45-65] lists some of the important nano-anticancer drugs along with their brand names, nanoparticulate type used in their synthesis and the types of cancers treated.

6. NANODRUG DELIVERY SYSTEMS AND ENHANCED SUCCESS OF CANCER TREATMENT

Drug delivery is thought by many workers as the greatest immediate impact of nanotechnology in cancer therapy. Nanotechnology based drug delivery systems can improve the therapeutic index of almost all the currently used drugs by ensuring their safe targeting to their sites of action [66, 67]. Drugs, previously failed in clinical trials might also be reinvestigated by the applications of nanotechnology approaches. Novel applications of nanodrug delivery may eradicate a number of obstacles those hinder the action of conventional anticancer drugs. For example, poorly water soluble [68, 69] drugs may be solubilised by trapping them into crystalline nano suspensions those are stabilized by surfactants

[70], or by their combination with organic or lipid nanoparticles to keep them in circulation for longer periods of time [71-73]. The half-lives of pharmacologically active compounds can be significantly increased by encasing them into nanosized liposomes [72].

Table 1: Nano-anticancer drugs in market and in clinical trials.

Drugs	Nanomaterial Used	Brand Names	Drug Status	Applications	References
Doxorubicin	Liposome	Myocet	Market	Metastatic breast cancer	[45-47]
Daunorubicin	Liposome	DaunoXome	Market	Kaposi's sarcoma	[48]
Cisplatin	Liposome	SPI-077	Phase II	Various cancers	[49-51]
Paclitaxel	Liposome	LEP ETU	Phase I/II	Advanced solid tumors	[52]
Oxaliplatin	Liposome	Aroplatin	Phase II	Advanced colorectal cancer	[53]
Lurtotecan	Liposome	OSI-211	Phase II	Recurrent ovarian cancer; re-current small cell lung cancer	[54]
Doxorubicin	Polymeric Dextran	AD-70,DOX-OXD	Phase I	Various cancers	[55]
Doxorubicin	PEG-aspartic acid	NK911	Phase I	Pancreatic cancer	[56, 57]
Paclitaxel	Albumin	Abraxane	Market	Metastatic breast cancer	[58-60]
Camptothecin	PEG	Prothecan	Phase II	Various cancers	[61, 62]
Doxorubicin	HPMA copolymer	PK1; FCE28068	Phase II	Various cancers, particularly lung and breast cancer	[63, 64]
Paclitaxel	HPMA copolymer	PNU166945	Phase I	Various cancers	[65]

Basically, nanoparticle drug delivery systems are nanometeric entities used to deliver drugs or biomolecules to specific sites in the body. Generally, nanometeric carriers comprise of sub-micron particles (100nm and below) with various morphologies, including nano capsules, nanospheres, nanoliposomes, nanomicelles and nanodrugs etc. [74-76]. Nanoparticle drug delivery systems have some outstanding advantages that increase the therapeutic index of the loaded drugs significantly [75], for example, due to their ultra-tiny volume; they can pass through the smallest capillary vessels. Moreover, they avoid rapid clearance by phagocytes so that their duration in blood stream is greatly prolonged; they arrive at target organs such as liver, spleen, lung, spinal cord and lymph by penetrating into cell and tissue gap. In addition, they exhibit controlled release of the trapped drug molecules due to their biodegradability, pH, ion and/or temperature sensibility. Finally, nano drug delivery systems have the potential to improve the utility of drugs and reduce toxic side effects.

Recently, Li *et al.* [77] reported the controlled release of quercetin (QC) via a novel drug delivery system. Quercetin with cancer chemopreventive effect and anticancer potential was successfully loaded into methoxy poly(ethylene glycol)-cholesterol conjugate (mPEG-Chol) polymeric micelles in order to increase its water solubility. QC-loaded micelles were observed to have good drug loading (3.66%) and entrapment efficiency (93.51%) and were found to release QC quite slowly. Besides, the release of QC from the nano polymeric micelles was slightly faster in PBS at pH 5 than that in PBS at pH 7.4, which implied that QC-loaded micelles might be pH-sensitive and, thereby, selectively deliver QC to tumor tissues (due to different pH inside cancer cells with respect to normal cells). Therefore, the study revealed that mPEG-Chol was a promising micellar vector for the controlled and targeted delivery of QC to tumor. QC-loaded micelles were also worth being further investigated as a potential formulation for cancer chemoprevention and treatment. Perez-Martinez *et al.* [78] developed a non-viral delivery system (f-CNH_3) for small interfering RNA (siRNA) by anchoring a fourth-generation polyamidoamine dendrimer (G4-PAMAM) to carbon nanohorns (CNHs). The authors delivered a specific siRNA to human prostate cancer (PCa) cells by using the reported delivery system. The carbon nanohorn derivative bound to siRNA and released it in the presence of an excess of the polyanion heparin *in vivo*. Synthetic siRNA delivered to PCa cells by f-CNH_3 decreased the cofilin-1 mRNA and protein levels to about 20% of those of control values. Docetaxel, the drug of choice for the treatment of PCa was reported to produce a concentration dependent activation of caspase-3, an increase in cell death, cell cycle arrest and inhibition of tumor cell proliferation. All these toxic effects were potentiated when cofilin-1 was down regulated in these cells by a siRNA delivered by the nanoparticle. The authors concluded that the knocking down of certain proteins involved in cancer cell survival and/ proliferation may enhance the cytotoxic actions of anticancer drugs and it might be a new therapeutic approach to treat tumors. Song and coworkers [79] recently, reported self-assembled plasmonic vesicles (vesicular nanomaterials which are sensitive to radiations) of SERS (Surface enhanced Raman spectroscopy)-encoded amphiphilic gold nanoparticles for cancer cell targeting and traceable intracellular drug delivery. pH-responsive disassembly of the plasmonic vesicle that was stimulated by the hydrophobic-to-hydrophilic transition of the hydrophobic brushes in acidic intracellular compartments triggered intracellular drug release. Self-assembled plasmonic vesicles exhibited significantly variant plasmonic properties and, therefore, greatly enhanced SERS intensity in comparison to single gold nanoparticles. The unique structural and optical properties of the plasmonic vesicle have made it a promising platform for targeted combination therapy and theranostic (proposed process of diagnostic therapy for individual patients) applications by taking advantage of recent advances in gold nanostructure based *in vivo* bioimaging and photothermal therapy and their loading capacity for both hydrophilic (nucleic acids and proteins) and hydrophobic (small molecules) therapeutic agents. Wu *et al.* [80] reported a nano-sized protein-derived micellar drug delivery system which was based on the polycationic albumin precursor protein cBSA-147. Efficient encapsulation of the doxorubicin (DOX) was ensured into nanosized micelles via hydrophobic interactions with the polypeptide scaffold. Attractive stabilities in various physiological buffers and a wide pH range and a quite efficient uptake into A549 cells after 1 hr incubation time was exhibited by the reported micelles. The loaded DOX had five-fold increased cytotoxicity as compared to free DOX *in vivo* indicating efficient intracellular drug release. As a result, this denatured albumin-based drug delivery system represented a highly attractive platform for nanomedicine approaches towards cancer therapy. Xu *et al.* [81] reported a paclitaxel (PTX)-loaded mixed micelles with Folate-Poly (ethylenimine)-Pluronic and Pluronic L121 copolymers. Nano-sized spherical morphology was observed for the mixed micelles. Due to the high solubilization capacity of L121 copolymers, the solubilization capacity of the mixed micelles was significantly higher than Folate-Poly (ethylenimine)-Pluronic micelles. Maximum anticancer activity was demonstrated by the PTX in Folate-Poly (ethylenimine)-Pluronic micelles. In addition, a markedly increased cellular accumulation of folate-modified Pluronic-poly(ethylenimine) micelles was observed as compared with Pluronic P123 micelles. Furthermore, Folate-Poly (ethylenimine)-Pluronic micelles exhibited enhanced pulmonary retention in rats after injection.

7. DIVERSITY OF NANODRUGS

The term "nanoparticles" covers a wide array of numerous engineered entities, architectures, and particulate systems. All the identities usually share a common feature, i.e. size, that ranges from a few nanometers to several nanometers [82, 83]. Several nanodrugs represent free polymeric nanoconjugates, but most of them are formed by self-assembly of their constituents and include dendrimers, micelles, polymeric nanoparticles, liposomes and cyclodextrins, by which therapeutic agents can be entrapped, encapsulated, covalently bound, or adsorbed to overcome various therapeutic issues of drugs including stability, solubility, activity, side effects, time of action, controlled release and specificity [84]. The various classes of nanoparticles those come our way during the design of nanodrugs are discussed in the following sections:

7.1. Polymeric Nanodrugs

Due to the diversity of surface characteristics and sizes of free polymeric nanoconjugates and of assembled polymeric materials, they are increasingly gaining importance [85] as nano drug carriers. Besides, the surface characteristics and sizes of polymeric material can be tuned and optimized for both passive and active transport, sustained and controlled drug release and the minimum degradation of drugs in blood. The biodegradability, biocompatibility and non-toxicity of the polymeric nanoparticles make them the most preffered vehicles for the delivery of therapeutic agents [86-88]. The drugs trapped into the nanoparticulate polymeric framework are generally released at a sustained rate through the diffusion of the drug and the degradation of the nanoparticles [89]. These exciting properties inspired scientists, pharmaceutical companies and oncologists towards the development of safe and efficient polymeric motors for drug delivery. The most common and important materials are nano-gels, albumin, polymer and lipid-like systems. Some of these materials are biodegradable and are, therefore, easily excreted after their job is done. The most useful materials for these types of nanoparticles are polylactic acid, polyalkylcyanoacrylate, poly(3-hydroxybutanoic acid), polyglycolic acid or polyethylene oxide and others [90, 91]. Biopolymers are polyamino acids, polymalic acid, polysaccharides peptides, proteins and nucleic acids. Amphotericin B, camptothecin (Fig. (**6**)), paclitaxel and etoposide are some of the commonly tested drugs by the use of these polymers. Some important and recent reports in this area are discussed in the following paragraph.

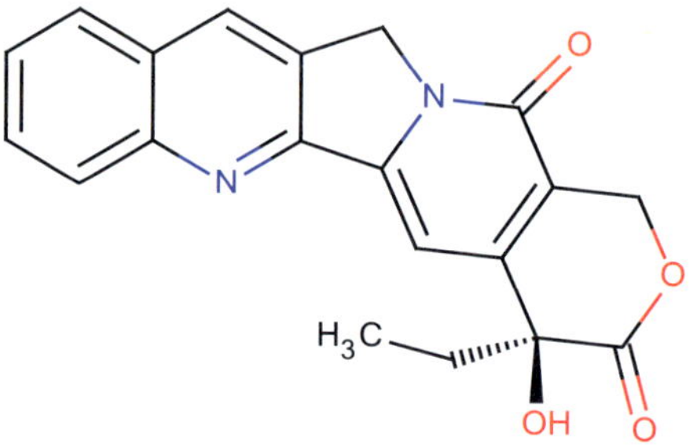

Figure 6: Chemical structure of camptothecin.

Targeting of anticancer drugs to tumor sites is a potential powerful approach for the selective treatment of cancer. For example, integrins are a class of heterodimeric transmembrane proteins that play important roles in cell adhesion and cell signaling. The expression of the essential proteins is commonly upregulated in cancers and inflammatory diseases. The $\alpha_v\beta_3$ integrin is usually differentially upregulated on the surfaces of angiogenic endothelial cells and many cancer cells. Graf *et al.* [92] described the differential targeting of cisplatin prodrug-encapsulated poly(D,L-lactic-co-glycolic acid)-block-polyethylene glycol (PLGA-PEG) nanoparticles to the $\alpha_v\beta_3$ integrin on cancer cells using the cyclic pentapeptide c(RGDfK). The RGD-targeted Pt(IV)-encapsulated nanoparticles displayed considerably enhanced cytotoxicity with respect to cisplatin administered in its conventional dosage form in model prostate and breast cancer epithelial cells *in vitro*. The RGD-targeted PLGA-PEG nanoparticles were more pharmacologically active and better tolerated in comparison to cisplatin in an orthotopic human breast cancer xenograft model *in vivo*. Recently, Wan *et al.* [93] reported two types of nanoparticles using diblock copolymer methoxy poly(ethylene glycol)-block-poly(caprolactone) (MePEG-b-PCL) employing either a short PCL block length forming micelles, or with a longer PCL block length forming kinetically frozen core structures (nanospheres). Both the paclitaxel (PTX)-loaded micelles and nanospheres were screened for their cytotoxicity, cellular polymer uptake, and drug accumulation in drug-sensitive (Madin-Darby Canine Kidney [MDCK]II) and multidrug-resistant (MDR) P-glycoprotein (P-gp)-overexpressing (MDCKII-MDR1) cell lines. It was observed that both types of PTX-loaded nanoparticles equally inhibited proliferation of MDCKII cells. However, PTX-loaded micelles were remarkably more cytotoxic as compared to nanospheres on MDCKII-MDR1 cells. Interestingly, intracellular accumulation of both PTX and the diblock copolymers were similar for both the types of nanoparticles indicating that the differential cytotoxicity might be due to the differential drug-release profiles. Moreover, enhancement of the cytotoxicity of these PTX-loaded nanoparticles was brought about by the combination of this nanoparticulate systems molecular-weight MePEG-b-PCL diblock copolymer. Dhar and coworkers [94] reported a significant enhancement in the *in vivo* pharmacokinetics, biodistribution, tolerability and efficacy of Pt-PLGA-b-PEG-Apt-NP (150 $\pm$ 15 nm encapsulating ~5% *w/w* Pt(IV) prodrug) in comparison to cisplatin administered in its conventional form in normal Sprague Dawley rats, Swiss Albino mice, and the PSMA-expressing LNCaP subcutaneous xenograft mouse model of PCa, respectively. Prolonged platinum persistence in systemic blood circulation and decreased accumulation of Pt in the kidneys was observed from pharmacokinetic studies with Pt-PLGA-b-PEG-NP. Pt-PLGA-b-PEG-Apt-NPs further displayed the significant dose-sparing characteristics of the drug, with equivalent antitumor efficacy in LNCaP xenografts at 1/3 the dose of cisplatin administered in its conventional form (0.3mg/kg vs. 1mg/kg). Due to the concomitant improvement in tolerability and efficacy, Pt-PLGA-b-PEG-Apt NP brings about a remarkable improvement in the therapeutic index of the drug. Shah and coworkers [95] determined the efficacy and bioavailability of cisplatin in the form of cisplatin-loaded self-assembled amphiphilic copolymer nanoparticles (NPs). Sustained release of the loaded cisplatin from the nanoconjugate was evident from its *in vitro* release profile. Besides, internalization of cisplatin-loaded NPs into the tumor cells was clearly evident from the TEM and confocal microscopy studies. The reported NPs significantly suppressed the tumor cell growth, and enhanced the apoptotic process of the tumor cells compared to free drug treated cells. Etrych *et al.* [96] described the biological activity of paclitaxel (PTX) and docetaxel (DTX) conjugated with a water-soluble *N*-(2-hydroxypropyl)methacrylamide (HPMA) copolymer as drug carrier. Derivatized drugs were attached to the backbone of the polymer via spacer (compounds with cleavable hydrazone bonds, e.g., 6-aminohexanoic acid residue and a hydrazone bond) stable under physiological conditions (pH 7.4) and hydrolytically degradable in mild acidic environments (e.g., endosomes, pH = 5). Quite faster release of drugs and their derivatives from the polymer at pH 5 than at pH 7.4 was observed on *in vitro* incubation of the conjugates in buffers. Besides, PTX-containing conjugate exhibited better antitumor efficacy in the 4T1 model of mammary carcinoma than the parent drug and its derivative. The DTX containing conjugate showed high activity for the treatment of EL4 T cell lymphoma and the treatment with the polymer conjugates was devoid of side toxicity. Elamanchili and coworkers [97] demonstrated that the diblock copolymer MePEG-b-PCL significantly enhanced the accumulation of various Pgp (P-glycoprotein) substrates in Pgp over-expressing MDR cells, however, there was no effect on the substrate accumulation in non-Pgp expressing cells. Besides, the treatment of MDR cells with the diblock copolymer significantly enhanced paclitaxel (PTX) and doxorubicin (DOX) accumulation. After uptake, PTX was immediately effluxed from MDR cells whereas diblock copolymer treatment retained DOX inside MDR cells. Reversal of drug resistance of MDR cells towards DOX on treatment with the diblock copolymer was observed but not towards PTX. However, verapamil reversed the resistance of MDR cells to PTX indicating that a sustained inhibition of Pgp (P-glycoprotein) was crucial for PTX to induce cytotoxicity in MDR cells. These results explore the potential of MePEG-b-PCL diblock copolymer for the reversal of reverse drug resistance in MDR cancer cells via inhibition of Pgp function, and therefore, making it a promising candidate for overcoming MDR.

7.2. Liposomal Nanodrugs

From the last fifty years, liposomes have been considered quite important in formulating novel and efficient drug delivery systems. Liposomes are capable to carry nucleic acids and some anti-neoplastic drugs. Due to biodegradability and non-toxicity of most liposomes, they can be safely used as drug carriers. The drug delivery process of liposomes is controlled by several parameters including their size (30 nm to 1000 nm), surface composition and charge. Liposomes are, generally, composed of lipids having a hydrophilic centre with special features [98]. Doxorubicin, daunorubicin, camptothecin, paclitaxel, cisplatin, some antibiotics (ciprofloxacin, amikacin and vancomycin) and nucleic acids can be easily sandwiched with liposomes for delivery into the cells [8, 99-106]. Normally, liposomes with the size of 30 nm deliver drugs at their targets without degradation during blood circulation [107]. Surface modifiers like dextrans [108], hydrophilic polymers such as PEG [109], poly-*N*-vinylpyrrolidones [110], gangliosides [111] and polyvinyl alcohol [112] avoid the degradation of large sized liposomes during blood circulation.

Lee *et al.* [113] reported tetraiodothyroacetic acid (tetrac) as a novel, efficient and safe moiety for the delivery of anticancer drugs to tumor tissues. Tetrac was covalently linked to the activated end of pegylated lipid and used to formulate tetrac-tagged pegylated liposomes (TPL). After incubation with TPL for 9 hr., cellular accumulation efficiency into A375 human melanoma cells was high (98.5% $\pm$ 0.5% of cells), whereas that in KB cells was much lower (35.1% $\pm$ 4.5%). TPL preferentially distributed into tumor tissues after systemic administration in mice as was evident from molecular imaging, whereas non-targeting pegylated liposomes were distributed to tumors at background levels. Treatment of A375 tumor cells with alkyl lysophospholipid anticancer drug edelfosine, encapsulated in TPL, significantly reduced their survival in comparison to cells treated with edelfosine in pegylated liposomes or with lysophosphatidylcholine encapsulated in TPL. Besides, the growth of tumors was significantly reduced by the intravenous administration of edelfosine in TPL. In addition, a prolonged survival of A375-xenografted mice with 100% protection against tumors for up to 50 days and some protection until 66 days (0% survival endpoint) was observed. All these results indicated the enormous potential of tetrac as a new ligand moiety for the delivery of anti-cancer drug-loaded nanoparticles to tumors. Recently, Mangiapia and coworkers [114] reported a new organometallic ruthenium complex, named AziRu, along with three amphiphilic nucleoside-based ruthenium complexes, ToThyRu, HoThyRu and DoHuRu, (Fig. (7)) incorporating AziRu in their skeleton (into the structure of complexes). The complexes were stabilized in POPC (1-Palmitoyl-2-oleoyl phosphate-dylcholine) formulations and investigated for their antineoplastic activity. The authors observed that the three AziRu derivatives formed liposomes, and, elongated micelles under specific conditions. The micellar formulations prepared in POPC were stable for months and exhibited high *in vitro* antiproliferative activity.

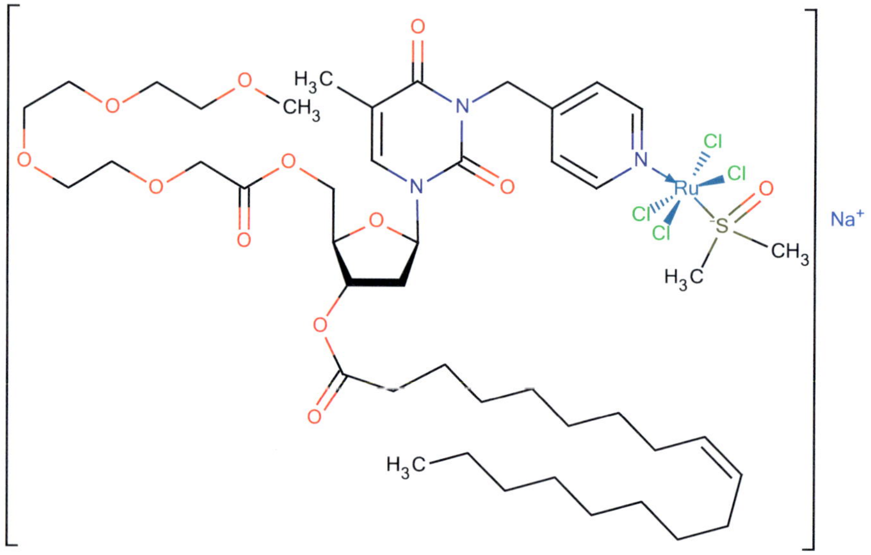

ToThyRu

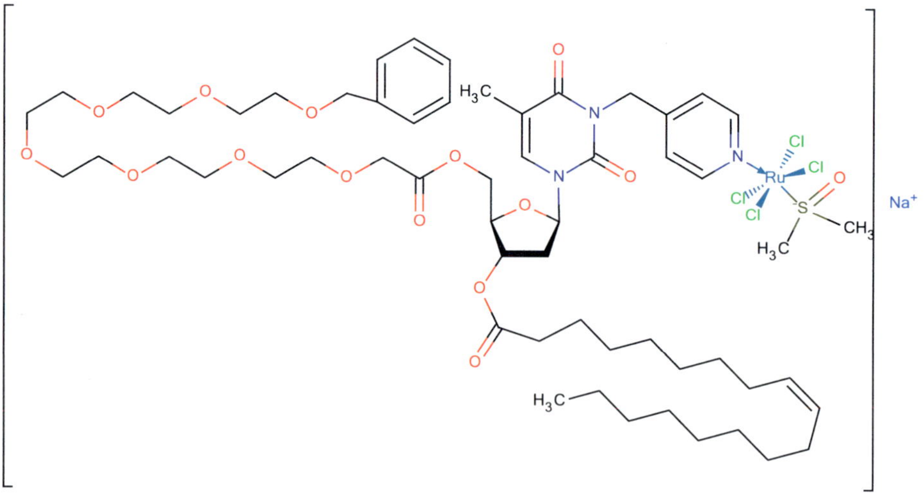

HoThyRu

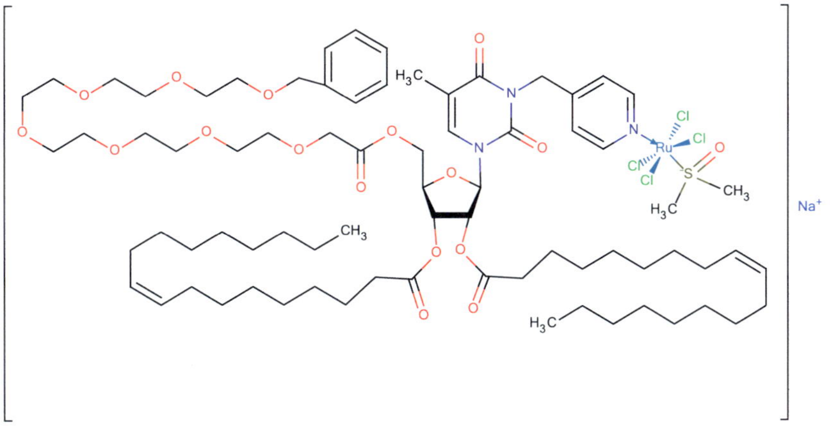

DoThyRu

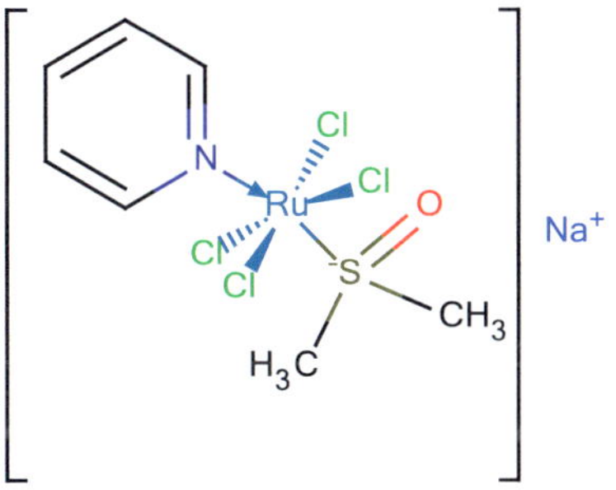

AziRu

Figure 7: Functional nucleolipids: ToThyRu, HoThyRu and DoHuRu incorporating the complex AziRu into their structure.

7.3. Micellar Nanodrugs

In certain cases, 100 nm or below sized drug delivery structures are required for targeting specific tissues. Micelles made of ampiphillic polymers efficiently do this job. The pluronic block copolymers, phospholipids, poly (L-aminoacid) and polyesters are commonly used as components for micelle formation. The various drugs including cisplatin, camptothecin, doxorubicin and paclitaxel are usually delivered via micelles with greater distribution efficiencies (distribution to their target sites). Circulation half lives of micellar systems are greater than the ones of free drugs resulting in their accumulation into cancer tissues [115]. Yoon *et al.* [116] reported a hydrotropic micelle (HM) which encapsulated superparamagnetic iron oxide nanoparticles (SPIONs) as magnetic resonance imaging (MRI) agent and paclitaxel (PTX) as the hydrophobic anti-cancer drug. HM effectively encapsulates both PTX and SPION via its hydrophobic inner core. It was observed that PTX was released from the micelles in a sustained manner. In addition, the bare HM and HM-SPION showed no toxicity to SCC7 (murine squamous carcinoma) cells, whereas HM-PTX and HM-SPION-PTX showed dose-dependent cytotoxicity that was lower than free PTX. Moreover, HM-SPION-PTX exhibited 8.1 fold higher magnetic relaxivity than HM-SPION, justifying the potential of HM-SPION-PTX as a contrast agent for MRI. HM-SPION-PTX was effectively accumulated at the tumor site, allowing its detection using MR imaging when administered to tumor-bearing mice. This study indicates that HM-SPION-PTX has potential as future candidate for combined diagnosis and treatment of cancer. Recently, Vetvicka *et al.* [117] documented pharmacological properties of a polymeric micellar conjugate containing doxorubicin (DOX) covalently bound to the micelle core through hydrolytically cleavable hydrazone bonds. The nanoparticulate system had a very low toxicity almost 20 times lower than free DOX and long circulation in the blood stream. The newly developed micellar system exhibited promising therapeutic activity against established murine EL-4 T-cell lymphoma. It was found to be able to cure 75% of tumor-bearing mice completely (with doses of either 1 x 150 mg DOX kg^{-1} or 2 x 75 mg DOX kg^{-1}, administered intraveinously). Tsallas *et al.* [118] reported the treatment of freshly excised pig bladder sections with anticancer drugs, paclitaxel (PTX) and docetaxel (DTX) formulated in diblock copolymer (methoxy poly(ethylene glycol)-block-poly (D,L-lactic acid) (MePEG-PDLLA) and methoxypoly(ethylene glycol)-block-poly(caprolactone) (MePEG-CL) nanoparticles for 2 h. It was observed that the PTX or DTX loaded in MePEG-PDLLA micelles caused significantly higher urothelial tissue levels and greater bladder wall exposures in comparison to their commercial formulations, Cremophor EL/ethanol (PTX) or Tween 80 (DTX). In conclusion, the use of diblock copolymer micellar PTX or DTX formulations are encouraged for the treatment of bladder tumors as compared to commercial formulations for taxane delivery to superficial bladder tumors. Malzert-Freon and coworkers [119] reported the effect of incorporation of a solubility enhancer on the formulation of lipidic nanoparticles with improved drug loading rates. A solubility enhancer (Labrasol) was incorporated in a formulation process based on a low-energy Phase inversion temperature method. The results of a partial least square analysis showed that these nanoparticles present a core-shell structure where Labrasol is well encapsulated and contributes to the formation of the oily liquid core of the nanoparticle. These nanoparticles were smaller than 200nm and spherical in shape were able to encapsulate a tripentone, a new anticancer agent, with drug loading rates up to 6.5% (w/w). So, highly drug-loaded lipidic nanocarriers were developed without using the slightest organic solvent trace, and making it easily possible dose adjustment.

7.4. Inorganic Material Containing Nanodrugs

Hard nanoparticles of very small sizes are essentially required for the synthesis of inorganic nanoparticle drugs. The most commonly used inorganic materials are metal ions of Au, Ag, Cu, Bi, Fe, Ge, Pb, Pd, Pt, Se, Si, Te and W [120] and their compounds (Ag_2Se, CdS, CdSe, CdTe, CuO, GaN, GaAs, GaP, Ga_2O_3, GeO_2, InAs, InP, In_2O_3, MgO, MnO_2, PbS, SiC, SnO_2, TiO_2, ZnO, ZnS and WO_3) [100]. Inorganic material is coated with or embedded in organic nanoparticle forming material. Due to the flexibility of tuning and optimization of size, morphology and spatial organization of such nanoparticles, their future seems to be quite bright [121-124].

Hu *et al.* [125] demonstrated the loading of a model hydrophobic anticancer drug, paclitaxel (PTX), and 4nm sized SPIO nanoparticles into micellar cores and hydrophilic coronas, respectively. The authors observed controlled and sustained release of PTX from hybrid micelles, exhibiting a cumulative release of 61% encapsulated drugs (loading content, 8.5w/w) over ~130 h. From the results of *in vivo* MR imaging, it was observed that amphiphilic block copolymer micelles surface embedded with SPIO nanoparticles at the hydrophilic corona may be a new generation of nanoplatform useful for targeted drug delivery, controlled release, and disease diagnostic functions. Balivada *et al.* [126] reported the effect of bimagnetic nanoparticles (MNPs) along with short external alternating magnetic field (AMF) on the growth of subcutaneous mouse melanomas (B16-F10). Bimagnetic Fe/Fe_3O_4 core/shell nanoparticles were designed for the targeting of cancer after intratumoral or intravenous administration. Organic dopamine-oligoethylene glycol ligands were used to protect their inorganic center against rapid biocorrosion. In addition, TCPP (4-tetracarboxyphenyl porphyrin) units were attached to the dopamine-oligoethylene glycol ligands. It was observed that micromolar concentrations of iron given within the modified core-shell Fe/Fe_3O_4 nanoparticles caused a significant anti-tumor effect on murine B16-F10 melanoma with three short 10-minute AMF exposures. Moreover, a decrease in tumor size after intravenous administration of the MNPs followed by three consecutive days of AMF exposure 24 hrs after the MNPs injection was reported. Leticia and coworkers [127] studied the effect of the conjugation of Kahalalide F (a novel anticancer drug of murine origin) (Fig. (**8**)) or its analogues with colloidal metal nanoparticles of gold on their antitumor activities against HeLa cells. For the study of the feasibility and biological properties of colloidal gold nanoparticles conjugated with Kahalalide F or an analogue thereof, synthetic epimer analogues of Kahalalide F (KF) were synthesised and separately conjugated to two different sized (20 nm and 40 nm) colloidal gold nanoparticles (AuNPs). It was observed that the functionalized gold nanoparticles showed an improved antitumoral activity against HeLa cells in comparison to the activity of the compounds administered alone. Interestingly, AuNP-40 (40 nm size gold nanoparticles) conjugates were slightly more cytotoxic than AuNP-20 (40 nm size gold nanoparticles) conjugates probably due to better cell uptake of the AuNP-40 conjugates. Depending on tumor types and the stage of the disease, the treatments of the invention promote tumor regression, stop tumor growth and prevent metastasis. Preferably, breast cancer, colon cancer, renal cancer, leukemia, melanoma, colorectal cancer, epithelial cancer, ovarian cancer, cervix cancer, pancreatic cancer, lung cancer, liver cancer and prostate cancer may be treated by the reported colloidal metal nanoparticle. The authors suggested that the increase in the antitumor activity of Kahalalide F and its analogues might be due to the nanoparticle acting as a presenter of the anti-tumor agent, and as a result concentrating numerous peptide molecules on its surface. Tuan *et al.* [44] reported functionalized nanoparticle, comprising of a core with a shell. Coatings of plasmonics active material on the surface of the core, most preferably a shell of gold or silver or other materials, which enhance or intensify either or both of the applied X-ray energy or emitted UV energy. The functionalized nanoparticles most preferably contained a rare-earth oxide (Y_2O_3) core and a noble metal (Au, Ag, etc.) shell. To the surface of the nanoparticles was anchored a cysteine-terminated cell penetrating/nuclear targeting peptide, that could demonstrate the ability to functionalize the peptide with a variety of fluorescent dyes. After the attachment of the dye molecules to the nuclear targeting peptide anchored to the gold shells, their ability to fluoresce retained which might indicate that these hybrid nanoparticles should remain visible within cells and taken up via endocytosis, phagocytosis, or a combination of these and other cellular uptake processes. Due to the ability to inhibit cell growth and/or induce apoptosis of the reported functionalized nanoparticle system, it may therefore, be used as non-invasive anti-cancer treatment modality for deep-tissue tumors in hypoxic environments. In addition, the functionalized nanoparticles can be well incorporated into pharmaceutical compositions suitable for administration. Kingston *et al.* [128] devised a strategy to deliver fully active sulphur-containing paclitaxel derivatives to their target sites by covalently linking them to gold nanoparticles. The attachment of the paclitaxel derivatives to the gold nanoparticles generated a substance capable of acting as a cancer chemotherapeutic agent directly, with paclitaxel still bound to the nanoparticle, or by release of paclitaxel from the nanoparticle. The release of the drug might be due to hydrolysis reaction or by some other release mechanism. The system ensured more efficient delivery of paclitaxel due to the fact that a nanoparticle can access a tumor more specifically due to the leaky vasculature associated with solid tumors while it is less able to access other cell types. The delivery of a fully active form of paclitaxel to a desired site is more efficient than when the paclitaxel is delivered by conventional means (when the drug is not attached to a nanoparticle). The compositions are used to treat various types of cancers, including ovarian cancer, lung cancer, head and neck cancer, breast cancer, prostate cancer, advanced forms of Kaposi's sarcoma, bladder cancer, melanoma, stomach cancer, colon cancer, pancreatic cancer, etc. An interesting advantage of the delivery system of paclitaxel reported herein is that the gold nanoparticles enable the delivery of the drug in greater concentration because of the delayed conversion of the drug to its active form until the target site is reached. Besides, paclitaxel release from analogs occurs via hydrolysis or reductive cleavage of the gold-sulphur bonds. Briefly, gold contributed to the stabilization of the paclitaxel analog and therefore, significantly decreased premature conversion or activation in plasma.

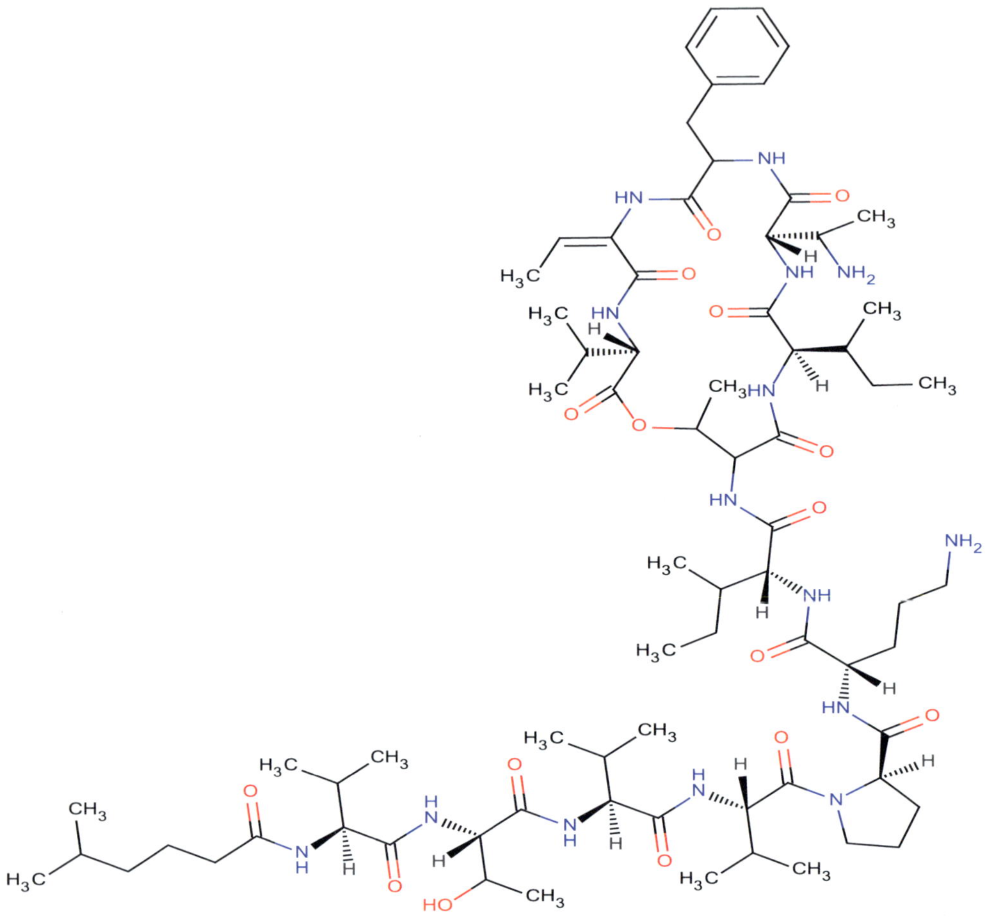

Figure 8: Kahalalide F: A novel anticancer drug of murine origin.

7.5. Organic Material Based Nanodrugs

Usually, a minute fraction of most of the drugs is released from their nano cages into the blood stream before reaching their target. Even this trace amount of drugs can cause certain side effects and toxicities to normal cells. In such cases nanoparticles with no drug leakage via blood circulation are required, and, this task is thought to be well served by clusters of carbon like C_{60} (fullerenes and buckyballs) [129, 130]. Carbon nano-tubes (CNTs) were first investigated in 1991 [131] and were found to have high thermal and electrical conductivities, rigidity and resilience; making them ideal for several applications including anticancer drug delivery systems to targeted tissues [132].

Li *et al.* [133] developed a method for the targeted delivery of 10-hydroxycamptothecin (HCPT)-loaded nanoparticles to cancer cells. Micronized HCPT (nHCPT) were prepared by a supercritical antisolvent process. Further, folate-conjugated human serum albumin (HSA) nHCPT-loaded NPs (FA-HSA-nHCPT-NPs) were prepared using a NP-coated method combined with a desolvation technique. FA-HSA-nHCPT-NPs were reported to show sustained-drug release characteristics for 120 hours *in vitro*, with a drug-loading content of 7.3% and an encapsulating efficiency of 79.1%. It was observed that FA-NPs were effective delivery systems for uptake by SGC7901 cells compared to folate-free NPs. These results suggested that a NP-coated method combined with a desolvation technique is effective for preparing NPs with drugs having poor solubility in water and most organic solvents, using albumin as the wall material. Gao *et al.* [134] described the encapsulation of quercetin (QU) into biodegradable monomethoxy poly(ethylene glycol)-poly(ε-caprolactone) (MPEG-PCL) micelles. The drug loading capacity and mean particle size of the developed QU loaded MPEG-PCL (QU/MPEG-PCL) micelles was 6.9% and of 36nm. The intravenous administration of QU/MPEG-PCL micelles was found to significantly suppress the growth of established xenograft A2780S ovarian tumors through cancer cell apoptosis and the inhibition of angiogenesis *in vivo*. Besides, the treatment with quercetin induced the apoptosis of A2780S cells associated with activating caspase-3 and caspase-9. MCL-1 down regulation, Bcl-2 down regulation, Bax upregulation and mitochondrial transmembrane potential change were observed, suggesting that quercetin may induce apoptosis of A2780S cells through the mitochondrial apoptotic pathway. Overall, the authors concluded that the QU/MPEG-PCL micelles were a novel nano-formulation and might have several clinical applications in ovarian cancer therapy. Gou and coworkers [135] reported the encapsulation of curcumin into monomethoxy poly(ethylene glycol)-poly(ε-caprolactone) (MPEG-PCL) micelles via a one-step nano-precipitation method, creating curcumin-loaded MPEG-PCL (Cur/MPEG-PCL) micelles. These Cur/MPEG-PCL micelles has a good solubility after freeze-drying with an encapsulation efficiency of $99.16 \pm 1.02\%$ and a drug loading of $12.95 \pm 0.15\%$. It was observed that the anticancer agent, curcumin was molecularly dispersed in the PCL core of MPEG-PCL micelles with the ability to be slowly released *in vitro*. The *in vivo* $t_{1/2}$ of curcumin was appreciably improved by its encapsulation in

MPEG-PCL micelles. Both Cur/MPEG-PCL micelles and free curcumin efficiently inhibited the angiogenesis on transgenic Zebra fish model. Intravenous application of Cur/MPEG-PCL micelles more efficiently inhibited the tumor cell-induced angiogenesis *in vivo* than that of free curcumin in alginate-encapsulated cancer cell assay. Besides, the cytotoxicity of curcumin on C-26 colon carcinoma cells *in vitro* was well maintained by MPEG-PCL micelle. Finally, the authors concluded that Cur/MPEG-PCL micelles represent an excellent intravenously injectable aqueous formulation of curcumin; which can inhibit the growth of colon carcinoma via the inhibition of angiogenesis and direct killing of cancer cells. Das *et al.* [136] encapsulated nutlin-3a and curcumin in PLGA nanoparticle (NPs) surface functionalized with folate for the enhancement of the therapeutic potential of nutlin-3a by modulating MDR (multi drug resistance). Curcumin has the potential to inhibit the expression of MRP-1 and LRP gene/protein in a concentration dependent manner in Y79 (human retinoblastoma cell line) cells. The authors reported that an increased therapeutic efficacy of targeted dual drug loaded NPs (Fol-Nut-Cur-NPs) over other formulations. Enhanced expression or down regulation of proapoptotic/antiapoptotic proteins, respectively and down-regulation of bcl2 and NFκB gene/protein by Fol-Nut-Cur-NPs fully confirm the above findings.

7.6. Dendrimers Nanodrugs

Dendrimers are branched polymeric nanoparticles with numerous arms extending from a center in a three dimensional fashion. They show a tendency towards toxicity and immunogenicity because of their positively charged surfaces. These types of nanoparticles are usually used for the delivery of 5-fluorouracil, indometacin and paclitaxel. Albumin nanoparticles loaded with paclitaxel have been used for the treatment of metastatic breast cancer [85]. Drugs can be loaded in different patterns within the core of dendrimer, either at dendrimer branches via network formation or through coupling of the drug on the dendrimer surface; due to amide and amine linkages [137]. Most often, biodegradable dendrimers are prepared by incorporating ester groups into the polymer backbone, which may be enzymatically cleaved or chemically hydrolyzed by esterases in physiological solutions [138-141]. Owing to their biodegradability and biocompatibility, polyester dendrimers have been and are being utilized for the delivery of anticancer drugs [139, 142, 143] and gene therapy [144-146] for treating different cancers.

During the last one decade polypropylenimine (PPI) dendrimers have been widely used for the effective delivery of drugs and nucleic acids. However, due to the serious cytotoxicity and low drug loading capacity of PPI dendrimers, their biomedical applications were limited. Recently, Wang and co-workers [147] carried out the acetylation of PPI dendrimers (ranging from 14.2% to 94.3%) which were then used to encapsulate drugs, including methotrexate sodium, sodium deoxycholate and doxorubicin. It was interesting to note that the acetylated PPI dendrimers with a degree of acetylation >80% showed a significantly decreased cytotoxicity (> 90% cell viability) on MCF-7 and A549 (adenocarcinomic human alveolar basal epithelial cells) cells. In addition, the drug loading capacity of acetylated PPI dendrimers was found to increase proportionally with the degree of acetylation on the dendrimer surface. Besides, 94.3% acetylated PPI dendrimers showed a pH-responsive release profile of anti-cancer drugs loaded within the nanoparticles. Moreover, significantly reduced cytotoxicities of methotrexate sodium and doxorubicin on MCF-7 and A549 cells were observed when they complexed with acetylated PPI dendrimers with high degrees of acetylation (>80%). These significantly reduced toxicities are obviously due to the sustained drug release from the dendrimers. Overall, the authors concluded that the cytotoxicity and anticancer drug loading capacity of cationic dendrimers can be fully optimized by surface acetylation and, therefore, acetylated PPI dendrimers are promising vehicles for anticancer drugs in clinical trials. Hu and coworkers [148] synthesized interior-functionalized fully acetylated dendrimers by the incorporation of functional groups into the interior pockets of fully acetylated dendrimers. COSY and 2D-NOESY studies indicated the encapsulation of guest molecules such as methotrexate within the interior pockets of dendrimers. The results of the study showed that the synthesized polymeric nanocarriers were therapeutically much more efficient than cationic dendrimers in terms of their much lower cytotoxicity on two cell lines and better performance than fully acetylated dendrimers in the sustained release of methotrexate. The findings provided a new strategy for the design of non-toxic dendrimers with high performance for the delivery of anticancer drugs to different tumor sites.

8. MECHANISM OF ACTION OF NANODRUGS

The basis for the development of nanodrugs rests on the fact that chemotherapeutic agents may be delivered to the cancerous cells exclusively without causing any disturbance to the normal cells. This allows for the little or no toxicities of the nanodrugs towards the normal cells. Besides, nanodrugs are able to circulate in blood for weeks in quest of tumors, without disturbing normal cells. Till now, the exact mechanism of action of nanodrugs is quite well understood. Scientists explain their targeting via active and passive transport processes. Blood vessels in tumor tissues have abnormalities like highly proliferating endothelial cells (endothelium) with aberrant underlying basement membrane, less pericytes and quite crooked blood vessels enhancing permeation and retention (EPR) and passive targeting by accumulating nanoparticles at higher concentration inside the tumor [149-153]. The permeability of blood vessels for nano drugs (10 to 100 nm) is increased by the abnormal secretion of vascular endothelium growth factors; bradykinin, nitric oxide, prostaglandins and matrix metalloproteinases [154-158]. In addition, cancerous cells are known to possess certain receptors that are not found on normal cells. As a result, nanoparticles adhered to antibodies get attracted towards these receptors which allows their selective entry into cancerous cells [159, 160]. Decreased lymphatic drainage does not allow these drugs to come out of cancerous cells and therefore, remain inside the cancerous cells for few days or even weeks i.e. an increase in therapeutic index [161, 162]. Cancer cells show increased cell surface expression of proteins (tumor specific overexpression of antigens) in comparison to normal cells in the case of active transport of the nanodrugs. Targeting of the drugs occurs by their physical attachment to the antigens (often receptors) at the surfaces of tumor cells and accumulation into tumor cells as the result of receptor mediated endocytosis. Due to the selective and specific nature of nanodrugs, they enter into the tumor cells and much less into healthy cell, which present only small amounts of receptor. After their entry into endosomes, nanodrugs would be trapped or degraded and thus worthless for treatment. Three possibilities account for continuing drug delivery into the cytoplasm: (i) nanodrugs are degraded in lysosomes releasing the degradation resistant active drug, usually hydrophobic that easily penetrates lysosomal membranes into the cytoplasm. (ii) Degradable drugs (like antisense oligonucleotides) prohibited to reach lysosomal maturation of endosomes are cleaved from the carrier platform by pH-sensitive spacer introduced during synthesis of the nanodrug and permeation of the hydrophobic drug through endosomal membranes into the cytoplasm. (iii) The nanodrug contains attached molecules, which actively destabilize the endosomal membranes allowing the release of the nanodrugs into the cytoplasm. Nanoconjugated drugs are delivered as inactive prodrugs. The prodrug can be cleaved either pH-dependently in the late endosome or after release in the cytoplasm by glutathione dependent cleavage of a disulphide spacer incorporated into the nanodrug between drug and platform during its chemical synthesis. Carrier platforms degrade during the course of time due to several factors like erosion of nanomaterials, pH changes, heat, light, diffusion and other cancer cell activities. Most often, nanoparticles are composed of biodegradable materials and are therefore, converted into small metabolites and finally egested out from tumor cells. After the drug is released from the drug carrier platform cells, the free drug works depending on its nature and the stage of cancer, for instance antisense oligonucleotides by targeted inhibition of mRNA directed protein synthesis.

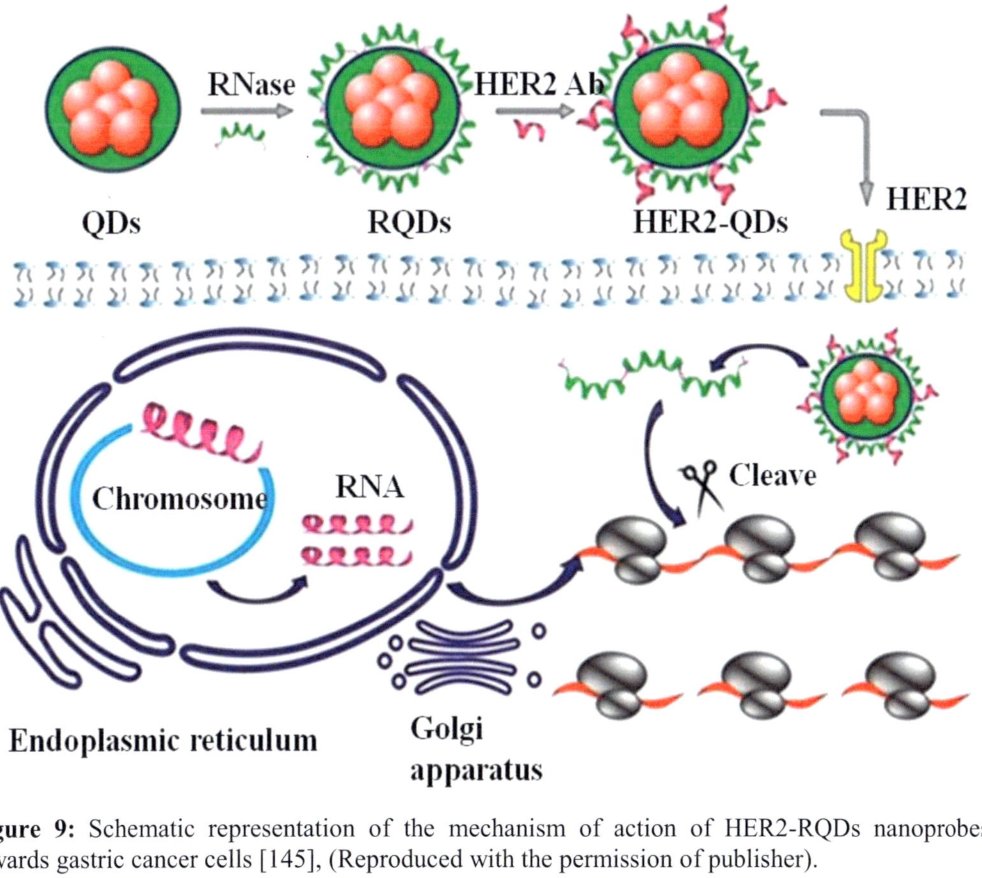

Figure 9: Schematic representation of the mechanism of action of HER2-RQDs nanoprobes towards gastric cancer cells [145], (Reproduced with the permission of publisher).

An interesting case is the treatment with a nanodrug that uses enzymatic RNA degradation. HER2 monoclonal antibody conjugated RNase A-associated CdTe quantum dot cluster (HER2-RQDs) nanoprobes ensure targeted imaging and therapy (so-called theranostic nanoparticles) of gastric cancer. Gastric cancer MGC803 cells are selectively killed by HER2-RQDs nanoprobes. RNase A has been used for the treatment of several diseases, and is known to play essential roles in host survival [163-165]. Herein, RNase A assisted the synthesis of the QDs, and is integrated into the RQDs. Partial RNase A peptides are located outside the RQDs and conjugate with HER2 monoclonal antibody, when the nanoprobes targeted the gastric cancer cells. Nanoprobes enter into the cytoplasm of tumor cells by endocytosis effects. Inside the cells, RNase A is released from the nanoprobes at low pH. The released RNase A then degrades cellular RNA, which results into the inhibition of the mRNA translation. This leads to the inhibition of the growth of tumor cells, inducing cell apoptosis (Fig. (**9**)) [166]. It is quite important to mention that nanodrugs act at supramolecular level and thus, as a result their normal properties and the mechanisms may vary for different drug molecules and various types of nano particle carriers.

9. NANODRUGS VERSUS CONVENTIONAL ANTICANCER DRUGS

The main ambitions of nanotechnology for anticancer drug development were; increasing bioavailability of drugs, ability to remain in blood circulation for longer time, releasing the incorporated drug in a controlled fashion and minimizing side-effects. Obviously, nanodrugs are able to penetrate easily into the tissues where they are taken up by cells, allowing efficient delivery of drugs to their target sites of action. The uptake of the delivered nanodrugs is known to be 15-250 times greater than that of microparticles in the 1-10 μm range [167]. Overall, nanotechnology improves the performance and acceptability of anticancer drugs by increasing their effectiveness, safety, patient adherence (degree to which a patient correctly follows medical advice) as well as ultimately reducing health care costs. Chemotherapeutics which are unable to pass clinical trial are expected to get benefited by nanotechnology [90].

Nanoanticancer drugs are superior to conventional anticancer drugs in terms of reduced treatment concentrations, low side effects, increased stability and efficient delivery to target sites. The therapeutic properties of conventional anticancer drugs are surprisingly altered when they are encapsulated into nanoidentities. For example, Verma and Sachin [168] developed drug polymer self folding nano-conjugates of pectin-cisplatin for enhancing the blood circulating levels of cisplatin. Bio-distribution and pharmacokinetic studies of the developed nanodrug formulation were carried out at various time points in normal, Balb-c mice. Pectin-cisplatin conjugate was found to be a stable, slow and sustained system with no burst effect. The immuno-fluorescence analysis of J-774 (a mouse macrophage cell line) was evaluated after the incubation of the cells with pectin chains tagged with FITC (fluorescein isothiocyanate) and pectin-cisplatin-FITC conjugates. It was observed that 40% of the cells showed uptake post 30 min of incubation. Besides, plasma proteins assist the release of cisplatin. 85-89% of the drug was released within 17 days, and only 57% of the drug was released in almost 30 days without plasma. In addition, cell uptake studies on J-774 cell line were indicative of the fact that the reduced negative charge on the conjugate helped in adhesion to the surface of cells and subsequent uptake by cells. Overall, long blood retention of nano-cisplatin was observed in mice and the drug was found in circulation even after 24 hrs. Pharmacokinetic study revealed that it could form a novel anticancer drug with good efficacy and safer profile than cisplatin. Ranjan *et al.* [169] recently, reported that curcumin loaded poly(lactic acid-co-glycolic acid) nanoparticles (PLGA-CURC) considerably improved the bioavailability of curcumin and therefore, making it suitable for cancer therapy. *In vitro* release study indicated a slow sustained release corresponding to 75% drug over a period of 10 days. Moreover, long term physiochemical stability of the PLGA-CURC formulation was observed. Lu *et al.* [170] reported significantly superior antimetastatic effect of pemetrexed-loaded gelatinase-responsive nanoparticles in a mouse metastasis model. The authors used a targeted delivery system to determine the potential of novel pemetrexed-loaded gelatinase-responsive nanoparticles for clinical therapy of malignant melanoma. Quite interesting antimetastatic effect in experimental lung metastasis models was reported by the application of pemetrexed-loaded PEG-peptide-PCL nanoparticles. The authors concluded that pemetrexed-loaded gelatinase-responsive nanoparticles may represent a potent drug delivery system for inhibiting pulmonary metastasis. Lopez-Gasco and co-workers [171] encapsulated paclitaxel in poly(DL-lactide-co-glycolide) and poly(ε-caprolactone) nano polymers by using double emulsion-solvent evaporation technique. The authors observed that poly(lactide-co-glycolide) nanoparticles showed more effective cellular uptake in comparison to those of poly(ε-caprolactone). Paclitaxel nano-formulations showed significantly higher efficacy in killing MCF-7 cells and induced the release of the drug-blocking cells in the G2/M Phase. Paclitaxel-loaded nanoparticles may therefore, be considered as a promising drug delivery system in the evaluation of an *in vivo* model. Kim *et al.* [172] in 2008 reported the synthesis of nano sized hydrophobically modified glycol chitosans (HGCs) encapsulating cisplatin. The nano formulation had 80% drug loading capacity with release of the drug in a sustained manner for a week. It was further reported that the nano encapsulated drug had less toxic side effects than pure cisplatin.

Of course, nanodrugs are improved modalities in terms of bioavailability, controlled release, rapidity, stability, prolonged action and side effects as compared to their conventional drug counterparts. Nano analogues of the well known anticancer drugs can simply reduce their side effects; improve stability and bioavailability with significantly enhanced bioactivity.

10. RECENT DEVELOPMENTS IN NANODRUG FORMULATIONS

Applications of nanotechnology have initiated the onset of quite significant advances in almost every field of science and technology, including newer drug delivery techniques. As a result, much attention has been paid by researchers all over the world for the development of nanodrugs, and their biocompatible, biodegradable submicron devices as drug delivery systems. Most preferably, drug delivery systems are prepared using natural polymers, because of their good availability, biocompatibility, biodegradability and are, generally, safe and non-immunogenic. Earlier research in this field indicates that these polymers are being made into colloidal particles that act as carriers for both large and small drugs and enhancing their delivery actively or passively [173].

In the present scenario, nanodrug delivery systems are being designed and developed to selectively target cancer cells. However, there are only few papers those report the targeting of the cancer cells nuclei by nanodrugs. Nuclear-targeted drug deliveries seem to kill cancer cells more efficiently. Pan *et al.* [174] used TAT peptide (TAT is a cell membrane penetrating peptide) conjugated onto mesoporous silica nanoparticles (MSNs-TAT) with high payload for nuclear-targeted drug delivery for the first time. Monodispersed MSNs-TAT of varied particle sizes were synthesized to investigate the effects of particle size and TAT conjugation on the nuclear membrane penetrability of MSNs. MSNs-TAT had a diameter of 50nm or smaller. (MSNs-TAT) was observed to assist nuclear internalization and, therefore, efficiently delivered the active anticancer drug doxorubicin (DOX) into the targeted nucleus, killing these cancer cells with much enhanced efficiencies. This study might provide the necessary stimuli for the design and development of cell-nuclear-targeted drug delivery. Recently, Ditto *et al.* [175] reported the conjugation of folic acid to functionalized poly(ethylene glycol) and decorated the surface of L-tyrosine polyphosphate (LTP) nanoparticles. These nanoparticles were found to posses the appropriate size (100-500 nm) for internalization. LTP nanoparticles decorated with folic acid (targeted nanoparticles) showed a 10-fold greater attachment to HeLa (cervical cancer) cell line in comparison to control nanoparticles and human dermal fibroblasts. The interactions of the targeted nanoparticles to HeLa cells are likely a result of receptor-ligand binding. Finally, the targeted nanoparticles encapsulated with a silver based drug show increased efficacy in comparison to non-decorated (plain) nanoparticles and drug alone against HeLa cells. Thus, the authors concluded that the targeted nanoparticles are a promising delivery platform for developing anticancer therapies that over-express the folate receptors (FRs). Tang *et al.* [176] reported the enhanced drug delivery and anticancer efficacy of an amphiphilic diblock copolymer consisting of a hydrophilic poly(ethylene glycol) (PEG) block and a hydrophobic polymethacrylate block (PEYM) bearing acid-labile ortho ester side-chains. A stable core shell structure was assumed by the PEG-b-PEYM micelles in aqueous buffer at physiological pH with a low critical micelle concentration. The hydrolysis of the ortho ester side-chain was minimum at physiological pH but more at mildly acidic pH. At pH 7.4, doxorubicin (Dox) was successfully loaded into the micelles and released at a higher rate in response to slight acidification to pH 5. The release of Dox at pH 5 consisted of an initial fast release of several hours followed by a sustained release for days. A rapid uptake of the Dox loaded into the micelles by human glioma (T98G) cells *in vitro* resulting into its accumulation in the endolysosome and subsequently into the nucleus within a few hours, in comparison to the very low uptake of free drug at the same dose. MTT assays indicated that the IC_{50} values of the Dox-loaded micelles were approximately ten-times (by 24h) and three-times (by 48 h) lower than the free drug. The much enhanced cell killing potency of Dox loaded in the micelles towards multi-drug-resistant human glioma cells was attributed to the high intracellular drug concentration and the subsequent pH-triggered drug release. Polymeric and other nanoplatforms as well as nanoparticles overcome drug resistance to DOX [177]. Taheri *et al.* [178] reported the decoration of methotrexate-human serum albumin conjugated nanoparticles with trastuzumab molecules for the targeted delivery to HER2 positive tumor cells. It was observed that the cytotoxicity of TMAB-MTX-HAS nanoparticles on HER2 positive cells was significantly higher than that for non-targeted MTX-HSA nanoparticles and also the free MTX after 24hr. However, it was further observed that when the number of attached TMAB molecules was very high, the cytotoxicity of TMAB-MTX-HSA nanoparticles was almost similar to that of the non-targeted MTX-HSA nanoparticles. In addition, TMAB-MTX-HSA nanoparticles showed significantly higher uptake to HER2 positive cells compared to non-targeted MTX-HSA nanoparticles when the optimized amount of TMAB was conjugated onto the surface of nanoparticles. Finally, the authors concluded that the conjugation of TMAB molecules onto the MTX conjugated HSA nanoparticles is an appropriate method for active tumor targeting of MTX. Kilic *et al.* [179] recently reported an apoferritin-doxorubicin complex which they prepared by opening and closing of the apoferritin sphere in the presence of doxorubicin. Encapsulation of doxorubicin was ensured by the direct and step-wise change of pH of the solution from 2.5 to 7.4. The authors reported that almost 28 doxorubicin molecules can be capsulated per apoferritin protein with no significant drug leakage during the first two days. Shin and coworkers [180] reported a novel pH-responsive HDL-like nanoparticle that selectively releases paclitaxel at acidic pH. The paclitaxel nanoparticle showed good stability over physiological and basic pH values, and a wide range of temperatures; an essential feature for efficient cancer chemotherapy. The homogeneous assembly had high paclitaxel loading capacity per nanoparticle (62.2% w/w). A molar ratio of 1:55 for the apolipoprotein A-I and paclitaxel suggested that a single nanoparticle contained approximately 110 paclitaxel molecules in a spherical structure with 9.2 nm diameter. The anticancer activity of both paclitaxel nanoparticles and PTX-PL-NP depended on the expression of scavenger receptor class B type I whereas the apoptotic efficacy of free paclitaxel does not depend on this receptor. Therfore, it might be speculated that the pH responsiveness of paclitaxel nanoparticles enabled efficient endosomal escape of paclitaxel before lysosomal break down. Lv *et al.* [181] reported the targeted delivery of insoluble cargo (paclitaxel) by PEGylated chitosan nanoparticles grafted with Arg-Gly-Asp (RGD) for better tumor growth inhibition and much lower side effects. The loading efficiency (LE) was improved by combining O/W/O (oil/water/oil) double emulsion method with temperature-programmed solidification technique and PTX was controlled within the matrix network as *in situ* nanocrystallite form. These CMC nanoparticles were further PEGylated for reducing their recognition by the reticuloendothelial system (RES) as a result of which their circulation time in blood could be prolonged. Furthermore, a graft of cyclic RGD peptide at the terminal of PEG chain enhanced the affinity of these nanoparticles towards *in vitro* Lewis lung carcinoma (LLC) cells and *in vivo* tumor tissue. These outstanding pharmacological properties enabled the designed nanodevice to exhibit a greater tumor growth inhibition effect and much lower side effects over the commercial formulation Taxol. Kwon [182] reported the encapsulation of paclitaxel, rapamycin (Fig. (**10**)) and 17-AAG (17-N-Allylamino-17-demethoxygeldanamycin) (Fig. (**11**)) encapsulated by poly(ethylene glycol)-block-poly(lactic acid) (PEG-b-PLA) micelles. The nanodrug delivery system provided effective solubilization of drug combinations. Overall, the reported nanodrug formulation was stable, biocompatible, and with good bioavailability. Furthermore, larger doses of individual drugs could be administered in micelle formulations as compared to non-micelle formulations. Yourong *et al.* [183] reported a nano drug delivery system of monomethoxypoly(ethylene glycol)-poly(lactic-co-glycolic acid)-poly-l-lysine (mPEG-PLGA-PLL) cationic polymer. The basic polymer skeleton of the delivery system was modified through the incorporation of side chains and targeting groups. This modification was found to improve the carrier performance. The reported drug delivery system was quite useful for tumor diagnosis and treatment, ultrasonic contrast and reversing or reducing drug resistance. Xiaohai and coworkers [184] reported a pectin-doxorubicin passive solid tumor-targeted anticancer prodrug with particle size of 100-200 nm. The cells inhibition ability of the pectin-doxorubicin conjugate was found equivalent to doxorubicin hydrochloride for humanized lung cancer cells NCI-H446 and A549.

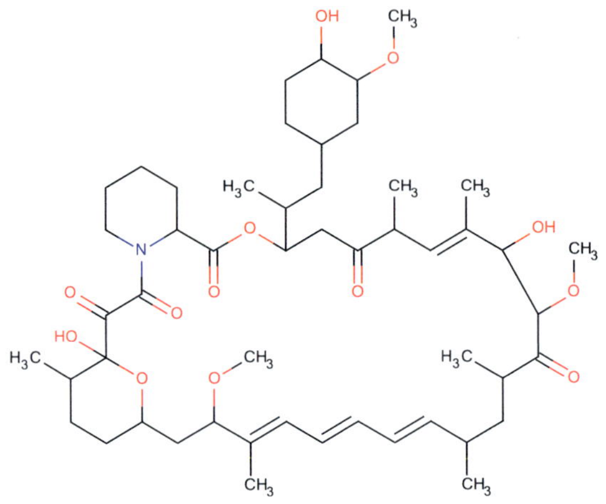

Figure 10: Chemical structure of Rapamycin.

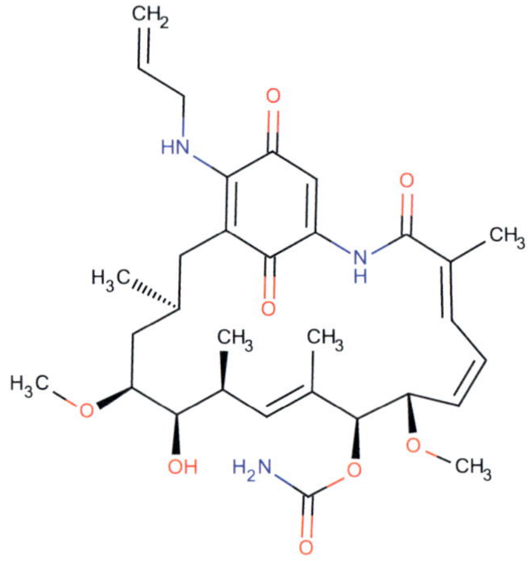

Figure 11: Chemical structure of 17-AAG (17-N-Allylamino-17-demethoxygeldanamycin).

11. CURRENT & FUTURE DEVELOPMENTS

Despite the progress made during past few years, there are many issues related to the safety profiles of nano anticancer drugs, those need to be addressed. In the present scenario, we do not have completely safe and non-toxic nanoparticles. The size, surface charge, intra-cellular degradation, cancer stage, cancerous cell size, etc. considerably affect the mechanism of action of nano anticancer drugs. Human friendly procedures including optimizing formulation steps, sterilization and storage, may be employed to prepare these drugs. In addition, nanoparticle formulations in hybrid based systems may be used to derive a synergistic efficacy as the pharmacokinetics of different loaded drugs are unified by simultaneous delivery to the target site leading to minimization of their limitations. Dendrimers with metallic cores may be used as contrast imaging agents and drug delivery systems simultaneously. Tuning the size and shape of nanoparticles can bring about great improvements in nanomedicine. Blood circulation time, controlled release, tumor cell specificity, stability etc. can be modulated by optimizing their size and shape. Nanoparticles larger than ~10nm, generally, avoid single pass renal clearance. In order to minimize non-specific interactions of the nanoparticles with proteins and cells, these should not be positively charged. Nanoparticles usually carry a large payload [185,186] and multivalent bindings to cell surface receptors [187], enabling them to carry multiple drug molecules with potential of bypassing multidrug resistance mechanisms. Bio-computational methods might be highly useful in investigating the fundamental physical principles affecting the delivery and degradation of nanoparticles in the treatment of cancer. A good insight into the *in vivo* drug delivery along with simulation of therapeutic effects of the delivery device can be had by means of the bio computation of targeted and controlled drug delivery system. This may lead to optimize and improve existing products and design and develop new products for better cancer chemotherapy. Presently, main focuss is being paid to the design and development of nanodrug delivery systems selectively targeting cancer cells and there are very few reports on drug delivery systems targeting nuclei and other cellular compartments of cancer cells. It seems that nuclear-targeted drug delivery systems might be killing cancer cells more efficiently. Therefore, research leading to the development of nuclear-targetted drug delivery should be encouraged for ensuring more effective cancer treatment. Moreover, drug delivery systems capable to sense different ionic strengths, pH values, temperatures, oxidative stresses etc. should be designed to selectively target cancer cells without causing any disturbance to the normal cells. Polymeric nanoparticles responsive to internal or external stimuli are of considerable interest because of their more efficient delivery of therapeutics to pathological regions. Stimulus-sensitive polymeric nanoparticles have been fabricated in the form of diverse nanostructures viz, vesicles, crosslinked nanoparticles, micelles and hybrid nanoparticles. In response to single, dual, or multiple stimuli, several changes are brought in the chemical and physical properties of polymeric nanoparticles. As a result, these nanoparticles retain the loaded drug molecules during circulation. These specifically target the pathological region, and release the loaded therapeutics after cell internalization. Therefore, it is the need of this era to develop stimuli-responsive nanoparticles for ensuring safe cancer chemotherapy.

The biological identities at nano scale are still not known exactly. Due to these hurdles it is not possible to determine exactly the target of nanodrugs and their associated toxicities [188]. Electron microscopy (SEM and TEM) and atomic force microscopy (AFM) techniques are good tools to assess the surface chemistry and approximate the applications of nanodrugs; even then nanotechnology for drug design and development requires extremely precise determination of biological systems at supra-molecular level. Nanodrugs are fantastic and promising, which need more focuss of scientists towards exploring their exact mechanism of action. Therefore, efforts should be made by oncologists all over the world for the development of safe, with no or least side effects, biodegradable, biocompatible, pH responsive, targetted action nanodrugs to ensure safer and cost effective treatment of cancer. No doubt, nano anticancer drugs are the bullet medications for the safe and cost effective cancer chemotherapy. These have a bright and promising future in cancer chemotherapy.

CONCLUSION

By keeping the above discussion into consideration, we are in the middle age of nanodrugs design and development. Interesting work has been carried out in this direction and, therefore, as a result some nanodrugs are available into the market. But, still they could not completely replace the conventional drugs. Of course, scientists have developed the mechanism of action of nanodrugs but could not fully design the exact size of nanodrugs for specific cancer cells. The targeted action of nanodrugs depends directly on the size of nanodrugs and the size and physiology of cancer cells. Therefore, more work is needed to develop a rationale between the size and shape of nanodrugs and the type of cancer cell. Besides, the various toxicities associated with the use of nanodrugs need to be eliminated to obtain safe nanodrugs (magic bullets) in near future. The future of nanodrugs is quite bright and, hopefully, these will replace the conventional drugs within coming decades.

ACKNOWLEDGEMENTS

The authors are thankful to UGC and CSIR for providing BSR Meritorious Fellowship to Waseem A. Wani and Senior Research Fellowship to Ashanul Haque.

CONFLICT OF INTEREST

There are no conflict of interest to declare.

ABBREVIATIONS

HPMA	=	*N*-(2-Hydroxypropyl) methacrylamide
RES	=	Reticuloendothelial system
GPs	=	Gelatin nanoparticles (GPs)
CDDP	=	cis-Diamminedichloroplatinum (II)
GPs (GP-Pt)	=	Gelatin nanoparticles (GPs) as carriers for cisplatin (CDDP)
bEGF	=	Biotinylated-endothelial growth factor
CDDP-GEL-PAA	=	(CDDP)-loaded gelatin-poly(acrylic acid)
LoVo	=	Human colorectal cancer cell line
PMLA	=	[Poly(β-L-malic acid)]

HER2/neu	=	Human Epidermal Growth Factor Receptor 2
Akt	=	Also known as Protein Kinase B (PKB), is a serine/threonine- specific protein kinase which plays an important role in metabolic processes like apoptosis, cell proliferation etc.
PEG-PLGA	=	Poly (ethylene glycol)-poly (lactic-co-glycolic acid)
mPEG-PLGA	=	Methoxy polyethylene glycol (mPEG), polylactic-co-glycolic acid
DOX	=	Doxorubicin
TAX	=	Hydrophobic paclitaxel.
QC	=	Quercetin
mPEG-Chol	=	Methoxy poly(ethylene glycol)-cholesterol conjugate
(f-CNH_3)	=	A carbon nanohorn derivative
siRNA	=	Small interfering RNA
G4-PAMAM	=	Fourth-generation polyamidoamine dendrimer
PCa	=	Human prostate cancer cell line
SERS	=	Surface Enhanced Raman Spectroscopy
cBSA-147	=	Cationic chemically modified plasma protein bovine serum albumin
PTX	=	Paclitaxel
DOX	=	Doxorubicin

αvβ3 integrin	=	A transmembrane receptors that mediate the attachment between a cell and the tissues that surround it. Integrin αvβ3 is an adhesion receptor expressed on angiogenic endothelial cells and highly aggressive tumors.
PLGA-PEG	=	Poly(D, L-lactic-co-glycolic acid)-block-polyethylene glycol
c(RGDfK)	=	A cyclic pentapeptide of arginine, glycine, aspartate.
Pt-PLGA-b-PEG-Apt-NP	=	Poly(D,L-lactic-co-glycolic acid)-b-poly (ethylene glycol) (PLGA-b-PEG) nanoparticles (NPs) encapsulating a Pt(IV) prodrug.
Pt-PLGA-b-PEG-NP	=	Poly(D, L-lactic-co-glycolic acid)-b-poly (ethylene glycol) (PLGA-b-PEG) nanoparticles (NPs)
LNCaP	=	Androgen-sensitive human prostate adenocarcinoma cells
TEM	=	Transition electron microscopy
Tetrac	=	Tetraiodothyroacetic acid
A375	=	Human melanoma cells
TPL	=	Tetrac-tagged pegylated liposomes.
ToThyRu, HoThyRu and DoHuRu	=	An amphiphilic nucleoside-based ruthenium complexes where:
ToThy	=	3-(4-Pyridylmethyl)-3-O-oleyl-50-O-monomethoxy)triethylene glycol-acetyl-Thymidine.

HoThy	=	(3-(4-pyridylmethyl)-30-O-oleyl-50-O-(benzyloxy)-hexaethylene glycol-acetyl-thymidine
DoHu	=	3-(4-pyridylmethyl)-20,30-di-O-oleyl-50-O-benzyloxy)hexaethylene glycol-acetyl-uridine.
POPC	=	1-Palmitoyl-2-oleoyl-sn-glycero-3-phosphocholine
HM	=	Hydrotropic micelle
SPIONs	=	Superparamagnetic iron oxide nanoparticles
MRI	=	Magnetic Resonance Imaging
MNPs	=	Magnetic nanoparticles
AMF	=	Alternating magnetic field
KF	=	Kahalalide F
AuNPs	=	Gold nanoparticles
nHCPT	=	Micronized 10-hydroxycamptothecin
HSA	=	Human serum albumin
QU	=	Quercetin
MCL-1	=	Myeloid cell leukemia sequence 1 (Mcl-1) is an antiapoptotic protein of the Bcl-2 family
Bcl-2	=	Bcl-2 (B-cell lymphoma 2) is the founding member of the Bcl-2 family of apoptosis regulator proteins encoded by the BCL2 gene
Bax	=	Bcl-2–associated X protein

Cur/MPEG-PCL	=	Curcumin-loaded methoxy polyethylene glycol and poly(ε-caprolactone) diblock copolymers
HER2-RQDs	=	HER2 monoclonal antibody conjugated RNase A-associated CdTe quantum dot cluster
QDs	=	Quantum dots
RNA	=	Ribonucleic acid
PLGA-CURC	=	Curcumin loaded poly (lactic acid-co-glycolic acid) nanoparticles
HGCs	=	Hydrophobically modified glycol chitosans
TAT peptide	=	Trans-activating transcriptional activator
MSNs-TAT	=	Mesoporous silica nanoparticles-TAT
PEYM	=	Hydrophilic poly(ethylene glycol) (PEG) block and a hydrophobic polymethacrylate block
T98G	=	Human glioma cells
TMAB	=	Trastuzumab molecules
MTX	=	Methotrexate
HDL-like nanoparticle	=	High density lipoprotein like nanoparticles
RGD	=	One letter abbreviations for the amino acids: arginine (R), glycine (G) and aspartate (D).
CMC nanoparticles	=	Carboxymethylated chitosan copolymer nanoparticles

LLC = Lewis lung carcinoma

NSCLC = Non-small-cell lung cancer

REFERENCES

[1] Cancer control: Knowledge into action. WHO Guide for effective programmes, www.who.int/cancer 2006.
[2] Siegel R, Naishadham D, Jemal A. CA Cancer J Clin 2013; 63: 11–30
[3] Mokarian F, Ramezani MA, Heydari K, Tabatabaeian M, Tavazohi H. Epidemiology and trend of cancer in Isfahan 2005-2010. J Res Med Sci 2011; 16(9): 1228-33.
[4] Ali I, Wani WA, Saleem K, Haque A. Platinum compounds: A hope for future cancer chemotherapy. Anti-Cancer Agents Med Chem 2012; 13(2): 296-306.
[5] Sikora K, Advani S, Koroltchouk V, Magrath I, Levy L, Pinedo H, *et al.* Essential drugs for cancer therapy: A World Health Organization consultation. Ann Oncol 1999; 10(4): 385-90.
[6] Ali I, Rahis-Uddin, Salim K, Rather MA, Wani WA, Haque A. Advances in nano drugs for cancer chemotherapy. Curr Cancer Drug Targets 2011; 11(2): 135-46.
[7] Leroux JC, Deolker E, Gurmy R, Nenita S. Micro encapsulations, methods and industrial application. New York, Dekker; 1996, 537-74.
[8] Kawasaki ES, Player A. Nanotechnology, nanomedicine, and the development of new, effective therapies for cancer. Nanomed 2005; 1(2): 101-9.
[9] Huang ZW, Laurent V, Chetouani G, Ljubimova JY, Holler E, Benvegnu T, Loyer P, Mariona SC. New functional degradable and bio-compatible nanoparticles based on poly(malic acid) derivatives for site-specific anti-cancer drug delivery. Int J Pharm 2012; 423(1): 84-92.
[10] Etrych T, Sírová M, Starovoytova L, Ríhová B, Ulbrich K. HPMA copolymer conjugates of paclitaxel and docetaxel with pH-controlled drug release. Mol Pharmaceutics 2010; 7(4): 1015-26.
[11] Wang F, Bronich TK, Kabanov AV, Rauh RD, Roovers J. Synthesis and evaluation of a star amphiphilic block copolymer from poly (epsilon-caprolactone) and poly (ethylene glycol) as a potential drug delivery carrier. Bioconjug Chem 2005; 16(2): 397-405.
[12] Mammen M, Choi SK, Whitesides GM. Polyvalent interactions in biological systems: Implications for design and use of multivalent ligands and inhibitors. Angew Chem Ed Eng 1998; 37: 2754-94.
[13] Allen TM, Cheng WW, Hare JI, Laginha KM. Pharmacokinetics and pharmacodynamics of lipidic nano-particles in cancer. Anticancer Agents Med Chem 2006; 6(6): 513-23.
[14] Simon M, Wittmar M, Bakowsky U, Kissel T. Self-assembling nano complexes from insulin and water-soluble branched polyesters, poly[(vinyl-3-(diethylamino)-propylcarbamate -co-(vinyl acetate)-co-(vinyl alcohol)]-graft-Poly(L-lactic acid): A novel carrier for trans mucosal delivery of peptides. Bioconjug Chem 2004; 15(4): 841-9.
[15] Goss I, Shu L, Schlute AD, Rabe JP. Molecular structure of single DNA complexes with positively charged dendronized polymers. J Am Chem Soc 2002; 124(24): 6860-5.
[16] Zeng F, Lee H, Allen C. Epidermal growth factor-conjugated poly (ethylene glycol)-block-poly (ä-valerolactone) copolymer micelles for targeted delivery of chemotherapeutics. Bioconjug Chem 2006; 17(2): 399-409.

[17] Esfand R, Tomalia DA. Poly (amidoamine) (PAMAM) dendrimers: From biomimicry to drug delivery and biomedical applications. Drug Disco Today 2001; 6(8): 427-36.
[18] Chamundeeswari M, Sastry TP, Lakhsmi BS, Senthil V, Agostinelli E. Iron nano particles from animal blood for cellular imaging and targeted delivery for cancer treatment. Biochim Biophys Acta 2013; 1830(4): 3005-10.
[19] Moshfeghi AA, Peyman GA. Micro- and nanoparticulates. Adv Drug Deliv Rev 2005; 57(14): 2047-52.
[20] Ali I, Wani WA, Saleem K. Cancer scenario in India with future perspectives. Cancer Ther 2011; 8(8): 56-70.
[21] Ali I, Rahis-ud-din, Saleem K, Aboul-Enein HY, Rather MA. Social aspects of cancer genesis. Cancer Ther 2011; 8(A): 6-14.
[22] Farin K, Graca MD, William FA. Patterns of cancer incidence, mortality and prevalence across five continents: Defining priorities to reduce cancer disparities in different geographical regions of the world. J Clin Oncol 2006; 24(14): 2137-50.
[23] WHO, 2006. Cancer. World Health Organisation. A Report. http://en.wikipedia.org/wiki/lungcancer (Accessed on: March 8, 2013).
[24] Pisani P, Parkin DM, Bray F, Ferlay J. Estimates of the worldwide mortality from 25 cancers in 1990. Int J Cancer 1999; 83(6): 870-3.
[25] Fox BD, Cheung VJ, Patel AJ, Suki D, Rao G. Epidemiology of metastatic brain tumors. Neurosurg Clin N Am 2011; 22: 1-6.
[26] D'Addario G, Fruh M, Reck M, Baumann P, Klepetko W, Felip E. Metastatic non-small-cell lung cancer: ESMO Clinical Practice Guidelines for diagnosis, treatment and follow-up. Annals Oncol 2010; 21(Supp 5): v116-v9.
[27] Ferlay J, Bray F, Pisani P. GLOBOCAN 2002, Cancer incidence, mortality and prevalence worldwide, IARC Cancer Base No. 5, version 2.0, IARC Press. Lyon, France. http://www.dep.iarc.fr/globocan/database.htm (Accessed on: August 10, 2012).
[28] Gilman A. The initial clinical trial of nitrogen mustard. Am J Surg 1963; 105(5): 574-8.
[29] Goodman LS, Wintrobe MM, Dameshek W, Goodman MJ, Gilman A, McLennan MT. Nitrogen mustard therapy. JAMA 1946; 132(3): 126-32.
[30] Ali I, Saleem K, Rahis-ud-din, Haque A, El-Azzouny A. Natural products: Human friendly anti-cancer medications. Egypt Pharm J (NRC) 2010; 9(2): 133-79.
[31] Cragg GM, Newman DJ. Plants as source of anticancer agents. J Ethnopharmacol 2005; 100(1-2): 72-9.
[32] Boisseau P, Bertrand Loubaton. Nanomedicine, nanotechnology in medicine. CR Physique 2011; 12: 620-36.
[33] Commission of the European Communities Communication, Towards a European Strategy for Nanotechnology, EU, DG Research, Brussels, 2004. www.cordis.lu /nanotechnology (Accessed on: August 10, 2012).
[34] ETP Nanomedicine: Nanomedicine, Nanotechnology for Health, Strategic Research Agenda, 2006.
[35] Patil R, Arias JP, Ding H, Konda B, Rekechenetskiy A, Inoue S, Black KL, Holler E, Ljubimova JY. Cellular delivery of doxorubicin via pH-controlled hydrazone linkage using multifunctional nano vehicle based on poly(β-L-Malic Acid). Int J Mol Sci 2012; 13(9): 11681-93.
[36] Kaminskas LM, Boyd BJ. Nanosized Drug Delivery Vectors and the Reticuloendo thelial System. Ed. Ferrari, Mauro. Fundamental Biomedical Technologies 5, 2011; 155-78.

[37] Chorny M, Hood E, Levy RJ, Muzykantov VR. Endothelial delivery of antioxidant enzymes loaded into non-polymeric magnetic nanoparticles. J Control Release 2010; 146(1): 144-51.

[38] Chekman IS. Pharmacological and pharmaceutical foundation of nanodrugs. Lik Sprava 2010; (1-2): 3-10.

[39] Anajwala CC, Jani GK, Swamy SMV. Current trends of nanotechnology for cancer therapy. Int J Pharm Sci Nanotech 2010; 3(3): 1043-56.

[40] Tseng CL, Su WY, Yen KC, Yang KC, Lin FH. The use of biotinylated-EGF-modified gelatin nanoparticle carrier to enhance cisplatin accumulation in cancerous lungs via inhalation. Biomaterials 2009; 30(20): 3476-85.

[41] Ding D, Zhu Z, Liu Q, Wang J, Hu Y, Jiang X, *et al.* Cisplatin-loaded gelatin-poly (acrylic acid) nanoparticles: Synthesis, antitumor efficiency *in vivo* and penetration in tumors. Eur J Pharm Biopharm 2011; 79(1): 142-9.

[42] Inoue S, Ding H, Portilla-Arias J, Hu J, Konda B, Fujita M, *et al.* Polymalic acid-based nanobiopolymer provides efficient systemic breast cancer treatment by inhibiting both HER2/neu receptor synthesis and activity. Cancer Res 2011; 71(4): 1454-64.

[43] Wang H, Zhao Y, Wu Y, Hu YL, Nan K, Nie G, *et al.* Chen H. Enhanced anti-tumor efficacy by co-delivery of doxorubicin and paclitaxel with amphiphilic methoxy PEG-PLGA copolymer nanoparticles. Biomaterials 2011; 32(32): 8281-90.

[44] Tamarkin, L., Paciotti, G.F., Huhta, M. Nanotherapeutic colloidal metal compositions and methods. US20090104114 (**2009**).

[45] Sapra P, Tyagi P, Allen TM. Ligand-targeted liposomes for cancer treatment. Curr Drug Deliv 2005; 2(4): 369-81.

[46] Charrois GJ, Allen TM. Drug release rate influences the pharmacokinetics, biodistribution, therapeutic activity, and toxicity of pegylated liposomal doxorubicin formulations in murine breast cancer. Biochim Biophys Acta 2004; 1663(1-2): 167-77.

[47] Allen TM, Cullis PR. Drug delivery systems: Entering the mainstream. Science 2004; 303: 1818-22.

[48] Fassas A, Anagnostopoulos A. The use of liposomal daunorubicin (DaunoXome) in acute myeloid leukemia. Leuk Lymphoma 2005; 46(6): 795-802.

[49] White SC, Lorigan P, Margison GP. Phase II study of SPI-77 (sterically stabilised liposomal cisplatin) in advanced non-small cell lung cancer. Br J Cancer 2006; 95: 822-8.

[50] Rosenthal DI, Yom SS, Liu L. A Phase I study of SPI-077 (Stealth liposomal cisplatin) concurrent with radiation therapy for locally advanced head and neck cancer. Invest. New Drugs 2002; 20(3): 343-9.

[51] Harrington KJ, Lewanski CR, Northcote AD. Phase I-II study of pegylated liposomal cisplatin (SPI-077) in patients with inoperable head and neck cancer. Ann Oncol 2001; 12(4): 493-6.

[52] Guo W, Johnson JL, Khan S. Paclitaxel quantification in mouse plasma and tissues containing liposome-entrapped paclitaxel by liquid chromatography-tandem mass spectrometry: Application to a pharmacokinetics study. Anal Biochem 2005; 336(2): 213-20.

[53] Dragovich T, Mendelson D, Kurtin SA. Phase 2 trial of the liposomal DACH platinum LNDDP in patients with therapy refractory advanced colorectal cancer. Cancer Chemother Pharmacol 2006; 58: 759-64.

[54] Seiden MV, Muggia F, Astrow A. A Phase II study of liposomal lurtotecan (OSI-211) in patients with topotecan resistant ovarian cancer. Gynecol Oncol 2004; 93(1): 229-32.
[55] Danhauser-Riedl S, Hausmann E, Schick HD. Phase I clinical and pharmacokinetic trial of dextran conjugated doxorubicin (AD-70, DOXOXD). Invest New Drugs 1993; 11(2-3): 187-95.
[56] Matsumura Y. Micelle carrier system in clinical trial. Nippon Rinsho 2006; 64(2): 316-21.
[57] Matsumura Y, Hamaguchi T, Ura T. Phase I clinical trial and pharmacokinetic evaluation of NK911, a micelle-encapsulated doxorubicin. Br J Cancer 2004; 91(10): 1775-81.
[58] Gradishar WJ. Albumin-bound nanoparticle paclitaxel. Clin Adv Hematol Oncol 2005; 3: 348-9.
[59] Ferrari M. Experimental therapies: Vectoring siRNA therapeutics into the clinic. Nat Rev Clin Oncol 2010; 7: 485-6.
[60] Gradishar WJ, Tjulandin S, Davidson N. Phase III trial of nanoparticles albumin-bound paclitaxel compared with polyethylated castor oil-based paclitaxel in women with breast cancer. J Clin Oncol 2005; 23: 7794-803.
[61] Greenwald RB, Choe YH, McGuire J, Conover CD. Effective drug delivery by PEGylated drug conjugates. Adv Drug Deliv Rev 2003; 55(2): 217-50.
[62] Rowinsky EK, Rizzo J, O`Choa LF. A Phase I and pharmacokinetic study of pegylated camptothecin as a 1 hour infusion every 3 weeks in patients with advanced solid malignancies. J Clin Oncol 2003; 21: 148-57.
[63] Thomson AH, Vasey PA, Murray LS. Population pharmacokinetics in Phase I drug development: A Phase I study of PK1 in patients with solid tumors. Br J Cancer 1999; 81(1): 99-107.
[64] Bilim V. Technology evaluation: PK1, Pfizer/Cancer Research UK. Curr Opin Mol Ther 2003; 5(3): 326-30.
[65] Terwogt M, Jetske M, Huinink TB, Wim W. Phase I clinical and pharmacokinetic study of PNU166945, a novel water soluble polymer-conjugated prodrug of paclitaxel. Anticancer Drugs 2001; 12(4): 315-23.
[66] Sahoo SK, Labhasetwar V. Nanotech approaches to drug delivery and imaging. Drug Discov Today 2003; 8(24): 1112-20.
[67] Vasir JK, Reddy MK, Labhasetwar V. Nanosystems in drug targeting: Opportunities and challenges. Curr Nanosci 2005; 1(1): 47-64.
[68] Kipp JE. The role of solid nanoparticle technology in the parenteral delivery of poorly water-soluble drugs. Int J Pharm 2004; 284(1-2): 109-22.
[69] Muller RH, Keck CM. Challenges and solutions for the delivery of biotech drugs-a review of drug nanocrystal technology and lipid nanoparticles. J Biotechnol 2004; 113(1-3): 151-70.
[70] Rabinow BE. Nanosuspensions in drug delivery. Nat Rev Drug Discov 2004; 3(9): 785-96.
[71] Horn D, Rieger J. Organic nanoparticles in the aqueous Phase-theory, experiment and use. Angew Chem Int Ed Engl 2001; 40(23): 4330-61.
[72] Torchilin VP. Recent advances with liposomes as pharmaceutical carriers. Nat Rev Drug Discov 2005; 4: 145-60.
[73] Wissing SA, Kayser O, Muller RH. Solid lipid nanoparticles for parental drug delivery. Adv Drug Deliv Rev 2004; 56(9): 1257-72.
[74] Gounko, K.I., Rakovich, Y., Volkov, Y., Dongegan, J., Kelleher, D., Mitchel, S. A delivery system. WO05105035 (**2005**).

[75] Jung T, Kamm W, Breitenbach A, Kaiserling E, Xiao JX, Kissel T. Biodegradable nanoparticles for oral delivery of peptides: Is there a role for polymers to affect mucosal uptake? Eur J Pharm Biopharm 2000; 50(1): 147-60.
[76] Reis CP, Neufeld RJ, Ribeiro AJ, Veiga F. Nanoencapsulation I. Methods for preparation of drug-loaded polymeric nanoparticles. Nanomedicine 2006; 2(1): 8-21.
[77] Li J, He Z, Yu S, Li S, Ma Q, Yu Y, *et al.* Micelles based on methoxy poly(ethylene glycol)-cholesterol conjugate for controlled and targeted drug delivery of a poorly water soluble drug. J Biomed Nanotechnol 2012; 8(5): 809-17.
[78] Perez-Martinez FC, Carrion B, Lucio MI, Rubio N, Herrero MA, Vazquez E, *et al.* Enhanced docetaxel-mediated cytotoxicity in human prostate cancer cells through knockdown of cofilin-1 by carbon nanohorn delivered siRNA. Biomaterials 2012; 33(32): 8152-9.
[79] Song J, Zhou J, Duan H. Self-Assembled Plasmonic Vesicles of SERS-encoded amphiphilic gold nanoparticles for cancer cell targeting and traceable intracellular drug delivery. J Am Chem Soc 2012; 134(32): 13458-69.
[80] Wu Y, Shih EK, Ramanathan A, Vasudevan S, Weil T. Nano-sized albumin-copolymer micelles for efficient doxorubicin delivery. Biointer Phases 2012; 7(1-4): 5.
[81] Xu W, Cui Y, Ling P, Li LB. Preparation and evaluation of folate-modified cationic Pluronic micelles for poorly soluble anticancer drug. Drug Deliv 2012; 19(4): 208-19.
[82] Wang X, Yang L, Chen ZG, Shin DM. Application of nanotechnology in cancer therapy and imaging. CA Cancer J Clin 2008; 58(2): 97-110.
[83] Haley B, Frenkel E. Nanoparticles for drug delivery in cancer treatment. Urol Oncol 2008; 26(1): 57-64.
[84] Moghimi SM, Hunter AC, Murray JC. Nanomedicine: Current status and future prospects. FASEB J 2005; 19: 311-30.
[85] Couvreur P, Gruslain L, Lenaerts V. Polymeric nanoparticles and microspheres. Boca Raton (FL): CRC Press 1986.
[86] Park TG. Degradation of poly(lactic-co-glycolic acid) microspheres: Effect of copolymer composition. Biomaterials 1995; 16; 1123-30.
[87] Panyam J, Labhasetwar V. Biodegradable nanoparticles for drug and gene delivery to cells and tissue. Adv Drug Deliv Rev 2003; 55: 329-47.
[88] Kataoka K, Harada A, Nagasaki Y. Block copolymer micelles for drug delivery: Design, characterization and biological significance. Adv Drug Deliv Rev 2001; 47: 113-31.
[89] Ikada Y, Tsuji H. Biodegradable polyesters for medical and ecological applications. Macromol Rapid Commun 2000; 21: 117-32.
[90] Koo OM, Rubinstein I, Onyuksel H. Role of nanotechnology in targeted drug delivery and imaging: A concise review. Nanomedicine 2005; 1(3): 193-212.
[91] Hughes AG. Nanostructure-mediated drug delivery. Nanomedicine 2005; 1(1): 22-30.
[92] Graf N, Bielenberg DR, Kolishetti N, Muus C, Banyard J, Farokhzad OC, *et al.* $\alpha_v\beta_3$ integrin-targeted PLGA-PEG nanoparticles for enhanced anti-tumor efficacy of a Pt(IV) prodrug. ACS Nano 2012; 6(5): 4530-9.
[93] Wan CP, Letchford K, Jackson JK, Burt HM. The combined use of paclitaxel-loaded nanoparticles with a low-molecular-weight copolymer inhibitor of P-glycoprotein to overcome drug resistance. Int J Nanomedicine. 2013; 8: 379-91.
[94] Dhar S, Kolishetti N, Lippard SJ, Farokhzad OC. Targeted delivery of a cisplatin prodrug for safer and more effective prostate cancer therapy *in vivo*. Proc Natl Acad Sci USA 2011; 108(5): 1850-5.

[95] Shah M, Ullah N, Choi MH, Kim MO, Yoon SC. Amorphous amphiphilic P(3HV-co-4HB)-b-mPEG block copolymer synthesized from bacterial copolyester via melt transesterification: nanoparticle preparation, cisplatin-loading for cancer therapy and *in vitro* evaluation. Eur J Pharm Biopharm 2012; 80(3): 518-27.
[96] Etrych T, Sırova M, Starovoytova L, Rhova B, Ulbrich K. HPMA copolymer conjugates of paclitaxel and docetaxel with pH-controlled drug release. Mol Pharm 2010; 7(4): 1015-26.
[97] Elamanchili P, McEachern C, Burt H. Reversal of multidrug resistance by methoxy polyethylene glycol-block-polycaprolactone diblock copolymers through the inhibition of P-glycoprotein function. J Pharm Sci 2009; 98(3): 945-58.
[98] Sethi V, Onyuksel H, Rubinstein I. Liposomal vasoactive intestinal peptide. Methods Enzymol 2005; 391: 377-95.
[99] Yang K, Chen SW, Chen R, Wan YM. Experimental study of cisplatin loaded polylactic acid-polyethylene glycol nanoparticles for targeting oral carcinoma. Hua Xi Kou Qiang Yi Xue Za Zhi 2005; 23(5): 445-8.
[100] Yu JY, Jun YJ, Jang SH, Lee HJ, Sohn YS. Nano particulate platinum(II) anticancer drug: Synthesis and characterization of amphiphilic cyclotriphosphazene-platinum(II) conjugates. J Inorg Biochem 2007; 101(11-12): 1931-6.
[101] Feng S, Huang G. Effects of emulsifiers on the controlled release of paclitaxel (Taxol) from nanospheres of biodegradable polymers. J Control Release 2001; 71(1): 53-69.
[102] Fonsece C, Simoes S, Gaspar RE. Paclitaxel-loaded PLGA nanoparticles: Preparation, physicochemical characterization and *in vitro* anti-tumoral activity. J Control Release 2002; 83(2): 273-86.
[103] Yan GP, Zong, RF, Li L, Fu T, Liu F, Yu XH. Anticancer drug-loaded nanospheres based on biodegradable amphiphilic ε-caprolactone and carbonate copolymers. Pharm Res 2010; 27(12): 2743-52.
[104] Yadav S, Van Vlerken LE, Little SR, Amiji MM. Evaluations of combination MDR-1 gene silencing and paclitaxel administration in biodegradable polymeric nanoparticle formulations to overcome multidrug resistance in cancer cells. Cancer Chemother Pharmacol 2009; 63(4): 711-22.
[105] Yang K, Wen Y, Li L, Wang C, Hou S, Li C. Preparation of cucurbitacin BE polylactic acid nano-particles for targeting cervical lymph nodes. Hua Xi Kou Qiang Yi Xue Za Zhi 2001; 19(6): 347-50.
[106] Koo O, Rubinstein I, Onyuksel H. Camptothecin in sterically stabilized phospholipid micelles: A novel nanomedicine. Nanomedicine 2005; 1(1): 77-84.
[107] Yavlovich A, Singh A, Blumenthal R, Puri A. A novel class of photo-triggerable liposomes containing DPPC: DC(8,9)PC as vehicles for delivery of doxorubcin to cells. Biochim Biophys Acta 2011; 1808(1): 117-26.
[108] Pain D, Das PK, Ghosh PC. Increased circulatory half-life of liposomes after conjugation with dextran. J Biosci 1984; 6(6): 811-6.
[109] Lasic DD, Martin FJ, Gabizon A. Sterically stabilized liposomes: A hypothesis on the molecular origin of the extended circulation times. Biochim Biophys Acta 1991; 1070(1): 187-92.
[110] Torchilin VP, Levchenko TS, Whitemman KR. Amphiphilic poly-*N*-vinylpyrrolid ones: Synthesis, properties and liposome surface modification. Biomaterials 2001; 22(22): 3035-44.
[111] Allen TM, Chonn A. Large unilamellar liposomes with low uptake in to the reticulo endothelial system. Fed Eur Biochem Soc Lett 1987; 223(1): 42-6.

[112] Takeuchi H, Kojima H, Yamamoto H. Evaluation of circulation profiles of liipososmes coated with hydrophilic polymers having different molecular weights in rats. J Control Release 2001; 75(1-2): 83-91.
[113] Lee S, Kim J, Shim G, Kim S, Han SE, Kim K, *et al.* Tetraiodothyroacetic acid-tagged liposomes for enhanced delivery of anticancer drug to tumor tissue via integrin receptor. J Control Release 2012; 164(2): 213-20.
[114] Mangiapia G, D'Errico G, Simeone L, Irace C, Radulescu A, Di Pascale A *et al.* Ruthenium-based complex nanocarriers for cancer therapy. Biomaterials 2012; 33(14): 3770-82.
[115] Brewer M, Zhang T, Dong W, Rutherford M, Tian ZR. Future approaches of nanomedicine in clinical science. Med Clin N Am 2007; 91(5): 963-1016.
[116] Yoon HY, Saravanakumar G, Heo R, Choi SH, Song IC, Han MH, *et al.* Hydrotropic magnetic micelles for combined magnetic resonance imaging and cancer therapy. J Control Release 2012; 160(3): 692-8.
[117] Vetvicka D, Hruby M, Hovorka O, Etrych T, Vetrik M, Kovar L, *et al.* Biological evaluation of polymeric micelles with covalently bound doxorubicin. Bioconjug Chem 2009; 20(11): 2090-7.
[118] Tsallas A, Jackson J, Burt H. The uptake of paclitaxel and docetaxel into *ex vivo* porcine bladder tissue from polymeric micelle formulations. Cancer Chemother Pharmacol 2011; 68(2): 431-44.
[119] Malzert-Freon A, Saint-Lorant G, Hennequin D, Gauduchon P, Poulain L, Rault S. Influence of the introduction of a solubility enhancer on the formulation of lipidic nanoparticles with improved drug loading rates. Eur J Pharm Biopharm 2010; 75(2): 117-27.
[120] Xia Y, Yang P, Sun Y, Wu Y, Mayers B, Gates B, *et al.* One-dimensional nano structures: Synthesis, characterization, and applications. Adv Mater 2003; 15(5), 353-89.
[121] Shimizu T, Masuda M, Minamikawa H. Supramolecular nanotube architectures based on amphiphilic molecules. Chem Rev 2005; 105(4): 1401-43.
[122] Tian ZR, Voigt James A, Jun L. Complex and oriented ZnO nanostructures. Nat Mater 2003; 2: 821-6.
[123] Tian ZR, Voigt JA, Liu J. Biomimetic arrays of oriented helical ZnO nanorods and columns. J Am Chem Soc 2002; 124(44), 12954-5.
[124] Tian ZR, Voigt JA, Liu J. Large oriented arrays and continuous films of TiO_2-based nanotubes. J Am Chem Soc 2005; 125(41): 12384-5.
[125] Hu J, Qian Y, Wang X, Liu T, Liu S. Drug-loaded and superparamagnetic iron oxide nanoparticle surface-embedded amphiphilic block copolymer micelles for integrated chemotherapeutic drug delivery and MR imaging. Langmuir 2012; 28(4): 2073-82.
[126] Balivada S, Rachakatla RS, Wang H, Samarakoon TN, Dani RK, Pyle M, *et al.* A/C magnetic hyperthermia of melanoma mediated by iron(0)/iron oxide core/shell magnetic nanoparticles: A mouse study. BMC Cancer 2010; 10: 119.
[127] Hosta, L., Pla, M., Cruz, L.J., Kogan, M., Albericio, F. Antitumoral treatments. US20100323021 (**2010**).
[128] Kingston, D.G.I., Cao, S., Zhao, J., Hodge, M., Paciotti, G.F., Huhta, M.S. Thiolated paclitaxels for reaction with gold nanoparticles as drug delivery agents. WO2009062138 (**2009**).
[129] Lavan DA, Lynn DM, Langer R. Moving smaller in drug discovery and delivery. Nat Rev Drug Discov 2002; 1(1): 77-84.

[130] Agrawal A, Tripp Ralph A, Anderson LJ. Real-time detection of virus particles and viral protein expression with two-color nanoparticle probes. J Virol 2005; 79(13): 8625-8.
[131] Ijiima S. Helical microtubules of graphitic carbon. Nature 1991; 354: 56-8.
[132] Kostarelos K, Lacerda L, Partidos CD. Carbon nanotube mediated delivery of peptides and genes to cells: Translating nanobiotechnology to therapeutics. J Drug Deliv Sci Technol 2005; 15(1), 41-7.
[133] Li Q, Liu C, Zhao X, Zu Y, Wang Y, Zhang B, *et al.* Preparation, characterization and targeting of micronized 10-hydroxycamptothecin-loaded folate-conjugated human serum albumin nanoparticles to cancer cells. Int J Nanomedicine 2011; 6: 397-405.
[134] Gao X, Wang B, Wei X, Men K, Zheng F, Zhou Y, *et al.* Anticancer effect and mechanism of polymer micelle-encapsulated quercetin on ovarian cancer. Nanoscale 2012; 4(22): 7021-30.
[135] Gou M, Men K, Shi H, Xiang M, Zhang J, Song J, *et al.* Curcumin-loaded biodegradable polymeric micelles for colon cancer therapy *in vitro* and *in vivo*. Nanoscale 2011; 3(4): 1558-67.
[136] Das M, Sahoo SK. Folate decorated dual drug loaded nanoparticle: Role of curcumin in enhancing therapeutic potential of nutlin-3a by reversing multidrug resistance. PLoS One 2012; 7(3): 32920.
[137] Quintana A, Raczka E, Piehler L, Lee I, Myc A, Majoros I, *et al.* Design and function of a dendrimer-based therapeutic nanodevice targetted to tumor cells through the folate receptor. J Pharmacol Res 2002; 19(9): 1310-6.
[138] Morgan MT, Nakanishi Y, Kroll DJ, Griset AP, Carnahan MA, Wathier M, *et al.* Dendrimer-encapsulated camptothecins: Increased solubility, cellular uptake, and cellular retention affords enhanced anticancer activity *in vitro*. Cancer Res 2006; 66: 11913-21.
[139] Grinstaff MW. Biodendrimers: New polymeric biomaterials for tissue engineering. Chem Eur J 2002; 8(13): 2838-46.
[140] Goodwin AP, Lam SS, Frechet JMJ. Rapid, efficient synthesis of hetero bifunctional biodegradable dendrimers. J Am Chem Soc 2007; 129(22): 6994-5.
[141] Padilla De Jess OL, Ihre H, Gagne L, Frechet JMJ, Szoka FC Jr. Polyester dendritic systems for drug delivery applications: *In vitro* and *in vivo* evaluation. Bioconj Chem 2002; 13: 453-61.
[142] Stover TC, Kim YS, Lowe TL, Kester M. Thermo responsive and biodegradable linear-dendritic nanoparticles for targeted and sustained release of a pro-apoptotic drug. Biomaterials 2008; 29(3): 359-69.
[143] Galie KM, Mollard A, Zharov I. Polyester-based carborane-containing dendrons. Inorg Chem 2006; 45: 7815-20.
[144] Ou M, Wang XL, Xu R, Chang CW, Bull DA, Kim SW. Novel biodegradable poly(disulfide amine)s for gene delivery with high efficiency and low cytotoxicity. Bioconj Chem 2008; 19: 626-33.
[145] Russ V, Elfberg H, Thoma C, Kloeckner J, Ogris M, Wagner E. Novel degradable oligoethylenimine acrylate ester-based pseudodendrimers for *in vitro* and *in vivo* gene transfer. Gene Ther 2008; 15(1): 18-29.
[146] Lee JS, Huh J, Ahn CH, Lee M, Park TG. Synthesis of novel biodegradable cationic dendrimers. Macromol Rapid Commun 2006; 27: 1608-14.
[147] Wang F, Cai X, Su Y, Hu J, Wu Q, Zhang H, *et al.* Reducing cytotoxicity while improving anti-cancer drug loading capacity of polypropylenimine dendrimers by surface acetylation. Acta Biomater 2012; 8(12): 4304-13.

[148] Hu J, Su Y, Zhang H, Xu T, Cheng Y. Design of interior-functionalized fully acetylated dendrimers for anticancer drug delivery. Biomaterials 2011; 32(36): 9950-9.

[149] Less JL, Skalak EM, Sevick EM, Jain RK. Microvascular architecture in a mammary carcinoma: Branching patterns and vessel dimensions. Cancer Res 1991; 51: 265-73.

[150] Intaglietta M, Myers RR, Gross JF, Reinhold HS. Dynamics of microvascular flow in implanted mouse mammary tumors. Bibl Anat 1977; 15(1), 273-6.

[151] Chaplin DJ, Olive PL, Durand RE. Intermittent blood flow in a murine tumor: Radiobiological effects. Cancer Res 1987; 47: 597-601.

[152] Chaplin DJ, Trotter MJ, Durand RE, Olive PL, Minchinton AI. Evidence for intermittent radiobiological hypoxia in experimental tumor systems. Biomed Biochim Acta 1989; 48: 255-9.

[153] Dewhirst MW, Braun RD, Lanzen JL. Temporal changes in PO2 of R3230AC tumors in Fischer-344 rats. Int J Radiat Oncol Biol Phys 1998; 42: 723-6.

[154] Senger DR, Galli SJ, Dvorak A, Perruzzi C, Harvey V, Dvorak F. Tumor cells secrete a vascular permeability factor that promotes accumulation of ascites fluid. Science 1983; 219: 983-5.

[155] Maeda H, Noguchi Y, Sato K, Akaike T. Enhanced vascular permeability in solid tumor is mediated by nitric oxide and inhibited by both new nitric oxide scavenger and nitric oxide synthase inhibitor. Jpn J Cancer Re 1994; 85: 331-4.

[156] Maeda H, Akaike T, Wu J, Noguchi Y, Sakata Y. Bradykinin and nitric oxide in infectious disease and cancer. Immunopharmacology 1996; 33: 222-30.

[157] Wu J, Akaike T, Maeda H. Modulation of enhanced vascular permeability in tumors by a bradykinin antagonist, a cyclooxygenase inhibitor, and a nitric oxide scavenger. Cancer Res 1998; 58: 159-65.

[158] Wu J, Akaike T, Hyashida K, Okamoto T, Okuyama A, Maeda H. Enhanced vascular permeability in solid tumor involving peroxynitite and matrix metalloproteinases. Jpn J Cancer Res 2001; 92: 439-51.

[159] Torchilin VP, Levchenko TS, Lukyanov AN, Khaw BA, Klibanov AL, Rammohan R, *et al.* p-Nitrophenylcarbonyl-PEG-PE-liposomes: Fast and simple attachment of specific ligands, including monoclonal antibodies, to distal ends of PEG chains via p-nitrophenylcarbonyl groups. Biochim Biophys Acta 2001; 1511(2): 397-411.

[160] Elbayoumi TA, Torchilin VP. Enhanced accumulation of long-circulating liposomes modified with the nucleosome-specific monoclonal antibody 2C5 in various tumors in mice: Gamma-imaging studies. Eur J Nucl Med Mol Imaging 2006; 33(10): 1196-205.

[161] Matsumura Y, Maeda H. A new concept for macromolecular therapeutics in cancer chemotherapy: Mechanism of tumoritropic accumulation of proteins and the antitumor agent Smancs. Cancer Res 1986; 46: 6387-92.

[162] Maeda H. The enhanced permeability and retention (EPR) effect in tumor vasculature: The key role of tumor-selective macromolecular drug targeting. Adv Enzyme Regul 200; 41: 189-207.

[163] Walberer M, Tschernatsch M, Fischer S, Ritschel N, Volk K, Friedrich C, *et al.* RNase therapy assessed by magnetic resonance imaging reduces cerebral oedema and infarction size in acute stroke. Curr Neurovasc Res 2009; 6(1): 12-9.

[164] Altman S. RNA enzyme-directed gene therapy. Proc Natl Acad Sci USA 1993; 90: 10898-900.

[165] Lewin AS, Hauswirth WW. Ribozyme gene therapy: Applications for molecular medicine. Trends Mol Med 2001; 7(5): 221-8.

[166] Ruan J, Song H, Qian Q, Li C, Wang K, Bao C, *et al.* HER2 monoclonal antibody conjugated RNase-A-associated CdTe quantum dots for targeted imaging and therapy of gastric cancer. Biomaterials 2012; 33(29): 7093-102.

[167] Panyam J, Labhasetwar V. Biodegradable nanoparticles for drug and gene delivery to cells and tissue. Adv Drug Deliv Rev 2003; 55(3): 329-47.

[168] Verma AK, Sachin K. Novel hydrophilic drug polymer nanoconjugates of cisplatin showing long blood retention profile: Its release kinetics, cellular uptake and bio-distribution. Curr Drug Deliv 2008; 5(2): 120-6.

[169] Ranjan AP, Mukerjee A, Helson L, Vishwanatha JK. Scale up, optimization and stability analysis of Curcumin C3 complex-loaded nanoparticles for cancer therapy. J Nano biotechnology 2012; 10(1): 38.

[170] Lu N, Liu Q, Li R, Xie L, Shen J, Guan W, *et al.* Superior antimetastatic effect of pemetrexed-loaded gelatinase-responsive nanoparticles in a mouse metastasis model. Anti cancer Drugs 2012; 23(10): 1078-88.

[171] Lopez-Gasco P, Iglesias I, Benedi J, Lozano R, Blanco MD. Characterization and *in vitro* bioactivity evaluation of paclitaxel-loaded polyester nanoparticles. Anticancer Drugs 2012; 23(9): 947-58.

[172] Kim JH, Kim YS, Park K, Lee S, Nam HY, Min KH, *et al.* Antitumor efficacy of cisplatin-loaded glycol chitosan nanoparticles in tumor-bearing mice. J Control Release 2008; 127(1): 41-9.

[173] Anwunobi AP, Emeje MO. Recent applications of natural polymers in nanodrug delivery. J Nanomed Nanotechnol 2011, S4: 002.

[174] Pan L, He Q, Liu J, Chen Y, Ma M, Zhang L, *et al.* Nuclear-targeted drug delivery of TAT peptide-conjugated monodisperse mesoporous silica nanoparticles. J Am Chem Soc 2012; 134(13): 5722-5.

[175] Ditto AJ, Shah KN, Robishaw NK, Panzner MJ, Youngs WJ, Yun YH. The interactions of L-tyrosine based nanoparticles decorated with folic acid and cervical cancer cells under physiological flow. Mol Pharm 2012; 9(11): 3089-98.

[176] Tang R, Ji W, Panus D, Palumbo RN, Wang C. Block copolymer micelles with acid-labile ortho ester side-chains: Synthesis, characterization, and enhanced drug delivery to human glioma cells. J Cont Rel 2011; 151(1): 18-27.

[177] Pramanik D, Campbell NR, Das S, Gupta S, Chenna V, Bisht S, *et al.* A composite polymer nanoparticle overcomes multidrug resistance and ameliorates doxorubicin-associated cardiomyopathy. Oncotarget 2012; 3(6): 640-50.

[178] Taheri A, Dinarvand R, Atyabi F, Ghahremani MH, Ostad SN. Trastuzumab decorated methotrexate-human serum albumin conjugated nanoparticles for targeted delivery to HER2 positive tumor cells. Eur J Pharm Sci 2012; 47(2): 331-40.

[179] Kilic MA, Ozlu E, Calis S. A novel protein-based anticancer drug encapsulating nanosphere: Apoferritin-doxorubicin complex. J Biomed Nanotechnol 2012; 8(3): 508-14.

[180] Shin JY, Yang Y, Heo P, Lee JC, Kong B, Cho JY, *et al.* pH-responsive high-density lipoprotein-like nanoparticles to release paclitaxel at acidic pH in cancer chemotherapy. Int J Nanomedicine 2012; 7: 2805-16.

[181] Lv PP, Ma YF, Yu R, Yue H, Ni DZ, Wei W, *et al.* Targeted delivery of insoluble cargo (paclitaxel) by PEGylated chitosan nanoparticles grafted with Arg-Gly-Asp (RGD). Mol Pharm 2012; 9(6): 1736-47.

[182] Kwon, G.S. Micelle encapsulation of therapeutic agents. US8383136 (**2013**).
[183] Yourong, D., Peifeng, L., Ying, S., Ming, S., Mingjie, Z., Yanming, S., Qi, W., Zelai, H., Liubin, Q., Hui, Y., Xiaoyu, L., Xuelian, Q., Xiaoyan, C., Qiufen, S., Bingwu, W. PEG-PGLA-PLL polymer and method for preparing and using the same as the drug and gene carrier. US20130052134 (**2013**).
[184] Xiaohai, T., Yu, Q., Xin, S. Passive solid tumor targeting anticancer prodrug and preparation method thereof. US20120244193 (**2012**).
[185] Bartlett DW, Davis ME. Physicochemical and biological characterization of targeted, nucleic acid-containing nanoparticles. Bioconjug Chem 2007; 18(2): 456-68.
[186] Song E, Zhu P, Lee SK, Chowdhury D, Kussman S, Dykxhoorn DM, *et al.* Antibody mediated *in vivo* delivery of small interfering. RNAs via cell-surface receptors. Nat Biotechnol 2005; 23: 709-17.
[187] Hong S, Leroueil PR, Majoros IJ, Orr BG, Baker JR Jr, Banaszak Holl MM. The binding avidity of a nanoparticle-based multivalent targeted drug delivery platform. Chem Biol 2007; 14(1): 107-15.
[188] Faure J, Lachenal G, Court M, Hirrlinger J, Chatellard-Causse C, Blot B, *et al.* Exosomes are released by cultured cortical neurones. Mol Cell Neurosci 2006; 31(4): 642-8.

Topics in Anti-Cancer Research, Vol. 2, 2013, 495-521

CHAPTER 14

Chemotherapy of Nano-Sized Camptothecin-Derived Drugs

Nguyen-Van Cuong [1], Chi-Hui Guo[2] and Ming-Fa Hsieh[2,*]

[1]Department of Chemical Engineering, Ho Chi Minh City University of Industry, 12 Nguyen Van Bao, Ho Chi Minh, Vietnam; [2]Department of Biomedical Engineering, Chung Yuan Christian University, 200, Chung Pei Rd., Chung Li, Taiwan 32023, R.O.C.

Abstract: DNA topoisomerase is one of drug targets in cancer therapy. Camptothecin is a plant alkaloid derived from the Chinese tree *Camptotheca acuminate.* It has been demonstrated that the plant alkaloid camptothecin (CPT) and its analogs caused DNA damage by specifically targeting DNA topoisomerase, effectively devastating a broad spectrum of tumors. Although the anti-tumor activities of CPT and its analogs have been intensively studied for nearly fifty years, recent advances in drug delivery systems of CPT have considerably improved this drug's efficiency and prevented drug resistance. However, CPT and its analogs showed extremely low water solubility, inactivation of carboxylate salt, undesired interaction with human serum albumin and short half-life, therefore, the development of new and effective CPT-derived products is ongoing. In this chapter, we will summarize the current status of CPT-derived anti-cancer drugs in literatures, patents and highlight their clinical application.

Keywords: Aminocamptothecin, anti-tumor efficacy, belotecan, bioavailability, Camptothecin, cancer, clinical trial, drug delivery system, irinotecan, liposomal camptothecin, micelles, nanomedicine, nanoparticles, 9-nitrocamptothecin, pharmaceutical dosage form, pharmacokinetics, poly(ethylene glyclol), polymeric therapeutics, serum stability, topoisomerase I inhibitor, topotecan, water solubility.

INTRODUCTION

Naturally occurring bases, Camptothecin (CPT) was discovered by Wall *et al.* from the bark of Chinese tree *Camptothecaacuminata Decne* [1]. Some CPT

*Address correspondence to Ming-Fa Hsieh:** Department of Biomedical Engineering, Chung Yuan Christian University, 200, Chung Pei Rd., Chung Li, Taiwan 32023, R.O.C.; Tel: 886-3-265-4550; Fax: 886-3-265-4599; E-mail: mfhsieh@cycu.edu.tw

Atta-ur Rahman and Khurshid Zaman (Eds)

analogs, either semi-synthetic or synthetic drugs have been applied in clinical therapy of cancers. The drawbacks of CPT were its extremely low water solubility, inactivation of carboxylate salt, undesired interaction with human serum albumin and short half-life. The chemical structures of CPT and its analogs have been developed to overcome these drawbacks and increase anti-tumor activity such as 9-Nitrocamptothecin (9-NC), Irinotecan (CPT-11), 9-aminocamptothecin (9-AC), topotecan and etc. [2-6]. CPT and its analogs have proved to be effective in killing various cancer cells such as small and non-small cell lung cancer, ovarian cancer, pancreatic cancer, myelomonocytic leukemia and relative disorders. CPT has been identified as DNA topoisomerase I (Topo I) poison and stabilized the CPT-Topo I-DNA complex during S-Phase of cell cycle. The formation of this complex leads to reversible and single strand nicks.

The clinical application of CPT requires the targeting of the lactone form of CPT to the site of action. However, as-administered CPT in blood vessels can be easily transformed into predominate carboxylate form at physiological pH Fig. (**1**), then being bound by serum albumin which is preferentially eliminated. This disadvantage remains the clinical hurdle of CPT in which low therapeutic efficacy and severe toxicity were displayed. In order to overcome the poor water solubility of lactone form and instability at physiological pH, the derivatives (or called pro-drugs) of CPT have been synthesized by modifying at quinolone, E-ring [7] and 20-hydroxy sites [8] and being used in clinical cancer treatment. Figure **2** shows the chemical structures of these CPT-derived compounds.

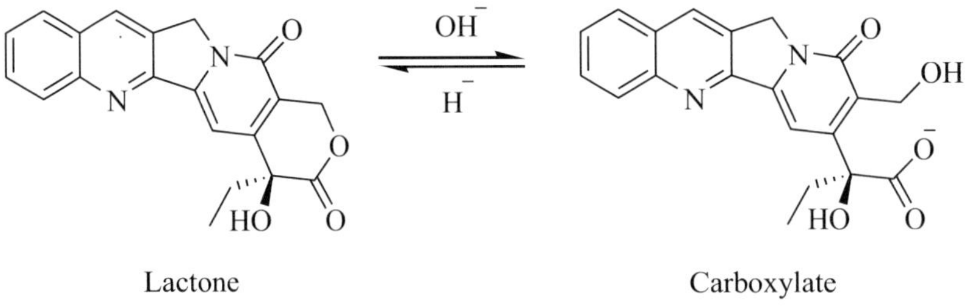

Figure 1: Camptothecin hydrolysis at physiological pH.

Extending the idea of pro-drugs into conjugating CPT to polymer, the polymeric therapeutics has been investigated to improve the lactone stability and water

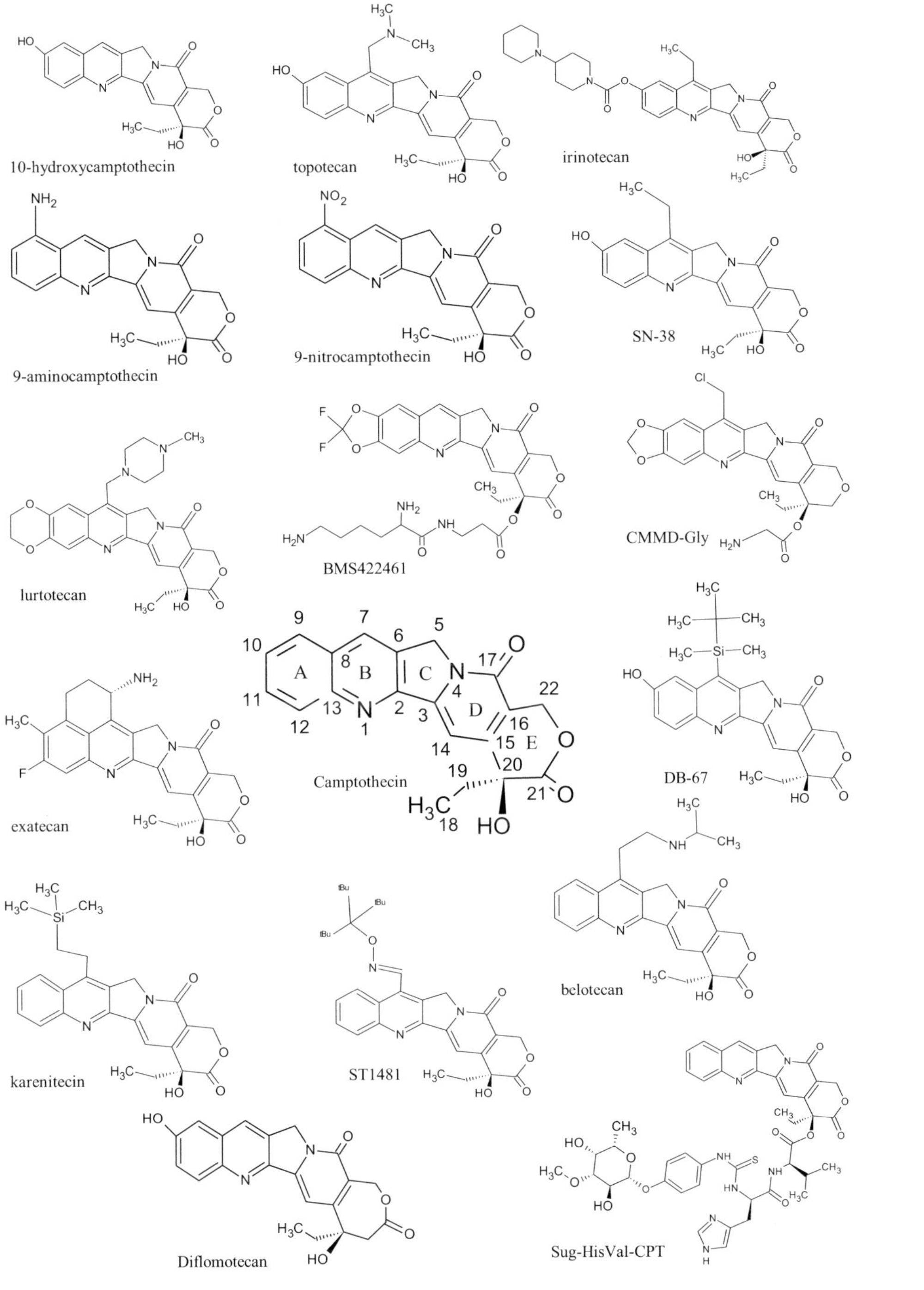

Figure 2: The chemical structures of the camptothecin-derived drugs. The rings in the chemical structure of CPT are also numbered from A thru E.

solubility of CPT. In this type of drugs, the stoichiometric ratio of drug to polymer is important for dosage form design. The percentage of active ingredient in a macromolecular drug can be much higher when CPT is attached to the pendant groups of the polymer. Figure **3** shows the chemical structures of polyethylene glycol (or cyclodextrin)-conjugated CPT. Macromolecular drugs were designed to be released into blood circulation by enzymatic cleavage and/or pH-dependent hydrolysis. To name a few, these macromolecular drugs are micelles [9], pegylated CPT [10], cyclodextrin-PEG CPT [11], poly (L-glutamic acid) CPT [12], poly (*N*-2-hydroxypropyl) methacrylamide CPT [13], carboxymethyl dextran CPT [14], respectively. This approach definitely endows more freedom of clinical therapy of cancers. The following paragraph will discuss more about this approach.

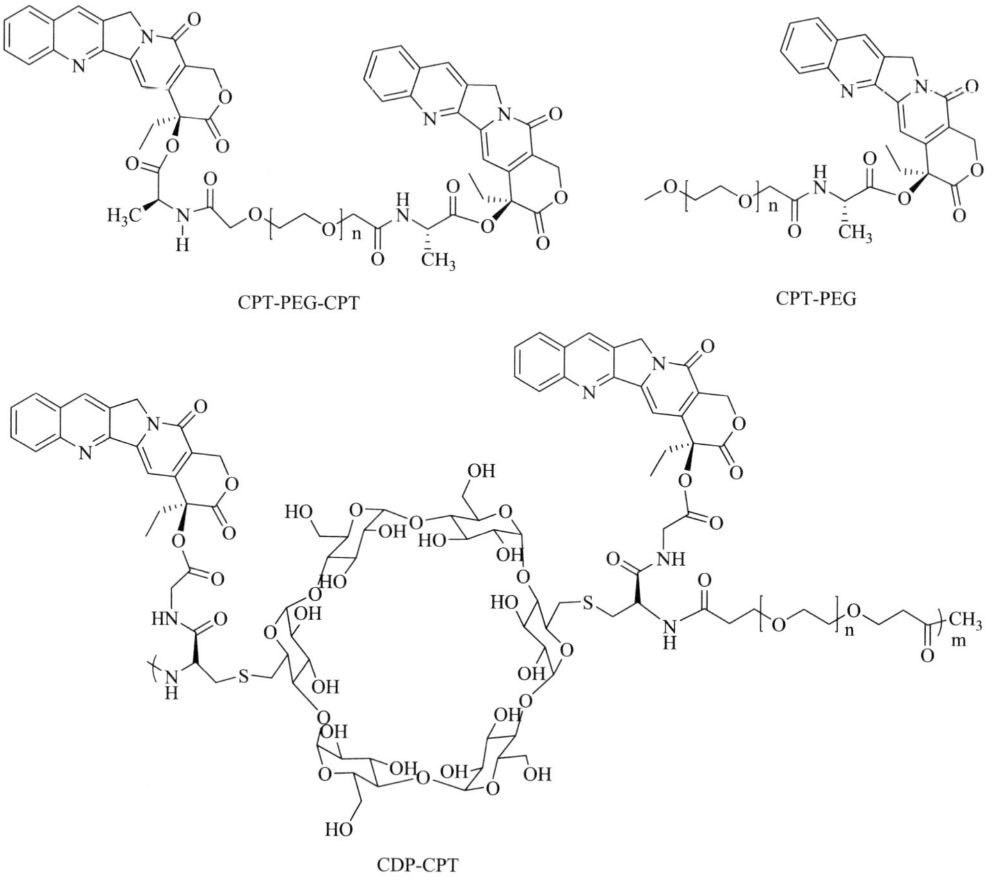

Figure 3: Structures of macromolecular drugs of CPT.

However, some of these analogs are time-consuming in chemical synthesis as well as unsatisfactory in the potency of anti-tumor activity [5, 15]. Consequently, the development of the particle-based delivery systems of CPT is of potential for medical and pharmaceutical practitioners. An ideal drug delivery system can prevent CPT from being rapidly hydrolyzed from the lactone to inactive carboxylated form and prolong the circulation time in blood pool [16]. The aim of this chapter is to summarize the inventions and papers related to nanoparticles-based drug delivery systems for CPT and its derivatives.

HYDROPHILIC CAMPTOTHECIN-DERIVED DRUGS

Camptothecin is anti-cancer reagent which is known to inhibit topoisomerase I. However, CPT and some of its analogs are associated with poor water-solubility, unfavorable pharmacokinetic profile, and rapid inactivation through lactone ring hydrolysis at physiological pH. Conjugation of CPT with polymers to increase their solubility is considered animportant therapeutic goal. These types of polymeric drugs hold several advantages such as improvement of aqueous solubility of CPT, bioavailability of drug and pharmacodynamic and pharmacokinetic properties. Especially, conjugation of polymer to CPT reduces side effect and increases the CPT accumulation in solid tumors through the enhanced permeability and retention (EPR) effect [17-20]. Most of these recent approaches employed PEG-modified CPT and its derivatives. PEGs are non-toxic and water-soluble as well as organic solvent-soluble polymer. PEG has been approved by FDA for human intravenous injection, oral and dermal applications. CPT and its derivatives were conjugated to linear PEG or multi arm-PEG of molecular weight ranging from hundreds to thousands Dalton through hydrolyzable or enzymatically cleavable bonds such as esters, carbonates, carbamates, amide and hydrazones [21]. PEG-CPT prodrugs increased the solubility, blood retention time and stability of the active lactone form. Additionally, PEG-CPT exhibited various advantages over CPT including higher cell uptake and tumor accumulation (30 folds), the lower efflux through EPR effect, longer tumor retention time (72h) and enhancement of apoptosis induction in tumor cells, resulting higher anti-tumor activity [9, 12]. In one invention, Zhao *et al.* demonstrated the conjugation of multiarm-PEG to irinotecan and SN-38 [22]. The molecular weight of multiarms PEG was 20kDa and 40kDa, resulting in

4-arm PEG-GLY-Irino-20K, 4-arm PEG-GLY-Irino-40K, 4-arm PEG-GLY-SN-38-20K and 4-arm PEG-GLY-SN-38-40K, respectively. The antitumor activity of 4-arm PEG-GLY-Irinotecan was studied in human HT29 colon and NCI-H460 lung tumor xenografts. The mice-bearing tumors were administered intravenously at doses of 40, 60, and 90mg/kg (irinotecan and SN-38 equivalent) every four days for three cycles. As results indicated the group of animals administered with 4-arm-PEG-GLY-Irino and 4-arm PEG-GLY-SN-38 showed significant reduction of tumor size when compared to the group of animals administered unconjugated active agents. Additionally, multiarm PEGylated CPT improved significantly tumor retention time when compared to unmodified parent drug. Moreover, this system was also an effective way to treat a resistant or refractory cancer in a mammal [23]. For a CPT/polymer dual Phase drug release system, Rolke *et al.* [24] invented formulations using poly(1-hydroxymethylethylene hydroxymethyl-formal) which was conjugated to CPT via a succinamidoester linker. Stability of aqueous solution of CPT-polymer conjugate was pH and temperature dependence and preferred storage in low pH and temperature.

Recently, cyclodextrin-contaning polymer (CDP) was conjugated to topoisomerase inhibitors (CPT, SN-38, irinotecan, topotecan and *etc.*) for treatment of human carcinomas and autoimmune diseases such as CDP-CPT conjugate, CDP-irinotecan conjugate, CDP-SN-38 conjugate, CDP-topotecan conjugate, CDP-lurotecan conjugate, etc. [11, 25]. The CPT and its derivatives can attach to CDP polymer though the hydroxyl group or amino group. In brief, cyclodextrin was modified with L-cysteine (named as CD-Bis-Cys), followed by conjugating to PEG derivatives (Mw: 3400) to give CD-Bis-Cys-PEG copolymer with different bonds between PEG and CD (propanoicamid bond, butanoicamid bond and carbamate bond), and then glycinated CPT or SN-38 (Gly-CPT) was attached to CD-Bis-Cys-PEG copolymer to form Poly (CD-Bis-Cys-PEG)-CPT conjugates. These conjugates named as HGGG6, LGGG10, HG6, HGGG10 with the different glycine linkers and different molecular weights (97kDa and 35kDa for H and L copolymer, respectively) [11, 25]. The CPT conjugation (lactone form) was 6.1, 10.2, and 9.6 w% for HGGG6, LGGG10, HG6, HGGG10, respectively. The released profile of CPT from conjugations exhibited the longer half-life in PBS when compared with human serum and mouse serum ($t_{1/2}$= 57 h for PBS *vs.* $t_{1/2}$ = 1.7 and 2.6 h for human serum and mouse serum, respectively). Additionally, the results indicated the more glycine linkers was residence, the longer half-life was observed [6]. pH presented a significant effect on the release of CPT from conjugations, as results, the released amount of CPT was less than 7% with pH range of 1.1-6.4. However, when pH increased to 13.1, most of CPT was released from conjugation after 24h at 37°C (HG6 and HGGG6). The *in vitro* cytotoxicity was tested on human ovarian carcinoma A2780, human colorectal adenocarcinoma HT29, human prostate carcinoma PC-3, and human colonic adeoncarcinoma LS174T cell lines. As results, the free CPT showed highest toxicity to all carcinoma cell lines in comparison with HG6 and HGGG6. For example; IC_{50} values of CPT were 10-fold and 2-fold lower than that of HG6 and HGGG6, respectively in LS174T cell line. More interesting, HGGG6 displayed lower IC_{50} values than that of HG6 in all cell lines. It may be due to a longer half-life of HGGG6 than that of HG6. The *in vivo* toxicity and antitumor efficacy was also investigated. The maximum tolerable dose for LGGG10, HG6, and HGGG10 were 36, 9, and 9mg CPT/kg with dose ranging from 2.25 to 54mg CPT/kg. The antitumor efficacy was performed using female Charles River nude mice bearing human LS174T colon carcinoma tumor. As results, three conjugates (LGGG10, HG6, and HGGG10) administered at their MTDs showed more prolonged tumor growth inhibition when compared to CPT and irinotecan. Additionally, tumor growth inhibitor of three conjugates indicated a dose dependent manner (a dosed of 9mg CPT/kg displayed higher antitumor activity than a dosed of 4.5mg CPT/kg). It has been also shown that the tumor growth inhibitor of the high MW polymer-drug conjugates has greater antitumor effect compared to the low MW conjugates which probably due to the enhanced accumulation (EPR effect) and reduced renal clearance [11, 25].

CAMPTOTHECIN DELIVERY USING LIPOSOMAL DELIVERY SYSTEMS

Liposomes are organized phospholipid vesicles that have been extensively used as carriers for many anti-cancer drugs and protein such as doxorubicin and ricin toxoid vaccine [26, 27]. However, liposome has been rapidly taken up by the reticuloendothelial system in the liver and spleen leading to a short circulation time. Various modifications of liposomes have been developed such as polymeric conjugation on liposome surface and polymer fixation [28-30] to avoid this clinical problem. Of the most successful compound to obtain a long circulation stability is to coat the surface of liposome with hydrophilic and flexible poly (ethylene glycol). As a result, PEG-liposome could reduce binding with the plasma protein, prevent oposonization and, therefore, long circulation is reached [31-33].

Small particle liposome aerosols for delivery of CPT, 9-NC and 9-AC, 10, 11-methylenedioxycamptothecin was demonstrated in the patents of Knight and co-workers [34-36]. In these inventions, the preparation methods of small particle aerosol delivery system and the administration of aqueous dispersions of dilauroylphosphatidylcholine (DLPC) liposomes carrying anti-cancer drugs to the lung were disclosed. In the invention, anti-tumor activity against various human tumors xenograftes in mice was compared. The concentration of 9-NC in the aerosol formulation was not exceeded 10% of total prepared volume and the preferred ratio of the anticancer drug to solvent was in the range of 1:10 to 1:50 wt: wt. In the embodiment of the invention, the particularly preferred ratio of 9-NC to DLPC was about 1:50 (wt: wt). The mechanical stability of liposome 9-NC-DLPC under vortexing before and after nebulizaion was studied. The results showed that the lowest concentration of 9-NC, for example 0.1mg 9-NC: 5.0mL DLPC lead to the most stable particle size. In addition, the particle size decreased ten-fold due to the shear force during the nebulization process, e.g. 332nm vs. 3μm.

The antitumor effect of 9-NC-DLPC was tested in human breast cancer, human colorectal cancer and human lung carcinoma xenografts in mice. Daily dosing of 8.1μg/kg 9-NC-DLPC was given to the mice for five days per week. At day 17 of the treatment, a five-fold increase of the 9-NC liposome aerosol was given to the mice. The result showed that human breast tumor mass was invisible after the treatment of 85th days. In human colorectal tumor xenograft in nude mice, 9-NC-DLPC formulation could suppress the rate of tumor growth 7-11 times to the control. However, there was no significant difference in suppressing tumor growth when the escalating doses were employed. The anti-tumor growth of 9-NC-DLPC was also tested in human lung carcinoma xenograft in nude mice via liposome aerosol and oral administration. The tumor size was decreased with an increase of dosage via aerosol. In contrary, oral administration did not present the same efficacy of the reduction of tumor size. This could be attributed to rapid entry of aerosol to circulation without the first pass effect. The drug transports to the left heart, and then to the aorta and peripheral circulation. The deposition of drug-liposome aerosol into the central airway could be further altered by modulation of respiratory physiology through the addition of 7.5% to 10% by volume of CO_2 gas to the air source. By this approach, an increase of inspired air along with aerosol was markedly achieved. After administration of new generation of CPT-liposome aerosol, the higher concentration of CPT was found in organs of treated mice and the highest concentration of CPT was detected in the lung [37]. An earlier study of Perez-Soler showed the preparation of several CPT-phospholipid complexes for intravenous administration. The fatty acids attached to the head group of the phospholipid were selected from oleic, linoleic, linoleoleic, eicosenoic, myristoleic, palmitoleic, etc. The *in vitro and in vivo* results of CPT-phospholipid formulation has anti-tumor activity similar to that of lactone form of CPT and shows similar cytotoxicity against both MDR-1 negative and positive tumor cells [38].

Fundamental pharmacokinetic data of 9-NC-DLPC was obtained in the Phase I study. Six patients of 18 years old or older with primary or metastatic cancers in lung were recruited in the study [39, 40]. Patients treated twice with a daily dose of 6.7μg/kg 9-NC-DLPC per nebulization in 30 min and then followed by an observation of 2 weeks. Afterward, a cohort of 3 to 6 patients received escalating doses and stopped at 26.6μg/kg/day. Pharmacokinetic data showed that peak plasma concentration of lactone form was found at 2hr post the aerosol exposure. In addition, a comparable area under curves (AUC) of the lactone form and total 9-NC in two patients indicated liposome was effective in the protection of lactone form of 9-NC.

To stabilize the lactone form of 9-NC, Chen *et al.* had published a formulation of 9-NC-encapsulated liposome for intravenous injection to rat [41]. The formulation enhances the lactone stability of 9-NC *in vivo* after intravenous administration. The lactone form was significantly stabilized in liver. The improvement was attributed by introducing another formulation agent, hydrogenated soybean phosphatidylcholine to increase affinity of 9-NC to lipid membrane of liposome [42].

While very successful advancements of liposomal delivery system of 9-NC were reported, the trials of the CPT pro-drugs were also being developed by a vast population of pharmaceutical scientists. Irinotecan, also known as CPT-11, is a CPT derivative. This pro-drug is converted to 7-ethylene-10-hydroxy-CPT (SN-38) by carboxylesterases. CPT-11 has been investigated against a variety of tumor types. When inserted between DNA and Topo I, it is a weak stabilized cleavable complex and required to convert to its active form SN-38. Therefore, development of CPT-11 and SN-38 formulation has been attempted. Rahman *et al.* [43] was granted an invention of liposomal formulation of CPT-11. This invention claimed a method for making CPT-11-liposome formulation in order to increase stability of CPT-11 and CPT-11-liposome formulation, increase drug payload, reduce the side effects and increase drug efficiency, and overcome the multi-drug resistance (MDR) of CPT-11 in cancer cells. The invention described CPT-11-liposome formulation utilized in treatment of human lymphoma, ovarian, breast, lung and colon cancers and disease caused by abnormal cellular proliferation. The formulation can prevent the MDR effect in cancer cells when the formulation is administered alone or in combination with other anti-cancer reagents (Doxorubicin, Taxol and CPT). Moreover, the pharmacokinetic parameters showed that the CPT-11 of inventive formulation has accumulated in cardiac tissue three fold less than that of conventional CPT-11. A higher AUC of CPT-11 and a longer plasma half-life than that of conventional CPT-11 were also achieved.

Recently, Yoshino *et al.* [44] has provided a liposome formulation of CPT-11 and SN-38. The invention disclosed the new remote loading method for fabrication of CPT-11-liposome formulation which had higher drug payload (at least 0.07mol drug/mol lipid) and drug encapsulation efficiency ($\geq$ 90%) than conventional passive method. The remote loading method based on an ion gradient is created across the liposomal membrane, and the drug can permeate through the vesicle membrane. Moreover, prolonged circulation of CPT-11 and SN-38 in plasma was displayed. In this system, the average size of 0.02 to 250μm of the stable formulation can be maintained for 14 days at 37°C and six months at 4°C. The extend stability was bestowed on liposomal surface modified with hydrophilic polymer PEG. The anti-tumor effects were studied in various mouse xenografts of human cancer cells. The details of the anti-tumor effects were summarized in Table **1**.

Table 1: Comparison of the Anti-Tumor Effect of Various CPT-11-Liposome Against Human Tumors Xenografted in Mice. The Inhibition Rate is Shown with Respect to the Dose Administrated [36].

CPT-11 Formulation	**Cancer Cell Lines**	**Drug Payload (mg/mL)**	**Dose (mg/kg)**	**Tumor Weight (g, mean ± S.D)**	**Inhibition Rate (%)**
HSPC:Chol:PEG-DSPE	PC-3	4.92	25 50 100	1.26 ± 0.18 0.03 ± 0.01 0.02 ± 0.00	97.9 98.3 99.0
HSPC:Chol:TRX-20:PEG-DSPE	HCT-116	4.66	18.75 37.5 75	0.61 ± 0.11 0.36 ± 0.07 0.14 ± 0.03	51.1 70.8 88.7
HSPC:Chol:TRX-20:PEG-PE	HT-29	3.22	25 50 100	0.18 ± 0.15 0.09 ± 0.06 0.05 ± 0.03	69.4 84.1 92.0
HSPC:Chol:TRX-20:PEG-PE	QG-56	3.28	25 50 100	0.03 ± 0.02 0.02 ± 0.00 0.03 ± 0.02	99.0 99.3 99.2

HSPC: Hydrogenated soybean phosphatidylcholine; Chol: cholesterol; TRX-20: 3,5-Dipentadecyloxybenzamidine hydrochloride; PEG-PE: Polyethylene glycol-phosphatidyl ethanolamine; PEG-DHPE: Polyethylene glycol-dihexadecanoyl phosphatidyl ethanolamine

The formulation showed the improved inhibition of tumor growth. Nano vesicles having surfaced PEG are generally regarded as stealth drug carrier indicating low macrophage recognition in blood stream [33]. This structural advantage can reflect the improved pharmacokinetic properties. In the pharmacokinetic data of CPT-11-liposome formulation for treating human colon cancer cells (HT-29) in rat, a 302-fold increase in the AUC of plasma concentration and a mean residue time up to 4.4-fold were seen as compared with similar dose of free CPT-11. Recently, cationic liposomes represent an alternative liposomal delivery system and displayed a specific targeting effect to neo-angiogenic areas in blood vessel. Mundus *et al.* [45] formulated cationic CPT-liposomes according to the film method in the pH range between 3-7 with improvement of physicochemical stability and pharmaceutical applicability. The liposome composed of one cationic lipid, such as DMTAP, DOTAP, DPTAP, DSTAP, DOTMA, and DDAB or mixture of cationic lipid such as DOTAP/DOPC = 1:1 and DOTAP/Chol 1:1, The cationic liposome was dehydrated and a stabilizing agent in an amount of about

0.1% (m/v) to about 20% (m/v) was added during drying process. The particle size was 156 nm with a PDI of 0.15.

CAMPTOTHECIN-POLYMER CONJUGATES AS NANOPARTICLE SYSTEMS

Nanoparticles are defined as the particles having its diameter in nanometer range. Nanoparticles are functional materials that can undergo surface modification for targeting to cancer cells of cellular membrane, cytoplasmic or nuclei. Furthermore, the encapsulation of anti-cancer drugs in the nanoparticles can prevent the multi-drug resistance and prolong the circulation half-life of drugs in the bloodstream [46, 47]. The nanoparticles consist of dendrimers, polymeric micelles, nanospheres, nanocapsules, fullerenes, nanotubes, and liposome [39], and can be different in material composition, drug loading capacity, drug stability, drug release rate, and target ability. Among these characteristic properties, the drug-carrying particles having defined particle diameter have been proven to preferentially accumulate in tumor mass because of the leaky vasculature of tumors which is so called enhanced permeability and retention effect [39].

IT-101 (now CRLX101) is a nanoparticle conjugated with CPT and a cyclodextrin based polymer. CPT was conjugated to the cyclodextrin at the 20-OH position which prevents the ring open of the lactone linkage of CPT [48-52]. The molecular weights of polymers used were 35kDa or 97kDa and CPT was linked to the cyclodextrin with the peptide spacer of triglycine [49]. The mean particle size of IT-101 was in the range of 54nm to 78nm depending upon the CPT loading [51]. In their report, CPT loading contents were 5.03wt% and 7.36wt%. The stability study showed no carboxylate form detected throughout a period of 7hr. Time for one half CPT released from IT-101 at 37°C was dramatically decreased from 59hr in PBS to 1.7hr in human plasma. This result inferred that the plasma proteins can de-stabilize the IT-101 and resulted in higher release rate. In the pharmacokinetic study of the camptothecin-polymer conjugate (IT-101) in rats, after intravenous injection, plasma concentration of CPT released from IT-101 are 100-fold higher than that of free CPT. Moreover, IT-101 presented greater CPT concentration in tumor site than that of free CPT or irinotecan. Anti-tumor activity of IT-101 in human LS174T colon tumor-bearing nude mice [50, 51] showed that the maximum tolerated dose (MTD) of IT-101 is 9mg/kg and significant anti-tumor activities were observed as well when compared to the administration of free CPT.

Clinical survey of IT-101 in human subject: A dose-finding pharmacokinetic study of IT-101 in the treatment of refractory solid tumors investigated by Insert Therapeutics (now Calando Pharmaceuticals) had been reported in American Society of Clinical Oncology Meeting in 2008 [52]. According to the meeting abstract, IT-101, having a particle size of 5-40nm, was administered intravenously every week of a 28-days cycle in 12 patients. The doses were from 6mg/m^2/week to 18mg/m^2/week with escalation of Simon's design. It was found that hematologic toxicity was dose limiting toxicity (DLT). This study concluded that the doses of 6 to 9mg/m^2/wk were safe and an outcome of stable disease was reached in patients completed 6 cycles of drug administration every other week. A Phase I trial was completed in October, 2008 with a positive safety profile and indications of efficacy. In June, 2009 Calando licensed IT-101 to Cerulean Pharma Inc, named as CRLX101.

The human Phase I study of CRLX101 was performed to determine the safety, toxicity, and the maximum tolerated dose in the treatment of advanced solid tumors. This study had 2 parts with 24 patens. In part 1, patients with metastatic or unresectable solid tumors were administered intravenously at 6, 12, or 18mg/m^{2}weekly for 3 consecutive weeks per month. CRLX101 is administered intravenously over 90 minutes on days 1, 8, and 15 for 28 day cycle. In part 2, after the first twelve patients were enrolled, CRLX101 was administered intravenously at doses of 12, 15 or 18mg/m^2 over 90 minutes as once biweekly, every 28 days. The last six patients were administered intravenously over 60 minutes as once for two weeks. It is has been shown that the MTD was approximately 9mg/m^2 and 15mg/m^2 for first dosing schedule (weekly) and second dosing schedule (biweekly), respectively. The DLTs of first dosing schedule were hematologic toxicity and cystitis. Non-hematologic grade 3/4 adverse events included fatigue was observed in 3 patients (25%). Additionally, the hematuria/dysuria, the elevated creatine phosphokinase and dehydration were observed in 2 patients (17%), 1 patient (8%), 1 patient (8%), respectively. However, in biweekly schedule, the DLT was only grade 3 neutropenia in one patient, which means the conjugated CPT reduced significantly cumulative toxicity than that of unconjugated CPT, resulting in the prevention of toxicities normally associated with CPT analogs.

According to the pharmacokinetic analysis, conjugated-CPT exhibited a shorter mean elimination half-life (31.8 ± 5.7 hr *vs.* 43.8 ± 9.7 hr for conjugated and unconjugated CPT), and a lower volume of distribution (4.2 ± 1.1 liter) than that of unconjugated CPT. In general, CRLX101 shown improvement in DLT, significantly increased the plasma concentrations of conjugated CPT, increased release of active CPT from the conjugate, and resulting in higher accumulation of CRLX101 in tumors [53, 54]. Recently, Cerulean Pharma Inc. processed a Phase 2 study of CRLX101 in patients with advanced non-small cell lung cancer in order to compare median overall survival of patients with advanced non-small cell lung cancer (NSCLC) treated with CRLX101 to patients treated with best supportive care. The patents were administered intravenously at a dose of 15mg/m^2 every other week.

Chemical modification is a highly effective approach to improve the pharmacokinetic characteristics of CPT-derived compounds as described above. However, the development of novel formulations without chemical modification of drugs shines a new way to small business of pharmaceutical industry because of shorter lead time, lower regulatory barrier and the most importantly, lower entry barrier into the market of cytotoxic chemotherapy. Recently, many Phase III studies of CPT-11 alone or in combination with other cytotoxic chemotherapeutics has been approved by FDA [55]. CPT-11 itself is a pro-drug and is converted to SN-38 at physiological pH. SN-38 exhibits enhanced cytotoxic activity against various cancer cells than that of CPT-11 [40]. In an effort to encapsulate the drugs, the nano-sized micellar delivery systems of CPT-11 or SN-38 have already gained a great deal of interest because of its excellent *in vivo* efficacy. Among the formulations being clinically studied [56], Nanocarrier's NK012 performed very well in the treatment of solid tumors. NK012 is SN-38-

conjuagted polymeric micelles (PEG-PGlu (SN-38)) formed by self-assembly of amphiphilic block copolymers in an aqueous solution [57-59] where PGlu is the abbreviation of poly (gluatmic acid). The particle size and drug loading content were 20nm and 20% (w/w), respectively. The cytotoxicity against non-small cell lung and colon cancer cells, pharmacokinetic analysis, anti-tumor activity and tissue distribution of NK012 in human tumor bearing-nude mice were reviewed [56]. The significant anti-tumor activity and low side effects were investigated under preclinical studies [57-58]. These results suggest a merit of clinical application of NK012.

In Phase I study, NK012 was administered intravenously as oncefor three weeks at a starting dose of 2mg/kg with escalating by acceleration titration method [59]. The MTD determined in the study is higher than 28mg/m^2. DLT was found to be grade 3 febrile neutropenia. Polymer-bound SN-38 and polymer-unbound SN-38 were prolonged in the circulation time in plasma with half-lives of approximately 121 hr and 205 h(at a dose of 28mg/m^2), respectively. In addition, the AUC of polymer-bound SN-38 and polymer-unbound SN-38 at dose of 28mg/m^2 were 307 $\pm$ 68μg.hr/mL and 2.42 $\pm$ 1.24μg.hr/mL, respectively [60]. Recently, Hamaguchi *et al.* conducted a human Phase I study in order to determine the dose-limiting toxicity; evaluate the pharmacokinetic profile, and antitumor activity of NK012. 24 adult patients with solid tumors were administered at dose of 2mg/m^{2}to 28 mg/m^{2}as a 30-minute infusion every 3 weeks [61]. The toxicity study indicated that NK012 was generally well tolerated. DLT was found to be grade 1 to 2 in severity: nausea, anorexia, vomiting, fatigue, elevated AST/ALT, elevated γ-glutamyltranspeptidase (γ-GTP), and thrombocytopenia. Additionally, the most common grade 3 to 4 events were leukopenia and neutropenia (fifteen patients) at a dose level of 28mg/m^2. No grade 3 or 4 diarrhea was observed, resulting in recommended Phase II dose was determined to be 28mg/m^2 with at least a 3-week interval between treatment cycles. The DLT and MDT of this study were also correlated with previous Phase I study [59]. The PK analysis of NK012 indicated CL_{tot} and V_{ss} of NK012 were approximately 150-and 80-fold lower than those of CPT-11, respectively. A significant decreased distribution in normal tissue and increased accumulation in tumor tissue, was due to the enhanced permeability and retention effect.

In an invention by Liu *et al.* [62, 63], a method for loading of SN-38 in PEGylated nano graphene oxide (NGO-PEG) has been described. It is interesting to learn that the authors utilized the principle of chemical π-π stacking to trap SN-38 to NGO-PEG. The SN-38 formulation was formed by simple mixing of SN-38 dissolved in DMSO with a NGO-PEG water solution, followed by removal of un-trapped drug and DMSO. The drug loading content was estimated to be 0.1g SN-38 loaded in 1.0g NGO-PEG. The present formulation was more water soluble than free SN-38 because of the presence of PEG. The stability of inventive SN-38-loaded NGO-PEG was investigated in PBS and mouse serum at 37°C. The results indicated that the faster release rate of SN-38 was observed in mouse serum (30%) than PBS (negligible release) for a period of three days. The IC_{50}values of NGO-PEG-SN38 for HCT-116, OVCAR-3, U-87MG and MDA-MB-45 cell lines were 6, 0.12, 50 and 2nM, respectively. This indicated that NGO-PEG-SN38 exhibited high potency of anti-tumor cells as compared to that of free SN-38.

In addition to CPT-conjugated nanoparticles, physical entrapment of CPT in amphiphilic block copolymers constitutes a drug delivery system of poorly soluble anti-cancer drugs. These kinds of copolymers have appropriate molecular weights and the property of self-assembly of nano-sized micelles. Notably, block copolymers of polylactides and PEG were preferentially claimed. We have investigated the patents granted in the world. A general keyword "polymeric micelles" was searched, and the results displayed an interesting outcome that linear and biodegradable amphiphilic block copolymers consisting of PEG, poly(DL-lactide-co-glycolide (PLGA), poly(ε-caprolactone) were claimed. Further analysis indicated that some pharmaceutical companies dominated the intellectual properties in the early development Phase of anticancer drugs-loaded nanoparticles. Table **2** displays these pioneer patent owners and properties of amphiphilic block copolymers [64-69]. After the latent period of patent application, a great number of patent applications showing various chemical structures of block copolymers emerged in recent years. Moreover, successful formulations have been entered Phase II clinical trial, such as Genexol-PM (Samyang, a Korean company). The following paragraphs review the most recent publications and patents disclosing block copolymers carrying CPT-derived drugs.

Table 2: United States Patents Granted for Amphiphilic Block Copolymers as Anti-Cancer Drug-Encapsulated Nanoparticles.

Assignee	**Properties of the Block Polymer**			**Ref.**
	No. of Block*	**Hydrophilic Block**	**Major Hydrophobic Block****	
Samyang Corp.	AB	Poly(alkylene oxide)	PLA, poly(p-dioxanone)	[56]
Samyang Corp.	AB	Poly(alkylene oxide)	PLA, PGA, PLGA, PCL	[57]
Samyang Corp.	AB, ABA, BAB	Poly(alkyleneglycol), PEG	PLA, PLGA, PCL	[58]
Samyang Corp.	AB	Poly(ethylene oxide)	PLA, PGA, PCL	[59]
Nektar Therapeutics Al, Corp.	ABCD	PEG	Poly(hydroxyester), poly(alkylene oxide)	[60]
Labopharm Inc.	AB	PVP	Polyester, polyorthoester, polyanhydride	[61]

* Number of hydrophilic and hydrophobic blocks in a polymeric chain; AB stands for di-block copolymers while ABA, BAB or ABCD is multi-block copolymer with alternating hydrophilicity.

** Only common hydrophobic segments are listed. PLA: poly(lactide), PGA: poly(glycolide), PCL: poly(ε-caprolactone), PVP: poly(vinyl pyrrolidone)

The invention of Kang *et al.* [70] disclosed a method of preparation and the composition of nanoparticles consisting of poorly soluble CPT analog that can prolong the stability of lactone form in the blood. The disclosed nanoparticles composed of SN-38, solid PEG, an anti-associative agent mPEG-PLA; a block copolymer of methoxy poly(ethylene glycol) and poly (D,L-lactic acid) and a solid surfactant (polyethyleneglycol tocopherol succinate). The loading yield of SN-38 was approximately 98%. SN-38-loaded nanoparticles were stable at 25°C for 6 months. In preclinical study, SN-38-loaded nanoparticles have demonstrated cytotoxic effect against human cancer cells (HT-29 and MIA-Paca-2) in xenografted nude mice when drug was administered with a dose of 10mg/kg. SN-38-loaded nanoparticle showed considerable tumor growth inhibition compared with control group and free CPT-11.

Other nanoparticles composed of PLA and poly (ethyleneglycol)-block-poly(propylene glycol)-block-poly(ethylene glycol) copolymers (PEG-PPG-PEG) which were used to carry the CPT-11. The nanoparticles exhibited a good anti-tumor activity and prolonged the retention of CPT-11 in bloodstream [71, 72]. CPT-loaded PLA/PEG-PPG-PEG nanoparticles have been investigated in an attempt to overcome the drawbacks of the high dose and frequent dosing. The preparation, anti-tumor effects and biodistribution of CPT-loaded PLA/PEG-PPG-PEG nanoparticles has been reported [73, 74]. Encapsulation of 9-NC in biodegradable PLGA nanoparticles has been described by Derakhshandeh *et al.* [75]. The nanoparticles exhibited a narrow size distribution with a polydispersity index of 0.01%, an average diameter of 207 $\pm$ 26nm, and a drug loading content of more than 33.5%. 3.63-fold and 5.40-fold increases in AUC were seen with 9-NC-nanocarriers for lactone and total 9-NC, respectively [76]. Other biodegradable copolymers that have been used as nanocarrier for CPT and its analogs include amphiphilic block copolymer of PLA, trimethylene carbonate and mPEG [77], mPEG-PLA [78], PLA-PEG-PLA [79] and methoxy poly(ethylene glycol)-*b*-poly(valerolactone) [80]. To summarize the present review, Table **3** shows the clinical trials of nano-sized drugs found in the literatures for the readers. Recently, combinatorial drug delivery, or combination therapy (use of multiple drugs) has been widely utilized to treat diseases or disorders in patients such as various cancers. In 2011, Zhang and co-worker reported the method for preparation lipid-polymer hybrid nanoparticles using DSPE-PEG and phospholipids to coat the polymeric nanoparticle core (DOX-PLA: CPT-PLA) for dual-drug delivery (DOX and CPT) [81]. The resulting lipid-polymer hybrid nanoparticles are highly stable in water, PBS and serum and have high drug loading yield (over 90% of drug). The particle size was around 100nm for molar ratio of DOX-PLA: CPT-PLA = 1:1 with narrow PDI value. The cytotoxicity of this dual-delivery system was tested against MDA-MB-435 breast cancer cells. The results indicate that the dual-delivery systems exhibited 3.5, 2.5, and 1.1-fold higher than those of single delivery system in the 3:1, 1:1 and 1:3 DOX-PLA:CPT-PLA combinations, respectively. This improvement of cytotoxicity of dual-delivery system can be explained by the fact that dual-drug loaded nanoparticles can deliver more consistent combination drug payloads to cells.

Recently, formulating poorly soluble drugs as nano suspensions can improve their bioavailability, reduce their large injection volume for intravenous administration, and also reduced undesired side effects. The CPT was prepared by supercritical anti-solvent process-high pressure homogenization technique resulting in mean diameter of nano-CPT was 125.1nm. The *in vitro* cytotoxicity of nano-CPT was

6-fold higher than that of topotecan against MCF-7 cell line. However, this nano-CPT exhibited higher IC_{50} values than those of CPT in DMSO against HCT-8, PC-3, and MCF-7 cell lines. Additionally, nano-CPT showed a similar antitumor activity topotecan [82].

Table 3: A summary of clinical trails of CPT and its analogs formulated in nano-sized dosage forms.

Formulation	**Administration Schedule**	**No. of Patients**	**Drug Limiting Toxicity**	**Dose Used in Phase II Trial ($mg/m^2/day$)**	**Ref.**
Liposomal-belotecan CKD-602	Once in three weeks	45	Bone marrow suppression febrile neutropenia and anemia	2.5 2.1	[75]
Liposomal-lurtotecan NX 211	Once in three weeks	29	Neutropenia and thrombocytopenia	3.8	[76]
Liposomal-lurtotecan (OSI-211)	Days 1st, 2nd, and 3rd in three weeks	81	Neutropenia and febrile neutropenia	1.8 2.4	[77]
Aerosolized liposomal-9-NC	5 Consecutive days every 8 week and 10 weeks a cycle	25	Chemical pharyngitis	0.5	[33, 78]
Liposome irinotecan.HCl: floxuridine CPX-1	90 Minutes every 14 days and 28 days a cycle	33	Diarrhea, neutropenia and hypokalemia	210mg Irinotecan +76mg floxuridine	[79]
Cyclodextrin-based polymer conjugate of IT-101	Days 1st, 8th, and 15th in a cycle of 28 days	12	Hematologic toxicity	< 30mg/m^2/month	[44]
NK012 SN-38-loaded (PEG-PEGlu) polymeric micelles	Once for three weeks	25	Grade 4 neutropenia	28mg/m^2/cycle	[51]

So far this article has reviewed various nano-sized dosage forms of CPT for cancer therapy. However, the therapeutic efficacy varies in different *in vivo* studies because of the nature of the multiple variances in the chemotherapy. To narrow down our discussion, here, we use dendrimer-based CPT drugs as an example to compare the differences for polymrer-CPT conjugate and CPT-encapsulated nanoparticles. In

Kaminskas *et al.*'s review article, they showed that CPT with covalent linkage dendrimers can stabilize the CPT, improve biodistribution and therapeutic efficacy, while that of CPT encapsulation displayed better aqueous solubility of CPT [83]. Therefore, the lactone stability and aqueous solubility of CPT are critical issues when developing an ideal drug delivery system.

CURRENT & FUTURE DEVELOPMENTS

The advancements in the nanotechnology are widely penetrating to biomedical sciences and technology. Since the discovery of the enhanced permeation and retention effect in 1986, a great variety of nano-sized dosage forms have been developed. Among tumorcidal agents classified in the cytotoxic chemotherapeutics, camptothecin (CPT) was proved to be effective in preclinical trials. Therefore, it is a great opportunity to overcome the current limitations of camptothecin and its derivatives. CPT-liposome formulations are known to stabilize active lactone form that hydrolyzes to inactive carboxylate form at physiological pH and increase the residence time in the bloodstream. Liposome-CPT has shown higher accumulation in tumors than free CPT and increases the therapeutic effectiveness. In addition, nanoparticle technology and development for anticancer drug delivery are being investigated. Although the present article reviews of the advancements in pharmaceutical dosage forms and associated drug carriers, there remains clinical unmet needs which hinder the freedom of chemotherapy. Therefore, the pharmaceutical practitioners are required to get into the insights of the clinical trials and discover the mechanistic findings to improve the drug delivery systems for CPT and its derivatives [84-88]. Finally, it is foreseeable that the clinical studies of nano-sized dosage forms of CPT and its derivatives will be expanding.

ACKNOWLEDGEMENTS

This work was supported by the National Science Council, Republic of China under grant NSC-99-2221-E-033-010.

CONFLICT OF INTEREST

The author's state no conflict of interest related to this publication.

DISCLOSURE

The chapter submitted for Patent eBook Series "Topics in Anti-Cancer Research", Volume 2 is an update of our article "Recent Development in Nano-Sized Dosage Forms of Plant Alkaloid Camptothecin", published in the journal 'Recent Patents on Anti-Cancer Drug Discovery', Volume 4, Number 3, November, 2009, Page 254 to 261 with modified title, additional text and references.

ABBREVIATIONS

9-AC	=	9-Amino camptothecin
9-NC	=	9-Nitrocamptothecin
mPEG	=	Monomethoxy poly(ethylene glycol)
A2780	=	Human ovarian adenocarcinoma
AUC	=	Area under the curve
CPT	=	Camptothecin
CPT-11	=	Irinotecan
DLPC	=	Dilauroylphosphatidylcholine
DOTAP	=	1,2-Diacyloxy-3-trimethylammonium propane
DDAB	=	Dimethyldioctadecylammonium bromide
DLT	=	Dose-limiting toxicity
H1299	=	Non-small lung carcinoma
H69	=	Small lung carcinoma
HCT-116	=	Human colon carcinoma
HT-29	=	Human colorectal adenocarcinoma

IT-101	=	Camptothecin-polymer conjugate
LS174T	=	Human colonic adenocarcinoma
MIA-Paca-2	=	Human pancreatic carcinoma
MDA-MB-231	=	Human breast adenocarcinoma
MDA-MB-45	=	Human breast carcinoma
MDR	=	Multi-drug resistance
MTD	=	Maximum tolerated dose
NGO-PEG	=	Pegylated nano-graphene oxide
OSI-211	=	Liposomal lurtotecan
OVCAR-3	=	Human ovarian carcinoma
Panc-1	=	Human pancreatic carcinoma
PC-3	=	human prostate adenocarcinoma
PEG	=	Poly(ethylene glycol)
PLA	=	Poly(D,L-lactic acid)
PLGA	=	Poly(D,L-lactide-co-glycolide)
QC-56	=	Human lung carcinoma
SN-38	=	7-Ethylene-10-hydroxy-camptothecin
TC71	=	LucEwing's sarcoma
Topo I	=	Topoisomerase I
U-87MG	=	Human malignant glioma

CL = Clearance

V_{ss} = Volume of distribution

REFERENCES

[1] Wall ME, Wani MC, Cook CE, Palmer KH, McPhail AT, Sim GA. Plant Antitumor agents. I. The isolation and structure of camptothecin, a novel alkaloidal leukemia and tumor inhibitor from *Camptotheca acuminata*. J Am Chem Soc 1966; 88(16): 3888-90.

[2] Verma RP, Hansch C. Camptothecins: A SAR/QSAR study. Chem Rev 2009; 109: 213-35.

[3] Zhang L, Bao Y, Knang Y, Chen F. Synthetic studies on camptothecins part 1: An improved asymmetric total synthesis of (20S)-camptothecin. Helv Chim Acta 2008; 91: 2057-61.

[4] Niizuma S, Tsukazaki M, Suda H, Murata T, Ohwada J, Ozawa S, *et al*. Synthesis of new camptothecin analogs with improved antitumor activities. Bioorg Med Chem Lett 2009; 19: 2018-21.

[5] Norbedo S, Dinon F, Bergamin M, Bosi S, Aroulmoji V, Khan R, *et al*. Synthesis of 6-amino-6-deoxyhyaluronan as an intermediate for conjugation with carboxylate-containing compounds: Application to hyaluronan-camptothecin conjugates. Carbohyd Res 2009; 344: 98-104.

[6] Kusari S, Zuehlke S, Spiteller M. An endophytic fungus from *Camptotheca acuminata* that produces camptothecin and analogues. J Nat Prod 2009; 72: 2-7.

[7] Lavergne O, Lesueur-Ginot L, Rodas FP, Kasprzyk PG, Pommier J, Demarquay D, *et al*. Homocamptothecins: Synthesis and antitumor activity of novel E-ring- modified camptothecin analogues. J Med Chem1998; 41(27): 5410-9.

[8] Lerchen H-G, Baumgarten J, von dem Bruch K, Lehmann TE, Sperzel M, Kempka G, *et al*. Design and optimization of 20-O-Linked camptothecin glycoconjugates as anticancer agents. J Med Chem 2001; 44(24): 4186-95.

[9] Koizumi F, Kitagawa M, Negishi T, Onda T, Matsumoto SI, Hamaguchi T, *et al*. Novel SN-38-incorporating polymeric micelles, NK012, eradicate vascular endothelial growth factor-secreting bulky tumors. Cancer Res 2006; 66(20): 10048-56.

[10] Greenwald RB, Pendri A, Conover C, Gilbert C, Yang R, Xia J. Drug delivery systems. 2. Camptothecin 20-*O*-poly (ethylene glycol) ester transport forms. J Med Chem 1996; 39(10): 1938-40.

[11] Cheng J, Khin KT, Davis ME. Antitumor activity of beta-cyclodextrin polymer-camptothecin conjugates. Molpharmaceut 2004; 1(3): 183-93.

[12] Zou Y, Wu QP, Tansey W, Chow D, Hung MC, Charnsangavej C, *et al*. Effectiveness of water soluble poly (L-glutamic acid)-camptothecin conjugate against resistant human lung cancer xenografted in nude mice. Int J Oncol 2001; 18(2): 331-6.

[13] Caiolfa VR, Zamai M, Fiorino A, Frigerio E, Pellizzoni C, d'Argy R, *et al*. Polymer-bound camptothecin: Initial biodistribution and antitumor activity studies. J Control Release 2000; 65(1-2): 105-19.

[14] Harada M, Sakakibara H, Yano T, Suzuki T, Okuno S. Determinants for the drug release from T-0128, camptothecin analogue-carboxymethyl dextran conjugate. J Control Release 2000; 69(3): 399-412.

[15] Thomas CJ, Rahier NJ, Hecht SM. Camptothecin: Current perspectives. Bioorg Med Chem 2004; 12: 1585-604.

[16] Ali I, Rahis-Uddin SK, Rajora AK, Rather MA, Wani WA, Haque A. Advances in nano drugs for cancer chemotherapy. Curr Cancer Drug Tar 2011; 11(2): 135-46.

[17] He C, Hu Y, Yin L, Tang C, Yin C. Effects of particle size and surface charge on cellular uptake and biodistribution of polymeric nanoparticles. Biomaterials 2010; 31: 3657-66.

[18] Zhao H, Rubio B, Sapra P, Wu DC, Reddy P, Sai P, *et al.* Novel prodrugs of SN38 using multi arm poly (ethylene glycol) linkers. Bioconjugate Chem 2008; 19: 849-9.

[19] Yu D, Peng P, Dharap SS, Wang Y, Mehlig M, Chandna P, *et al.* Antitumor activity of poly(ethylene glycol)-camptothecin conjugate: The inhibition of tumor growth *in vivo*. J Control Release 2005; 110: 90-102.

[20] Fang J, Nakamura H, Maeda H. The EPR effect: Unique features of tumor blood vessels for drug delivery, factors involved, and limitations and augmentation of the effect. Adv Drug Deliv Rev 2011; 63: 136-51.

[21] Cheng, J., Davis, M.E., Khin, K.T. Cyclodextrin-based polymers for therapeutics delivery. US7270808 (**2007**).

[22] Zhao, X., Bentley, M.D., Ren, Z., Viegas, T.X. Multi-arm polymer prodrugs. US7744861 (**2010**) & US20090074704 (**2009**).

[23] Zhao, H., Sapra, P. Treatment of resistant or refractory cancers with multi-arm polymeric conjugates of 7-ethyl-10-hydroxycamptothecin. US7928095 (**2011**).

[24] Rolke, J., Petter, R.C., Yin, M., Yurkovetskiy, A., Liu, G., Farhan, E. Pharmaceutical formulations of biodegradable biocompatible camptothecin-polymer conjugates. US20100179181 (**2010**).

[25] Eliasof, S. Compositions and methods for treatment of autoimmune and other disease. US20110300150 (**2011**) & US20120064107 (**2012**).

[26] Eliaz R, Nir S, Marty C, Szoka F. Determination and modeling of kinetics of cancer cell killing by doxorubicin and doxorubicin encapsulated in targeted liposomes. Cancer Res 2004; 64: 711-8.

[27] Griffiths GD, Bailey SC, Hambrook JL, Keyte M, Jayasekera P, Miles J, *et al.* Liposomally-encapsulated ricin toxoid vaccine delivered intratracheally elicits a good immune response and protects against a lethal pulmonary dose of ricin toxin. Vaccine 1997; 15: 1933-9.

[28] Auguste D, Prud'homme R, Ahl P, Meers P, Kohn J. Association of hydrophobically-modified poly(ethylene glycol) with fusogenic liposomes. BBA-Biomembranes 2003; 1616: 184-95.

[29] Xiong X, Huang Y, Lu W, Zhang H, Zhang X, Zhang Q, *et al.* Enhanced intracellular uptake of sterically stabilized liposomal doxorubicin *in vitro* resulting in improved antitumor activity *in vivo*. Pharm Res 2005; 22: 933-9.

[30] Han HD, Lee A, Song CK, Hwang T, Seong H, Lee CO, *et al. In vivo* distribution and antitumor activity of heparin-stabilized doxorubicin-loaded liposomes. Int J Pharmceut 2006; 313: 181-8.

[31] Calvo P, Gouritin B, Chacun H, Desmaile D, D'Angelo J, Noel JP, *et al.* Long-circulating PEGylated polycyanoacrylate nanoparticles as new drug carrier for brain delivery. Pharm Res 2001; 18: 1157-66.

[32] Immordino ML, Dosio F, Cattel L. Stealth liposomes: Review of the basic science, rationale, and clinical applications, existing and potential. Int J Nanomed 2006; 1: 297-315.

[33] Hsieh MF, Lin TY, Gau RJ, Chang HT, Lo YL, Lai CH. Biodegradable polymeric-nanoparticles bearing stealth PEG shell and lipophilic polyester core. J Chin Inst Chem Engrs 2005; 36: 609-15.

[34] Koshkina N, Gilbert B, Waldrep J, Seryshev A, Knight V. Distribution of camptothecin after delivery as a liposome aerosol or following intramuscular injection in mice. Cancer Chemoth Pharm 1999; 44: 187-92.

[35] Knight, J.V., Koshkina, N., Gilbert, B., Waldrep, J.C., Wellen, C.W., Giovanella, B. Small particle liposome aerosols for delivery of anti-cancer drugs. WO9915153 (**1999**).

[36] Koshkina NV, Knight V, Gilbert BE, Golunski E, Roberts L, Waldrep JC. Improved respiratory delivery of the anticancer drugs, camptothecin and paclitaxel, with 5% CO_2-enriched air: Pharmacokinetic studies. Cancer Chemoth Pharm 2001; 47(5): 451-6.

[37] Waldrep, J.C., Knight, J.V., Koshkina, N. Carbon dioxide enhancement of inhalation therapy. US6440393 (**2002**).

[38] Perez-Soler, R., Sugarman, S.M., Poirot, K.R. Lipid complexed topoisomerase I inhibitors. US5834012 (**1998**).

[39] Knight, J.V., Koshkina, N., Gilbert, B., Verschraegen, C.F. Small particle liposome aerosols for delivery of anticancer drugs. US7348025 (**2008**) & US20060204447 (**2006**).

[40] Verschraegen, C.F., Knight, J.V., Koshkina, N., Gilbert, B. Small particle liposome aerosols for delivery of anti-cancer drugs. US20080248096 (**2008**).

[41] Chen J, Cai B, Ping Q, Liu M, Guo J. Lactone stability and tissue distribution of free and liposomal encapsulated 9-nitrocamptothecin in rats following intravenous injection. Drug DevInd Pharm 2008; 34: 853-9.

[42] Chen J, Ping QN, Guo JX, Chu XZ, Song MM. Effect of phospholipid composition on characterization of liposomes containing 9-nitrocamptothecin. Drug DevInd Pharm 2006; 32: 719-26.

[43] Rahman, A., Ahmad, I. Liposomal formulation of irinotecan. US20050019387 (**2005**).

[44] Yoshino, K., Nozawa, S., Isozaki, M., Sawada, S., Kato, I., Matsuzaki, T. Irinotecan preparation. US20080069868 (**2008**).

[45] Mundus, C., Welz, C., Schramel, O., Haas, H., Fichert, T., Schulze, B., Peymann, T., Michaelis, U., Teifel, M., Gruber, F., Winter, G. Method of producing a cationic liposomal preparation comprising a lipophilic compound. US20120087975 (**2012**).

[46] Reis CP, Neufeld RJ, Ribeiro AJ, Veiga F. Nanoencapsulation I. Methods for preparation of drug-loaded polymeric nanoparticles. Nanomedicine NBM 2006; 2: 8-21.

[47] Matsumura Y, Maeda H. A new concept for macromolecular therapeutics in cancer-chemotherapy - mechanism of tumoritropic accumulation of proteins and the antitumor agent smancs. Cancer Res 1986; 46: 6387-92.

[48] Cheng J, Khin KT, Jensen GS, Liu A, Davis ME. Synthesis of linear, β-cyclodextrin-based polymers and their camptothecin conjugates. Bioconjugate Chem 2003; 14: 1007-17.

[49] Cheng J, Khin KT, Davis ME. Antitumor activity of β-cyclodextrin polymer-camptothecin conjugates. Mol Pharm 2004; 1: 183-93.

[50] Schluep T, Cheng J, Khin K, Davis M. Pharmacokinetics and biodistribution of the camptothecin-polymer conjugate IT-101 in rats and tumor-bearing mice. Cancer Chemoth Pharm 2006; 57: 654-62.

[51] Schluep T, Hwang J, Cheng J. Preclinical efficacy of the camptothecin-polymer conjugate IT-101 in multiple cancer models. Clin Cancer Res 2006; 12: 1606-14.

[52] Oliver JC, Yen Y, Synold TW, Schluep T, Davis M.A dose-finding pharmacokinetic study of IT-101, the first *de novo* designed nanoparticle therapeutic, in refractory solid tumors. J Clin Oncol 2008; 26(15S): 14538.
[53] Ryan, J., Schluep, T., Yun, Y., Oliver, J.C., Davis, M. Treatment of cancer. US20110245201(**2011**).
[54] Ryan, J. Treatment of cancer. US20120064071 (**2012**).
[55] Saltz LB, Cox JV, Blanke C, Rosen LS, Fehrenbacher L, Moore MJ, *et al.* Irinotecan plus fluorouracil and leucovorin for metastatic colorectal cancer. New Engl J Med 2000; 343: 905-14.
[56] Matsumura Y. Poly (amino acid) micelle nanocarriers in preclinical and clinical studies. Adv Drug Deliver Rev 2008; 60: 899-914.
[57] Sumitomo M, Koizumi F, Asano T, Horiguchi A, Ito K, Asano T, *et al.* Novel SN-38-incorporated polymeric micelle, NK012, strongly suppresses renal cancer progression. Cancer Res 2008; 68(6); 1631-5.
[58] Saito Y, Yasunaga M, Kuroda J, Koga Y, Matsumura Y. Enhanced distribution of NK012, a polymeric micelle-encapsulated SN-38, and sustained release of SN-38 within tumors can beat a hypovascular tumor. Cancer Sci 2008; 99: 1258-64.
[59] Burris HA, III, Infante JR, Spigel DR, Greco FA, Thompson DS, Matsumoto S, *et al.* A Phase I dose-escalation study of NK012. J Clin Oncol 2008; 26(15S) (May 20 Suppl; abstr 2538).
[60] Nakajima TE, Yanagihara K, Takigahira M, Yasunaga M, Kato K,Hamaguchi T, *et al.* Antitumor effect of SN-38-releasing polymeric micelles, NK012, on spontaneous peritoneal metastases from orthotopic gastric cancer in mice compared with irinotecan. Cancer Res 2008; 68: 9318-22.
[61] Hamaguchi T, Doi T, Eguchi-Nakajima T, Kato K, Yamada Y, Shimada Y, *et al.* Phase I study of NK012, a novel SN-38-incorporating micellar nanoparticle, in adult patients with solid tumors. Clin Cancer Res 2010; 16: 5058-66.
[62] Liu Z, Robinson JT, Sun X, Dai H. PEGylated nanographene oxide for delivery of water-insoluble cancer drugs. J Am Chem Soc 2008; 130: 10876-77.
[63] Dai, H., Liu, Z., Lin, X., Sun, X. Supramolecular functionalization of graphitic nanoparticles for drug delivery. WO2009018092 (**2009**).
[64] Seo, M.H., Choi, I.J. Biodegradable poly (alkylene oxide)-poly (p-dioxanone) block copolymer soluble in organic solvents, and drug delivery composition comprising same. US6599519 (**2003**).
[65] Kim, S.C., Chang, E.O., Song, I.S., Pai, C.M. Biodegradable polymeric micelle-type drug composition and method for the preparation thereof. US6322805 (**2001**).
[66] Seo, M.H., Choi, I.J. Polymeric composition for solubilizing poorly water soluble drugs and process for the preparation thereof. US6616941 (**2003**)
[67] Kim, H.H., Yeo, G.D., Yi, Y.W. Biodegradable copolymer as drug delivery matrix comprising polyethyleneoxide and aliphatic polyester blocks. US5548035 (**1996**).
[68] Zhao, X. Multi-arm block copolymers as drug delivery vehicles. US6730334 (**2004**).
[69] Leroux, J.C., Benahmed, A.S. Polymeric micelle compositions. US6338859(**2002**).
[70] Kang, H.W., Yim, E.Y., Seo, M.H. Submicron nanoparticle of poorly water soluble camptothecin derivatives and process for preparation thereof. WO2008038944 (**2008**).
[71] Miura H, Onishi H, Sasatsu M, Machida Y. Antitumor characteristics of methoxypolyethylene glycol-poly(DL-lactic acid) nanoparticles containing camptothecin. J Control Release 2004; 97: 101-13.

[72] Onishi H, Machida Y, Machida Y. Antitumor properties of irinotecan-containing nanoparticles prepared using poly (DL-lactic acid) and poly(ethylene glycol)-block-poly(propylene glycol)-block-poly(ethylene glycol). Biol Pharm Bull 2003; 26: 116-9.

[73] Kunii R, Onishi H, Machida Y. Preparation and antitumor characteristics of PLA/(PEG-PPG-PEG) nanoparticles loaded with camptothecin. Eur J Pharm Biopharm 2007; 67: 9-17.

[74] Onishi H, Machida Y. Macromolecular and nanotechnological modification of camptothecin and its analogs to improve the efficacy. Curr Drug Discovery Technol 2005; 2: 169-83.

[75] Derakhshandeh K, Erfan M, Dadashzadeh S. Encapsulation of 9-nitrocamptothecin, a novel anticancer drug, in biodegradable nanoparticles: Factorial design, characterization and release kinetics. Eur J Pharm Biopharm 2007; 66: 34-41.

[76] Dadashzadeh S, Derakhshandeh K, Shirazi FH. 9-Nitrocamptothecin polymeric nanoparticles: Cytotoxicity and pharmacokinetic studies of lactone and total forms of drug in rats. Anti-Cancer Drug 2008; 19: 805-11.

[77] Gao J, Ming J, He B, Fan Y, Gu Z, Zhang X. Preparation and characterization of novel polymeric micelles for 9-nitro-20(S)-camptothecin delivery. Eur J Pharm Sci 2008; 34: 85-93.

[78] Gao JM, Ming J, He B, Gu ZW, Zhang XD. Controlled release of 9-nitro-20(S) camptothecin from methoxy poly (ethylene glycol)-poly(D,L-lactide) micelles. Biomed Mater 2008; 3 (doi: 10.1088/1748-6041/3/1/015013).

[79] Lee W, Li Y, Chu I. Amphiphilic poly (D, L-lactic acid)/poly (ethylene glycol)/poly(D,L-lactic acid) nanogels for controlled release of hydrophobic drugs. Macromol Biosci 2006; 6: 846-54.

[80] Chang Y, Chu I. Methoxypoly (ethylene glycol)-b-poly(valerolactone) diblock polymeric micelles for enhanced encapsulation and protection of camptothecin. Eur Polym J 2008; 44: 3922-30.

[81] Zhang, L., Aryal, S., Hu, C.M. Ratiometric combinatorial drug delivery. WO2011143201 (**2011**).

[82] Yao L, Zhao X, Li Q, Zu Y, Fu Y, Zu B, *et al. In vitro* and *in vivo* evaluation of camptothecin nanosuspension: A novel formulation with high antitumor efficacy and low toxicity. Int J Pharm 2012; 423: 586-8.

[83] Kaminskas LM, McLeod VM, Porter C, Boyd BJ. Association of chemotherapeutic drugs with dendrimer nanocarriers: An assessment of the merits of covalent conjugation compared to non covalent encapsulation. Mol Pharmaceut 2012; 9(3): 355-73.

[84] Zambon WC, Ramalingam S, Friedland DM, Edwards RP, Stoller RG, Strychor S, *et al.* Phase I and pharmacokinetic study of pegylated liposomal CKD-602 in patients with advanced malignancies. Clin Cancer Res 2009; 15(4): 1466-72.

[85] Kehrer DFS, Bos AM, Verweij J, Groen HJ, Loos WJ, Sparreboom A, *et al.* Phase I and pharmacologic study of liposomal lurtotecan, NX 211: Urinary excretion predicts hematologic toxicity. J Clin Oncol 2002; 20(5): 1222-31.

[86] Dark, GG, Calvert AH, Grimshaw, R, Poole, C, Swenerton, K, Kaye S, *et al.* Randomized trial of two intravenous schedules of the topoisomerase I inhibitor liposomal lurtotecan in women with relapsed epithelial ovarian cancer: A trial of the National Cancer Institute of Canada Clinical Trials Group. J Clin Oncol 2005; 23(9): 1859-66.

[87] Verschraegen CF, Gilbert BE, Loyer E, Huaringa A, Walsh G, Newman RA, *et al.* Clinical evaluation of the delivery and safety of aerosolized liposomal 9-Nitro-20(S)-camptothecin in patients with advanced pulmonary malignancies. Clin Cancer Res 2004; 10(7): 2319-26.

[88] Batist G, Gelmon KA, Chi KN,Miller WH, Chia SKL, Mayer LD, *et al.* Safety, pharmacokinetics, and efficacy of CPX-1 liposome injection in patients with advanced solid tumors. Clin Cancer Res 2009; 15(2): 692-700.

Send Orders of Reprints at reprints@benthamscience.net

Topics in Anti-Cancer Research, Vol. 2, 2013, 522-552

CHAPTER 15

Onconutrition: Redox Chemoprevention by Functional Biomolecules and Biomarker Assessment

María D. Defagó and Elio A. Soria*

Escuela de Nutrición e Instituto de Biología Celular, Facultad de Ciencias Médicas, Universidad Nacional de Córdoba, Argentina

Abstract: Cancer, a leading cause of death, can be prevented by different nutrients, in accordance to epidemiological and experimental data. Cancer chemoprevention might involve different dietary substances, which can counteract genetic damage and modulate the acquisition of a neoplastic phenotype. Critical to this process is redox cellular homeostasis, with antioxidants and essential biomolecules being the most promising functional compounds of the diet. Nutritional interventions require accurate biomarkers in order to evaluate their appropriateness. Such parameters may be biological targets involved in the oncogenetic process, and biochemical changes deriving from the organic response to tumors, which can be considered as endpoints of dietary interventions. This chapter reviews the patents on recent progress in the development of redox-related anticancer nutritional interventions involving lipophilic compounds, and of scientific-based biological markers for evaluating them.

Keywords: Antioxidant, bioassay, biomarker, cancer, carcinogenesis, cellular differentiation, chemoprevention, chronic disease, clinical biochemistry, cytotoxicity, diet, fatty acid, immunity, inflammation, lipid, oxidative stress, phytochemical, polyphenol, synergy, tissue homeostasis.

INTRODUCTION

Many dietary compounds might be able to modulate and control the evolution of oncological diseases [1], such as liposoluble biomolecules closely related to cellular redox homeostasis (e.g., fatty acids and polyphenols). Regarding this, we have proposed the term Onconutrition to assess the biomedical role of nutrients as

***Address correspondence to Elio A. Soria:** Instituto de Biología Celular, Enrique Barros S/N, Ciudad Universitaria, Córdoba 5014, Córdoba, Argentina; Tel: +543514334020; Fax: +543514334023; E-mails: easoria@fcm.unc.edu.ar; danieladefago@hotmail.com

Atta-ur Rahman and Khurshid Zaman (Eds)

epigenetic modulating agents of the processes involved in cancer pathogenesis. This kind of approach enables different health strategies to be developed for preventing tumor appearance and progression [2]. In order to confirm this in humans, suitable biological parameters are required, among which the properties of transformed malignant cells and systemic responses to neoplastic disease might be used as biomarkers of cancer development. Regarding this, criteria to define a biomarker were taken from McCarthy and Shugart [3], which are classically accepted for scientific works. In this line, onconutritional biomarkers can represent exposition (e.g. nutrient metabolite dosage in plasma) or effect (e.g. lost of cancer viability by a determined nutrient).

I. NUTRITIONAL CANCER CHEMOPREVENTION BY REDOX-REGULATION

Involvement of Oxidative Stress in Cancer Development

Cancer is a multistage process with increasing failures in the mechanisms involved in cellular differentiation and proliferation. Clones are therefore able to invade and colonize various tissues [4]. The successive stages are:

1. Initiation (a normal cell is transformed): Rapid and irreparable damage occurs in the DNA.

2. Promotion (the initiated cell becomes pre-neoplastic): Over the years, the clone suffers various biological changes.

3. Progression (the pre-neoplastic cell become malignant): Finally, a neoplastic phenotype appears (self-promoted growth, inhibition and death resistance, unlimited replicating potential, angiogenic induction, and capacity for tissue invasion and metastasis) [5]. The complexity of this process is increased by the heterotypic microenvironment created within the tumor, with both malignant sub-clones and normal connective cells conditioning illness evolution [6, 7].

In this regard, there is a close relation between oxidative stress and neoplastic transformation involving different altered biochemical pathways and apoptosis-resistant clone selection due to hostile extracellular conditions [8]. Oxidative stress involves a loss of balance between the positive and negative effects of free radicals, with all responses being aimed at resetting the cell basal state. Nonetheless, these responses acquire pro-neoplastic properties when they become persistent [9]. Furthermore, free radicals can induce the three oncogenetic stages (initiation, promotion and progression) by oxidative damage of crucial molecules, such as DNA. Finally, tumor cells can exhibit different oxidation-induced genetic abnormalities [10], as follows:

- Increased oncogene activity (e.g., tyrosinases, embryonic products) and/or loss of tumor-suppressor gene protein products (e.g. p53, apoptotic molecules) as a consequence of chromosomal aberrations

- Unregulated production of growth factors (e.g., insulin-like growth factor 2), and tumor angiogenesis factors (e.g., haematopoietic growth factors) by alterations in DNA methylation patterns and genetic imprinting errors

- Genetic instability leading to progressive loss of regulated cell proliferation, increased invasiveness, and increased metastatic potential

- Alteration in enzyme patterns (e.g., increased levels of enzymes involved in nucleic acid synthesis, antioxidant defence, and macromolecular lysis)

The most important free radicals derive from oxygen (reactive oxygen species -ROS-; e.g., superoxide anion, hydroxyl radical) and nitric oxide (reactive nitrogen species -RNS-; e.g., peroxynitrite), with their effects being mediated by enzymatic and non-enzymatic derivates that in the former are more strongly oxidizing than molecular oxygen itself. The formation of these intermediates must steadily be controlled by the cell in order to maintain a redox homeostasis, which is involved in mechanisms of cellular signaling, regulation and survival in tissues [11], with high amounts of these being deleterious [12].

Cancer Chemoprevention by Redox-Modulating Nutrients

The effects of reactive species therefore depend on the extent to which their formation leads to homeostatic recovery (normal stress response) or to chronic deregulation and cellular transformation. Within this frame, nutrition plays an important role in these processes because different essential micronutrients and other dietary compounds are able to modulate free radical production due to both their intrinsic redox activity and their systemic bioavailability, given certain cases in which the availability of a micronutrient does not necessarily follow increased consumption [13]. Thus, dietary antioxidant compounds such as lipids, trace elements (selenium, zinc), vitamins (A, C, E), thiols and polyphenols (flavonoids, curcumin), among others may act as cancer modulating agents [14, 15], which can be general (for many cancer types) or specific (for a determined tumor) [16], and they have been thoroughly evaluated in cancer chemoprevention. Different compounds may be provided in food, supplements, pharmaceutical compositions, or cosmetics.

Cell susceptibility to nutrients depends on genetic information and epigenetic regulation, and the resultant phenotype may be modulated by nutrients. As a result, the expression of many genes is firmly regulated by the availability and quality of dietary compounds [17]. Moreover, the DNA damage caused by genotoxic and mutagenic insults (e.g., lipoperoxyl radicals) may be counteracted by cytoprotective agents found in foods and plants [18]. Another important aspect highly considered is the existence of nucleotide polymorphisms which determine human susceptibility to xenobiotic cancer modulators and potential pro-neoplastic phenotypes. Consequently, these polymorphisms must also be evaluated [19].

Among different nutrients, these two groups with relevant biomedical potential for cancer chemoprevention have given their multi-target redox-related activity:

- **Unsaturated fatty acids:** The chemical composition of biological membranes can be manipulated by exogenous lipid intake to change their physiological properties [20]. The function of proteins associated with membrane rafts (e.g., some kinase species) may be compromised, with malignant parameters being affected. Thus, lipid integrity and membrane markers could be useful markers. In this regard, oxidative damage of polyunsaturated fatty acids causes the formation of lipid peroxides and other secondary products, which may deregulate cellular pathways and modulate the tumor redox resistance [21]. These metabolites have already been proposed as redox biomarkers in nutritional interventions [22], with molecular basis about their involvement in carcinogenesis having been already elaborated [16]. The carbon chains of polyunsaturated fatty acids can present two or more double bonds, with the omega family depending on the first double bond position from the last carbon [23].

- **Polyphenols:** In recent years, a group of dietary compounds, the plant polyphenols (organic molecules characterized by the presence of large multiples of phenol structural units), such as flavonoids, has been proposed for cancer prevention [24], given their antioxidant activity and their affinity for biological membranes and other molecular targets [25, 26]. Also, they can change *in vivo* the bioavailability and the bioactivity of other substances, such as nutrients and drugs [27], which in turn can alter cell polyphenol activity [28]. In this regard, cancer chemopreventive and therapeutic methods based on the administration of phenolic compositions have recently been developed [29].

Also, both groups of bioactive molecules can interact in the organism given their lipophilicity. For example, triterpene saponins, constituents of many folk remedies and some of the more recently developed plant drugs, are known to form complexes with cholesterol by binding plasma lipids [30]. Thus, polyphenols compounds might change cellular response to lipid intake and, as a result, they modify fatty acid bioactivity Fig. (**1**).

Molecular Redox-Related Pathways in Cancer Development

The carcinogenetic involvement of redox metabolism has been confirmed by the fact that metal-associated compounds are able to modulate cancer progression. For example, cupredoxins are chemopreventive agents leading to cancer death by compromising endocytosis. This effect depends on the use of protein transduction domains derived from them (including p18 and p28 truncations) [31]. Moreover, expression of antioxidant genes is one of the most important criteria, together with DNA repair and transcription factor genes, for assessing cancer risk, with the transcript determination as a suitable means [32].

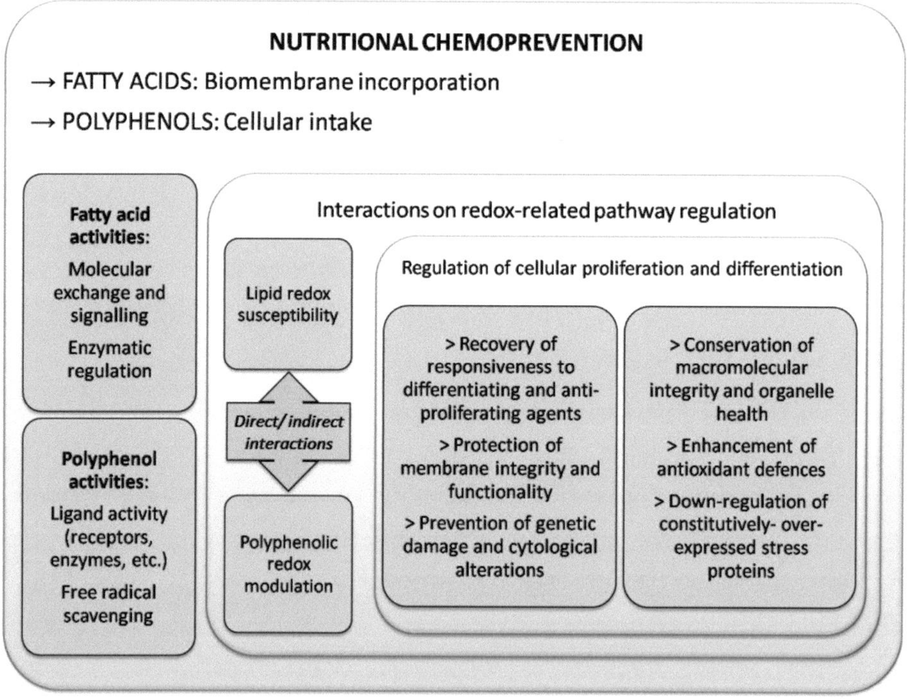

Figure 1: Onconutritional potential of dietary organic redox-related compounds: Fatty acids (essential unsaturated fatty acids) and polyphenols (flavonoids and related compounds).

Concerning this, the described dietary compounds are able to inhibit oxidative stress-sensitive pro-carcinogenetic pathways. Among them, the NF-κB activity is crucial, as is one of the central regulators of an organism's responses to various stress signals [33]. It is a ubiquitous transcription factor that regulates the transcription of a number of genes involved in immune pathways, such as pro-inflammatory cytokines and adhesion molecules and cellular proliferation, since it is an anti-apoptotic factor [34]. Deregulation of NF-κB contributes to a variety of pathological conditions such as septic shock, acute inflammation, viral replication, and malignant promotion [35]. Because of its role in inflammation and carcinogenesis, NF-κB inhibition has relevant implications for anticancer therapy. Furthermore, some downstream effects due to inhibition of NF-κB activity are such as a decrease in levels of inducible nitric oxide synthase (iNOS, a lipid membrane-bound enzyme) and cyclooxygenase-2 (COX-2, an eicosanoid-related enzyme) expression. Both iNOS and COX-2 have critical roles in the response of tissues to oxidative injury, and promote carcinogenesis [36].

In addition to the redox modulating effects of nutrients, macromolecular pathways can be affected by direct oxidative damage, of which protein biomarkers may be any amino acid that has undergone oxidation (or other modification, e.g. chlorotyrosine, dityrosine), and in this case especially, oxidized sulphur- or selenium-containing amino acids. They can be detected with an antibody that binds to them, which could aid in assessing the efficacy of environmental, nutritional and therapeutic interventions [37].

Biological Effects on Neoplastic Cells

Neoplastic cells have lost their differentiation grade to varying extents, but they have unlimitedly increased their proliferating capacity. Thus, biomedical approaches aim at inducing cytodifferentiation or cytotoxicity, respectively, and in this regard, nutrients can act as cytodifferentiating or cytotoxic agents in cancer therapy, whereas they should be cytoprotective for normal cells [38]. Cell protection and differentiation are thus crucial for cancer chemoprevention, and involve various actions intended to conserve or restore normal features in cells. For example, different regulators of the non-genomic action of progesterone have been developed in order to attenuate progesterone's inhibition of ovarian cancer apoptosis so that the neoplastic tissue recovers its responsiveness to therapeutic agents [39]. Among the polyphenols, 2-oxadiazolechromone derivatives are inhibitors of tyrosine kinase and can be employed for the treatment of tumors, for neuroprotection and for protection of the stress proteins of the skin [40].

When cells are initiated and acquire neoplastic characteristics, another kind of approach is necessary in which the induction of cytotoxicity in tumor cells is the main resource, although cytodifferentiation may still be involved in controlling some malignant properties [41]. In this regard, cytotoxicity involves the loss of cellular viability (cytolethality), the control of cellular proliferation (cytostasis), and pro-lethal injuries at different subcellular levels leading to cellular dysfunction (cytocompromise) (Tables **1** & **2**).

The modulation of cell proliferation by a determined polyphenol composition (e.g., polyphenol compounds extracted from *Olea europaea, Caiazzana* olives) comprises the induction of cell cycle arrest and apoptosis [42]. Polyphenols can control cancer proliferation by inducing apoptosis, which is frequently inhibited in tumor cells. These molecules can interact with specific regulating steps of cell death depending on their concentration, the cell system, the type or stage of the pathological process [43]. Proteomic studies in prostate cancer have shown that anticancer biological effects of polyphenols depend on their interaction with deregulated pathways, which participate in cytoskeletal functions, apoptosis, proteasome activity, NF-κB signaling, cancer cell proliferation, invasion and angiogenesis [44]. These effects can also be induced by extracellular modulation of cell interactions with tissue environment. Indeed, the tea polyphenol (-)-epigallocatechin-3-*O*-gallate stop with cancer progression by interacting with the 67-kDa laminin receptor (metastasis-related cell adhesion molecule), inhibiting the cellular proliferation [45]. Another example of an anticancer nutrient is genistein, a naturally occurring isoflavonoid isolated from soy products, being a tyrosine kinase inhibitor which has been shown to inhibit the proliferation of oestrogen-positive and oestrogen-negative human breast cancer cell lines, which depended on inhibition of the HER2 proto-oncogene (member of the epidermal growth factor receptor family, which is over-expressed in 20-30% of breast cancers) [46]. These authors proved that genistein delays mammary tumor onset *in vivo* (transgenic mice that over-express HER2 gene) and *in vitro* (BT-474 cells that are ERα- and ERβ+), by restraining HER2 protein expression and phosphorylation. Some plant triterpene aglycones exhibit cytotoxic or cytostatic properties against human carcinoma cells [47].

Table 1: Biological objectives of anticancer nutrition*.

A. Cytodifferentiation	
Cellular Responses	**Examples (Potential Biomarkers)**
Cytological Parameters:	
➢ Conservation of cell morphology	Cytoskeleton arrangement and membrane limits by immunocytofluorescence
➢ Prevention of cytological alterations	Cytoplasmic basophilia, nuclear number and size, nucleus/cytoplasm ratio, cell clusters and cords by optical microscopy.
➢ Secretion of cellular products	Lipid vesicles by Nile red staining
Plasma Membrane Biology:	
➢ Regulation of molecular exchange	Glucose transporters or multidrug resistance protein expression by Western-blotting
➢ Recovery of cell-cell and cell-extracellular matrix interactions	E-cadherin and major histocompatibility complex protein expression by immunhistochemistry
➢ Disappearance of tumor antigens	Carcinoembryonic antigen expression by ELISA
➢ Normal glycosilation	Ganglioside content by lipid extraction, cell surface glycoprotein expression by immunhistochemistry
➢ Lipid profile improvement	Content of n-3, n-6 and n-9 fatty acids, saturated/unsaturated fatty acid relation by gas chromatography

Table 1: contd…

Molecular Response and Growth Regulation:	
➢ Down-regulation of over-expressed antioxidant enzymes	Superoxide dismutase and γ-glutamyltranspeptidase by *kinetic* analysis
➢ Recovery of response to differentiation-inducing agents	Retinoic acid receptor expression by Western-blotting
➢ Recovery of regulating mechanisms of cellular proliferation	Proliferation assessment under metabolic restriction by vital staining, contact inhibition and anchorage dependence by migration systems
➢ Down-regulation of stress-related proteins and altered signal-transduction mechanisms constitutively activated	Heat shock protein 72, activated c-Jun *N*-terminal kinase, growth factor receptor expression by Western-blotting
B. Cytotoxicity	
Cellular Responses	Examples (Potential Biomarkers)
Growth Inhibition and Programmed Cell Death:	
➢ Cell cycle arrest	Cyclin inhibition by immunocytochemistry, mitotic spindle disruption by miscrocopy
➢ Up-regulation of death receptors and oncosuppressor proteins	FAS and p53 expressions by immunohistochemistry
➢ Down-regulation of anti-apoptotic proteins	Bcl-2 expression by Western blotting
➢ Apoptosis	Caspase activity by inhibitory tests, phosphatidylserine exteriorization by annexin-V assay
Free Radical Activity:	
➢ Reactive oxygen species	Superoxide anion, hydrogen peroxide by nitro blue tetrazolium staining.
➢ Reactive nitrogen species	Nitric oxide by Griess method, peroxinitrite by oxidizable detectors (i.e. dichlorofluorescin) or immunocytochemistry
➢ Reactive sulphur species	Sulphates by turbidimetry, thioradicals and sulfanilamides by high-performance liquid chromatography
Stress-related Responses and Intracellular Signaling:	
➢ Cytoskeleton re-arrangement	Actin stress fibres and granules and tubulin polymerization by immunocytochemistry
➢ Activity of redox-related pathways which regulate apoptosis	MAPK induction and NF-kB inhibition by interference RNA technology
Oxidative Macromolecular Damage:	
➢ Proteins and peptides	Oxidized sulphur groups (SS-bounds), glutathione deprivation, oxidized aromatic amino acids (nitrotyrosine), and carbonyl derivates by colorimetric assays
➢ Lipids	Conjugated dienes, hydroperoxides and short-chain fragments and adducts with other biological molecules by high-performance liquid chromatography
➢ Nucleic acids	Oxidized bases (8-oxo-guanidine, thyminglycol) by high-performance liquid chromatography. DNA adducts by UV-absorption.
➢ Sugars	Malondialdehyde by spectrophotometry

* Mentioned parameters constitute a non-limiting list.

II. BIOMARKER DEVELOPMENT

Clinical-Epidemiological Framework

The role of nutritional biomarkers was described in 1983 by Solomons and Allen, who emphasized their crucial role in the assessment of nutritional status [48]. In recent times, technological advances in bioengineering, molecular biology and physiology have enabled the development of different tests to identify parameters which directly reflect food consumption [49]. Thus, nutritional biomarkers have been developed to evaluate and validate different types of dietary surveys and interventions, and the future seems promising because the methodologies applied have been progressively improved, reducing technical and analytical errors [50]. On the other hand, while biomarkers are frequently used as surrogate efficacy endpoints to expedite the process, biomarker assessment and validation have proven to be difficult because dietary agents exert multiple actions with an unknown hierarchy of biological importance [51]. A valid nutritional biomarker should present a specific, appropriate half-life and a good biomarker-intake correlation [52].

The use of biochemical markers for assessing nutritional status in clinical practice involves the identification of compounds [53], such as:

- Proteins: albumin, transferrin, retinol-bound protein, etc.
- Carbohydrates: glucose, etc.
- Lipids: cholesterol, triglycerides, etc.
- Vitamins: vitamin C, vitamin E, etc.
- Minerals: zinc, iron, copper, sodium, potassium, etc.

These molecules and elements have been studied extensively in risk assessment of different chronic illnesses (e.g., heart ischemia, dementia and cancer) [54].

Blood is the most commonly used biological fluid for biomarker determination. Although some tests can be conducted in whole blood, plasma (serum) is considered more appropriate, as it is more sensitive to dietary intake [55]. An example of plasma parameter directly related to cancer development is the plasma cholesterol level, with detection of this nutrient being proposed to study various tumors, such as breast cancer. Moreover, recent technical advances, such as the differential scanning calorimetry, allow the assessment of blood proteomic profile in cancer diagnosis. Another sample is urine, which is considers as a good indicator of the intake of hydrosoluble compounds, since their concentration in urine depends on the degree of saturation of nutrients in tissues [56]. Recently, the use of saliva for analysis of biological compounds to evaluate the nutritional status has expanded, as this is easily obtained by non-invasive methods and presents suitable levels of lipids (e.g., cholesterol, unsaturated fatty acids) and other dietary compounds [57].

One of the most significant advances is the development of biomarkers designed to minimize methodological inaccuracies in dietary studies, to be used as additional measures of environmental exposure and as tools to test the effects of diet in chronic diseases [58]. Such biomarkers emerge from the existing interactions between diet, lifestyle, genetics, and the risk of many chronic diseases [59], with nutritional epidemiology becoming a strong support for oncological approaches [60, 61]. Nowadays, a combination of biomarker measurements with long-term dietary intake parameters is considered to measure exposure data [62]. This was the scientific rationale for designing and developing the European Prospective Investigation into Cancer and Nutrition (EPIC), which combines epidemiological and laboratory studies on healthy people, with the assessment of biochemical markers and genetic susceptibility [63]. Among the evaluated nutrients, fatty acids, carotenoids, tocopherols, vitamin D, folate, vitamin B12 and trace elements, were assayed in plasma [64].

For oncological risk assessment, genetic studies must be associated with specific biochemical activities to identify individuals with increased or decreased risk of some cancer types, involving the use of biochemical (e.g., hormones, enzymes) and genetic profiles of specific alleles of different genes [65]. For example, the methylation status of the COX-2 gene promoter region can be a prognostic therapeutic biomarker [66]. This kind of approach has increased in risk evaluation given the development of molecular marker detection by RNA microarrays [67].

Nonetheless, cytological methods of detecting progression from pre-cancer to cancer are still valuable, utilizing toluidine blue staining as well as detecting allelic variation at microsatellite loci, with an allelic variation in one or more loci being indicative of that progression [68]. Between cellular parameters and molecular markers, ultrastructural biomarkers from a given biological sample can also be identified. Thus, the image generated of them can be utilized for screening and monitoring diseases, evaluating drug and therapeutic efficacy, and assessing risks associated with a determined therapeutic candidate [69].

Biochemical Assessment of Lipid-Related Biomarkers

The implications and effects of dietary compounds on oxide-reduction processes can be evaluated through several specific biomarkers. These indicators mainly include the oxidative products of lipids, proteins and nucleic acids induced by free radical activity, and the complex of antioxidant molecules which appears as a response [70]. As regards lipids, radicals attack compounds with the structural element $-CH=CH-CH_2-CH=CH-$. Thus, in theory, they may act on all polyunsaturated fatty acids (PUFAs), either in free or conjugated forms, although some PUFAs are better ROS substrates than others. Radicals induce the generation of peroxyl radicals, which oxidize a great variety of biological molecules including proteins and nucleic acids. In tumors, non-enzymatic lipoperoxidation processes can be induced artificially by the treatment of pure PUFAs with bivalent metal ions. Then, lipid products can be separated by gas chromatography and identified by electron impact mass spectrometry [71].

Lipids are thus one of the most important molecular groups involved in oxidative stress because they are sensitive to oxidation and are then able to initiate a chain reaction with other macromolecules [72]. They can also interact with several hydrophobic substances of the diet, such as various unsaturated fatty acids and polyphenols [73]. In oxidative lipid derivates, underlying mechanisms involve a sequence of reactions which are measurable. The presence of free radicals can be assayed in biological samples by different colorimetric tests [74]. Then, conjugated dienes (an up-stream lipid oxidative state) can be obtained by a Fölch extraction followed by a UV-spectrophotometric assessment [75]. Although this parameter is classically used for lipid peroxide determination, the possibility cannot be discarded that an important proportion of conjugated dienes may be conjugated as linoleic acid, which can be incorporated by diet. Nonetheless, their *in vitro* levels may be attributed to changes in the redox membrane state, since mammalian cells are not able to synthesize that fatty acid [76]. This hypothesis is supported by the fact that directly quantified lipid hydroperoxides have a strong correlation with conjugated dienes in cells treated with arsenite and flavonoids [77]. Lastly, final derivates of lipid oxidation are short-chain peroxide compounds, such as OH-nonenal [78]. Although the presented biochemical markers can adequately reflect the lipid oxidation state, they have not been proposed as mandatory biomarkers of dietary intervention effects.

The lipid biomarkers chosen to be assessed in humans might include:

- Malondialdehyde (MDA): This is an end-product of lipid peroxidation, which is normally present in urine and blood, and can be quantified directly by different methods, such as spectrophotometry, high performance liquid chromatography and gas chromatography with mass spectrometry [79]. Its urinary levels are associated with a person's whole redox state, and two colorimetric tests have been recently developed to measure MDA in this fluid. They are easily performed and involve fuchsine or pararosaniline HCl [80, 81]. Also, MDA levels can be measured spectrophotometrically by a reaction with thiobarbituric acid (TBARS assay), which are generally used as an indicator of lipid peroxide generation [82]. TBARS can be measured in tissues, but are generally measured in plasma [83].

- Oxidized low density lipoprotein (LDL-ox): Oxidative damage to cholesterol-carrying molecules has been hypothesized to be a causative agent in the development of various pathologies, such as cardiovascular diseases [84] and certain types of cancer [85, 86]. LDL-ox forms a complex with β2-GPI within the body. This should be measured preferably in blood, and the resulting product from an immune reaction is assayed spectrophotometrically [87]. This technique enables various human diseases to be detected [88].

- F2 isoprostanes (F2-iso): These compounds are a family of prostaglandin F2-like compounds, which are formed by free radical-catalyzed peroxidation of arachidonic acid [89]. The most abundant F2 isoprostane is 8-isoprostaglandin F2a (8-iso-PGF2a), which has been suggested to be a promising marker for oxidative injury [90]. Isoprostanes may be measured in a plurality of human body fluids such as urine, blood, tears and saliva, but urine is generally considered the best matrix for quantifying isoprostane levels *in vivo* [91], with immunoassays or gas chromatography/mass spectrometry being generally used [92, 93].

- Breath hydrocarbons (BHC): Carcinogenesis is accompanied by increased production of ROS which degrade membranes by lipid peroxidation. The process involves the formation of volatile organic compounds, which are excreted in the breath. Volatile oxidation products of n-3 and n-6 fatty acids, such as ethane and pentane, are commonly used. This is a non-invasive approach for estimating lipid peroxidation *in vivo* [94]. BHC concentrations are quantifiable by solid phase micro-extraction and gas chromatography/mass spectrography techniques [95], or by electronic sensors [96].

- Hydroperoxides (HP): In order to study lipid peroxidation in human pathology, there is a simple and sensitive method for direct hydroperoxide measurement, the ferrous xylenol orange (FOX) assay, which has been previously validated and probed to be better than other techniques to measure hydroperoxide *per se* [97]. Moreover, FOX assay has been efficient for the measurement of 5-lipoxygenase activity at the stage of primary anticancer inhibitor screening [98]. Furthermore, they might be used as cancer biomarkers when are increased in urine [99]. Recently, the method was automated to improve stability and accuracy, getting a precision value lower than 3% [100]. Also, the reactivity between HP and ferrous ion can be revealed accurately by chemoluminiscence [100]. The assessment of HP is very relevant given their widespread presence in different samples, such as tissues, cells and biological fluids [101], including within plasma LDL-ox molecules [102].

Although, the list of potential lipid biomarkers has increased [103], data which validate their predictive use in human cancer is really scarce. For example, predictive assessments of lung cancer, which is one of the commonest cancers in both males and females [104], mainly derive from genomics and proteomics [105], with lipidomic markers ensuing in a small number [106].

For the prevention of lipid oxidation, polyphenolic antioxidant activity may depend on the lipophilicity of these compounds. Indeed, quercetin is a better antioxidant agent against lipid hydroperoxide overproduction than counteracting aqueous hydroperoxide increase in cells [77]. Moreover, flavonoids are more effective antioxidants than other commonly used substances, such as selenium, when oxidative lipid damage is assayed [107]. It is also important to keep in mind that aqueous and lipid hydroperoxides have different generation kinetics [21]. This is very relevant due to the participation of these lipid metabolites in oxidative chain reactions and their role as ligands of cellular receptors involved in cell proliferation and differentiation [108]. Furthermore, they co-modulate other cancer-related pathways which can be regulated by nutrients. For example, eicosanoid binding to peroxisome proliferating activating receptors is a key point of regulation for epigenetic actions of different liposoluble compounds on cancer development, such as vitamin A [16].

Nonetheless, it is important to keep in mind that biomarkers are surrogate endpoints, i.e. measures of effect of a certain treatment that may correlate with a real clinical endpoint, but they do not necessarily possess a guaranteed relationship [109]. Another analytical option is the direct measurement of polyphenolic compounds (or metabolites of) in human specimens (bioavailability), although it reflects exposure but not effect. In this regard, there are efficient validated immunoassays for phytoestrogen determination in epidemiological studies. This is important given the close relation between phytoestrogen intake and the risk of breast and prostate cancers [62]. Indeed, systematic information about the involvement of phytochemicals in cancer risk has consistently revealed protective effects of β-carotene in renal cell cancer, flavonoides, β-cryptoxanthin and isothiocyanates in lung cancer, isothiocyanates in gastrointestinal cancer, and lignans in postmenopausal breast cancer [110].

On the other hand, fatty acids themselves might be used as tumor biomarkers. Chromatographic lipid profile of erythrocytes and platelets from non-small cell lung cancer patients have revealed that some fatty acids are related to this cancer type (22:0 and 18:2n6 in erythrocytes, and 16:0, 18:0, and 18:2n6 in platelets), with platelet linoleic acid (18:2n6) being the best biomarker [111]. Also, both cell types showed essential PUFA decrease, which are correlated with the illness and with their susceptibility to oxidative stress with changes in the fluorescence of lipid extracts [112]. Nonetheless, given the insufficient studies and meta-studies of lipidomic biomarkers, comparisons of their accuracy in order to develop diagnostic criteria are encouraged. Considerations about sensitivity, specificity and predictive values of markers are pivotal, but still limited, even for the commonest cancers, as that of lung [113].

III. TRANSLATIONAL CONCERNS FOR PATENT DEVELOPMENT

Onconutrition and Patient Status

The challenge is to translate nutrition knowledge into strategies and health policies. Nutrition professionals trying to influence dietary selection must take into accounts both personal preferences and healthy foods to be chosen. As these challenges are faced, environmental factors and science-based tools also need to be considered. In this regard, nutritional standardization is pivotal, since vegetable food intake and consumption fortification differ worldwide [114]. Moreover, dietary interventions require a metabolomic assessment [115]. A dietary modification that includes anticancer nutrients represents one of the best ways to prevent cancer. This lifestyle change is simply trying to highlight the importance of food in everyday life. For example, the promotion of a high intake of sources food of omega 3 fatty acids, such as fish and seafood, and phenolic compounds, such as cruciferous, turmeric and green tea, may have a high impact on the risk of being affected by cancer (Table **2**) [116-129]. On the other hand, stop smoking, a low intake of calories and red meat, avoid foods that contain high potential carcinogenic products and daily exercise, are measures related to lifestyle that influencing prevention of cancer and other chronic diseases [116].

Table 2: Potential cancer chemopreventive nutrients*.

	Main Referents with Chemical Structure	Principal Mechanisms of Potential Chemopreventive Effects
Omega-3 Fatty Acids	α-Linolenic acid (α-LNA, 18:3n–3) 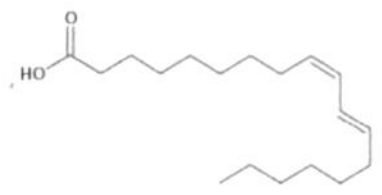 Eicosapentaenoic acid (EPA, 20:5n–3) 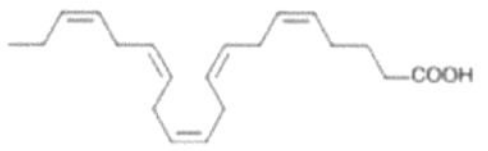 Docosahexaenoic acid (DHA, 22:6n–3) 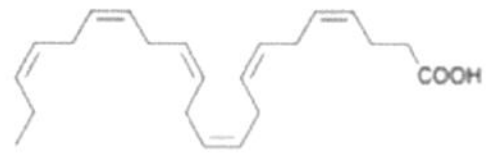	• Inhibition of arachidonic acid-derived eicosanoid biosynthesis [117] • Influence on transcription factor activity, gene expression, and signal transduction molecules [118] • Alteration of oestrogen metabolism, with decrease endogenous oestrogen production [119] • Perturbation on production of free radicals and reactive oxygen species [120]
Polyphenols	Flavonoids (e.g. quercetin, myricetin) 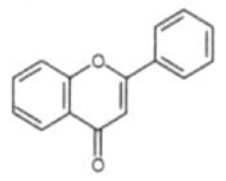 Phenolic acids (e.g. cinnamic, chlorogenic) 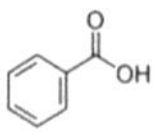 Polyphenolic amides 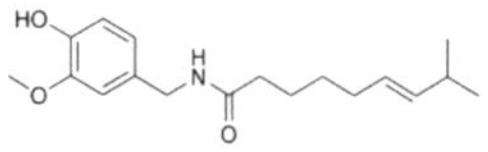 Others (e.g. resveratrol, tannins) 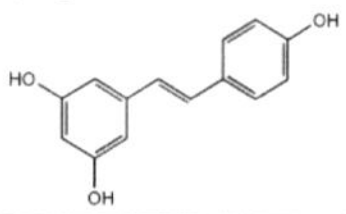	• Direct free radical scavenging [121], modulation of oxidative stress-related enzymes [122] • Inhibiting phase I drug metabolism enzymes [123], modulating the gene expression of phase II conjugating-enzymes [124] • Perturbation of cell cycle tumor-related proteins [125] • Apoptosis induction through cytochrome c release [126] • Inhibition of survival/proliferation signals such as NF-κβ [127] • Decreased cell proliferation [128] • Cyclooxygenase-2inhibition [129]

* Mentioned parameters constitute a non-limiting list.

Onconutritional interventions in humans should be thought in order to contribute to the general improvement of physical conditions and organic function [130], being not only focused to tumor mitigation, since it is not an isolated entity from the subject. In this regard, the immune enhancement is by itself a potent preventive and therapeutic resource. For example, fruit polyphenol-enriched extracts have shown to boost both humoral and cellular immunity, with these immuno enhancing activities resulting from an inhibition of inflammation leading to balanced immune function [131]. Therefore, tissue biomarkers of antioxidant chemoprevention also demonstrate the interrelation between oxidative stress, chronic inflammation and cancer development [132]. Meanwhile, fatty acids can also be used as immunoregulating compounds, given their multifaceted bioactivity [133]. It is important to keep in mind that anticancer strategies should be more selective as possible, without impairing general status by compromising normal cells and healthy tissues. This belief has motivated several researches intended for improving organic response [134].

Although, nutrition is a major determinant in patient evolution, there are not sufficient well-designed studies to define appropriate nutritional practices. Potential strategies have been developed to improve translational research: increase funding, foster physician training, and attract researchers to nutrition meetings, involving academic and professional integration [135].

Modulation of Age-Related Chronic Conditions

The age-related declining function in all organic systems is due to, at least in part, oxidative stress-induced cellular senescence with organelle dysfunction. Thus, antioxidant compounds have pharmaconutritional potential [136]. In this line, recent oral formulations with plant extracts might counteract aging deleterious effects by their redox-modulating activity, with polyphenols being central for such biomedical properties [137]. Moreover, these antioxidant phytochemicals delay progression of chronic tumor-predisposing diseases, with this chemopreventive activity being closely related to synergistic effects of plant micronutrients on cellular differentiation and proliferation [138].

A growing field of biomedical aging research investigates the role of chronic pro-inflammatory states as predisposing factors in the oncogenetic process. Again, oxidative stress is involved given that chronic inflammation produces high amounts of free radicals, which in turns are tumor initiators and promoters [139]. Thus, nutritional formulations have been developed with plant compounds and essential fatty acids in order to improve the physical condition of patients with chronic and wasting illnesses [140], where overproduction of inflammation-induced reactive intermediates is triggered. This type of invention considers optimal percentages of ω-6 and ω-3 fatty acid for oral intake, which are thought to be immunomodulator. Moreover, plasmatic biomarkers revealed organic nutritional responsiveness to them [140]. Phenolic compound-enriched compositions have also been formulated to prevent and treat the mentioned interrelation between redox unbalance and inflammation, which might be used in certain chronic degenerative diseases [141].

This biochemical network underlies many pathological events, which are related to lipid metabolism, such as obesity, diabetes mellitus, etc., among others [142]. This integrative view allows developing bioactive molecules with beneficial potential for the common treatment of several diseases through an epigenetic mechanism. Therefore, herbal polyphenol-containing pharmaceuticals (e.g. genistein, plumbagin, luteolin, rutin, forskolin, quercetin, epigallocatechin-3-gallate and azharone from *Glycine max, Plumbago zeylanica, Terminalia arjuna, Trigonella-foenum-graceum, Coleus forskohlii, Commiphora mukul, Camellia sinensis,* and *Azadirachta indica*, respectively), which are antioxidant, cytoprotective and anti-inflammatory, are potential adjuvants to conventional drugs for treating a wide range of organic dysfunctions, such as the above mentioned [143, 144].

Furthermore, exogenous incorporation of certain nutrients could enhance endogenous antioxidant defences [145]. In addition, nutrients and their derivates can bind nuclear receptors of the described pathways [146]. This nutrigenomic approach is completed by other epigenetic anti-genotoxic activities of food substances. For example, dietary plant extract-based supplements, such as those derived from *Cinnamonum* sp., might be useful to prevent some of genetic abnormalities found in cancer cells [147].

Biomarkers and Selective Cytotoxic Chemotherapy

Potential therapeutic compounds can be identified by high throughput screening methods, which provide a chemical library as an outcome of a large number of them (ligand libraries), with transcriptome and cell phenotype being assayed [148]. The efficient development of biomarkers depends on advances in reactive chemicals and technical improvement. For example, new synthetic markers allow kinetics of oxidative and nitrosative intermediates to be measured [149]. In addition to direct appraisal of reactive species, high throughput tests allow evaluating the biological response to these oxidizing intermediates, and their modulation by bioactive molecules [150]. Therefore, cellular systems can be used to quantify antioxidant activity of phytochemicals, food extracts and dietary supplements, by a fluorescent redox-sensing probe tested *in vitro*, accounting for free radical uptake, metabolism, and location within cells [151].

Beyond being used as biomarkers, specific biological parameters of neoplasias also represent treatment targets of functional biomolecules, thus chemotherapeutic interventions become selective [152, 153]. Furthermore, given that they represent biochemical outcomes of the carcinogenetic process, biomarkers allow assessing the effect of epigenetic factors and their modulations along such process [154]. A particular case of cellular target of anticancer polyphenols is the proteasome activity, which is associated with tumor behaviour. These compounds are thought to control tumor progression by inhibiting the mentioned protein complex [155].

Current & Future Developments

Onconutritional researchers suggest that dietary compounds and their chemical derivates might be used as anti-tumor compounds, mainly in cancer chemoprevention. In view of these concerns, the organic redox-modulating unsaturated fatty acids and polyphenols are promising given their capacity to control oxidative oncogenesis. This might depend on their physical-chemical properties, at least in part, as these lipids are redox-sensitive linear molecules (or chains), and the others are redox-modulating cyclic molecules (or rings). Specifically, polyphenolic compounds, such as antioxidant flavonoids, might be considered, since they possess multi-target and multi-stage actions [156], and they can reciprocally interact with lipids to regulate redox homeostasis and cell biology. Those may well constitute the only class of molecules which can modulate every stage of cancer development with a wide spectrum of regulatory activities.

In accordance to translational medicine criteria, polyphenol-based dietetic approaches require well-established biomarkers as predictors of cancer nutritional modulation against oxidative stress-induced oncogenesis. Among them, MDA and

TBARS (thiobarbituric acid reactive substances) are measurable by simple available techniques in organic fluids and tissues, and both represent the whole body status of lipid peroxidation. Nonetheless, they do not necessarily represent the nutritional status. On the other hand, LDL-ox does represent oxidative and nutritional status, since it depends on lipid and protein intake, while F2-iso assessment is useful to determine enzymatic lipid oxidation, and to evaluate cancer-regulating pathways (i.e., eicosanoids). But, assays for its determination are not already available in every clinical laboratory. This might be excelled by the inclusion of HP quantification, given its technical efficiency. Finally, given the promotion of non-invasive diagnostic methods, breath constitutes an incipient option, together with saliva, to evaluate lipid oxidation by-products *in vivo*, such as the BHC. Beyond the promising development of lipid biomarkers, further studies are required to validate their utilization in human cancer monitoring. Lipids also reflect the polyphenolic bioactivity given their redox interactions, which underlay the effects on both normal (cytoprotection) and neoplastic cells (cytodifferentiation and cytotoxicity).

Finally, biomarkers derived from biochemical studies should be developed into a clinical-epidemiological framework, with appropriate statistical techniques being required for outcome analysis. Thus, further long-term prospective studies in humans are required. Certainly, nutritional biomarker assessment and validation have proven difficult because dietary agents exert multiple actions with biological importance. Although, clinical epidemiology and related fields have improved understanding of individual treatment effects by analyzing subgroup effects and developing clinical prediction rules, appropriately-designed studies are required. Indeed, sanitary community has little guidance about which patients were most likely to benefit from a clinical-nutritional strategy. Furthermore, biomarker value suffers from the same limitation. Thus, the comparative-effectiveness research appears as a possible resource, since its most important goal is to broaden and deepen such information, providing tools for matching health care much more precisely to individual patients [157].

This work is based on a narrative review done with valid scientific criteria [158], including the current bibliography about features of the described dietary compounds, which can be identified by modern chromatographic techniques

[159]. Nonetheless, given the current limitations for nutritional translation, there is insufficient information to include nowadays dietary compounds as alternative to well-proved cytotoxic drugs, but there is growing evidence that this may be the case in future with ongoing developments. Thus, it is completely unsafe to replace or modify conventional anticancer therapies by natural compounds, since potential bioactivities need to be studied more extensively.

ACKNOWLEDGEMENTS

The authors would like to thank SECYT-UNC support and researchers of the Institute of Cell Biology (National University of Cordoba, Argentina) for their very valuable contributions in the critical reading of this chapter.

CONFLICT OF INTEREST

The authors declare that there are no conflicts of interest, and would like to clarify that cited patents were selected with descriptive criteria in accordance to the thematic adjustment and updating, without impairment of non-included ones or compulsory recommendation of those mentioned.

DISCLOSURE

The chapter submitted for Patent eBook Series "Topics in Anti-Cancer Research", Volume 2, is an update of our article "Biomarker Assessment in Nutritional Modulation of Oxidative Stress-Induced Cancer Development by Lipid-Related Bioactive Molecules", published in the journal 'Recent Patents on Anti-Cancer Drug Discovery', Volume 5, Number 3, November, 2010, Page 188 to 196 with modified title, additional text and references.

REFERENCES

[1] Ong TP, Moreno FS, Ross SA. Targeting the epigenome with bioactive food components for cancer prevention. J Nutrigenet Nutrigenomics 2011; 4(5): 275-92.

[2] Ramos EJ, Middleton FA, Laviano A, Sato T, Romanova I, Das UN, *et al.* Effects of omega-3 fatty acid supplementation on tumor-bearing rats. J Am Coll Surg 2004; 199(5): 716-23.

[3] McCarthy JF, Shugart LR. Biological markers of environmental and ecological contamination: An overview. Risk Anal 1992; 12(3): 353-60.
[4] Burnworth B, Arendt S, Muffler S, Steinkraus V, Bröcker EB, Birek C, *et al.* The multi-step process of human skin carcinogenesis: A role for p53, cyclin D1, hTERT, p16, and TSP-1. Eur J Cell Biol 2007; 86(11-12): 763-80.
[5] Abbott RG, Forrest S, Pienta KJ. Simulating the hallmarks of cancer. Artif Life 2006; 12(4): 617-34.
[6] Comba A, Maestri DM, Berra MA, Garcia CP, Das UN, *et al.* Effect of ω-3 and ω-9 fatty acid rich oils on lipoxygenases and cyclooxygenases enzymes and on the growth of a mammary adenocarcinoma model. Lipids Health Dis 2010; 9: 112.
[7] Moses, M.A., Pories, S., Zurakowski, D. Method to assess breast cancer risk. US20090215102 (**2009**).
[8] Orzechowski A. Possible implications of redox-sensitive tumor cell transformation; lessons from cell culture studies. Pol J Vet Sci 2007; 10(2): 123-6.
[9] Arya R, Mallik M, Lakhotia SC. Heat shock genes - Integrating cell survival and death. J Biosci 2007; 323(3): 595-610.
[10] Ruddon RW. Cancer Biology. 4th ed. Oxford University Press: Oxford, 2007.
[11] Trachootham D, Lu W, Ogasawara MA, Nilsa RD, Huang P. Redox regulation of cell survival. Antioxid Redox Signal 2008; 10(8): 1343-74.
[12] Valko M, Leibfritz D, Moncol J, Cronin MT, Mazur M, Telser J. Free radicals and antioxidants in normal physiological functions and human disease. Int J Biochem Cell Biol 2007; 39(1): 44-84.
[13] Krämer, K., Schweden, J. Method of increasing the content of flavonoids and phenolic substances substances inplants. US8105980 (**2012**).
[14] Steiner, M.S., Raghow, S. A method for chemoprevention of prostate cancer. EP2277514 (**2011**).
[15] Quiroga A, Quiroga PL, Martínez E, Soria EA, Valentich MA. Anti-breast cancer activity of curcumin on the human oxidation-resistant cells ZR-75-1 with gamma-glutamyltranspeptidase inhibition. J Exp Ther Oncol 2010; 8(3): 261-6.
[16] Quiroga PL, Eynard AR, Soria EA, Valentich MA. Interaction between retinoids and eicosanoids: Their relevance to cancer chemoprevention. Curr Nutr Food Sci 2009; 5: 126-33.
[17] Nichols JA, Katiyar SK. Skin photoprotection by natural polyphenols: Anti-inflammatory, antioxidant and DNA repair mechanisms. Arch Dermatol Res 2010; 302(2): 71-83.
[18] Cox, D., Ballinger, D., Ponder, B., Easton, D. Markers for breast cancer. US20090239763 (**2009**).
[19] Escribá Ruiz, P.V., Busquets Xaubet, X., Terés Jiménez, S., Barceló Coblijn, G., Lladó Cañellas, V., Marcilla Etxenike, A., Martín, M.L., Higuera Urbano, M., Álvarez Martínez, R., López, D.H. Use of derivatives of polyunsaturated fatty acids as medicaments. EP2409963 (**2012**).
[20] Lindskog M, Gleissman H, Ponthan F, Castro J, Kogner P, Johnsen JI. Neuroblastoma cell death in response to docosahexaenoic acid: Sensitization to chemotherapy and arsenic-induced oxidative stress. Int J Cancer 2006; 118(10): 2584-93.
[21] Soria EA, Goleniowski ME, Cantero JJ, Bongiovanni GA. Antioxidant activity of different extracts of Argentinian medicinal plants against arsenic-induced toxicity in renal cells. Hum Exp Toxicol 2008; 27(4): 341-6.

[22] Conselvan, P., Falanga, G. Antioxidant composition for reducing oxidative stress in dogs. EP2388011 (**2011**).

[23] Tvrzicka E, Kremmyda LS, Stankova B, Zak A. Fatty acids as biocompounds: Their role in human metabolism, health and disease--are view. Part 1: Classification, dietary sources and biological functions. Biomed Pap Med Fac Univ Palacky Olomouc Czech Repub 2011; 155(2): 117-30.

[24] Khan N, Mukhtar H. Multitargeted therapy of cancer by green tea polyphenols. Cancer Lett 2008; 269(2): 269-80.

[25] Scalbert A, Manach C, Morand C, Remesy C, Jimenez L. Dietary polyphenols and the prevention of diseases. Crit Rev Food Sci Nutr 2005; 45(4): 287-306.

[26] Rodeiro I, Donato MT, Lahoz A, Garrido G, Delgado R, Gómez-Lechón MJ. Interactions of polyphenols with the P450 system: Possible implications on human therapeutics. Mini Rev Med Chem 2008; 8(2): 97-106.

[27] Auger C, Mullen W, Hara Y, Crozier A. Bioavailability of polyphenon E flavan-3-ols in humans with an ileostomy. J Nutr 2008; 138(8): 1535S-42S.

[28] Galdi, A., Foltis, S.P., Shah, A. UV Protecting composition and methods of use. US20120015016 (**2012**).

[29] Matsui Y, Kobayashi K, Masuda H, Kigoshi H, Akao M, Sakurai H, *et al.* Quantitative analysis of saponins in a tea-leaf extract and their antihypercholesterolemic activity. Biosci Biotechnol Biochem 2009; 73(7): 1513-9.

[30] Gutterman, J.U., Haridas, V. Inhibition of NF-kappaB by triterpene compositions. US20060148732 (**2006**).

[31] Willey, J.C., Blomquist, T.M., Crawford, E.L., Mullins, D.N. Cancer risk biomarker. US20090181383 (**2009**).

[32] Ricciardiello, L., Boland, C.R., Romano, M., Fogliano, V. Chemopreventive, anticancer and anti-inflammatory effects of pinoresinol-rich olives. US20090048187 (**2009**).

[33] Pasparakis M. Regulation of tissue homeostasis by NF-kappaB signaling: Implications for inflammatory diseases. Nat Rev Immunol 2009; 9(11): 778-88.

[34] Kiessling MK, Klemke CD, Kaminski MM, Galani IE, Krammer PH, Gülow K. Inhibition of constitutively activated nuclear factor-kappaB induces reactive oxygen species- and iron-dependent cell death in cutaneous T-cell lymphoma. Cancer Res 2009; 69(6): 2365-74.

[35] Pan MH, Chang YH, Tsai ML, Lai CS, Ho SY, Badmaev V, *et al.* Pterostilbene suppressed lipopolysaccharide-induced up-expression of iNOS and COX-2 in murine macrophages. J Agric Food Chem 2008; 56(16): 7502-9.

[36] Kwon KH, Barve A, Yu S, Huang MT, Kong AN. Cancer chemoprevention by phytochemicals: Potential molecular targets, biomarkers and animal models. Acta Pharmacol Sin 2007; 28(9): 1409-21.

[37] Taylor, B.N., Mehta, R., Yamada, T., Beattie, C., Das Gupta. T. Compositions and methods to prevent cancer with cupredoxins. US20090202441 (**2009**).

[38] Peluso, J.J., Avon, C.T. Regulators of the non-genomic action of progesterone and methods of use. US20090226917 (**2009**).

[39] Mujica-fernaud, T., Buchholz, H. 2-Oxadiazolechromone derivatives. US7354945 (**2008**).

[40] Garattini E, Gianni' M, Terao M. Cyto differentiation by retinoids, a novel therapeutic option in oncology: Rational combinations with other therapeutic agents. Vitam Horm 2007; 75: 301-54.

[41] Kinkade, Jr, J.M., Shapira, R., Jensen, P.E., Le, N., Pohl, J., Brown, V.W. Biomarkers for oxidative stress. US6953666 (**2005**).

[42] Sakla MS, Shenouda NS, Ansell PJ, MacDonald RS, Lubahn DB. Genistein affects HER2 protein concentration, activation, and promoter regulation in BT-474 human breast cancer cells. Endocrine 2007; 32(1): 69-78.

[43] Giovannini C, Masella R. Role of polyphenols in cell death control. Nutr Neurosci 2012; 15(3): 134-49.

[44] Lee ST, Wu YL, Chien LH, Chen ST, Tzeng YK, Wu TF. Proteomic exploration of the impacts of pomegranate fruit juice on the global gene expression of prostate cancer cell. Proteomics 2012; [In press].

[45] Fujimura Y, Sumida M, Sugihara K, Tsukamoto S, Yamada K, Tachibana H. Green tea polyphenol EGCG sensing motif on the 67-kDa laminin receptor. PLoS One 2012; 7(5): e37942.

[46] Calabria LM, Piacente S, Kapusta I, Dharmawardhane SF, Segarra FM, Pessiki PJ, *et al.* Triterpene saponins from *Silphium radula*. Phytochemistry 2008; 69(4): 961-72.

[47] Solomons NW, Allen NH. The functional assessment of nutritional status: Principles, practice, and potential. Nutr Rev 1983; 41(2): 33-50.

[48] McKeown NM, Day NE, Welch AA, Runswick SA, Luben RN, Mulligan AA, *et al.* Use of biological markers to validate self-reported dietary intake in a random sample of the European Prospective Investigation into Cancer United Kingdom Norfolk cohort. Am J Clin Nutr 2001; 74(2): 188-96.

[49] Boaventura BC, DiPietro PF, deAssis MA, Ambrosi C, Nesello LA, DaSilva FO, *et al.* Antioxidant biomarkers and food intake in elderly women. J Nutr Health Aging 2012; 16(1): 21-5.

[50] Scott EN, Gescher AJ, Steward WP, Brown K. Development of dietary phytochemical chemopreventive agents: Biomarkers and choice of dose for early clinical trials. Cancer Prev Res (Phila Pa) 2009; 2(6): 525-30.

[51] Zamora-Ros R, Urpí-Sardà M, Lamuela-Raventós RM, Estruch R, Vázquez-Agell M, Serrano-Martínez M, *et al.* Diagnostic performance of urinary resveratrol metabolites as a biomarker of moderate wine consumption. Clin Chem 2006; 52: 1373-80.

[52] Ryan PB, Burke TA, Cohen Hubal EA, Cura JJ, McKone TE. Using biomarkers to inform cumulative risk assessment. Environ Health Perspect 2007; 115(5): 833-40.

[53] Ginter E. Vegetarian diets, chronic diseases and longevity. Bratisl Lek Listy 2008; 109(10): 463-6.

[54] Langley-Evans SC. Nutritional programming of disease: Unravelling the mechanism. J Anat 2009; 215(1): 36-51.

[55] Kato I, Ren J, Heilbrun LK, Djuric Z. Intra- and inter-individual variability in measurements of biomarkers for oxidative damage *in vivo*: Nutrition and Breast Health Study. Biomarkers 2006; 11(2): 143-52.

[56] Henríquez-Sánchez P, García-Closas R, Serra-Majem L. Indicadores bioquímicos de la ingesta dietética. In: Serra-Majem L, Aranceta-Bartrina J. Nutrición en salud pública. Métodos, bases científicas y aplicaciones. 2nd ed. Masson SA: Barcelona 2006.

[57] Defagó MD, Valentich MA, Actis AB. Lipid characterization of human saliva. J Calif Dent Assoc 2011; 39(12): 875-80.

[58] Bingham SA. Biomarkers in nutritional epidemiology. Public Health Nutr 2002; 5(6A): 821-7.

[59] Jenab M, Slimani N, Bictash M, Ferrari P, Bingham SA. Biomarkers in nutritional epidemiology: Applications, needs and new horizons. Hum Genet 2009; 125(5-6): 507-25.

[60] Maruvada P, Srivastava S. Biomarkers for cancer diagnosis: Implications for nutritional research. J Nutr 2004; 134(Suppl 6):1640-5.
[61] Defagó MD. Perfil lipídico de saliva humana según hábitos alimentarios: Un posible indicador de riesgo para el desarrollo de tumores salivales, mamarios y prostáticos. PhD Thesis, Universidad Nacional de Córdoba, Córdoba, Argentina, June 2010.
[62] Linseisen J, Rohrmann S. Biomarkers of dietary intake of flavonoids and phenolic acids for studying diet-cancer relationship in humans. Eur J Nutr 2008; 47 (Suppl 2): 60-8.
[63] González CA, Navarro C, Martínez C, Quirós JR, Dorronsoro M, Barricarte A, *et al.* The European prospective investigation about cancer and nutrition (EPIC). Rev Esp Salud Publica 2004; 78(2): 167-76.
[64] Bingham S, Luben R, Welch A, Low YL, Khaw KT, Wareham N, *et al.* Associations between dietary methods and biomarkers, and between fruits and vegetables and risk of ischaemic heart disease, in the EPIC Norfolk Cohort Study. Int J Epidemiol 2008; 37(5): 978-87.
[65] Parl, F.F., Crooke, P.S., Ritchie, M.D., Hachey, D.L., Dawling, S., Roodi, N. Biochemical and genetic analysis for prediction of breast cancer risk. US20090068653 (**2009**).
[66] Hoon, D.S.B., De Maat, M. Epigenetic silencing of cyclooxygenase-2 affects clinical outcome in gastric cancer. US20090061441 (**2009**).
[67] Dmitrovsky, E., Liu, X.I., Freemantle, S., Sempere, L., Cole, C., Kauppinen, S., Bak, M. MicroRNA biomarkers for human breast and lung cancer. US20070299030 (**2007**).
[68] Burkett, D.D., Sidransky, D., Allen, A.C.P., Chiafari, F.A., Bride, M., Maguire, Y.P. Oral cancer markers and their detection. US0090023138 (**2009**).
[69] Bose, A., Aziz, N. Systems and methods of identifying biomarkers for subsequent screening and monitoring of diseases. US7507533 (**2009**).
[70] Barbosa KB, Bressan J, Zulet MA, Martínez Hernández JA. Influence of dietary intake on plasma biomarkers of oxidative stress in humans. An Sist Sanit Navar 2008; 31(3): 259-80.
[71] Geromanos, S., Dongre, A.R., Opiteck, G., Silva, J. Method of mass spectrometry. US20080286764 (**2008**).
[72] Mayne ST. Antioxidant nutrients and chronic disease: Use of biomarkers of exposure and oxidative stress status in epidemiologic research. J Nutr 2003; 133(Suppl. 3): 933-40.
[73] Vivancos M, Moreno JJ. Effect of resveratrol, tyrosol and beta-sitosterol on oxidised low-density lipoprotein-stimulated oxidative stress, arachidonic acid release and prostaglandin E2 synthesis by RAW 264.7 macrophages. Br J Nutr 2008; 99(6): 1199-207.
[74] Pruche, F., Nguyen, Q.L., Hirt, J. Method of evaluating the potential of the skin for scavenging free radicals. US20060194333 (**2006**).
[75] Evans, G.S., Grochoski, G., Randolph, R., Connor, L.M., Scimeca, J.V., Gellenbeck, K.W., Mayne, J.R., Roh-Schmidt, H., Slaga, T.J., Hanausek-Walaszek, M., Walaszek, Z. Methods and kits for reducing cellular damage, inhibiting free radical production and scavenging free radicals. US7588785 (**2009**).
[76] Delmonte P, Roach JA, Mossoba MM, Losi G, Yurawecz MP. Synthesis, isolation, and GC analysis of all the 6, 8- to 13, 15-cis/trans conjugated linoleic acid isomers. Lipids 2004; 39(2): 185-91.
[77] Soria EA. Modulación del efecto citotóxico del arsénico por moléculas bioactivas. PhD Thesis, Universidad Nacional de Córdoba, Córdoba, Argentina, March 2009.
[78] Blair, I., Mesaros, C., Jian, W., Lee, S.H., Oe, T. GSH adducts and uses thereof. US20080280319 (**2008**).

[79] Abels, R.D. Agent for detecting malondialdehyde, method of making the same, and test kit for use thereof. US20040023402 (**2004**).
[80] Halstead, B.W. Methods for testing oxidative stress. US6165797 (**2000**).
[81] Yoon, M.J., Lee, J.C., Ku, Y.S. Aldehyde detection kit and method thereof. US7514265 (**2009**).
[82] Taylor, K., Mesaros, J. Accelerators for increasing the rate of formation of free radicals and reactive oxygen species. US20030082101 (**2003**).
[83] Zelkha, M., Sedlov, T., Nir, Z. Anti-atherosclerosis composition containing carotenoids and method for inhibiting LDL oxidation. US20080114074 (**2008**).
[84] Nilsson J, Fredrikson GN, Björkbacka H, Chyu KY, Shah PK. Vaccines modulating lipoprotein autoimmunity as a possible future therapy for cardiovascular disease. J Intern Med 2009; 266(3): 221-31.
[85] Wang Y, Li H, Diao Y, Li, H, Zhang Y, Yin C, *et al.* Relationship between oxidized LDL antibodies and different stages of esophageal carcinoma. Arch Med Res 2008; 39(8): 760-67.
[86] Scoles DR, Xu X, Wang H, Tran H, Taylor-Harding B, Li A, *et al.* Liver X receptor agonist inhibits proliferation of ovarian carcinoma cells stimulated by oxidized low density lipoprotein. Gynecol Oncol 2010; 116(1): 109-16.
[87] Witztum, J.L., Tsimikas, S., Palinski, W., Shaw, W.P. Methods for diagnosing, imaging and treating atherosclerotic disease. US7556927 (**2009**).
[88] Matsuura, E. Method of measuring oxidized LDL/β2-glycoprotein I complex occurring in the living body. US7455976 (**2008**).
[89] Bastani NE, Gundersen TE, Blomhoff R. Determination of 8-epi PGF (2alpha) concentrations as a biomarker of oxidative stress using triple-stage liquid chromatography/tandem mass spectrometry. Rapid Commun Mass Spectrom 2009; 23(18): 2885-90.
[90] Schwedhelm E, Tsikas D, Durand T, Gutzki FM, Guy A, Rossi JC, *et al.* Tandem mass spectrometric quantification of 8-iso-prostaglandin F2alpha and its metabolite 2,3-dinor-5,6-dihydro-8-iso-prostaglandin F2alpha in human urine. J Chromatogr BBiomed Sci Appl 2000; 744(1): 99-112.
[91] Epplein M, Franke AA, Cooney RV, Morris JS, Wilkens LR, Goodman MT, *et al.* Association of plasma micronutrient levels and urinary isoprostane with risk of lung cancer: The multiethnic cohort study. Cancer Epidemiol Biomarkers Prev 2009; 18(7): 1962-70.
[92] Cobain, M.R., Powell, J.R., Talbot, D.C.S. Psychological stress in humans. US20040054265 (**2004**).
[93] Singh, R., Zhou, H. Mass spectrometry of prostaglandins. US6939718 (**2005**).
[94] Knutson MD, Handelman GJ, Viteri FE. Methods for measuring ethane and pentane in expired air from rats and humans. Free Radic Biol Med 2000; 28(4): 514-9.
[95] Regev-Shoshani G, Shoseyov O, Kerem Z. Influence of lipophilicity on the interactions of hydroxy stilbenes with cytochrome P450 3A4. Biochem Biophys Res Commun 2004; 323: 668-73.
[96] Machado RF, Laskowski D, Deffenderfer O, Burch T, Zheng S, Mazzone PJ, *et al.* Detection of lung cancer by sensor array analyses of exhaled breath. Am J Respir Crit Care Med 2005; 171(11): 1286-91.
[97] Jiang ZY, Woollard AC, Wolff SP. Lipid hydroperoxide measurement by oxidation of Fe^{2+} in the presence of xylenol orange. Comparison with the TBA assay and an iodometric method. Lipids 1991; 26(10): 853-6.

[98] Cho YS, Kim HS, Kim CH, Cheon HG. Application of the ferrous oxidation-xylenol orange assay for the screening of 5-lipoxygenase inhibitors. Anal Biochem 2006; 351(1): 62-8.

[99] Banerjee D, Madhusoodanan UK, Nayak S, Jacob J. Urinary hydrogen peroxide: A probable marker of oxidative stress in malignancy. Clin Chim Acta 2003; 334(1-2): 205-9.

[100] Seya K, Ohkohchi N, Shibuya H, Satoh M, Oikawa K, Fukumori T, *et al.* A chemiluminescent assay for hydroperoxide level of phosphatidylcholine hydroperoxide fraction purified by two Sep-Pak cartridges in biological samples. J Pharm Biomed Anal 2000; 23(2-3): 515-20.

[101] Fukuzawa K, Fujisaki A, Akai K, Tokumura A, Terao J, Gebicki JM. Measurement of phosphatidylcholine hydroperoxides in solution and in intact membranes by the ferric-xylenol orange assay. Anal Biochem 2006; 359(1): 18-25.

[102] Handelman GJ. High-performance liquid chromatography analysis of cholesterol linoleate hydroperoxide in oxidized low density lipoproteins: Calibration by conjugated diene internal standard. Methods Enzymol 1999; 300: 43-50.

[103] Meagher EA, Fitzgerald GA. Indices of lipid peroxidation *in vivo*: Strengths and limitations. Free Rad Biol Med 2000; 28(12): 1745-50.

[104] De Groot P, Munden RF. Lung cancer epidemiology, risk factors, and prevention. Radiol Clin North Am 2012; 50(5): 863-76.

[105] Wang, T., Fan, L., Kalos, M.D., Bangur, C.S., Hosken, N.A., Fanger, G.R., Li, X.S., Wang, A., Skeiky, Y.A.W., Henderson, R.A., Mcneill, P.D., Fanger. N. Methods for diagnosis of lung cancer. US7049063 (**2006**).

[106] Uzun K, Vural H, Öztürk T, Özer F, Imecik I. Diagnostic value of lipid peroxidation in lung cancer. East J Med 2000; 5: 48-51.

[107] Bongiovanni GA, Soria EA, Eynard AR. Effects of the plant flavonoids silymarin and quercetin on arsenite-induced oxidative stress in CHO-K1 cells. Food Chem Toxicol 2007; 45(6): 971-6.

[108] Obinata H, Hattori T, Nakane S, Tatei K, Izumi T. Identification of 9-hydroxyoctadecadienoic acid and other oxidized free fatty acids as ligands of the G protein-coupled receptor G2A. J Biol Chem 2005; 280(49): 40676-83.

[109] Cohn JN. Introduction to surrogate markers. Circulation 2004; 109(25): 20-1.

[110] Miller PE, Snyder DC. Phytochemicals and cancer risk: A review of the epidemiological evidence. Nutr Clin Pract 2012; 27(5): 599-612.

[111] De Castro J, Rodríguez MC, Martínez-Zorzano VS, Llanillo M, Sánchez-Yagüe J. Platelet linoleic acid is a potential biomarker of advanced non-small cell lung cancer. Exp Mol Pathol 2009; 87(3): 226-33.

[112] De Castro J, Hernández-Hernández A, Rodríguez MC, Llanillo M, Sánchez-Yagüe J. Comparison of changes in erythrocyte and platelet fatty acid composition and protein oxidation in advanced non-small cell lung cancer. Cancer Invest 2006; 24(4): 339-45.

[113] Defagó MD, Soria EA. Biomarker assessment in nutritional modulation of oxidative stress-induced cancer development by lipid-related bioactive molecules. Recent Pat Anticancer Drug Discov 2010; 5(3): 188-96.

[114] Innocenzi, M.A. Methods for quantifying the complete nutritional value of a standard equivalent unit of the nutritional value. US20120027897 (**2012**).

[115] Paetau-Robinson, I., Brockman, J. Methods of promoting or maintaining an anabolic state in a female animal. US20120028891 (**2012**).

[116] Béliveau R, Gingras D. Los alimentos contra el cáncer. 1st ed. El Ateneo: Buenos Aires 2007.

[117] Pauwels EK, Kairemo K. Fatty acid facts, part II: Role in the prevention of carcinogenesis, or, more fish on the dish? Drug News Perspect 2008; 21(9): 504-10.

[118] Comba A, Lin YH, Eynard AR, Valentich MA, Fernandez-Zapico ME, Pasqualini ME. Basic aspects of tumor cell fatty acid-regulated signaling and transcription factors. Cancer Metastasis Rev 2011; 30(3-4): 325-42.

[119] Kim JY, Park HD, Park E, Chon JW, Park YK. Growth-inhibitory and proapoptotic effects of alpha-linolenic acid on estrogen-positive breast cancer cells. Ann NY Acad Sci 2009; 1171:190-5.

[120] Schubert R, Reichenbach J, Koch C, Kloess S, Koehl U, Mueller K, *et al.* Reactive oxygen species abrogate the anticarcinogenic effect of eicosapentaenoic acid in Atm-deficient mice. Nutr Cancer 2010; 62(5): 584-92.

[121] Alvarez-Suarez JM, Dekanski D, Ristić S, Radonjić NV, Petronijević ND, Giampieri F, *et al.* Strawberry polyphenols attenuate ethanol-induced gastric lesions in rats by activation of antioxidant enzymes and attenuation of MDA increase. PLoSOne 2011; 6(10): e25878.

[122] Rodrigo R, Miranda A, Vergara L. Modulation of endogenous antioxidant system by wine polyphenols in human disease. Clin Chim Acta 2011; 412(5-6): 410-24.

[123] Srinivasan P, Suchalatha S, Babu PV, Devi RS, Narayan S, Sabitha KE, *et al.* Chemopreventive and therapeutic modulation of green tea polyphenols on drug metabolizing enzymes in 4-nitroquinoline 1-oxide induced oral cancer. Chem Biol Interact 2008; 172(3): 224-34.

[124] Wenzel U, Schoberl K, Lohner K, Daniel H. Activation of mitochondrial lactate uptake by flavone induces apoptosis in human colon cancer cells. J Cell Physiol 2005; 202(2): 379-90.

[125] Halder B, Das Gupta S, Gomes A. Black tea polyphenols induce human leukemic cell cycle arrest by inhibiting Akt signaling: Possible involvement of Hsp90, Wnt/β-catenin signaling and FOXO1. FEBSJ 2012; 279(16): 2876-91.

[126] Karna P, Gundala SR, Gupta MV, Shamsi SA, Pace RD, Yates C, *et al.* Polyphenol-rich sweet potato greens extract inhibits proliferation and induces apoptosis in prostate cancer cells *in vitro* and *in vivo*. Carcinogenesis 2011; 32(12):1872-80.

[127] Ho HH, Chang CS, Ho WC, Liao SY, Wu CH, Wang CJ. Anti-metastasis effects of gallic acid on gastric cancer cells involves inhibition of NF-kappaB activity and downregulation of PI3K/AKT/small GTPase signals. Food Chem Toxicol 2010; 48(8-9): 2508-16.

[128] Mouria M, Gukovskaya AS, Jung Y, Buechler P, Hines OJ, Reber HA, *et al.* Food-derived polyphenols inhibit pancreatic cancer growth through mitochondrial cytochrome C release and apoptosis. Int J Cancer 2002; 98(5): 761-9.

[129] Wang J, Chen X, Hou L, Li L, Lu H, Liu W. Effects of tea polyphenols on the expression of NF-κB, COX-2 and survivin in Lewis lung carcinoma xenografts in C57BL/6 mice. Zhongguo FeiAiZaZhi 2012; 15(5): 271-6.

[130] Howard, C. Dietary supplement. US20120003378 (**2012**).

[131] Cowan, F.M. Phytochemical combinations that regulate pathological immunity. US20110305779 (**2011**).

[132] Basu, H.S., Zarling, D. Methods and kits for determining oxygen free radical (OFR) levels in animal and human tissues as a prognostic marker for cancer and other pathophysiologies. WO2010124257 (**2011**).

[133] Pacioretty, L.M., Babish, J.G. Methods for the treatment of HIV-1 related fat maldistribution, fasting hyperlipidemia and modification of adipocytes. US8093292 (**2012**).
[134] Longo, V.D., Lee, C. Methods and nutritional formulations to increase the efficacy and reduce the side effects of cancer treatment. US20110118528 (**2011**).
[135] Moore FA, Ziegler TR, Heyland DK, Marik PE, Bistrian BR. Developing research programs in clinical and translational nutrition. JPEN J Parenter Enteral Nutr 2010; 34(6): 97S-105S.
[136] Graves, D.J., Lew, J. Proanthocyanidins from cinnamon and its water soluble extract inhibit tau aggregation. US20110263696 (**2011**).
[137] Mastaloudis, A., Wood, S., Weindruch, R., Prolla, T.A., Barger, J.L., Bartlett, M., Ferguson, S.B., Chang, J. Oral formulations for counteracting effects of aging. WO2011149981 (**2011**).
[138] Bui, C.V., Bui, C.Q. Nutraceutical for the prevention and treatment of cancers and diseases affecting the liver. US20120034310 (**2012**).
[139] Vara Messler M, Cremonezzi DC, Soria EA, Eynard AR. Nutritional chemoprevention of urinary tract tumors (UTT) induced by lithogenic agents: Risk for UTT in children exposed to melamine-contaminated milk formulae. J Environ Sci Health C Environ Carcinog Ecotoxicol Rev 2012; 30(2): 174-87.
[140] Somekawa. S., Mine, T., Hayashi, N. Nutrient composition. EP2374452 (**2011**) & US20110288012 (**2011**).
[141] Rupasingue, H.P.V., Robertson, G.S. Phenolic compositions derived from apple skin and uses thereof. WO2011140655 (**2011**).
[142] Daín A, Repossi G, Das UN, Eynard AR. Role of PUFAs, the precursors of endocannabinoids, in human obesity and type 2 diabetes. Front Biosci (Elite Ed) 2010; 2: 1432-47.
[143] Managoli, N.B. Herbal composition for treatment of hyperlipidemia and the inhibition of myocardial infarction. US8067043 (**2011**).
[144] Sinclair, D.A., Alexander-Bridges, M. Compositions for treating or preventing obesity and insulin resistance disorders. US20120029065 (**2012**).
[145] Middleton, R.P., Impanbutr, N. Methods for increasing the production or activity of catalase. WO2011149513 (**2011**).
[146] Narayanan, R., Yepuru, M., Dalton, J.T. Nuclear receptor binding agents. WO2011140228 (**2011**).
[147] Miller, P.J., Romero, T., Qin, B., Romero, A. Dietary supplements containing extracts of cinnamon and methods of using same to promote enhanced sirtuin, cell and telomere integrity. WO2011150229 (**2011**).
[148] Morris, M., Ng, S.F. Inheritance of metabolic dysfunction. WO2012000058 (**2012**).
[149] Vaya, J., Tamir, S. Exogenous markers for oxidative stress. US20080311667 (**2008**).
[150] Zhang, B., Ng, S.C., Au, Q. Screening methods for heat-shock response modulators. US20110166038 (**2011**).
[151] Liu, R.H., Nehmer, K.L. Cellular antioxidant activity (CAA) assay. US20110313672 (**2011**).
[152] Das, K.M., Lin, J.C.C. Chemoprevention of colorectal cancer by mesalamine/sulfasalazine. US20110059924 (**2011**).
[153] Yu, X.X., Bhanot, S. Compositions and methods for the modulation of JNK proteins. US8101585 (**2012**).

[154] Pass, H.I., Wali, A. Asbestos exposure, pleural mesothelioma, and osteopontin levels. US7901896 (**2011**).

[155] Dou, Q.P., Chan, T.H., Smith, D.M. Polyphenol proteasome inhibitors, synthesis, and methods of use. US20120029067 (**2012**).

[156] Cossio, F.P., Arevalo Aldalba, E., Salazar Vara, Y.I., Olascoaga Zubia, A., Amato Vivanco, S., Arteche Mendoza, M.L., Pogonza Salado, C., Escobal Gallot, N., Vanaclocha Vidal, F. Nitrogenated trans-stilbene analogs, method for the obtention and medical applications thereof. US20110060038 (**2011**).

[157] Garber AM, Tunis SR. Does comparative-effectiveness research threaten personalized medicine? N Engl J Med 2009; 360: 1925-7.

[158] Atkins D, Best D, Briss PA, Eccles M, Falck-Ytter Y, Flottorp S, *et al.* Grading quality of evidence and strength of recommendations. BMJ 2004; 328(7454): 1490.

[159] Canalis AM, Defagó MD, Soria EA. Perfil farmaconutricional de azafrán y cúrcuma: Identificación de compuestos lipídicos y fenólicos con potencial xenohormético. 1st ed. Editorial Académica Española: Saarbrücken, 2012.

Author Index

Atta-ur Rahman and Khurshid Zaman (Eds)

Made in the USA
Las Vegas, NV
03 November 2026

57424110R00335